Herbal Drugs

and Phytopharmaceuticals

Herbal Drugs

and Phytopharmaceuticals

A handbook for practice on a scientific basis

Edited and translated
from the second
German edition by
Norman Grainger Bisset,
London

German edition edited
by **Max Wichtl**, Marburg

With contributions from
F.-C. Czygan
D. Frohne
C. Höltzel
A. Nagell
H.J. Pfänder
G. Willuhn
W. Buff

With a foreword
by J. David Phillipson, London

medpharm

Scientific Publishers
Stuttgart 1994

CRC Press
Boca Raton   Ann Arbor   London   Tokyo

Editors: English edition

Prof. Norman Grainger Bisset †
King's College London
University of London
Chelsea Department of Pharmacy

Original German edition

Prof. Dr. Max Wichtl
Institut für Pharmazeutische Biologie
der Philipps-Universität Marburg
Deutschhausstr. 17$^1/_2$
D-35032 Marburg/Lahn

Title of original German edition:

Teedrogen. Ein Handbuch für die Praxis auf wissenschaftlicher Grundlage / Hrsg. von Max Wichtl

© 1984, 1989 Wissenschaftliche Verlagsgesellschaft mbH, Birkenwaldstrasse 44, D-70191 Stuttgart, Germany

Translated from the 2nd German edition by Prof. N.G. Bisset

Cataloguing-in-Publication Data available from the Library of Congress

Sole distribution rights for North America granted to CRC Press, 2000 Corporate Blvd., N.W., Boca Raton, FL 33431, USA

ISBN 3-88763-025-4 medpharm Scientific Publishers, Stuttgart
ISBN 0-8493-7192-9 CRC Press, Boca Raton, Ann Arbor, London, Tokyo

Die Deutsche Bibliothek — CIP-Einheitsaufnahme
Herbal drugs and phytopharmaceuticals
a handbook for practice on a scientific basis / ed. and transl. from the 2. German ed. by Norman Grainger Bisset. With contributions from F.-C. Czygan ...
With a foreword by J. David Phillipson. —
Stuttgart : medpharm Scientific Publ. ; Boca Raton ; Ann Arbor ; London ; Tokyo : CRC Press, 1994
    Einheitssacht.: Teedrogen <engl.>
    ISBN 3-88763-025-4 (medpharm Scientific Publ.)
    ISBN 0-8493-7192-9 (CRC Press)
NE: Bisset, Norman Grainger [Hrsg.] ; Czygan, Franz-Christian ; EST

English language edition:
© 1994 medpharm GmbH Scientific Publishers, Birkenwaldstrasse 44, D-70191 Stuttgart, Germany.
Printed in Germany
Cover Design: Hans Hug, Stuttgart
Reproductions: Eder-Repros, Ostfildern
Composition, Printing and Binding: Universitätsdruckerei H. Stürtz AG, Würzburg

Authors: Prof. Dr. Franz-Christian Czygan
Lehrstuhl für Pharmazeutische Biologie
Institut für Botanik und Pharmazeutische Biologie
der Universität Würzburg
Mittlerer Dallenbergweg 64
D-97082 Würzburg

Prof. Dr. Dietrich Frohne
Institut für Pharmazeutische Biologie
der Christian-Albrechts-Universität Kiel
Grasweg 9
D-24118 Kiel

Dr. Christoph Höltzel
Rosen-Apotheke
Dresdnerplatz 1
D-72760 Reutlingen

Dr. Astrid Nagell
Addipharma GmbH
Wandalenweg 24
D-20097 Hamburg

Dr. Hans Jürgen Pfänder
Institut für Pharmazeutische Biologie
der Christian-Albrechts-Universität Kiel
Grasweg 9
D-24118 Kiel

Prof. Dr. Günter Willuhn
Institut für Pharmazeutische Biologie
der Universität Düsseldorf
Universitätsstraße 1
D-40225 Düsseldorf

Dr. Wolfram Buff
Schlehenhang 13/1
D-88400 Biberach/Riß

Foreword
to the English Edition

This book is of interest to all who are involved with plants as medicines whether they be physicians, pharmacists, herbalists, botanists, chemists or manufacturers. Even the general public cannot fail but to be impressed by the wealth of information it encompasses. The current interest in and demand for herbs to treat disease is a worldwide phenomenon. It was forecast not so many years ago that single drug substances resulting from rational design and synthesis would replace the old fashioned herbal plants which had been the mainstay of medicinal treatment for many centuries. In fact the subject of Pharmacognosy, which deals with medicinal plants and the pharmacologically active substances which they contain, has disappeared from, or has been markedly reduced in the undergraduate curriculum of many degree courses in Pharmacy of universities in the USA and the UK. The general population, knowing little about such changes within the curricula of Pharmacy Schools, has not only continued to use herbal remedies but has increased their usage. Why should this have happened? There is no simple answer and opinions vary but there can be little doubt that there is a widespread distrust of potent medicines and particularly a fear of the adverse reactions which patients may experience. There is a general, and mistaken belief, that anything which is natural is inherently safe (conveniently forgetting compounds such as strychnine and ricin) whereas anything that is synthetic is unnatural and probably toxic (ignoring many of the excellent pharmaceutical preparations which are lifesaving). Fast life styles, overcrowded urban environments engender the feeling that life must have been better in the old days and that as far as medicine is concerned surely grandmother knew best. Many people in developed countries are able to travel and in many ways we are living in a shrinking world. Imagine the shock of the British traveller having braved the sea crossing to France and finding that pharmacies stock many medicinal herbs and their products whilst some Phytopharmacies specialise entirely in medicinal plants. In Germany and European countries further east the English speaking traveller will quickly realise that medicinal plants and their preparations are popular items of commerce. Television programmes, family magazines, newspapers and again travel make us appreciate that China and other countries have maintained a long tradition in the use of plants for the treatment of disease. In fact we are constantly aware that the majority of the World's population relies almost entirely on traditional medicines which are mainly plant based.

Whatever the reasons may be, there can be no doubt that the public's interest in plant medicines is considerable. Pharmacists and physicians are asked for advice and their undergraduate education is often lacking in this type of information. Of course education is on-going and as there is such a wealth of literature on medicinal plants it might be thought that it should be a relatively simple matter to locate the answers to such questions as to which herb should be used for a particular illness, what doses are needed and can we rely on the authentication and quality of medicinal herbs. It is not always easy to obtain these answers quickly but there is one book, Teedrogen, which does give clear answers to such questions. Sadly it has been available only in a German

Foreword to the English Edition

edition so that there has been a barrier for many of the English speaking world.

This volume is a new edition of Teedrogen which for the first time is available in English. It has detailed monographs on 181 medicinal herbs and maintains its high standard of clearly presented information. Colour prints of the actual dried part of the plant which is used medicinally as well as colour photographs of the whole plant growing in its natural habitat are available with most monographs. The text for each herb gives references to pharmacopoeial monographs, sources, synonyms, constituents (often with chemical structures), indications, side effects, preparation of a tea, commercially available phytomedicines, regulatory status, authentication using macroscopical, microscopical and chromatographic techniques. Many of the herbs have photographs or drawings to aid the process of authentication and quality assurance. Quantitative studies, likely adulterations and storage requirements complete the text which is supplemented by references to original scientific publications.

Teedrogen was prepared for the Germanic countries and the English translation has been prepared by the late Professor Norman Bisset of the Department of Pharmacy, King's College, University of London. As with other translations made by Norman Bisset the English is of a high standard but not being content solely with translation he has added to the text for the benefit of English readers. Thus, extra references are included to the British Pharmacopoeia, British Herbal Pharmacopoeia and US Pharmacopoeia, the work of scientists in the English language and most importantly to phytomedicines available in the UK. Some monographs have been included which are the subject of a British monographs and not of a German one (e.g. Artemisiae herba, Mugwort; Bardanae radix, Burdock). Thus although the main text is aimed at the position in Germany, the modified translation is skilfully blended with a wealth of information for the U.K. As I write this foreword to the English edition it is exactly one year from the untimely death of Norman Bisset, my former colleague and good friend. He laboured conscientiously over this translation and would have loved to have seen the finished volume.

Professor J. David Phillipson
The School of Pharmacy
Department of Pharmacognosy
University of London

Preface

to the English Edition

Writing the preface to the English edition of Herbal Drugs and Phytopharmaceuticals fills me with joy and, at the same time, with sorrow.

Herbal Drugs was designed for practical use and has enjoyed great success in German-speaking countries. I am pleased that it will now be available to English-speaking readers as well, but I am saddened by the fact that its translator, Prof. Norman Bisset, did not live to see the appearance of the English edition. He died unexpectedly on 12 February 1993.

I was in constant contact with Prof. Bisset during the last few years and, indeed, he was much more than a mere translator of the edition you have before you. He adapted the text for the United Kingdom and in part for the USA and also incorporated recent work up to about 1992 into this English edition. It was typical of his noble character that he always sought my consent for changes but seldom called on my assistance. In any case it is difficult to overstate his contribution to the making of this book. My great debt of gratitude to Prof. Bisset continues beyond his death. His wish would have been that this English edition proves to be just as useful as the German edition.

Marburg, December 1993   Max Wichtl

From the Prefaces

to the First and Second German Editions

These days, those telling words from the Austrian poet Waggerl almost seem to have been turned around. The modern aversion to pills and tablets, for whatever reason (and often unfoundedly), is coupled with a desire on the part of many to attain or maintain their health with "natural" remedies. And thus pharmacists and physicians feel the effects of the ecology movement even in the field of pharmaceuticals. The demand for herbal drugs has risen considerably in the last few years. But are pharmacists and physicians prepared for it? Are they trained to answer all the questions this demand brings with it about uses, constituents, indications and side effects, authentication and adulterations of herbal drugs?

These questions prompted us to consider publishing a book about herbal drugs.

After carefully examining the available literature we tried to treat all aspects of the topic, i.e., constituents, indications and side effects, testing, storage and, of course, the making of the tea, herbal preparations and phytopharmaceuticals, in as up-to-date a fashion as possible. In listing indications we paid particular attention to clearly distinguishing between medically substantiated use and purely empirical, folk medicinal use. Drugs whose efficacy is unsubstantiated are clearly identified as such in this book without passing a final, negative judgment on them. Research on the active substances in herbal drugs is at least partially reflected by numerous references to pharmacological tests on isolated constituents. Of course, the efficacy of one single constituent cannot automatically be equated with the effectiveness of an herbal tea against a specific human illness.

In addition, this book is intended to help the pharmacist, who must bear the responsibility for the authenticity and quality of the drugs he dispenses, by providing instructions for testing even those drugs which are not officinal.

This project would not have been possible without the willing assistance of colleagues, active in universities, pharmacies and medical practice.

Besides my own contributions to the text, I had the editor's task of striking a balance between sections which were too short or too lengthy as they came from the pens of the authors (Prof. Dr. F.-C. Czygan, Prof. Dr. D. Frohne, Dr. A. Nagell, and Prof. Dr. G. Willuhn). Dr. A. Nagell was responsible for the information regarding the plant sources of the drugs and adulterations commonly seen today. Dr. Chr. Höltzel contributed the text for the headings "Making the Tea" and "Herbal Preparations". Dr. H.J. Pfänder had the vital task of making the black-and-white and coloured photographs which contributed so substantially to achieving the goals set for this book.

As the reader can see by the fact that the second edition is considerably larger than the first, several significant changes were made in the contents. After numerous requests by our readers, especially the pharmacists, 39 drugs were added to the original 142 of the first edition, so that the book now provides information about 181 herbal drugs. The second edition also gave us the opportunity to follow the suggestion made repeatedly while the first edition was being prepared and include photographs of the plants from which the drugs are obtained. As you can readily see from leafing through the second edition, there are now many more illustrations. Another significant addi-

From the Prefaces to the First and Second German Editions

tion was the – albeit only partial – inclusion of monographs of the German Commission E (Prepared Monographs for Human Medicine, Section of Phytotherapy). These texts were edited by the Federal Ministry of Health (BGA) and represent, as it were, the official position on the indications claimed for the herbal drugs. This makes them interesting not only for doctors and pharmacists but also for the manufacturers of phyto-pharmaceuticals.

It goes without saying that all of the monographs from the first edition of <u>Herbal Drugs</u> have been thoroughly revised and updated. Literature is now cited more often, which will hopefully enhance this book's usefulness as a reference work. Every effort has been made to include stereochemical structure when giving the formulas of the constituents. The number of illustrations of thin layer chromatograms (now in original size) has been expanded considerably. For the most part they were made by Dr. Nagell, who also gave the corresponding analytical procedures. German standard licenses have been included, as have the German-language pharmacopoeias which have appeared in the meantime, the DAB 9* and Ph. Helv. VII.

The division of labour amongst the authors which worked so well in the first edition was retained in the second. We were able to welcome a new colleague to the team, Dr. W. Buff, who contributed most of the photographs of the plants in their natural habitats. The microscopical pictures of the newly added drugs were made by my wife with the assistance of Mr. R. Ochs.

The authors and editor are indebted to a number of colleagues for their help, hints and suggestions, in particular to Prof. Dr. C.H. Brieskorn (Würzburg), Dr. Rita Jaspersen-Schib (Zurich), Prof. Dr. K.H. Kubeczka (Hamburg), Dr. W. Schier (Bad Salza), Prof. Dr. O. Sticher (Zurich), Pharmacist Dr. M. Veit (Würzburg), Prof. Dr. O.H. Volk (Würzburg) and Dipl.-Handelslehrer Mr. F. Wiedemann (Frankfurt/Main).

I would like to take this opportunity to thank my wife for our many stimulating discussions and for her tireless help in correcting the manuscript.

I would like to thank our publisher, and in particular Dr. W. Wessinger and Mr. W. Studer, for the excellent collaboration and their willingness to fulfil special wishes. The editor and authors hope that this second edition will also prove to be a helpful reference work in day-to-day use. We would welcome any ideas, criticism and suggestions for improvement.

Marburg, August 1984 and October 1988
M. Wichtl

---

* DAB 10 in this English Edition

Table of Contents

Important Indications for the Reader of This Book

General Part

Monographs

Table of Contents

Table of Contents

Table of Contents

Table of Contents

Table of Contents

List of Abbreviations

AB-DDR	Arzneibuch der DDR (Pharmacopoeia of the (former) German Democratic Republic), 6 volumes, 1985.
BAN	British Approved Name
BAnz	Bundes-Anzeiger (German Federal Gazette), edited by the Federal Minister of Justice.
BP 1988	British Pharmacopoeia 1988; Addendum 1989; Addendum 1991; Addendum 1992.
Berger	F. Berger, Handbuch der Drogenkunde, 7 volumes. Verlag W. Maudrich, Vienna 1949–67.
BHP 1983	British Herbal Pharmacopoeia 1983.
BHP 1/1990	British Herbal Pharmacopoeia, Volume 1, 1990.
DAB 6	Deutsches Arzneibuch (German Pharmacopoeia), Sixth edition 1926.
DAB 7	Deutsches Arzneibuch (German Pharmacopoeia), Seventh edition 1968.
DAB 8	Deutsches Arzneibuch (German Pharmacopoeia), Eighth edition 1978; First Supplement 1980, Second Supplement 1983.
DAB 9	Deutsches Arzneibuch (German Pharmacopoeia), Ninth edition 1986; First Supplement 1989, Second Supplement 1990.
DAB 10	Deutsches Arzneibuch (German Pharmacopoeia), Tenth edition 1991; First Supplement 1992; Second Supplement 1993.
DAC 1986	Deutscher Arzneimittel-Codex (German Drug Formulary) 1986; First-Fourth Supplement 1986–1992.
Erg. B. 6	Ergänzungsbuch zum Deutschen Arzneibuch (Supplement Volume to German Pharmacopoeia, Sixth edition 1926). Reprinted 1953.
Hager	Hager's Handbuch der Pharmazeutischen Praxis. Edited by L. Hörhammer (†) and P.H. List. Fourth edition, Volumes 1–8. Springer Verlag, Berlin – Heidelberg – New York 1967–1980. Fifth edition, Volumes 1–5; next Volumes in preparation. Springer Verlag, Berlin – Heidelberg – New York 1990–1993.
Kommentar DAB 10	K. Hartke, H. Hartke, E. Mutschler, G. Rücker and M. Wichtl (Eds.), DAB 10 – Kommentar. Wissenschaftliche Erläuterungen zum Deutschen Arzneibuch, 10. Ausgabe. (German Pharmacopoeia, Tenth edition – Commentary), 6 volumes. Wissenschaftliche Verlagsgesellschaft mbH, Stuttgart, and Govi-Verlag, Frankfurt/M., 1991 ff.
Kommentar Ph. Eur. I/II	H. Böhme and K. Hartke, Europäisches Arzneibuch Band I and Band II, Kommentar (European Pharmacopoeia, Volume I and Volume II – Commentary), Third edition. Wissenschaftliche Verlagsgesellschaft mbH, Stuttgart, and Govi-Verlag, Frankfurt/M., 1983.
Kommentar Ph. Eur. III	H. Böhme and K. Hartke, Europäisches Arzneibuch Band III – Kommentar (European Pharmacopoeia, Volume III – Commentary). Wissenschaftliche Verlagsgesellschaft mbH, Stuttgart, and Govi-Verlag, Frankfurt/M., 1982.
ÖAB	Österreichisches Arzneibuch (Austrian Pharmacopoeia), 2 volumes, 1981; First Supplement 1983.
Ph. Eur. 2	European Pharmacopoeia. Second edition 1980–1992.
Ph. Helv. VII	Pharmacopoeia Helvetica, 4 volumes. Seventh edition 1987.
St.Zul.	Standardzulassung (Standard Licence)
TLC	Thin-layer chromatography

List of Abbreviations

USAN	United States Adopted Name
USP XXII	Pharmacopoeia of the United States XXII-NF XVII 1990–1992
UV 254	Ultraviolet light, 254 mm.
UV 365, 366	Ultraviolet light, 365 resp. 366 mm.
Solvent System (80 + 18 + 2)	The figures in brackets give volume parts.

Important Indications
for the Reader of This Book

What the Reader Will Find in This Book

In this book 181 drugs are described which (almost without exception) are used for the preparation of teas or are components of herbal mixtures. They are arranged in the order of their Latin names. The selection is based on an enquiry carried out in 180 pharmacies [1] and takes into account the many requests made to the (German) editor by readers of the first edition. The selection comprises particularly those drugs for which Standard Licences are available (see p. 39). Drugs which in practice have little importance, or which are not intended to be components of herbal teas (horse-chestnut seeds, belladonna leaves, etc.), are not included. Even so, it may be that readers will miss certain drugs.

Use is made of modern Latin names, but older ones which may be more familiar to some people are also included, as well as a selection of English, German, and French names. Appropriate references are inserted where the drugs are included in certain English language pharmacopoeias (EP, BP, USP). In the same way, references are given to the appropriate sources where the drugs are only to be found in the German language pharmacopoeias (DAB, ÖAB, Ph.Helv., etc.). Where a Standard Licence exists, the corresponding number is cited, e.g. for arnica flowers: St.Zul. 8199.99.99.

The rest of the text in the monographs is arranged as follows:

Illustration and Description: A coloured illustration of the chopped drug is shown, and the accompanying text gives the essential features by which the drug can be recognized. Where appropriate, odour and taste are indicated.

Plant source: The scientific name is given, based primarily on the Flora Europaea or the Index Kewensis, followed by the common English name and the plant family. Pictures of many of the plant sources are included, and sometimes also pictures of the characteristic parts of the plants, e.g. flowers or fruits, while a brief explanatory text supplies appropriate information.

Synonyms: Here, the common English names of the drug are given, as well as the principal Latin, German, and French names. These are not synonyms in a taxonomic sense.

Origin: This section furnishes details of the natural distribution of the plants, indications regarding their cultivation and the occurrence, if any, of market forms of the drug. The exporting countries are listed in the current (1988) order of their importance, the main exporting country being given first. It should, however, be noted that in this respect there may be changes from year to year.

Constituents: The substances mainly responsible for the use of the drug are mentioned first, and these are followed by other compounds. Wherever possible, quantitative data are given, and any pharmacopoeial requirements are indicated. The composition of different groups of substances (essential oil, flavonoids, saponins, bitter substances) is set out in greater or lesser detail: this mirrors current knowledge, but in addition also reflects the individual author's assessment of the significance of such facts (and in this respect the German editor has on occasion had to exercise his judgement). Frequently, attention is drawn to characteristic properties of the constituents: haemolytic activity, ready oxidation, solubility, distribution in the drug, etc.

What the Reader Will Find in This Book

Indications: Particular emphasis has been laid on distinguishing the clinically or pharmacologically based therapeutic use of the drug from the purely empirical, *folk medicinal*, application. As far as possible, the more significant investigations into the activity or action of the drug are cited. Reference is also made to the pharmacology of individual constituents, though only in order to give the pharmacist and doctor an idea of the present situation regarding phytochemical and medicinal research. *Since these data refer to isolated constituents, no conclusions whatsoever should be drawn regarding corresponding activity of a tea prepared from the drug*, as long as it has not been demonstrated that the constituent concerned gets into the tea (infusion) and is absorbed in sufficient amounts from the gastrointestinal tract. (Many people – authors of books on medicinal plants, journalists in the lay press, etc. – fail to appreciate this basic fact; the following is a typical example: a report in a weekly declares, "Saffron keeps the arteries clean", although only the blood lipid-lowering effect of an isolated constituent [crocetin] on rabbits is reported [2]).

Information regarding the use in *folk medicine* has been purposely kept low-key. In this second edition, information from the Commission E of the German Federal Health Office (see p. 40) regarding the indications, side effects, interactions, mode of administration, and effects, is also included; see the relevant explanatory notes on pp. 40–41.

Side effects: Undesirable, and indeed toxic, effects are also possible when herbal drugs are used. These, as far as known, are described under this heading, even though they are not expected to occur when the drug is taken properly according to instructions.

Making the tea: This section gives details of the individual dose (per teacup of ca. 150 ml), the degree of comminution of the drug, and the way in which it is prepared; the weight of a spoonful of the drug is also given. (Since the spoons in use nowadays are smaller, they are not equivalent to the "normal" spoonful of the pharmacopoeias. We have followed current practice, so that differences from the Standard Licences are thus possible.)

Standard Licence: Wherever available, the text of the package insert is reproduced. This text is obligatory in Germany for prepared remedies of the particular drugs concerned (see p. 39).

Herbal preparations: This section lists prepared remedies that can mostly be taken directly by the consumer e.g. tea bags, instant teas, or paste teas. See further, pp. 22 et seq.

Phytomedicines: To give the pharmacist and the doctor an idea of the extent to which and of the range of indications in which the drug is used in the manufacture of prepared remedies; this information is often supplemented by figures and the names of available preparations. This, of course, does not in any way imply an assessment of these products.

Inclusion (or omission) of particular German preparations is not to be taken as a value judgement. The manufacturers bear no responsibility for the selection of products named, nor was it intended that the list should influence them in any way. In the same way, the UK and other products included are merely to give an idea of the

What the Reader Will Find in This Book

types of preparations that may be encountered on the UK market.

Authentication: This section points out diagnostic features of the drug which are essential for a reliable identification. Wherever appropriate, besides the microscopical examination, details of thin-layer chromatographic (TLC) methods are included. References to pharmacopoeias and other readily available standard literature are also given. In this section, throughout the book the "TLC test of identification" is presented under the following headings:

1. [Preparation of the] Test solution
2. [Preparation of the] Reference solution
3. Loadings
4. Solvent system [and height of run]
5. Detection
6. Evaluation.

The methods that have been worked out specifically for this book make use of 4×8 cm silica-gel GF_{254} foil, which can be either obtained as such or simply cut from larger sheets of TLC foil. This very convenient format enables the development to be carried out with a few ml of the solvent system in small separating tanks [3]. The coloured illustrations, which are natural size, allow a direct comparison with one's own TLC.

An additional subsection has been included here, viz **Quantitative Standards**. For many of the drugs included in this book, there is no literature in English dealing with their analytical standards. It is appropriate, therefore, to indicate the standards which are required in those (German-language) pharmacopoeias which include them.

Adulteration: Here, an attempt is made to present the current situation. Much of the information to be found in textbooks and handbooks no longer reflects present-day conditions. It is hoped that this will enable the pharmacist to detect cases of adulteration with certainty.

Storage: In general, drugs should be stored with protection from light and moisture. Where no other conditions than these are required, this section is omitted. It is therefore only included in the monographs on those herbal drugs for which additional indications are required. However, for the sake of completeness, in these cases the necessity for the exclusion of light and moisture is mentioned.

Literature: In accordance with the original purpose of this book, preference was given to literature that is readily available to pharmacists and doctors in Germanophone countries, but publications in other journals were also cited, in order to let the reader know that the data have been published and can be checked. For this edition of the book, literature available up to the middle of 1992 has been consulted.

[1] M. Wichtl, Dtsch. Apoth. Ztg. **124**, 60 (1984).
[2] F.-C. Czygan, Dtsch. Apoth. Ztg. **124**, 1069 (1984); die "Safran-Story".
[3] M. Wichtl, Prüfung von Drogen in Apotheken (Schriftenreihe der Bundesapothekerkammer, Davos 1984. Dokumentation der Vorträge).

General Part

Fundamentals of Herbal Drugs and Herbal Teas

Introduction

Day after day, patients appear in the pharmacy asking for a herbal tea for a particular kind of condition. When the pharmacist asks the routine question whether a "simple" herbal tea or a special mixed tea or a tea bag or an instant tea is wanted, mostly the stereotyped answer comes back "You know which is the best one. Give me that one!"

This trust in the pharmacist must not be disappointed, but – with his hand on his heart – what pharmacist has not sometimes wondered whether he has recommended the right one?

Whoever wants to get rid of such doubts looks in the literature, but which literature? Textbooks of pharmacognosy or pharmaceutical biology do give information on some herbal drugs [1, 2], but they do not tell how to prepare a tea correctly. Hager's *Handbuch der Pharmazeutischen Praxis*, if available, is a mine of information, but the manuscript for some drugs was finished about 20 years ago. The commentaries on the pharmacopoeias, on the other hand, set out the current position, but do not mention many herbal drugs that are important in daily practice (nettle herb, yarrow, mistletoe, etc.).

The present book is an attempt to fill this gap and to make available to the pharmacist and doctor a coherent discussion of everything to do with herbal drugs.

First of all, in the general part, the supply of herbal drugs and herbal mixtures, the indications and possible treatments, are dealt with, as well as explaining herbal preparations, how to make the tea, storage, and authentication. Short sections are devoted to the Standard Licences and the contamination of drugs (microbiological, heavy metal, fumigation, radioactive substances).

In the main part of the book, detailed monographs of 181 drugs are set out; concerning the arrangement of these monographs, see the section: Important Indications for the Reader of This Book (pp. 3 et seq.).

[1] G. Schneider, Pharmazeutische Biologie, B.I.-Wissenschaftsverlag Mannheim-Wien-Zürich 1975. In the 2nd edition (1985) the corresponding chapter is omitted.

[2] E. Steinegger and R. Hänsel, Lehrbuch der Pharmakognosie und Phytopharmazie. 4th completely revised edition by R. Hänsel, Springer Verlag 1988.

Herbal Teas and Herbal Mixtures

Drugs obtained by drying parts of plants can be used medicinally in various ways: they may simply be the raw material for isolating the constituents, e.g. digitalis leaves or horse-chestnut seeds, extracts may be prepared from them, e.g. hawthorn fruit or milk thistle fruit, or they are used directly for the preparation of teas. It is this last group, the herbal drugs, that will be discussed below.

An essential feature of herbal teas – as a rule used medicinally – is that the patient sees himself as his own pharmacist and uses them to prepare a tea, which is usually intended to be drunk. In rare cases, however, the aqueous extract is also used externally, for dressings, or the drugs are put into pot pourri. The only herbs that are suitable as drugs are those which have constituents or active principles with a relatively large therapeutic latitude; otherwise, they could not be employed for self-medication, e.g. belladonna leaves, rauvolfia root, etc. Exceptions, such as ipecacuanha root or celandine, go to prove the rule.

Herbal drugs are available in coarsely to finely chopped forms, as cut or *"concis"* drugs; leaves often appear on the market cut into four-sided fragments; woods, roots, and barks as chips; most fruits and seeds usually unbroken, in the whole or *"toto"* condition, and they are sometimes crushed before being used. The extent of comminution plays an important part in the preparation of herbal infusions (see below: Making the Tea).

There is a series of herbal drugs that are used on their own – they are called "mono-" or "monovalent" drugs; examples of these are: chamomile flowers, peppermint leaves, wormwood, etc. This book described 181 such individual drugs.

Besides these single herbal drugs, a few of which may also be intended for internal use in powdered form, e.g. cucurbita seeds, ratanhia root, etc., in practice herbal mixtures also have a major role to play. These are mixtures which are either prepared in the pharmacy or industrially, comprising several drugs often belonging to the same indication group, to which are added other drugs which assist the action or are included to correct the taste. Among the Standard Licences (see p. 39), there are several monographs for herbal mixtures used for a variety of different conditions [1]; in them, a distinction is made between the principal drug (of major relevance for the treatment of the condition concerned), supplementary drugs (listed according to their importance for the condition concerned) and adjunct drugs (important for the smell and taste; but drugs which improve the appearance of the mixture also belong here). It is a good pharmaceutical rule that a herbal mixture should consist of only a few, about 4–7, drugs. The composition of a herbal mixtures with 20–30 drugs, which are prepared by a number of manufacturers, represents an attempt at treatment with many drugs below therapeutically useful levels, which is likely to be of little help. Some pharmacopoeias, as well as the Standard Licences, offer good examples of appropriately composed herbal mixtures. The Standard Licences aim to give the maker a certain leeway, distinguishing between the "active components" (or principal drugs of major importance for the indication) and "other components" (supplementary and adjunct drugs), as for example in cough tea I and the examples below.

Herbal Teas and Herbal Mixtures

Although neither the Standard Licences nor the pharmacopoeias (except Ph.Helv. VII) include indications of the degree of comminution, correct choice of the size of the cut is of crucial importance. On storage, and especially during transport, separation into several distinct layers with different compositions may occur [3]. See further, the sections Making the Tea, Degree of comminution of the drugs (pp. 24 et seq.).

Species sedativae
= Sedative tea (Ph.Helv. VII)

10 Parts Balm
10 Parts Peppermint leaves
25 Parts Valerian root
20 Parts Orange flowers
15 Parts Aniseed
20 Parts Passiflora

Species sedativae
= Nerve tea (ÖAB)

10 Parts Balm
10 Parts Peppermint leaves
60 Parts Valerian root
10 Parts Orange flowers
10 Parts Bitter-orange peel

Species anticystiticae
= Bladder tea (Ph. Helv. VII)

25 Parts Birch leaves
45 Parts Uva ursi
30 Parts Liquorice

Species carminativae
= Carminative tea (ÖAB)

25 Parts Peppermint leaves
25 Parts Matricaria flowers
25 Parts Calamus rhizome
25 Parts Caraway (crushed)

Species amaricantes
= Bitter tea (ÖAB)

20 Parts Wormwood
20 Parts Lesser centaury
20 Parts Bitter-orange peel
10 Parts Bogbean
10 Parts Calamus rhizome
10 Parts Gentian
10 Parts Cinnamom

Species laxantes
= Laxative tea (Ph.Helv. VII)

50 Parts Tinnevelly Senna fruit
15 Parts Aniseed (crushed)
15 Parts Fennel (crushed)
10 Parts Liquorice
10 Parts Elder flowers

Herbal Teas and Herbal Mixtures

Sedative tea I
(St. Zul. 1949.99.99)

40 Parts Valerian root
20 Parts Hops
15 Parts Balm
15 Parts Peppermint leaves
10 Parts Bitter-orange peel

Wording of the package insert according to the Standard Licence:

8.1 **Uses**

Nervous excitement, disturbances of sleep.

8.2 **Dosage and manner of use**

Boiling water (ca. 150 ml) is poured over a tablespoonful of tea, covered and allowed to draw for 10–15 min., and then passed through a tea strainer. If not otherwise prescribed, a cup of the freshly prepared tea is drunk 2–3 times a day and before going to bed.

8.3 **Note**

Store protected from light and moisture.

Bladder and kidney tea I
(St. Zul. 1959.99.99)

20 Parts Birch leaves
20 Parts Couch-grass root
20 Parts Early golden-rod herb
20 Parts Restharrow root
20 Parts Liquorice

Wording of the package insert according to the Standard Licence:

8.1 **Uses**

To increase the amount of urine in renal and bladder catarrh; to prevent the formation of urinary gravel and calculi.

8.2 **Contraindications**

Accumulation of water (oedema) arising from impaired heart or kidney function.
In cases of chronic kidney diseases, a doctor should be consulted before using Bladder and kidney tea.

8.3 **Dosage and manner of use**

Boiling water (ca. 150 ml) is poured over 2–3 teaspoonfuls of tea, covered and allowed to draw for 15 min., and then passed through a tea strainer.
If not otherwise prescribed, a cup of the freshly prepared tea is drunk 3–4 times a day between meals.

8.4 **Note**

Store protected from light and moisture.

Herbal Teas and Herbal Mixtures

Chest Tea
(St. Zul. 1969.99.99)

10 Parts Aniseed
10 Parts Liquorice
20 Parts Iceland moss
30 Parts Marshmallow root
30 Parts Coltsfoot

Wording of the package insert according to the Standard Licence:

8.1 **Uses**

To alleviate irritation in catarrh of the upper respiratory passages with a dry cough.

8.2 **Dosage and manner of use**

Boiling water (ca. 150 ml) is poured over about one tablespoonful of the tea, covered and allowed to draw for ca. 10 min., and then passed through a tea strainer.
If not otherwise prescribed, a cup of the freshly prepared tea is drunk several times a day, especially in the morning after waking and at night before going to bed.

8.3 **Note**

Store protected from light and moisture.

Cough tea I
(St. Zul. 1979.99.99)

30 Parts Elder flowers
30 Parts Lime tree flowers
20 Parts Meadowsweet
(these 3 drugs are the so-called "active components")
20 Parts Rose hips
(they are considered as "other components")

Wording of the package insert according to the Standard Licence:

8.1 **Uses**

For feverish colds, when a sweat cure is desired.

8.2 **Dosage and manner of use**

Boiling water (ca. 150 ml) is poured over ca.one tablespoonful of the tea, covered and allowed to draw for ca. 10 min., and then passed through a tea strainer.
If not otherwise prescribed, a cup of the freshly prepared tea is drunk several times a day.

Herbal Teas and Herbal Mixtures

Bile tea I
(St. Zul. 1989.99.99)

10 Parts Caraway
20 Parts Javanese turmeric
30 Parts Dandelion
20 Parts Milk-thistle herb
20 Parts Peppermint leaves

Wording of the package insert according to the Standard Licence:

8.1 **Uses**

In supportive treatment of non-inflammatory disorders of the bile duct and in disorders of bile production; gastrointestinal troubles, such as bloating, flatulence, and dyspepsia.

Contraindications Inflammation or occlusion of the bile duct; intestinal occlusion.

8.3 **Dosage and manner of use**

Boiling water (ca. 150 ml) is poured over about one tablespoonful of the tea, covered and allowed to draw for 10–15 min., and then passed through a tea strainer.
If not otherwise prescribed, a cup of the freshly prepared infusion is drunk 3–4 times a day half-an-hour before meals.

8.4 **Note**

Store protected from light and moisture.

Cough tea
(St. Zul. 2009.99.99)

25 Parts Marshmallow root
10 Parts Fennel
10 Parts Iceland moss
15 Parts Plantain herb
10 Parts Liquorice
30 Parts Thyme

Wording of the package insert according to the Standard Licence:

8.1 **Uses**

In symptoms of bronchitis and catarrh of the upper respiratory passages.

8.2 **Dosage and manner of use**

Boiling water (ca. 150 ml) is poured over about one tablespoonful of the tea, covered and allowed to draw for 10 min., and then passed through a tea strainer.
If not otherwise prescribed, a cup of the freshly prepared tea is drunk several times a day.

8.3 **Note**

Store protected from light and moisture.

Herbal Teas and Herbal Mixtures

Stomach tea I
(St. Zul. 2019.99.99)

20 Parts Gentian
20 Parts Bitter-orange peel
25 Parts Lesser centaury
25 Parts Wormwood
10 Parts Cinnamom

Wording of the package insert according to the Standard Licence:

8.1 **Use**

For stomach disorders, such as insufficient formation of gastric juice; for stimulating the appetite.

8.2 **Contraindications**

Stomach and intestinal ulcers.

8.3 **Side effects**

Occasionally, headaches may be caused in people who are sensitive to bitter substances.

8.4 **Dosage and manner of use**

Boiling water (ca. 150 ml) is poured over two teaspoonfuls of the tea, covered and allowed to draw for 5–10 min., and then passed through a tea strainer. If not otherwise prescribed, a cup of the fresh and moderately warm infusion is drunk several times a day half-an-hour before meals.

8.5 **Note**

Store protected from light and moisture.

Stomach and bowel tea I
(St. Zul. 2029.99.99)

25 Parts Valerian root
25 Parts Caraway
25 Parts Peppermint leaves
25 Parts Matricaria flowers

Wording of the package insert according to the Standard Licence:

8.1 **Uses**

Troubles such as a feeling of being bloated, flatulence, and mild cramp-like gastrointestinal upsets; nervous heart-stomach troubles.

8.2 **Dosage and manner of use**

Boiling water (ca. 150 ml) is poured over a tablespoonful of the tea, covered and allowed to draw for ca. 10 min., and then passed through a tea strainer. If not otherwise prescribed, a cup of the freshly prepared tea is drunk warm several times a day between meals.

8.3 **Note**

Store protected from light and moisture.

Herbal Teas and Herbal Mixtures

The Standard Licences currently being prepared deal with herbal mixtures in which the proportions of the individually active components can be varied within certain limits by the manufacturer; it is required that the active components make up at least 70% of the mixture. The other components (mostly to improve the appearance of the tea or to make it more pleasant, but also as adjunct drugs important for the taste and aroma) can be selected from a list of the appropriate drugs. The monographs proposed are: Sedative teas (II–VIII), Bladder and kidney teas (II–VII), Chest and cough teas (I–VIII), Cold teas (II–V), Stomach teas (II–VI), and Stomach and bowel teas (II–XII).

Occasionally, in addition to the drugs, inorganic or organic water-soluble substances are incorporated into herbal teas. These are first dissolved in an inert solvent (usually water) and then certain components of the tea are impregnated with the solution and dried at 30–40° C. Only those drugs are chosen to be impregnated whose constituents are not affected by the treatment. An example of this is the following laxative tea (ÖAB):

Species laxantes
= Laxative tea (ÖAB)

50 Parts Senna leaves
20 Parts Elder flowers
 5 Parts Chamomile flowers
15 Parts Fennel (crushed)
 6 Parts Potassium sodium tartrate
 4 Parts Tartaric acid

Besides the medicinally used herbal mixtures, there are also the so-called household teas which are preferred by people who are sensitive to coffee or who do not wish to drink a caffeine-containing beverage on a regular basis. Household teas are made up from drugs which, apart from small amounts of tannins, have only aroma substances and possibly also plant acids: bramble leaves, raspberry leaves, hibiscus flowers, hips and haws, and apple skins are frequent components of such teas [4].

[1] R. Braun, in: „Qualität pflanzlicher Arzneimittel", Herausg. G. Hanke, Wiss. Verlagsgesellschaft, Stuttgart 1984.
[2] Standardzulassungen für Fertigarzneimittel. Text und Kommentar. Ed. R. Braun, Deutscher Apotheker Verlag Stuttgart and Govi-Verlag Frankfurt, 1987.
[3] Chr. Höltzel, Dtsch. Apoth. Ztg. 124, 2479 (1984).
[4] M. Pahlow, Dtsch. Apoth. Ztg. 124, 1117 (1984).

Indications and Possible Treatments

It is one of the peculiarities of herbal drugs that their indications have for the most part been determined empirically. The reason is easily understood: most herbal drugs have been used for a very long time to alleviate or cure illnesses and more especially disorders. Their introduction in therapeutics happened at a time when pharmacodynamics and pharmacokinetics were unknown concepts, when there was no Medicines Act to require proof of the quality, efficacy, and innocuity of herbal medicines. Today, when introducing a new medicine, extensive investigations are required in the interest of safety. To many the requirement of the proof of activity of such a drug as chamomile appears to be superfluous; but nevertheless, as a representative of a scientifically oriented pharmaceutical science, one strives to pluck herbal drugs out of their present level of pure empiricism and by elucidating their active principles give their application a more secure basis.

The missing proof of active constituents certainly taints the reputation of many herbal drugs in the minds of many doctors, especially younger doctors (who during their medical education learn almost nothing about them) and pharmacologists (herbal drugs are not discussed in pharmacology textbooks); this tendency is worsened by the use of many expressions from years gone by which nowadays are really no longer appropriate, e.g. "for stimulating the appetite", "for purifying the blood", "for the lungs", or "for the nerves". It should be the common purpose of all who are interested in medicines, to change this unsatisfactory situation. True, the patient is not helped very much when (s)he is assured that the molecular mechanism of action and the metabolism of the drug (s)he is taking are known, while on the other hand the same cannot be said of a nerve tea of a given composition. The result of a treatment is crucial, but the patient's bare statement that "the tea has helped", of course, does not meet present-day scientific requirements. It will be necessary to develop methods for the pharmacologically less obviously active constituents by which their effects can be determined more precisely. Another possibility is so-called scientific evidence which in many cases has been deemed sufficient to allow recognition in the form of a Standard Licence. Perhaps some of the difficulties associated with demonstrating activity in herbal drugs in the same way as is required for medicines is connected with the fact that only for some of the constituents of herbal drugs is it possi-

Indications and Possible Treatments

ble to claim them as direct active principles, e.g. the sennosides in senna leaves and senna fruits. In these cases, the use does not pose any problems (rapidity of effect and dose-dependent action) and neither does the demonstration of activity.

For many of the drugs, however, the active constituents are not (yet) known; the examination of their activity is thus often rendered more difficult in that experience of its administration over a long period of time is required. In these cases, it is often said that the drug concerned stimulates the body's own defence mechanisms: formerly, the administration of such drugs was called non-specific stimulant therapy, nowadays the concept of immunostimulation is used or paramunity inducers [1–6].

Finally, it may also be understood that certain herbal drugs are (or can be) used more as psycho-therapeutic agents: the simple act of preparing a tea, the stirring, the slow sipping of the tea throughout the day can bring about a change in the psychological condition of the patient. This approaches a placebo effect, which indeed is put forward by many pharmacists and doctors, who look upon themselves as particularly critical, as being "characteristic of herbal drugs". That may perhaps sometimes be the case, but the placebo effect is by no means confined to herbal drugs: in series of tests dealing with analgesics or sedatives, high rates of effectiveness have been observed with placebos.

There are already many publications that deal with various aspects of the use of herbal drugs and of the ideas about the ways in which they work; some of these are listed in the accompanying bibliography [7–12].

Unencumbered by theoretical considerations, indications belonging to certain areas may perhaps indeed be considered as typical:

Gastrointestinal upsets: Here, herbal drugs are very widely used, not only to stimulate the secretion of gastric juice and the appetite (drugs containing bitter substances), but also to alleviate constipation (drugs that swell, like linseed; drugs that contain anthracene glycosides) and diarrhoea (tannin-containing drugs). Drugs that have a carminative action (with essential oil) or have spasmolytic activity are often included in this group.

Biliary disorders: The number of drugs used for these is also very large, but only a few of them have proved activity; a critical attitude towards "bile teas" containing 15 or more components is advisable.

Psychological disturbances: With nervousness, disturbances of sleep, and similar symptoms, herbal drugs are often, and often justifiably, used. It is noteworthy that mostly aromatic constituents (essential oil) are present.

Coughs and colds, etc.: In this group, there are numerous secretolytic and secretomotor expectorants, containing saponins and/ or essential oil, and drugs containing mucilage, which alleviate irritation of the throat.

Kidney and bladder disorders: Herbal drugs with this indication are usually only for supportive treatment, since their effects as urinary disinfectants and as diuretics are mostly slight, a point which is mentioned under the individual drugs.

Indications and Possible Treatments

Most of the herbal drugs that are used medicinally are comprised in these five groups of indications. Relative few are employed in a limited number of other areas: occasionally in skin remedies, liver remedies, coronary remedies, blood circulation remedies, and in other groups of medicines.

Summarizing, it can be said that the possibilities of treatment with herbal drugs are limited for a number of reasons: for a series of illnesses like severe cardiac insufficiency, tumours, infectious diseases, diabetes, etc., herbal drugs are not adequate remedies, even though, in contravention of the law, such claims are made in many publications. In a series of further cases, they only find use in support of the actual medical treatment; they are nevertheless of value.

The domain of herbal drugs is undoubtedly situated in the grey area between health and illness; but it is fundamentally wrong to uphold a totally negative opinion of herbal drugs on that basis; they are an important supplement to highly active medicines and for minor conditions (as far as they can be unequivocally identified as such!) a means of reducing the requirement of medicines which may have an element of risk attached to them.

[1] A. Mayr et al., Fortschr. Med. **97**, 1159 (1979).
[2] A. Mayr, Sandorama **1**, 9 (1983).
[3] H. Raettig, Fortschr. Med. **100**, 792 (1982).
[4] U. Lindequist and E. Teuscher, Pharmazie **40**, 10 (1985).
[5] R. Hänsel, Dtsch. Apoth. Ztg. **125**, 155 (1985).
[6] H. Wagner, Z. Phytother. **7**, 91 (1986).
[7] R. Mohr, Österr. Apoth. Ztg. **36**, 472 (1982).
[8] H. Schilcher, Pharm. Ztg. **127**, 2174 (1982).
[9] R.F. Weiß, Z. Phytother. **4**, 573 (1983).
[10] H. Brüggemann, Z. Phytother. **4**, 577 (1983).
[11] G. Vogel, Dtsch. Apoth. Ztg. **124**, 639 (1984).
[12] V. Fintelmann, Z. Phytother. **6**, 169 (1985); **8**, 1 (1987).

Herbal Preparations

All those types of preparations for which no measurement of the amount needful for a cup is required, thus, for example, a tea bag, or products which contain prepared, mostly directly soluble extracts, as for example instant or tube teas.

Tea bags offer many advantages, but also have certain disadvantages. The patient undoubtedly finds it an advantage that a priori the correct amount (dose) is to hand; other advantages are that because of the considerable degree of comminution which is always required for drugs to be put into tea bags, there is usually a better extraction of the constituents (exception: drugs with essential oil, see next section) and the tendency of the components to separate, during transport or on storage, is abolished.

Disadvantages are related particularly to the degree of comminution of drugs containing essential oil, since damage to the glandular trichomes or oil glands results in loss of a considerable proportion of the oil. Our own studies on tea bags containing chamomile, fennel, and peppermint have shown that, especially in food shops, they may have an essential-oil content far below the minimum required by the pharmacopoeia. Another disadvantage of tea bags is that, since the consumer does not see the contents, foreign matter may be present to a greater or lesser extent. In an extensive investigation, Franz et al. [1] found that in chamomile tea bags, quite often chamomile herb (instead of just the flowers), and in peppermint tea bags pieces of stem (instead of only leaves), could be present. This is permissible in the food industry, since medicinal use is not envisaged and flavour plays a dominant role (chamomile flowers on their own taste somewhat bitter and chamomile herb spicy); the tea is correspondingly cheaper. In the pharmacy, the contents of the tea bags must correspond to the requirements of the pharmacopoeia, so that the pharmacist must make sure that the supplier guarantees pharmacopoeial quality and (s)he must make spot checks to ensure that this is so.

Tea bags which are available in the pharmacy must conform to the following quality standards:

- Starting material of pharmacopoeial quality
- Double-thickness bags, not glued, with thread and marking (so as to make identification of the drug batch possible)
- Better protection of the aroma and against moisture, and in special cases protection of the aroma for individual tea bags
- Recognizable date of manufacture or, better, sell-by date

The higher price of such tea bags is justified by the higher quality of the product. Every pharmacist should be in a position to make clear this essential advantage to his clients.

Instant teas offer the consumer the convenience of rapid preparation – it is sufficient to dissolve the product in hot water – to allow it to draw and to strain it is unnecessary – coupled with a uniform and constant composition.

Mostly, instant teas are manufactured by exhaustive extraction of drugs, using not only water but also water/ethanol mixtures, which can lead to the enrichment of certain constituents or active principles. The industrial manufacture of such extracts also enables batches of drug which are not of pharmacopoeial quality to be used, since they can be adjusted with extracts from drugs of higher quality. This aspect is not only of interest industrially, but is also of significance with regard to the possible exhaustion of naturally-occurring resources (protection of plants!). By controlling the manufacturing process in this way, it is possible to achieve standardization of certain active substances or groups of active substances in the final product.

In making his (her) recommendations, the pharmacist must realize that two types of instant teas are available, which, as a result of the manufacturing process and the resulting quality characteristics, are very different from each other:

Spray-dried extract: The solutions containing the drug extracts, which are sprayed through a nozzle, sink in the form of fine droplets in the current of warm air, losing their moisture and reaching the separator as dry and hollow pellets of extract which can be recognized with a hand lens. The spray-

Herbal Preparations

dried extract requires little in the way of a carrier, so that the proportion of carbohydrate not originating from the drug (and which have to be taken into account in calculating dietary requirements) is relatively small. Essential oils which have been lost during the drying can be added again as active substances, either simply by grinding or, better, in micro-encapsulated form. The resulting product is a low-density powder which is easily soluble in water: because it is somewhat hygroscopic, occasionally there are complaints because of the caking of the package contents or patients take out the powder with wet spoon or in making the tea (vapour!) leave the vessel open for a while or after use they do not shut it properly.

Tea granules: In granulation or agglomeration processes, the fluid drug extracts are sprayed on to a carrier (mostly saccharose or other carbohydrate) and dried with heating. The dried mass is crushed in a suitable mill to granular or cylindrical aggregates. These granular products, of average density, are very readily soluble in water with only a slightly hygroscopic tendency, and caking of the contents of the package is rarely observed. Because of the ease of manipulation and its initial sweet taste, this type of instant tea is often preferred by patients; however, the pharmacist must bear in mind, particularly for diabetics, the number of bread units; in teas intended for children, the saccharose (which promotes caries!) is replaced by other carriers.

In comparing the content of drug extract in the final product, teas in granule form are usually very much inferior to instant teas which are prepared from spray-dried extracts: teas in granular form, in addition to 97–98% filler and carrier substances often contain only 2–3% dry extract, while in spray-dried products almost ten times as much, viz on average 20%, drug extract is present.

[1] Ch. Franz, D. Fritz and E. Ruhland, Planta Med. **42**, 132 (1981).

On looking at all the facts presented, the patient will attain, comparatively speaking, the least satisfactory outcome with the classical tea or tea mixture, because the preparation of the tea encompasses the largest number of uncertain factors. Rather better results are to be expected from tea bags (outside pharmacies, nowadays this is the form of tea which has by far the largest part of the market), provided that the requirements of quality of content and packaging are satisfied. Spray-dried instant teas are the nearest approach to the ideal of a tea for medicinal purposes: particularly with drugs which contain lipophilic and hydrophilic active principles, e.g. chamomile flowers, in which water is not *a priori* the optimal extraction solvent, standardized preparations of herbal drugs may be better – a point of view that in advising clients in the pharmacy merits more attention.

Making the Tea

The preparation of a tea, even for medicinal purposes, is largely carried out according to experience which is based on the preparation of an infusion of black tea: boiled water is poured over the dried herbal drugs, in chopped form, and after "being allowed to draw" for 5–10 min. strained.

There are many variations of this simple procedure which in pharmacopoeias are called and described as decoctions, infusions, and macerates (thus, for example, in the DAB 8 [but no longer in DAB 9], ÖAB) and consist of the short (infusions) or longer (decoctions) heating of the drug with water or extraction with cold water (macerates). While in DAB 8 details of the extraction of drugs were only given for bearberry leaves, marsh-mallow root, and linseed, in the ÖAB, under the heading "Dosierung" (dosage), information regarding the preparation of an infusion is given for all drugs for which that is appropriate, e.g. "Usual single dose as infusion":1.5 g to a teacup (gentian root) or "Usual single dose as decoction": 1 g to a teacup (alder buckthorn bark).

There are several general rules which apply to these procedures, though they are essentially empirical; even with drugs which have constituents of known structure and pharmacology, studies are lacking aimed at optimizing the making of the tea; it is therefore not surprising to find in books dealing with folk medicine or medicinal plants very different statements on how to make the tea.

In making a tea, the following information should be noted:

- Amount of drug (a single dose) and amount of liquid
- Extent of comminution of the drug
- Method of extraction (temperature, length of time)

Amounts of drug and liquid

The single dose of a drug is mostly derived from experience; it is only possible in a very few cases to calculate it from the activity of the constituents. However, as many herbal drugs are only weakly active and contain non-toxic substances, i.e. the therapeutic index is large, exceeding the dose is usually only of minor significance; nevertheless, the pharmacist must know what the exceptions are: in this book, the sections on "Side effects" and "Making the tea" draw particular attention to such cases, e.g. arnica flowers, liquorice root, etc.

For a teacup (150 ml (ÖAB) to 250 ml – statements in the Standard Licences relate mostly to 150 ml), the amount required is given in grams or – which is more practicable – as spoonfuls (normally 1 teaspoonful = ca. 5 ml, 1 tablespoon = ca. 15 ml; but there is considerable variation! The spoons normally used today generally have a much smaller volume.). In this book, due note has been taken of some of the pharmacopoeias (ÖAB, Erg.B. 6) and their commentaries in indicating the dosages; for other drugs, information has been taken from the technical literature (Haffner/Schultz: "Normdosentabelle" (Tables of standard doses), etc.). In quite a few books on medicinal plants, the recommended doses (teaspoons or tablespoons) converted to the weight of drug are considerably greater than those given in the pharmacopoeias.

Degree of comminution of the drug

In extracting the constituents of a drug, the degree of comminution is of crucial importance, as has been shown in some of our own

Making the Tea

(so far unpublished) investigations; as would be expected, the amount of the constituents in the tea increases as the degree of comminution increases, and the highest "yields" are obtained with powdered drugs. Apart from a few exceptions, however, the consumer expects the tea in more or less finely chopped form rather than as a powder.

For some drugs (but not mixed teas), the following fragment sizes have been derived on a purely empirical basis and found to be effective:

Leaves, flowers, herbs – coarsely to moderately finely chopped (particle size ca. 4 mm);
Woods, barks, and roots – finely chopped to coarsely powdered (particle size ca. 2.5 mm);
Fruits and seeds crushed or coarsely powdered immediately before use (particle size ca. 2 mm);
Alkaloid- and saponin-containing drugs, as well as bearberry leaves, as a moderately fine powder (particle size ca. 0.5 mm).

The definitions "coarsely chopped" to "finely powdered", which formerly in the pharmacopoeias were given as mesh sizes, are mostly nowadays indicated without such a requirement; in the DAB 10, V. 4.N6, only "coarsely chopped" (4000 to 2800 sieve), "finely chopped" (2000 sieve), and "powdered" (710 to 180 sieve) are distinguished. The wide particle-size ranges have rightly been criticized [1, 2], partly on the basis of extensive investigations.

Especially with mixed herbal teas, attention must be paid to ensuring that the particle size of the components is as uniform as possible; otherwise, separation will occur just on storage and to a greater extent during transport. In preparing small amounts of a mixed tea, it is certainly worth while to pass the weighed-out portions of the components together through the selected sieve, e.g. 4000 ro 2800, and to further reduce the residue [2].

It must be remembered that during comminution oil glands and oil cells are broken which not only accelerates loss of the volatile essential oil, e.g. peppermint leaves, chamomile flowers, fennel, aniseed, bitter orange peel, etc., but also favours oxidation processes, e.g. formation of insoluble phlobaphenes from tannins. On the other hand, as the example of fennel has shown, the volatile oil of apiaceous (umbelliferous) fruits is very inefficiently extracted from the whole drug, whereas with crushed or powdered fruits several times as much is present in the tea made from them. It is therefore expedient to keep the supply of such drugs in the whole form and each time to comminute the amount corresponding to the use expected. Very generally, of course, the constituents are better extracted from more highly comminuted drugs, so that the degree of comminution is a compromise between the parameters content of active substances (whole drug) and optimal extraction (highly comminuted drug).

That the degree of comminution on its own is not the only factor involved in the kinetics of the release of the active principles, but that evidently the nature and amount of the accompanying substances also play an essential part, has been demonstrated in the case of the sennosides in aqueous preparations (hot extractions and cold macerates) from senna fruits and senna leaves [3].

Method of extraction

There are three different methods to be considered, of which the infusion is the most often used. If no well-established special di-

Making the Tea

rections need to be followed, the following general rules can be applied:

Infusion: Boiling water (150–250 ml) is poured over the prescribed amount of drug in a heat-resistant glass or porcelain vessel, which is then covered; if necessary, the contents are stirred occasionally. If no other indication is given, the contents are strained after 5–10 min. This method can be used for most leaves, flowers, and herbs and also for many correspondingly comminuted barks and roots.

Decoction: The required amount of drug is placed in cold water and heated to boiling; it is allowed to boil for a short while (mostly 5–10 min.) and after standing for a short while strained. This procedure is particularly suitable for hard to very hard drugs (woods, roots, barks), especially when they contain tannins., e.g. ratanhia root, etc.

Maceration: The required amount of cold water is poured over the prescribed amount of drug and allowed to stand at room temperature for several hours; finally, it is passed through a tea strainer. The macerate can be drunk cold or it can be warmed. The method of preparation is particularly appropriate for mucilage-containing drugs (marsh-mallow root, linseed, Icelandic moss, etc.). Preparing a macerate rather than a tea is preferred for some other drugs when undesirable constituents, which are less soluble in cold water, have to be excluded (tannins in bearberry leaves; viscotoxins in mistletoe); thus a decoction of bearberry leaves contains 600 mg tannin and 600 mg arbutin, while a cold extract contains only 300 mg tannin and 800 mg arbutin; thus, the cold extract is to be preferred [4]. The end result of this method of preparation is improved by occasional stirring or shaking.

Objections have more than once been raised against cold extracts. Hameister [5], for example, reported that brewing a microbially unsatisfactory drug with boiling water yielded a bacteriologically harmless tea; in contrast, however, in extracts which had been prepared with warm water at only 60° C there were higher, and in cold extracts very high, bacterial counts. In the meantime, several drug importers and suppliers have emphasized to their trade buyers the necessity of indicating in their instructions to consumers that the drug should always be brewed with boiling water.

Brewing drugs usually reduces the germ count to one-tenth of the original figure and kills any enterobacteria present [6, 7]. Reduction of the germ count can be achieved by brief boiling of the (strained) extract – a matter that the pharmacist should, if appropriate, point out.

Attention should be drawn to a very interesting possibility, viz subjecting drugs before their use as *teas* to pressure, followed by rapid release of the pressure (so-called PEX procedure), in order to achieve a kind of "opening up" and thereby improving the liberation of many constituents during the preparation of the tea. The use of supercritical carbon dioxide in this connection is particularly suitable [8].

The result of taking into account the three factors mentioned – dose – degree of comminution – method of extraction – should be a tea that has an optimal amount of active constituents. But, at present there are very few studies which answer the often posed question: What proportion of the active principles in the drug pass over into the tea? With a hot-water infusion of chopped senna

Making the Tea

fruits ca. 85% of the sennosides A and B are extracted within 5 min., but from chopped senna leaves, under the same conditions, only ca. 65% sennosides A and B [3].

The large influence that the degree of comminution of the drug has on the liberation of active principles during preparation of the tea has been domonstrated in investigations with alder buckthorn bark and cascara bark:

Using the powdered drugs, almost 90% of the anthracene derivatives are found in the tea, while with coarsely chopped drugs only ca. 30% [9].

A tea made with chopped lime flowers had ca. 60% of the flavonoids in the infusion, but ca. 80% when prepared with the powdered drug [9].

It is also known that during the usual procedure for making teas, in the marc left after straining in the case of fennel ca. 70% of the essential oil present in the original drug is left behind, in the case of chamomile as much as 50–70% (with 60–70% of the chamazulene), and in the case of peppermint ca. 30%. Even though these data refer to lipid-soluble but poorly water-soluble constituents, they nevertheless show that water is not always the ideal solvent or extractant for making a tea. Even just considering these drugs is enough to pose the question of the extent to which preference should be given to the use of standardized herbal tea preparations (see also the section on: Herbal preparations).

[1] Chr. Höltzel, Dtsch. Apoth. Ztg. **124**, 2479 (1984).
[2] U.H.T. Hagenström and G. Bleske, Dtsch. Apoth. Ztg. **125**, 1597 (1985).
[3] H. Miething, W. Boventer and R. Hänsel, Dtsch. Apoth. Ztg. **127**, 2587 (1987).
[4] D. Frohne, Planta Med. **18**, 1 (1970).
[5] W. Hameister, in: „Qualität pflanzlicher Arzneimittel", Ed. G. Hanke, Wiss. Verlagsgesellschaft, Stuttgart 1984.
[6] Chr. Härtling, Pharm. Ztg. **128**, 1006 (1983).
[7] R. Leimbeck, Dtsch. Apoth. Ztg. **127**, 1221 (1987).
[8] W. Carius and E. Stahl, Dtsch. Apoth. Ztg. **127**, 901 (1987).
[9] So far unpublished findings carried out in connection with literature studies directed by M. Wichtl (A. Gerlach, D. Hüttner, B. Bozek, Th. Fingerhut).

Storage, Packaging, Keeping Properties

Assuming that herbal drugs are going to be used medicinally, the same care will be taken regarding their storage and packaging as with any other medicine. There are not many indications to be found in the pharmacopoeias as to how drugs should be stored.

Important factors to which attention should be paid in regard to the storage of drugs and to how they should be kept, e.g. by patients, include:

- Light
- Temperature
- Humidity
- Degree of comminution

Nearly all drugs require protection against light and this is specifically directed; this requirement arises, on the one hand, from the circumstance that leaf, flower, and herb drugs rapidly fade in light and become poor looking and, on the other hand, light accelerates numerous chemical processes which may bring about degradation of or changes in the constituents of the drug.

Temperature is another parameter in maintaining the quality of a drug. According to a rule formulated by van't Hof in 1884, a temperature rise of 10° C causes a doubling of the reaction rate, i.e. changes in drug constituents can be accelerated not only by light but also by heating; the content of volatile constituents (essential oil) diminishes more rapidly with increasing temperature. This leads to the necessity of storing drugs under the coolest conditions possible. Preference should definitely be given to storage in a dry cellar over a warm or hot (but also dry) loft. The formerly very popular hay lofts belong to the past!

Too high a humidity has two disadvantageous effects on the keeping properties of drugs. Moisture allows certain enzymes to become active, especially glycosidases, and hence to start degradation of the constituents. High humidity also brings with it increased danger of attack by moulds or other microorganisms. It is therefore advisable to keep or store drugs dry, i.e. in conditions of relative humidity below 60%.

Last but not least, the degree of comminution also plays a part in keeping drugs in the best possible condition: too fine a degree of comminution increases the surface area and allows disadvantageous factors to operate more strongly and rapidly than in the case of the whole drug.

This needs to be taken into account particularly with drugs containing essential oils, tannins, and bitter substances [1, 2]. Herbal drugs with these active constituents should not be stocked in the powdered state.

The containers in which drugs are kept or stored should ensure that the foregoing conditions are met. In some pharmacopoeias, the relevant details are more precisely defined, e.g. in the ÖAB "in well-closed containers" = adequate protection against being contaminated or affected by other substances; further, "in tightly closed containers" = additional protection against the effects of the moisture in the air. For some drugs, the addition "with a suitable desiccant" can be indicated, e.g. for mullein flowers, to prevent discoloration or other changes. It is recommended to select containers with a double bottom, in which, e.g. silica gel, can be placed and the drug on a layer of dry humus spread over the perforated plate. In the ÖAB, there is also the indication "protected from insect attack", in which the drug is first fumigated with chloroform and then well aired – a procedure which has attracted much criticism, owing

Storage, Packaging, Keeping Properties

to the use of a chlorinated solvent, but which is difficult to replace by other techniques (see also the section Contamination with plant protection products).

In the pharmacy, tinplate boxes as storage containers are perfectly satisfactory, as long as they can really be tightly closed; for small amounts of drugs (with the exception of those containing essential oil), plastic containers are also suitable, as well as tightly closed boxes made of wood or heavy cardboard. Small amounts of essential-oil drugs are best kept in brown glass containers or also in polyamide containers; on the other hand, those made of polyethylene, polypropylene, or polyvinylchloride are unsuitable, since they rapidly absorb essential oil from the drug itself as well as from the atmosphere above it which usually soon becomes saturated with volatile substances.

For delivering herbal drugs to patients, paper bags cannot be wholeheartedly recommended. It is better to pack herbal teas in pergamyn (glassine, imitation parchment) or cellophane bags, while aromatic drugs can be packed in the somewhat more expensive bags with aluminium foil. Storage jars for tea made of polyamide or Hostalen® when they are tinted as a protection against light are also suitable. The importance of the label needs to be emphasized. Not only must it offer correct information, but it should also have an attractive appearance [3, 4].

There are few investigations into the stability of herbal drugs [5–7] which take into account all the relevant parameters (light, temperature, humidity, degree of comminution, material of the storage container), and no general rules concerning the period during which they can be used. While in the AB-DDR, maximum periods of storage for practically all the drugs have been prescribed (3 years or sometimes only 18 months, and for a few drugs in the powdered state 24 hours), such indications are absent from the Ph.Eur., DAB 10, ÖAB, and Ph.Helv. VII. Nevertheless, more attention should be paid to the length of storage of herbal drugs, also in regard to drug safety. In the Standard Licences, appropriate indications concerning the stability are provided for a whole series of drugs. The length of time an essential-oil drug can be kept can be calculated from the initial value (content at the time of packaging) and the (percentage) decrease per unit of time. For other drugs, the length of time they can be kept is indicated directly in years. The pharmacist should therefore only buy drugs from the last harvest (but not all drug wholesalers make such declarations) and should only stock such amounts as are likely to be disposed of before the next harvest.

[1] H. Flück, Pharm. Acta Helv. **43**, 1 (1968).
[2] M. Wichtl, Pharmazie **25**, 692 (1970).
[3] U.H.T. Hagenström and A. Schmidt, Pharm. Ztg. **130**, 3102 (1985), inclusive comments of H. Morck.
[4] Anonym (schle), Dtsch. Apoth. Ztg. **127**, 875 (1987).
[5] D. Fehr and G. Stenzhorn, Pharm. Ztg. **124**, 2324 (1979).
[6] L. Kreutzig, Pharm. Ztg. **127**, 893 (1982).
[7] D. Fehr and G. Stenzhorn, Pharm. Ztg. **127**, 111 (1981).

Import Control and Testing

In the medicinal plant and drug wholesale trade

Herbal drugs are imported from various parts of the world, from overseas in containers, from eastern Europe usually in heavy lorries or by road, delivered not only as the whole drug, but also in the cut form in the most varied containers (bags made from jute, paper, polypropylene, etc.) [1]. The import control of the drug parcels, which are first put into quarantine, is carried out by visual examination – whether the labelling of the packing and the documents agree with the contents. In addition, attention is paid to damage during transport, insect and mould attack, as well as the weight. Samples are removed from each parcel according to a definite plan and these are examined macroscopically, microscopically, and phytochemically, as far as possible along the lines of the pharmacopoeias; often, tests are made for bacterial contamination and residues from plant protection substances, heavy metals, and radioactive residues.

If the drug passes all the requirements, the parcel – after retaining a reserve sample – is released for sale. If, on the other hand, it fails only a few of the tests (humidity, ash content, etc.), the drug is either reprocessed (dried, garbled) or appropriately relabelled, e.g. for industrial use (extraction). If a low content of active principles is the reason for rejecting the drug, depending on experience, the drug may either be released for extraction purposes or, if possible, standardizing it by mixing it with drugs having a higher content.

Import Control and Testing

In the pharmacy

Although according to the "Apotheken-betriebsordnung" (Regulations for the Management of Pharmacies) the pharmacist is allowed to have the testing of medicines carried out by organizations outside his/her pharmacy, e.g. by the "Zentrallaboratorium Deutscher Apotheker" (Central Laboratory of the German Pharmacists) which then gives the so-called ZL-Zeichen (Central Laboratory stamp) [2], this does not release him/her from personal responsibility for the quality of the drugs. A check on the drugs supplied must therefore be carried out even if they have already been tested; at the very least, to establish the identity is an activity of everyday practice. Very often it is possible simply by macroscopic examination to determine whether the drug is satisfactory: after some experience, linseed, chamomile flowers, and peppermint leaves can be exam-ined without any special means, i.e. they can be recognized as the genuine drug and un-contaminated; for this, a stereo hand lens is very handy.

On the other hand, for very many drugs, it is essential in order to identify them unequivo-cally or definitely to exclude falsification, to have recourse to the microscope. In this book, microscopy is highly valued means of examination, as can be seen from the many illustrations of drug diagnostic features. In doing so, particular attention has been paid to measurements, since these are not infre-quently crucial to the evaluation (see, e.g. Salvia/Threelobed Salvia – basal cells of the trichomes); for this reason, a scale is given in all microphotographs. Where the measure-ments allow for some variation, instead of calibrating a micrometer eyepiece with a micrometer scale, a little lycopodium can be added (a tiny spatula point is enough for a slide): the spores have a diameter which is very close to 30 μm and can thus serve as a "measuring rod".

Besides the microscopy, TLC plays a very important role in the identification and quality control of the drugs; it can be car-ried out in the pharmacy laboratory with the simplest of means, e.g. empty, well-cleaned baby food jars as "separating tanks", prespread 4 × 8 cm foil and, instead of spraying, dipping the developed chro-matogram in the diluted reagent and heat-ing on a hotplate covered with aluminium foil. This affords a surprising amount of in-formation with a minimum of test material and chemicals [3]. These methods are dis-cussed in many of the monographs in this book where microscopy on its own is diffi-cult or insufficient. There is a book on TLC which has been specially written for use in pharmacy practice [4], as well as a kind of

Import Control and Testing

illustrated atlas for the TLC identification of drugs [5]. There is also a very useful compendium of procedures for the examination of drugs [6].

[1] A. Nagell, in: „Qualität pflanzlicher Arzneimittel", Ed. G. Hanke; Wiss. Verlagsgesellschaft Stuttgart 1984.

[2] H. Blume, Pharm. Ztg. **132**, 1638; 2323 (1987).

[3] M. Wichtl, Prüfung von Drogen in Apotheken (Schriftenreihe der Bundesapothekerkammer, Davos 1984, Dokumentation der Vorträge).

[4] P. Pachaly, Dünnschichtchromatographie in der Apotheke, 2nd edition, Wiss. Verlagsgesellschaft, Stuttgart 1983.

[5] H. Wagner, S. Bladt and E.M. Zgainski, Plant drug analysis. Springer-Verlag, Berlin, Heidelberg, New York, Tokyo 1984.

[6] P. Rohdewald, G. Rücker and K.-W. Glombitza, Apothekengerechte Prüfvorschriften. Dtsch. Apoth. Verlag, Stuttgart 1986.

Residues in Plant Drugs (Contamination Problems)

Plants, including those used as drugs, during their growth are exposed to a multitude of environmental influences, of which the following are of interest in connection with herbal drugs: attack by microorganisms (bacteria, moulds), contamination by heavy metals (e.g. lead from motor exhausts), and treatment with plant protection substances (pesticides) and fumigation residues.

In drying the plant parts for the manufacture of drugs, the effects of the environmental factors just mentioned may be present in the form of residues, and this requires special attention on hygienic and toxicological grounds. While during the drying process, depending on their structure, pesticides may be at least partially decomposed and heavy metals may remain as such on the drugs, the number of microorganisms may, according to the method of drying, under certain circumstances, increase very considerably, so that drugs which have been dried slowly and at a relatively high humidity, e.g. in sheds during the rainy season, have a higher bacterial count than fresh plants.

Not only on hygienic grounds, but also because of the formation of toxins by moulds and bacteria, microbiological contamination is as toxicologically serious as the presence of heavy-metal and pesticide residues. These problems have long been known in the food industry and are partly covered by the regulations dealing with the maximum amounts of plant protection substances. As far as medicinal plants are concerned, these questions have only started to be considered in the last few years. Without denying the existence of these problems, it must be remembered that food is taken on a regular basis, but that herbal extracts are taken only now and then, except when they are part of a course of treatment. The problem has thus been of much greater importance in the food sector.

Residues in Plant Drugs

Microbial contamination

mind that human beings themselves are not sterile and they do not live in a sterile world [1]; the buccal flora has about 300 different organisms, especially ca. 10^9–10^{12} anaerobes/g and 10^5–10^{11} aerobes/g saliva [1], and these are to a large extent swallowed. On human skin, there are ca. 10^5–10^6 microbes/cm^2. The total germ count is therefore of relatively little significance. On the other hand, it is important to ensure the absence of pathogenic germs and to limit the number of enterobacteria, as is usual in the food industry. The limits of the germ counts has been much discussed in recent years; starting from the FIP guidelines [2] and up to the initial proposals of the DAB 9 regulations, fairly divergent data have been presented [3–5]. The proposals of B. Frank [1] are considered to be particularly well founded, since they have been made on extensive study of the literature and on his own researches on herbal drugs. In the meantime the following prescriptions are given in DAB 10, VIII.N5:

For herbal drugs which undergo a diminution of germ count before used (i. e. by making a tea) or externally used herbal drugs:

Aerobial bacteria	max. 10^7/g
Yeasts and moulds	max. 10^4/g
Escherichia coli	max. 10^2/g
Enterobacteria	max. 10^4/g
Salmonella	no

For herbal drugs used orally without diminution of germ count:

Aerobial bacteria	max. 10^5/g
Yeasts and moulds	max. 10^3/g
Escherichia coli	max. 10^1/g
Enterobacteria	max. 10^3/g
Salmonella	no

The richer a plant part is in nutrients and the slower the drying process, the higher the bacterial count of the resulting drug: root drugs, which of course are to begin with more heavily contaminated, always have a higher bacterial count than do flowers, for example, which are a less suitable as a nutrient medium.

The total germ count varies enormously from drug to drug [1, 2] and lies between 10^2/g and 10^8/g. It also has to be borne in

Residues in Plant Drugs

In this connection it is to be noted that in preparing an infusion or decoction there is a very considerable decrease in the germ count. In contrast, macerates, i.e. cold-water extracts of drugs, on standing for several hours can so change that they can no longer be considered hygienically reliable (see also the section: Making the Tea).

In regard to the specifications relating to the limits of germ counts, it must be realized that in effect there are practically no processes for reducing the germ count of a drug which at the same time do not adversely affect its constituents:

• Pasteurization or autoclaving is unsuitable;

• Dry heat can only be used for a very few drugs;

• Fumigation with ethylene oxide does indeed lead to a considerable reduction in the germ count (and at the same time destruction of insects), but the process, because of the formation of toxic reaction products (ethylene chlorhydrin, ethylene glycol) has been banned throughout the European Community since 01.01.1990;

• Ionizing irradiation: a declaration of the treatment is obligatory, but such drugs find little acceptance by the public who expect nature's products as such.

The high doses of irradiation required probably mostly also bring about changes in the constituents.

Residues in Plant Drugs

Contamination with heavy metals

In recent years, environmental contamination by lead, cadmium, and mercury has been repeatedly observed and has given rise to partly exaggerated reports.

There are a number of investigations on drugs [6–8]. In general, the figures established by the ZEBS (Zentrale Erfassungs- und Bewertungsstelle für Umweltchemikalien = Central Institute for the Study and Evaluation of Environmental Chemicals) form the basis. For foodstuffs, they are as follows:

- **Lead**
  max. 0.5 ppm* (fruit and root vegetables, cereals)
  max. 1.2 ppm (green vegetables)

- **Cadmium**
  max. 0.1 ppm (green and fruit vegetables, cereals)
  max. 0.05 ppm (root vegetables)

- **Mercury**
  max. 0.03 ppm (cereals)

Again, it is to be remembered that only a fraction of the heavy metals gets into the tea. Owing to the very low concentrations, analyses are only possible by means of atomic absorption spectroscopy, after digesting the drugs with perchloric acid/nitric acid (hence not in the pharmacy laboratory).

---

* 1 ppm = 1 part per million = 0.0001%.

Residues in Plant Drugs

Contamination with plant protection products

chlorinated hydrocarbons, carbamates, and many others. In investigating drugs according to the pharmacopoeia, pesticide residues fall into the category "unusual contaminants" and one follows the regulations dealing with pesticide residues in foodstuffs. It is to be noted that nowadays residues are always found both in foodstuffs and in medicinal plants, whether the living plants were treated with pesticides or not, since these environmental substance have spread more or less worldwide. The essential thing is to keep their amounts within limits, by, among other things, keeping to the indicated dates (period of time between the date of the last treatment and the date of harvesting). In an extensive study based on 2654 products, Schilcher [6] showed that a proportion did not conform to the regulations governing the maximum permissible amounts. But again, it should not be forgotten that only a fraction of the pesticides present will get into the infusion, viz only ca. 10% [6, 7].

Since a gas chromatograph and/or high-pressure liquid chromatograph is absolutely essential for analytical work, the required investigations cannot be carried out in the pharmacy laboratory. TLC is only possible using disproportionately large samples, and even then only usable for a very few pesticides (with higher limits of tolerance), so that in practice it is excluded. Reputable herbal drug wholesalers, however, examine their parcels of drugs for residues or have the examinations carried out in appropriate laboratories.

The problem of ethylene-oxide residues has already been pointed out in the section on "Microbial contamination".

As with food plants, so also with medicinal plants, it is not possible to cultivate them without making use of plant protection products: because of the expense, organic cultivation is only possible on a small scale (in a garden) – or one accepts the risk of severe to very severe attacks by pests.

While the use of plant protection products for food plants is regulated by law in many European and overseas countries, such legislation is lacking in many developing countries or in practice is largely ignored. It can therefore happen that drugs from these countries contain pesticides, e.g. DDT, which elsewhere have long been banned – a problem for the analyst, who already has to test for a range of the most widely differing substances, such as thiophosphoric esters,

Residues in Plant Drugs

Contamination with radioactive substances

Since the disaster with the reactor at Chernobyl in May 1986, the contamination of drugs with radioactive substances has regularly been the subject of research reports. In the meantime, in the European Community, the maximum value has been fixed at 600 Bq/kg, a figure which also guides the drug importers and suppliers. In the "months after Chernobyl", for some drugs considerably higher Bq values were reported, especially for those from eastern Europe. But for the tea drinker, there is hardly any real danger, since each time only a small part of the radionuclides goes into the tea; at that time, milk exhibited ca. 20 times higher Bq values than a tea prepared from contaminated drugs [9]. Studies carried out in 1987 came to similar conclusions [10].

[1] B. Frank, Keimreduzierung und mikrobiologischer Status von Drogen und Drogenzubereitungen, Vortrag auf dem APV-Seminar „Qualität pflanzlicher Arzneimittel IV.", Darmstadt 3. Mai 1988.
[2] FIP-Sektion Industrieapotheker, Pharm. Acta Helv. **51**, 41 (1976).
[3] W. Hameister, in: „Qualität pflanzlicher Arzneimittel", Ed. G. Hanke, Wiss. Verlagsgesellschaft Stuttgart 1984.
[4] R. Leimbeck, Dtsch. Apoth. Ztg. **127**, 1221 (1987).
[5] E. Schneider, Dtsch. Apoth. Ztg. **127**, 1683 (1987).
[6] H. Schilcher, Planta Med. **44**, 65 (1982).
[7] S.L. Ali, Pharm. Ztg. **130**, 1927 (1985).
[8] H. Schilcher, Fresenius Z. Anal. Chem. **321**, 325 (1985).
[9] H. Pratzel and D. Reinelt, Dtsch. Apoth. Ztg. **126**, 1957 (1986).
[10] S.L. Ali and M. Ihrig, Pharm. Ztg. **132**, 2537 (1987).

Standard Licenses

In the (then) Federal Republic of Germany, the Arzneimittelgesetz (Medicines Act) (AMG 78) required that from 1.1.1978 all prepared medicines require a special licence; only a few, mostly prescription-only, drugs made on a limited scale are excepted (§21 Para. 2 No. 1). This means that many equivalent or identical retail remedies, e.g. herbal drugs packaged in large numbers (more than 100), also require a licence. The expenditure connected with this (proposal and supporting documentation concerning quality, activity, and harmlessness) would be unreasonable both for the Bundesgesundheitsamt (BGA) (Federal Ministry of Health) as licensing authority and for the pharmacies. The legislator has therefore created the expedient of the Standard Licences (§35 AMG), the regulations requiring that monographs of the drugs concerned be published, in which the qualitative and quantitative characteristics of the drug, the marking (according to §10 AMG) and the information to be given in the package insert (according to §11 AMG) are included. In practice, such a monograph will go beyond that of a pharmacopoeia, since it must contain additional information on the stability and the container. At the time the manuscript was being finished (June 1988), there were outline monographs for Standard Licences for 83 drugs and these have been taken into account in writing the text, more particularly the wording of the package inserts of all these drugs has been included separately.

The Standard Licences allow the pharmacist to produce and make available these 83 drugs, as well as certain mixtures (see pp. 12 et seq.), as ready-made remedies, i.e. of uniform composition and prepared and packaged in advance for direct sale to the customer, without having to go through the lengthy licensing procedure required for ready-made remedies: all that is necessary is to adhere to the wording of the monograph of the Standard Licence. Further details are to be found in [1].

[1] Standardzulassungen. Text und Kommentar, Ed. R. Braun, Deutscher Apotheker Verlag and Govi-Verlag, Stuttgart and Frankfurt/M., 1987ff.

Prepared Monographs of the German Commission E for Human Medicine, Section of Phytotherapy

In the (then) Federal Republic of Germany, after the second Medicines Act (AMG) came into force, since 1978 all drugs in the licensing procedure are tested not only for their quality, but also for their activity and harmlessness (§22 AMG). The remedies which were on the market at that time could, in conformity with the transitional regulations (Art. III §7 AMNG), be notified and given a "fictitious" licence, i.e. a licence "as of right", which would expire on 31.12.1989. This twelve-year transition period would, according to the philosophy of the Medicines Act, be used to remove the split in the existing market between old and new preparations and to carry out the essential preliminary work for this. Of particular importance for this is the screening of the scientific evidence for drugs, as required by §25, Abs. 7 AMG, by the committee specially set up by the Federal Ministry of Health. The monographs resulting from this work form the foundations for the licensing and the so-called re-licensing.

Example of a Commission E Prepared Monograph

Valerianae Radix (Valerian Root)

Name of the drug

Valerianae radix, Valerian root.

Constituents of the drug

Valerian root, consisting of the underground parts of the collective species *Valeriana officinalis* Linné, fresh or carefully dried at or below 40° C, and its preparations in active doses.

The roots contain essential oil with mono- and sesquiterpenes (valerenic acids).

The thermo- and chemolabile genuine valepotriates are not present in the usual therapeutically used formulations (infusion, extract, fluid extract, tincture).

Uses

Restlessness, nervous disturbances of sleep.

Contraindications

None known.

Side effects

None known.

Interactions

None known.

Dosage

If not otherwise prescribed:

Infusion: 2–3 g drug to a cup, one or more times a day.

Tincture: $^1/_2 - 1$ teaspoonful (1–3 ml), one or more times a day.

Extracts: corresponding to 2–3 g drug, one or more times a day.

Manner of use

Internally: as expressed juice, tincture, extracts, and other galenical preparations.

Externally: as a bath additive.

Effects

Calming, promoting readiness to sleep.

Prepared Monographs of the German Commission E for Human Medicine, Section of Phytotherapy

Up till now (July 1988), over 200 monographs, including more than 140 *drug* monographs have been published and additional ones have been prepublished.

The results have not been entirely satisfactory. On the one hand, it would be expected that for many preparations a "relicensing" would be simplified and, on the other hand, it should not be overlooked that the opinions of the risks in the partly very schematic and uniform details regarding the indications take up a considerable amount of space. For combined drugs, including herbal mixtures, the second bill modifying the AMG, which came into force on 1.2.1987, led to further problems: now it has to be shown that each medicinally active component contributes to the positive evaluation of the remedy.

The Federal Ministry of Health (BGA) now publishes the drafts produced by the Commission E for consideration by people and bodies interested in the monographs and then publishes them in the Bundesanzeiger (BAnz) (Federal Gazette) after taking into account the views received. The form of such a monograph can be seen in the example given before (p. 40) (BAnz no. 90, dated 15.03.1985).

Although the information is important, especially for the manufacturer of phytopharmaceuticals, it should also interest the pharmacist and doctor which indications, contraindications, side effects, interactions, dosages, manner of use, and effects are, as it were, officially recognized; in some cases, where the evidence is insufficient, the Commission E came to the conclusion not to advocate therapeutic use – this, of course, in no way prohibits their use, but the pharmacist in his discussions with his clients will be hesitant in recommending or will inform them of the fact. Since the information regarding the constituents of the drugs in this book is mostly more detailed than in the monographs of the Commission E, as a rule this has been omitted here.

The reader will in each case find the corresponding text, specially marked and set apart, near the section Indications.

Monographs

Absinthii herba   (DAB 10), Wormwood, Artemisia absinthium (BHP 1983)

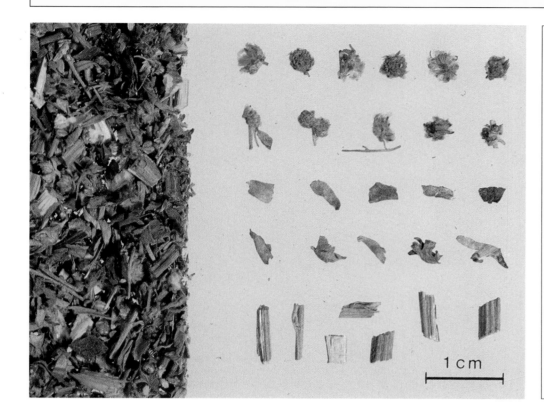

Fig. 1: Wormwood

Description: The drug consists of the dried flowering tops of branches from plants with stems that are not more than 4 mm thick. Leaf fragments, pubescent on both surfaces and therefore appearing matt silvery grey, predominate; their origin, up to three times pinnately divided leaves, can to some extent be recognized in the ca. 2 mm wide, lanceolate fragments with a blunt to pointed tip (Fig. 3). The yellow, subspherical flowering heads bear a few ray florets and many tubular disk florets (Fig. 3), partly still in bud. The stem fragments are angled, silvery grey on the outside, and with a pith inside.

Odour: Aromatic and characteristic.

Taste: Aromatic and intensely bitter.

Fig. 2: *Artemisia absinthium* L.
An up to 1 m tall subshrub having aromatic scented, 2–3 times pinnately divided leaves and – in contrast to *A. vulgaris*, mugwort – a dense silky pubescence on both surfaces; small, yellow, almost spherical, flowering heads arranged in much branched panicles.

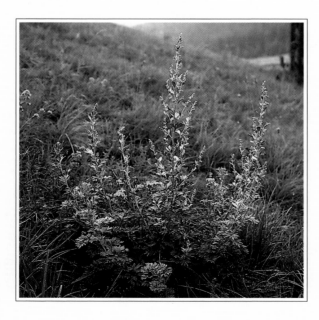

DAB 10: Wermutkraut
ÖAB: Herba Absinthii
Ph. Helv. VII: Absinthii herba
St.Zul. 1339.99.99

Plant source: *Artemisia absinthium* L. (Asteraceae).

Synonyms: Absinthium, Absinth (Engl.), Wermutkraut, Bitterer Beifuß, Wurmkraut (Ger.), Herbe d'absinthe (Fr.).

Origin: Native in the drier regions of Europe and Asia. The drug comes from the former USSR, Bulgaria, former Yugoslavia, Hungary, and Poland.

Constituents: 0.15–0.4% bitter substances and 0.2–1.5% essential oil are the most important components. The bitter substances are sesquiterpene lactones, with as the main component the dimeric guianolide absinthin (0.20–0.28%); there are also other sesquiterpene lactones, such as artabsin, matricin, anabsinthin, etc., and the pelenolides [1]; of these last, hydroxypelenolide can be detected during the TLC identification of the drug.

Absinthin

Artabsin

β-Thujone

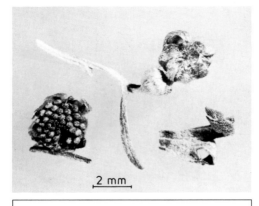

Fig. 3: Yellow flower-head (left), silvery grey flower bud (centre), and fragment of pinnately divided leaf (right)

The essential oil consists mainly of terpenes. The following components may dominate and form up to more than 40% of the oil, depending on the geographical source of the drug: *β*- or *α*-thujone ((1*S*,4*R*)-thujan-3-one or (1*S*,4*S*)-thujan-3-one) [2, 3, 12], *trans*-sabinyl acetate [3, 12], *cis*-epoxyocimene [2], or chrysanthenyl acetate [4]. Of the more than 50 other identified mono- and sesquiterpenes, thujan, thujyl alcohol, linalool, and cineole, as well as *α*-bisabolol, *β*-curcumene, and spathulenol, may be mentioned. Various flavonoids [5] occur in the drug, and caffeic and other phenolic carboxylic acids [6] have been detected; small amounts of polyacetylenes are probably also present; traces of a mixture comprising two diastereoisomeric homoditerpene peroxides (with *in vitro* antimalarial activity) [13]; some 24*ζ*-ethylcholesta-7,22-dien-3*β*-ol (antipyretic activity) [14].

Indications: As a bitter aromatic, to stimulate the appetite, for gastrointestinal complaints, e.g. gastritis with reduced formation of acid. On the basis of the *mild* hyperaemic action of the essential oil, also in chronic gastritis.
Further, as a carminative, a choleretic, and in spasmodic disorders of the intestines and biliary tract [7]. Wormwood also finds use as as an anthelmintic; see the BHP 1983.

Side effects: Only likely on overdosage, and due essentially to the effects of the (toxic) thujone. The symptoms are vomiting, stomach and intestinal cramps, retention of urine, and in serious cases renal damage,

vertigo, tremors, and convulsions. Thujone can be quantitatively removed from wormwood by high-pressure extraction with supercritical carbon dioxide [8, 9].
Owing to the toxicity of the thujone, alcoholic wormwood extracts and the use of the essential oil (in absinth liqueurs, etc.) has been banned in many countries. Aqueous extracts, on the other hand, contain relatively little thujone.

Making the tea: Boiling water is poured over 1–1.5 g of the finely chopped drug and after 10 min. passed through a tea strainer. To stimulate the appetite before eating and as a cholagogue after meals.

1 Teaspoon = ca. 1.5 g. The dose must not be exceeded!

Herbal preparations: The drug is also available in tea bags (0.9–1.8 g).

Phytomedicines: The drug and fluid and dry extracts are components of many prepared gastrointestinal remedies, cholagogues, and roborants.

Authentication: Macro- (see: Description) and microscopically, following the DAB 10. Besides the occurrence of asteraceous glandular trichomes (Fig. 4), the T-shaped trichomes (Fig. 5) present especially on the upper and lower leaf surfaces are characteris-

*Extract from the German Commission E monograph
(BAnz no. 228, dated 05.12.1984)*

Uses
Lack of appetite, dyspeptic troubles, dyskinesia of the biliary tract.

Contraindications
None known.

Side effects
None known.

Interactions
None known.

Dosage
Unless otherwise prescribed: average daily dose, 2–3 g drug as an aqueous infusion.

Mode of administration
Chopped drug for decoctions and infusions, powdered drug, also extracts or tinctures exclusively as fluid or solid formulations for oral use.

Warning
Combinations with other bitters or aromatics may be advantageous. In toxic doses, thujone, the active component of the oil, acts as a convulsant poison. Therefore, the essential oil must not be used on its own.

Effects
The action as a bitter aromatic is due to the content of bitter substances and essential oil.

There are no recent worthwhile experimental pharmacological data available.

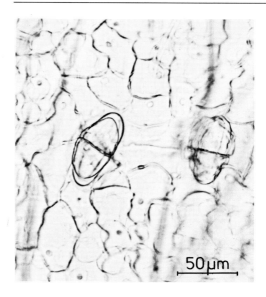

50 μm

Fig. 4: **Asteraceous glandular trichomes in surface view**

tic. The receptacles of the small flowering heads have tubular covering trichomes, with a multicellular stalk and a longer, thin-walled terminal cell, which are up to 1500 μm long (Fig. 6). Cf. the BHP 1983.
The drug should be checked for the presence of pollen grains. If none, or only a few, are present (in the powdered drug, they are quite common), then the material does not come from flowering plants, as is prescribed, and is therefore not of the proper quality.
The TLC examination set out in the DAB 10 (detection of bitter substances and components of the essential oil) is as follows:

Test solution: 1 g powdered drug shaken with 10 ml dichloromethane for 2–3 min., filtered, and the filtrate gently reduced to half the volume; the test solution must be freshly prepared and the solution spotted at once (decomposition of artabsin).

Reference solution: 50 μl thujone and 2.0 mg each of methyl red, phloroglucinol, and resorcinol dissolved in 10 ml methanol.

Loadings: 30 μl test solution and 10 μl reference solution, as 2-cm bands on silica gel G.

Solvent system: acetone + dichloromethane (10 + 90), 10 cm run.

Detection and Evaluation: sprayed with anisaldehyde reagent and evaluated without heating after 2–3 min. Test solution: at about the same Rf as the methyl red band of the reference solution, a bluish violet zone

becoming more intense on heating (artabsin); occasionally, below it a bluish grey zone (matricin).
Plate then heated at 100–110°C for 5–10 min. Test solution: brown zone (absinthin) with an Rf in between those of the yellowish orange reference resorcinol (upper) and phloroglucinol (lower) zones; a conspicuous reddish violet zone (hydroxypelanolide) with an Rf slightly greater than that of resorcinol; in the upper part of the chromatogram a reddish violet zone, fluorescing intense brick red (thujone) under UV 365 nm light, and above it, zones belonging

to esters of sabinyl and thujyl alcohols; additional, fainter reddish, bluish, or bluish violet zones present.
Other TLC systems are given in [10, 11]. The absinthin content can be determined photometrically [4].

Quantitative standards: DAB 10: *Volatile oil*, not less than 0.2%. *Bitterness value*, not less than 15 000. *Foreign matter*, not more than 2% and not more than 5% stem fragments with a diameter greater than 4 mm. *Loss on drying*, not more than 10.0%. *Ash*, not more than 12.0%.

Fig. 5: **T-shaped trichome from leaf and stem fragments**

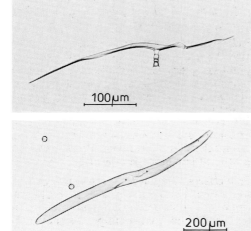

100 μm

200 μm

Fig. 6: **Smooth pollen grains and strap-shaped tubular covering trichome from the receptacle of the inflorescence**

<u>ÖAB</u>: *Volatile oil*, not less than 0.3%. *Bitterness value*, not less than 10,000. *Foreign matter*, not more than 5% stem fragments with a diameter greater than 3 mm. *Ash*, not more than 10.0%.

<u>Ph. Helv. VII</u>: *Volatile oil*, not less than 0.2%. *Bitterness value*, 250 Ph. Helv. units/g. *Foreign matter*, not more than 5% stems with a diameter greater than 4 mm. *Sulphated ash*, not more than 17%.

Adulteration: Seldom, but happens occasionally; mostly, it concerns admixture with *Artemisia vulgaris* L., mugwort (Artemisiae herba, q.v.). The leaves, which are similar to those of wormwood, are pubescent only on the lower surface and they are much less bitter in taste. The T-shaped trichomes have a slender, twisted transverse cell; the long covering trichomes are absent from the receptacle of the inflorescence.

Storage: Protected from light, and kept cool and dry in well-closed containers (not made of plastic).

Literature
[1] Kommentar DAB 10.
[2] O. Vostrowsky et al., Z. Naturforsch. **36c**, 369 (1981).
[3] F. Chialva, P.A.P. Liddle and G. Doglia, Z. Lebensm. Unters. Forsch. **176**, 363 (1983).
[4] G. Schneider and B. Mielke, Dtsch. Apoth. Ztg. **118**, 469 (1978) und **119**, 977 (1979).
[5] B. Hoffmann and K. Herrmann, Z. Lebensm. Unters. Forsch. **174**, 211 (1982).
[6] L. Swiatek and E. Dombrowicz, Farm. Pol. **40**, 729 (1984).
[7] H. Kreitmair, Pharmazie **6**, 27 (1951).
[8] E. Stahl and D. Gerard, Planta Med. **45**, 147 (1982).
[9] E. Stahl and D. Gerard, Z. Lebensm. Unters. Forsch. **176**, 1 (1983).
[10] H. Wagner, S. Bladt, and E. M. Zgainski, Plant drug analysis, Springer-Verlag, Berlin, Heidelberg, New York, Tokyo, 1984, p. 134.
[11] E. Stahl, Drug analysis by chromatography and microscopy, Ann Arbor Science, Ann Arbor MI, 1973, p. 158.
[12] T. Sacco and F. Chialva, Planta Med. **54**, 93 (1988).
[13] G. Rücker, D. Manns, and S. Wilbert, Phytochemistry **31**, 340 (1992).
[14] M. Ikram, et al. Planta Med. **53**, 389 (1987).

Agrimoniae herba

Agrimony, Agrimonia (BHP 1983)

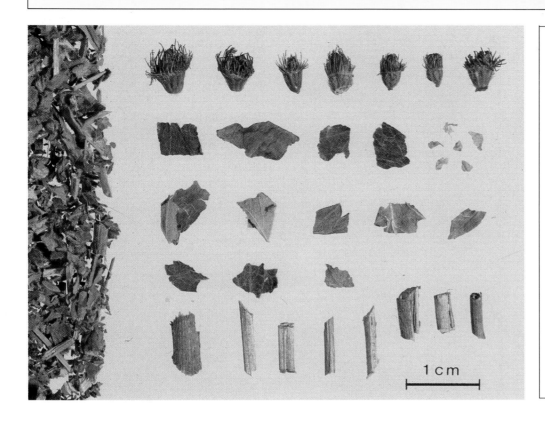
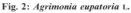

Fig. 1: Agrimony

<u>Description</u>: The 2–3 cm long pinnate leaflets have a coarsely serrate margin; the leaf fragments are green and they are covered with a grey velvety pubescence on the lower surface (Fig. 4) and a sparse pubescence on the upper surface. The pieces of stem have coarse stiff hairs. The occasional small syncarps with hooked bristles at the margin of the hypanthium (Fig. 3) are characteristic. Yellow flower fragments are rare.

<u>Odour</u>: Very faintly aromatic.

<u>Taste</u>: Somewhat bitter.

Fig. 2: *Agrimonia eupatoria* L.
A ca. 0.5–1.0 m tall chalk-loving herb with pinnate leaves comprising pairs of leaflets of different sizes and with leafy stipules; upper surface of the leaflets dark green, lower surface shaggy. Golden-yellow flowers, 5–8 mm in diameter, in long spikes; hypanthium, grooved and provided with small projecting hooked bristles.

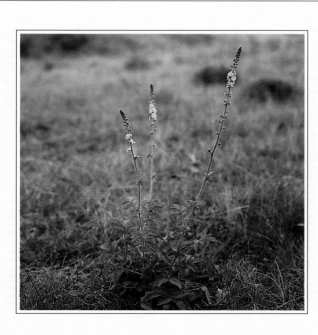

DAC 1986: Odermennigkraut
ÖAB: Herba Agrimoniae

Plant sources: *Agrimonia eupatoria* L., (common) agrimony, and more rarely *A. procera* WALLR. (syn. *A. odorata* auct. non MILLER), fragrant agrimony (Rosaceae).

Synonyms: Herba Eupatoriae (Lat.). Cocklebur, Stickwort, Liverwort (Engl.), Odermennigkraut, Fünffingerkraut, Ackerkraut (Ger.), Herbe d'aigremoine, Herbe de Saint-Guillaume (Fr.).

Origin: Distributed in the northern hemisphere. Imports come from Bulgaria, Hungary, and former Yugoslavia.

Constituents: In the aerial parts 4–10% condensed tannins, along with a little ellagitannins and traces of gallotannins [1, 3]. Ca. 20% polysaccharides [3]. Triterpenes, including ursolic acid; reportedly, up to 12% (?) silicic acid [2]; flavonoids, including luteolin and apigenin 7-*O*-β-D-glucosides [3]; traces of essential oil (but only when *A. pro-*

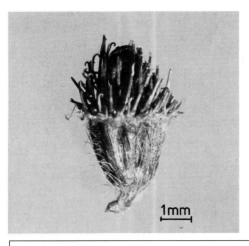

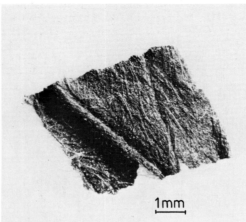

Fig. 3: *Agrimonia eupatoria* **fruit, showing the hooked bristles**

Fig. 4: Densely shaggy lower surface of the leaf

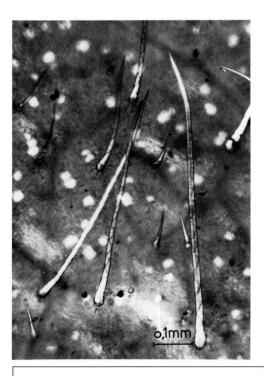

Fig. 5: Unicellular, thick-walled trichomes with spiral thickening and numerous calcium oxalate crystals (clusters, prisms) in the leaf tissue (polarized light)

component of phytomedicines, it should be regarded with scepticism.

Ethanolic extracts have antiviral properties [4].

Making the tea: 1.5 g of the finely chopped drug is put into cold water and boiled briefly, or boiling water is poured over it, and after 5 min. passed through a tea strainer. As an astringent for gargling or rinsing. Internally, for bowel complaints, a cup of the tea is taken two or three times a day.
1 Teaspoon = ca. 1 g.

Phytomedicines: The drug is present in a number of liver and bile teas; extracts of the drug are present, mostly in small amounts, in prepared cholagogues and stomach and bowel remedies, e.g. Divinal®-Bohnen (beans), Neo-Gallonorm®-Dragees, etc., and urological remedies, e.g. Rhoival®, etc.
Agrimony is a component of the UK product Potter's Piletabs.

Regulatory status (UK): General Sales List – Schedule 1, Table A.

Authentication: Macro- (see: Description) and microscopically, following the DAC 1986. The thick-walled stiff trichomes with spiral thickening (Fig. 5) and the calcium oxalate prisms and/or clusters occurring in the mesophyll (Fig. 5) are particularly diag-

Extract from the German Commission E monograph (BAnz no. 50, dated 13.03.1986)

Uses

Internally: mild, non-specific, acute diarrhoea; inflammation of the mucous membranes of the mouth and throat.
Externally: mild, superficial inflammation of the skin.

Contraindications

None known.

Side effects

None known.

Interactions with other remedies

None known.

Dosage

Unless otherwise prescribed:
Internal use: daily dose, 3–6 g drug; preparations correspondingly.
External use: poultices with a 10% decoction, several times a day.

Mode of administration

Finely chopped or powdered drug for infusions and other galenical preparations for internal and topical use.

Effect

Astringent.

cera is present in the drug); other data refer to ubiquitous plant substances.

Indications: As a mild astringent, internally and externally, against inflammation of the throat, gastroenteritis, and intestinal catarrh.

In *folk medicine,* in gall-bladder disorders, though the known constituents provide no grounds for this; insofar as the drug is a

nostic. Multicellular glandular trichomes are rare.

A detailed description of the macroscopy and microscopy of the drug is also to be found in the BHP 1983.

Quantitative standards: <u>DAC 1986</u>: *Tannins precipitable with hide powder*, not less than 5.5% calculated as pyrogallol (M_r 126.1). *Foreign matter*, not more than 2%; frag- ments of *Verbascum nigrum* can be recognized by their dense woolly pubescence. *Loss on drying*, not more than 10%. *Ash*, not more than 8%.

<u>ÖAB</u>: *Foreign matter*, not more than 5% stem fragments with a diameter greater than 3 mm. *Ash*, not more than 10.0%.

<u>BHP 1983</u>: *Water-soluble extractive*, not less than 12%. *Total ash*, not more than 10%. *Acid-insoluble ash*, not more than 2%.

Adulteration: In practice, does not occur.

Literature:
[1] F. von Gizycki, Pharmazie **4**, 276, 463 (1949).
[2] H.A. Hoppe, Drogenkunde, de Gruyter, Berlin – New York, 1975, vol. **1**.
[3] G.A. Drozd et al., Khim. Prir. Soedin. (1), 106 (1983); C. A. **98**, 194984 (1983).
[4] S.C. Chon et al., Med.Pharmacol. Exp. **16**, 407 (1987).

Alchemillae herba   (DAB 10), Alchemilla (BHP 1983), Lady's-mantle

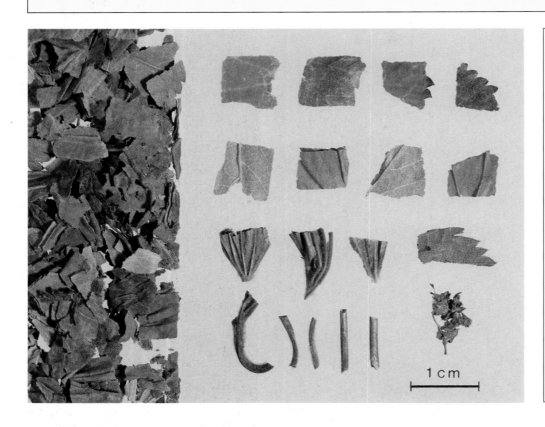

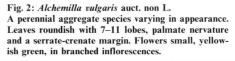

1 cm

Fig. 1: Lady's-mantle

Description: The leaves are up to 8 cm wide, reniform, 7–9-lobed, with a white silvery appearance because of the abundant pubescence; in the drug, less strongly pubescent fragments of older leaves occur as well (Fig. 3). The leaf margin is coarsely serrate (Fig. 4) and the main nerves are conspicuous on the lower surface. Pubescent pieces of stem and yellowish green clumps of flowers are also present.

Taste: Slightly bitter and astringent.

Fig. 2: *Alchemilla vulgaris* auct. non L.
A perennial aggregate species varying in appearance. Leaves roundish with 7–11 lobes, palmate nervature and a serrate-crenate margin. Flowers small, yellowish green, in branched inflorescences.

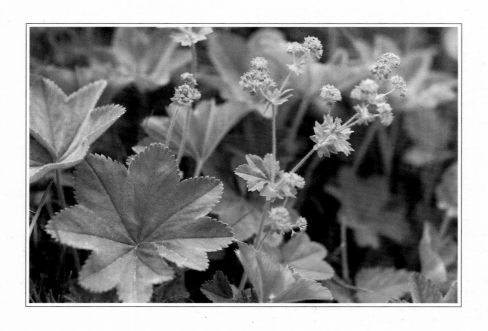

DAB 10: Frauenmantelkraut
St.Zul. 9499.99.99

Plant source: *Alchemilla xanthochlora* ROTHM. (syn. *A.vulgaris* auct. non L.), lady's-mantle (Rosaceae).

Synonyms: Herba leontopodii (Lat.), Lion's foot (Engl.), Frauenmantelkraut, Marienmantel, Löwenfuß, Silberkraut (Ger.), Feuilles d'alchemille (Fr.).

Origin: Distributed in Europe, North America, and Asia. The drug is imported from Poland, former Czechoslovakia, Bulgaria, and Hungary.

Constituents: 6–8% tannins (partly gallotannins?); Lund [1] has detected ellagitannins (pedunculagin, the dimeric alchemillin). A number of flavonoids has been obtained by Russian workers; and quercetin 3-O-β-D-glucuronide has been isolated and identified as the major flavonoid in leaves of French origin [2]. Other information relates only to ubiquitous substances.

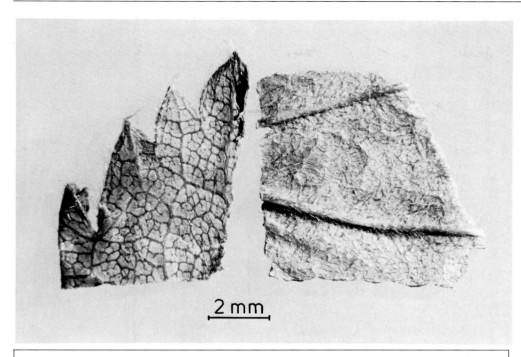

2 mm

Fig. 3: Older, only slightly pubescent leaf (left) with a dark-coloured, finely reticulate nervature; silky pubescence on the lower surface of a young leaf (right)

Authentication: Apart from the macroscopically recognizable characters, the essential microscopical diagnostic features are the unicellular, long, partly tortuous, thick-walled trichomes found on both leaf surfaces. There are occasional calcium oxalate clusters in the mesophyll.

The following is a suitable TLC identification test:

Test solution: 1 g powdered drug refluxed for 10 min. with 10 ml methanol at 60°C and filtered warm.

Reference solution: 10 mg rutin and 5 mg hyperoside dissolved in 10 ml methanol.

Loadings: 3μl test solution as a band, 1μl reference solution as a spot.

Solvent system: ethyl acetate + anhydrous formic acid + water (80 + 8 +12), 6 cm run.

Detection: after drying in a current of hot air, sprayed with 1% methanolic diphenylboryloxyethylamine, then oversprayed with 5% methanolic polyethylene glycol 400, and heated for a short while at 100–105 °C.

Evaluation: In UV 365 nm light. <u>Reference solution</u>: yellowish orange fluorescent zones, the lower one belonging to rutin, the upper one to hyperoside. <u>Test solution</u>: an intense orange fluorescent zone slightly higher than that of hyperoside and a faint orange fluorescent zone slightly below it; at about the same Rf as rutin, also a faint yellowish orange fluorescent zone; directly below the solvent front, a blue fluorescent

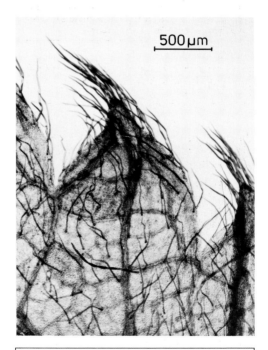

500μm

Fig. 4: Coarsely crenate and finely ciliate leaf margin of *Alchemilla xanthochlora*

Indications: On the basis of its tannin content, as an astringent against bleeding and diarrhoea, and as a remedy for healing wounds (?). As is also evident from the use of the drug in some phytomedicines (q.v.), gynaecological indications such as menorrhagia or "weakness of the lower abdomen", go back to *folk medicinal* (doctrine of signatures (?): *lady's-mantle*), and not to scientifically established, ideas [3]. See also the BHP 1983. The warning in the Standard Licence about possible liver damage appears to be exaggerated.

Making the tea: Hot water is poured over 1–2 g of the drug and allowed to stand for 10 min.; it is then poured through a tea strainer. Using cold water and allowing it to stand for several hours at room temperature is also recommended.
1 Teaspoon = ca. 0.9 g.

Herbal preparations: The drug is available in tea bags (0.9–1.6 g) and is also a component of some commercial herbal mixtures ("female teas").

Phytomedicines: A number of prepared gynaecological remedies, and, presumably on the basis of the tannin content, products for oral and pharyngeal hygiene, e.g. Salviathymol®, etc.

Extract from the German Commission E monograph (BAnz no. 173, dated 18.09.1986)

Uses
Mild, non-specific diarrhoea.

Contraindications
None known.

Side effects
None known.

Dosage
Unless otherwise prescribed: average daily dose, 5–10 g drug; preparations correspondingly.

Mode of administration
Chopped drug for infusions and decoctions, as well as other galenical preparations for internal use.

Duration of use
If the diarrhoea lasts for more than 3–4 days, a doctor should be consulted.

Effects
Astringent.

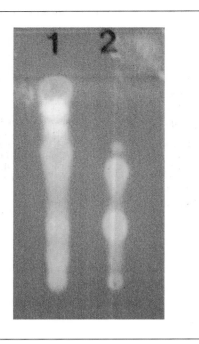

Fig. 5: TLC on 4 × 8 cm silica-gel foil

1: Lady's-mantle
2: Reference compounds

For details, see the text

zone; and below that a yellowish green fluorescent zone (Fig. 5); additional, faint fluorescent zones also present.

The DAB 10 method makes use of silica gel G and the solvent system: ethyl acetate + anhydrous formic acid + water (84 + 8 + 8); the reference compounds are chlorogenic and caffeic acids, and the spray is the same as that already indicated above.

Quantitative standards: <u>DAB 10</u>: *Foreign (vegetable and/or mineral) matter*, not more than 2%. *Loss on drying*, not more than 10%. *Ash*, not more than 15%.
<u>BHP 1983</u>: *Total ash*, not more than 6%.

Adulteration: Does not occur in practice.

Literature:
[1] K. Lund, Dissertation, Freiburg i. Br. (1986).
[2] J.L. Lamaison, A. Carnat, C. Petitjean-Freytet, and A. P. Carnat, Ann. Pharm. Franç. **49**, 186 (1991).
[3] P. Petcu et al., Clujul Med. **52**, 266 (1979); C. A. **93**, 843 (1980).

Alkannae radix   Alkanna root

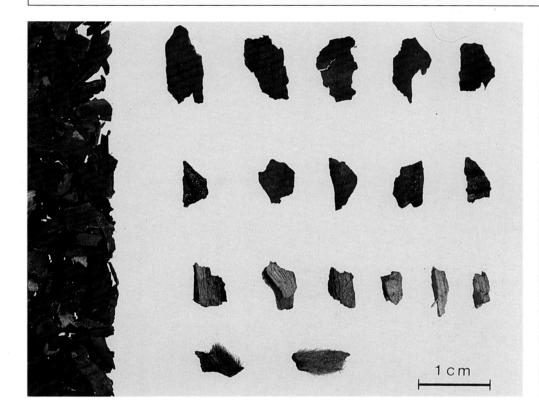

Fig. 1: Alkanna root

Description: The cylindrical, fissured rhizome has a dark purple, readily exfoliating, brittle bark on the outside and the remains of bristly leaves and stems near the crown (bottom row; see also Fig. 3). In broken pieces, or in the cut drug, below the bark there is a narrow white cortex and an irregularly radiate, light coloured xylem with a brownish pith.

Taste: Mucilaginous, somewhat bitter.

Fig. 2: *Alkanna tinctoria* (L.) TAUSCH

Mostly prostrate herbs up to 30 cm in height, occurring on sandy shores and cliff meadows. Bristly lanceolate leaves and stems, and flowers with glabrous, bright blue petals.

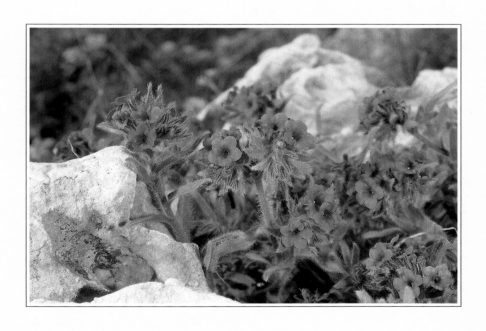

Erg. B. 6: Radix Alkannae

Plant source: *Alkanna tinctoria* (L.) TAUSCH (Boraginaceae).

Synonyms: Radix Anchusae (tinctoriae) (Lat.), Alkanet, Anchusa, Dyers's Bugloss, Orchanet (Engl.), Alkannawurzel, Schminkwurzel, Alkermeswurzel, Rote Ochsenzungenwurzel (Ger.), Racine d'orcanette, Racine d'alcanna (Fr.).

Origin: Native to southern Europe. The drug is cultivated in and imported from Turkey, India, and Albania.

Constituents: A mixture of red colouring matters (alkanna), which is present especially in the bark (up to 5–6%), consisting chiefly of lipophilic naphthazarin (5,8-dihydroxy-1,4-naphthaquinone) derivatives such as alkannin and its esters [1]. Alkanna is soluble in organic solvents, in fixed oils, and to some extent also in essential oils (hence the use of the tincture in microscopy for their histochemical detection). Being phe-

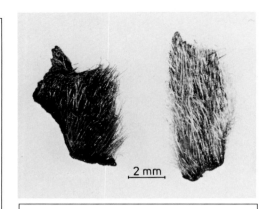

Alkannin R = —H
Alkannin esters, e.g.

R =

R =

R =   ---OCOCH₃

Fig. 3: Fragments of the bristly leaf and stem of *Alkanna tinctoria*

nols, the individual components of alkanna are soluble in solutions of alkali hydroxides, with a change in colour to green or blue. As is the case with many other Boraginaceae, pyrrolizidine alkaloids have also been detected in *Alkanna tinctoria*, but so far there is no information about the amounts present in the various parts of the plant and in extracts prepared from it [2].

Indications: The drug has *no medicinal importance* (it was formerly used as an astringent) and currently its only role is a modest one as a pigment. Nevertheless, in many countries, the use of alkanna for colouring food is prohibited, and nowadays it is utilized almost exclusively for colouring cosmetics. Antibiotic and wound-healing properties, e.g. for ulcus cruris (indolent leg ul-

cers), have been reported for some alkannin esters [3, 4].

Regulatory status (UK): General Sales List – Schedule 1, Table B; external use only.

Authentication: This can be limited to determination of the colour value: 2.5 g powdered drug is extracted with 100 ml toluene + ethanol (1 + 1) and the solution obtained is then diluted 1 in 25. At this dilution, the solution should have the same intensity of colour as a mixture of 20 ml 0.01% potassium permanganate solution and 5 ml 0.1% potassium dichromate solution.

Quantitative standard: Erg. B. 6: *Ash*, not more than 14%. *Drug with the bark partly removed must not be used.*

Adulteration: Nowadays, extremely rare, though formerly often described in the literature. Nevertheless, steps should be taken to verify that the drug has not lost all its bark – the colouring matters are only present in the outer parts.

Literature:
[1] V.P. Papageorgiou et al., Flavour Fragrance J. **1**, 21 (1985).
[2] E. Röder et al., Phytochemistry **23**, 2125 (1984).
[3] V.P. Papageorgiou, Planta Med. **31**, 390 (1977).
[4] V.P. Papageorgiou, Experientia **34**, 1499 (1978).

Allii ursini herba   Ramsons

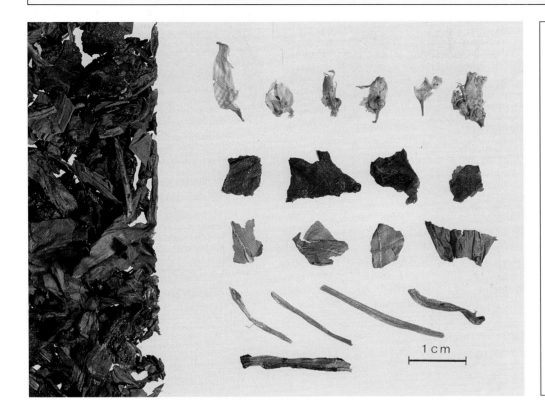

Fig. 1: Ramsons

<u>Description:</u> The leaf fragments, dark green on the upper surface and light green on the lower surface, show parallel venation in which the main nerve is very prominent on the lower surface and the lateral nerves are indistinct. The light yellow to yellowish brown flowers (top row) are 6-partite, with a short pedicel; the fruit, a small capsule, contains black seeds. Peduncles of the umbellate inflorescences are also present (bottom row).

<u>Odour:</u> Faintly spicy.

<u>Taste:</u> Somewhat pungent, reminiscent of garlic.

Fig. 2: *Allium ursinum* L.

Bulbous plants with broad lanceolate leaves. Umbels with white flowers. Garlic-like odour, especially on bruising.

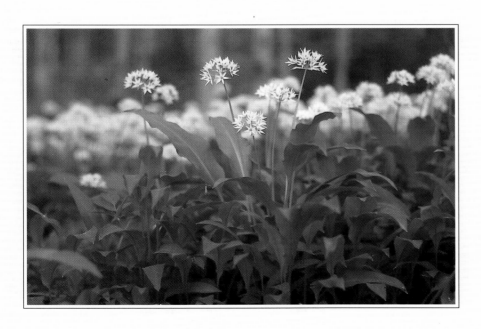

Plant source: *Allium ursinum* L., ramsons (Alliaceae; Liliaceae s.l.).

Synonyms: Wild or Wood or Bear's or Hog's garlic, Gipsy onion (Engl.), Bärlauchkraut, Waldknoblauch, Zigeunerlauchkraut, Ramsel, Hexenzwiebel (Ger.), Ail des ours, Ail des bois (Fr.).

Origin: Ramsons occurs scattered throughout Europe and northern Asia, but is also often found en masse covering the ground in moist, humus-rich deciduous and coniferous woods. It is imported from eastern European countries.

Constituents: The drug has been little investigated, and the older information available needs to be checked. On steam distillation, up to ca. 0.007% of an "onion" oil is obtained, which arises, as with garlic and other *Allium* species, from odourless precursors, e.g. alliin (= (+)-*S*-allyl-L-cysteine sulphoxide). On drying, much of this oil is lost, so that the fresh plant should be used.
The oil from ramsons contains principally vinyl disulphide, as well as vinyl polysulphides. Whether the allyl isothiocyanate, re-

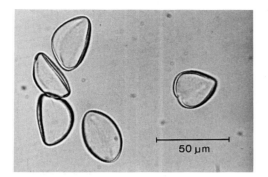

Fig. 3: Pollen grains from *Allium ursinum*

ported in 1963, really does occur in ramsons needs to be verified. Recent examination of an acetone/chloroform extract has shown the presence of ajoene and homologues, together with alliin (0.20%) and (+)-S-methyl-L-cysteine sulphoxide (0.40%) and a range of other sulphur-containing compounds; the overall qualitative composition is like that of *A. sativum* [5]. The drug also contains flavonoids [1] and traces of prostaglandins A, B, and F [2].

Indications: Like *Allium sativum*, in *folk medicine* it is used as a carminative in gastrointestinal upsets and, because of the antibacterial action, in dyspeptic complaints; it is further applied as an antihypertonic and anti-arteriosclerotic. It has been reported that ajoene inhibits thrombocyte aggregation, as well as the action of lipoxygenase, and that (+)-S-methyl-L-cysteine sulphoxide decreases blood cholesterol levels [5].

Side effects: Not expected with normal use; in excess, it may lead to gastric irritation.

Making the tea: Not usual. The fresh leaves are employed as a seasoning, in the same way as chives, onions, or garlic.

Herbal preparations: Ramsons is a component of the Künzle Herz- und Kreislauftee (heart and circulation tea), which is available in tea bags.

Phytomedicines: Only a few heart and circulation remedies, e.g. Lapidar 2®-Tabletten (tablets); homoeopathic dilutions are present in a few prepared remedies.

Authentication: Macro- (see: Description) and microscopically [3]. The leaf epidermis on both surfaces consists of elongated cells; stomata are present only on the lower surface and are large and roundish, with two subsidiary cells at each end. The mesophyll is not differentiated into palisade layer and spongy mesophyll. Trichomes and crystals are absent. The pollen is ovoid or hemispherical, 35–40 µm long and 20–25 µm broad, with an elongated pore and somewhat warty exine (Fig. 3).

Adulteration: Not known. Confusion is unlikely during collection because of the marked odour. However, the case of adulteration with Colchicum leaves, described not long ago, emphasizes the need for care [4].

Literature:
[1] C. Laracine, P. Lebreton, and P. Berthel, Lett. Bot. **1985**, 307; C. A. **105**, 57925 (1986).
[2] K. Proboszny et al., Herba Hung. **18**, 71 (1979); C. A. **92**, 211834 (1980).
[3] K. Kraus, Dissertation Univ. Innsbruck, 1985.
[4] D. Frohne and H. J. Pfänder, Giftpflanzen, 3rd ed., Wiss. Verlagsges., Stuttgart, 1987.
[5] A. Sendl and H. Wagner, Planta Med. **57**, 361 (1991).

| **Aloe** | **barbadensis** (DAB10, Ph. Eur. 2), Barbados aloes (BP 1988, BHP 1/1990), Aloe (USP XXII) |
| | **capensis** (DAB10, Ph. Eur. 2), Cape aloes (BP 1988, BHP 1/1990), Aloe (USP XXII) |

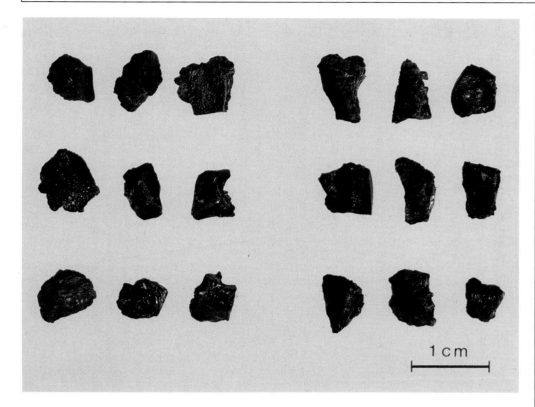

1 cm

Fig. 1: Barbados aloes (right) and Cape aloes (left)

Barbados aloes

<u>Description</u>: The drug consists of the juice from the secretory cells of the leaves of the aloe plant which has been concentrated and allowed to solidify. It is a dark brown, slightly shiny, opaque mass with a waxy conchoidal fracture. The powder is brown and soluble in warm ethanol, partly soluble in boiling water, and practically insoluble in ether and chloroform. The aqueous solution turns red after the addition of alkalis (Bornträger reaction).

<u>Odour</u>: Characteristic, strong.

<u>Taste</u>: Bitter, unpleasant.

Cape aloes

<u>Description</u>: The drug is the juice from the secretory cells of the leaves of the aloe plant which has been concentrated and allowed to solidify. It is a deep brown mass with a greenish reflex and a glassy conchoidal fracture. The powder is greenish brown and soluble in warm ethanol, partly soluble in boiling water, and practically insoluble in ether and chloroform. The aqueous solution turns red after the addition of alkalis (Bornträger reaction).

<u>Odour</u>: Characteristic, strong.

<u>Taste</u>: Bitter, unpleasant.

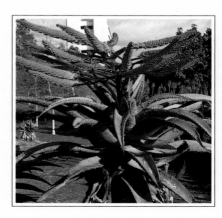

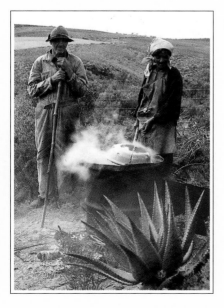

Fig. 2: *Aloe ferox* MILLER

A 2–3 m tall xerophyte with succulent leaves up to 50 cm long bearing spines along the edge.

Fig. 3: Preparation of aloes

The cell sap of the leaves is concentrated over an open fire for about four hours and then poured into tins in which the mass solidifies.

DAB 10: Curaçao-Aloe
          Kap-Aloe
ÖAB: Aloe (=Aloe capensis)
      Aloe barbadensis
Ph. Helv. VII: Aloe barbadensis
          Aloe capensis

Aloe barbadensis, Barbados Aloes

Plant source: *Aloe barbadensis* MILLER (Aloaceae or Asphodelaceae; formerly Liliaceae s.l.).

Synonyms: Curaçao aloes (Engl.), Curacao-Aloe, Venezuela-Aloe (Ger.), Aloès (Fr.).

Origin: Native in Africa, introduced into America. Cultivated particularly in the West Indies and in the coastal regions of Venezuela. The drug is mostly exported via Curaçao. There is little trade in it in **Central** Europe, but in Western Europe, including Great Britain, it is widely used. In recent years, cultivation of *Aloe barbadensis* (syn. *A. vera* (L.) WEBB et BERTH. non MILLER) in the subtropical regions of the United States (Florida, Texas, Arizona) has been increasing steadily, mainly for the exploitation of the "Aloe vera gel" used in cosmetics and beverages (see further: Phytomedicines).

Constituents [1–3]: Hydroxyanthracene derivatives: as the principal components (also in Aloe capensis, q.v.) 25–40% aloins A and B (= aloin, barbaloin = 10-*C*-β-D-glucosyl diastereoisomers of aloe-emodin anthrone; configurational and conformational

analysis [6, 7]); the 3–4% 7-hydroxyaloins A and B, and their 6'-*p*-coumaroyl and feruloyl esters, are also characteristic; in addition, small amounts of aloe-emodin and chrysophanol, but no aloinosides and no 5-hydroxyaloin (see: Aloe capensis). Chromone derivatives: the main component (up to 30%) is 8-*C*-glucosylchromone aloeresin B (=aloesin) and there are smaller amounts of the sugar-free compound aloesone, as well as its derivative aloeresin A (=2'-*p*-coumaroylaloesin) and aloeresin C (= 7-*O*-β-D-glucoside of aloeresin A). The bitter-substance glycoside aloenin is absent (but see: Aloe capensis).

Indications: Owing to the anthracene derivatives, as a powerful colonic laxative. Aloe-emodin anthrone, the presumed active substance, is formed in the colon by enzymic or bacterial reductive cleavage of the anthracene derivatives. The anthrones irritate the mucous membrane, leading to an increase in the secretion of mucus, thus stimulating peristalsis. At the same time, the reabsorption of water and electrolytes is inhibited. See also [5].

Aloins A and B (Barbaloin)

Aloinoside A

Aloenin A

Aloeresin B (=Aloesin) (R¹=R²=H)
Aloeresin A (R¹=p-Coumaric acid, R²=H)
Aloeresin C (R¹=p-Coumaric acid, R²=Glucose)
Aloesone = Aglycone of aloeresins A, B, C

Side effects: The mechanism of action of anthraquinone-containing laxatives is such that chronic use often upsets the electrolyte balance. In particular, there is loss of potassium and, at the same time, sodium ions are removed through the loss of water. The potassium depletion finally leads to paralysis of the intestinal musculature and the laxative becomes less active. The amount of drug taken then has to be raised in order to achieve the same effect. In patients with a heart condition, the potassium depletion may also disturb the cardiac rhythm. Moreover, the frequent use of anthraquinones causes damage to the epithelial membrane of and irreversible damage to the muscular coat of the intestine. Tenesmus with loss of mucus occurs; on the other hand, the brown coloration of the mucous membrane is harmless – it is due to the deposition of various anthraquinone reduction products. Finally, attention must also be drawn to the fact that aloes in large doses leads to the accumulation of blood in the pelvic region. In addition, as a result of the irritation of the large intestine, there is reflex stimulation of the musculature of the uterus, which in late pregnancy may bring about abortion or premature birth. Toxic doses of aloes cause severe haemorrhagic diarrhoea and kidney damage, and sometimes death. The lethal dose is stated to be 1 g/day taken for a period of several days. Indication for taking aloes must be very precisely worded: acute constipation. Contraindications: pregnancy, menstruation, kidney complaints. Note must be taken of the interference that hypokalaemia may cause with saluretics. The uncontrolled use of anthraquinones is not without its dangers and they are only suitable for self-medication under certain conditions [1, 4]; see also the literature in [5].

Making the tea: Not applicable.

Phytomedicines: Aloes is one of the strongest of the anthraquinone group of stimulant laxatives. It is present in many purgatives, often together with other anthraquinone drugs or with belladonna extract or chelidonium extract, etc., mainly in the form of dragees, tablets, and capsules. Often, instead of aloes itself, the standardized dry extract (Ph. Eur. 2, BP 1988, etc.: if necessary, adjusted by the addition of saccharose to contain 19.0–21.0% hydroxyanthracene derivatives, calculated as anhydrous aloin), a purified aloes obtained by treatment with boiling water, is used. This

Extract from the German Commission E monograph
(*BAnz. no.* 154, *dated* 21.08.1985)

Uses

Patients for whom an easy defaecation with a soft stool is desirable, e.g. in cases of anal fissures, haemorrhoids, after rectal or anal operations, constipation.

Contraindications

Ileus of whatever origin; during lactation, to be taken only after consultation with a doctor.
Owing to its abortifacient action, aloes should not be used during pregnancy.

Side effects

None known.
On chronic use or misuse: loss of electrolytes, especially potassium, and harmless deposition of pigment in the intestinal mucosa.

Interactions

None known.
Potassium depletion resulting from chronic use or misuse may potentiate the effects of cardiotonic glycosides.

Dosage

Unless otherwise prescribed: average daily dose, 0.05–0.2 g of powdered aloes or dry extract of aloes.

Mode of administration

Powdered aloes or dry extracts for liquid and solid oral formulations.

Duration of use

Anthraquinone-containing laxatives should not be taken over long periods of time.

Warning

During treatment, a harmless red coloration of the urine may occur.

Effects

The constituents bring about active secretion of electrolytes and water into the lumen of the intestine and inhibit their re-absorption from the colon. The resulting increase in volume of the contents of the intestine leads to a feeling of distension and stimulation of peristalsis.
The aloe resins are believed to be responsible for the undesirable effects.

---

has the advantage of reducing the proportion of amorphous resins, which are inactive but which occasionally lead to problems in some patients. Dose: 0.1–0.2 g aloes or 0.05–0.1 g aloes extract, taken in the evening for a period of several days.

Aloes is an ingredient of Compound Benzoin Tincture (Friars' Balsam) and it is also present in Opobyl (UK) and Nature's Remedy (US). Aloin (*BAN*), which contains not less than 70% anhydrous barbaloin, is a component of the UK preparations: Alophen, Aperient Dellipsoids D9, Purgoids, etc.

Regulatory status (UK): General Sales List – Schedule 1, Table A; maximum single dose 50 mg.

Note: In recent years, under the name "Aloe vera gel", the stabilized viscous juice from the mucilage-containing parenchyma in the inner part of the succulent aloe leaves has been an ingredient in cosmetic preparations (and in the United States also in the food industry, in so-called "fitness" preparations). A wide variety of products, including creams, is manufactured, since humectant, anti-inflammatory, and antibacterial actions are ascribed to the gel.

Authentication: Macro- and microscopically, and especially by TLC, the Ph. Eur. 2 (BP 1988) method being as follows:

Test solution: 0.5 g powdered drug boiled and shaken with 20 ml methanol for a few mins.; the supernatant decanted and kept at 4 °C and used within 24 hours.

Reference solution: 50 mg barbaloin in 10 ml methanol.

Loadings: 5 μl each of the test and reference solutions, as 2-cm bands on silica gel.

Solvent system: water + methanol + ethyl acetate (13 + 17 + 100), 10 cm run.

Detection and Evaluation: in UV 365 nm light after spraying with 10% methanolic potassium hydroxide. Barbados aloes: a yellow fluorescent zone at about the same Rf (0.4–0.5) as the aloin zone; in the lower part of the chromatogram, a light blue fluorescent zone corresponding to aloesin. Cape aloes: in the lower part of the chromatogram, two yellow fluorescent zones belonging to the aloinosides A and B and a blue fluorescent zone corresponding to aloesin.

Then heated at 110 °C for 5 min. Barbados aloes: just below the aloin zone, a violet fluorescent zone belonging to 7-hydroxyaloin [3]; aloinosides (below) should not be present on the chromatogram. See also [5]. Cape aloes: **no** violet fluorescent zone immediately below the level of the aloin zone.

Quantitative standards: Ph. Eur. 2, etc.: *Hydroxyanthracene derivatives*, not less than 28.0% calculated as anhydrous aloin (barbaloin) (M_r 418.4). *Loss on drying*, not more than 12.0%.
BHP 1/1990: The material has to comply with the requirements of the appropriate monographs in the Ph. Eur. 2 or BP 1988.

Adulteration: Nowadays, very rare. Particularly those varieties containing homonataloin, e.g. South African Natal aloes, used to be considered a serious adulteration. (Homonataloins are 10-*C*-glucosyl derivatives of 1,7-dihydroxy-8-methoxy-3-methylanthrone.) See also: Aloe capensis. Adulteration with other *Aloe* species can be recognized by the TLC method outlined.

Literature:
[1] Kommentar DAB 10.
[2] H.-W. Rauwald and R. Voetig, Arch. Pharm. (Weinheim) **315**, 477 (1982).
[3] H.-W. Rauwald, Pharm. Weekbl. (Sci. ed.) **9**, 215 (1987).
[4] E.O. Riecken and H. Leonhardt, Internist **22**, 733 (1981).
[5] A series of articles published by the *Zeitschrift für Phytotherapie* vol. **7** (1986) summarizes the current situation regarding the analysis, metabolism, action, pharmacology, and toxicology, as well the clinical relevance, of the anthraquinone laxatives:
H. Wagner and C. Ludwig: analysis, p. 123.
J. Lemli: metabolism, p. 127.
K. Ewe: action on intestinal transport, p. 130.
L. Maiwald: clinical relevance, p. 153.
C.-P. Siegers, M. Younes, and E.W. Herbst: toxicology, p. 157.
Ph. Gendre and Ph. Dufour: effects of chronic administration, p. 160.
[6] H.D. Höltje, K. Stahl, K. Lohse, and H.W. Rauwald, Arch. Pharm. (Weinheim) **324**, 859 (1991).
[7] H.-W. Rauwald, K. Lohse, and J.W. Bats, Angew. Chem. (Internat. ed.) **28**, 1528 (1989).
[8] G. Speranza, P. Manitto, D. Monti, and D. Pezzuto, J. Nat. Prod. **55**, 723 (1992).
[9] G. Speranza, A. Martignoni, and P. Manitto, J. Nat. Prod. **51**, 588 (1988).
[10] W.T. Mabusela et al., Phytochemistry **29**, 3555 (1990).
[11] W.C. Evans, Trease and Evans' Pharmacognosy, 13th ed., Baillière Tindall, London, 1989, p. 414.
[12] J.M. Conner, A. I. Gray, T. Reynolds, and P.G. Waterman, Phytochemistry **26**, 2995 (1987).

Aloe capensis, Cape aloes

Plant sources: *Aloe ferox* MILLER (Aloaceae or Asphodelaceae; formerly Liliaceae s.l.) and, according to the USP XXII, hybrids with *A. africana* MILLER and *A. spicata* MILLER. Formerly, the main source of the drug was *A. perryi* BAKER, but nowadays this species has almost ceased to be used.

Synonyms: Kap-Aloe, Afrikanische Aloe (Ger.), Aloès (Fr.).

Origin: Indigenous in Africa; cultivated in southern and eastern Africa; the commercial varieties may be classified according to their geographical origin: South Africa: Cape, Natal Aloes; East Africa/Arabia: Kenya, Uganda, Socotrine, Zanzibar, Mocha Aloes. Socotrine and Zanzibar aloes are no longer official drugs. Natal aloes is no longer being imported into the UK [12].

Constituents: Hydroxyanthracene derivatives: especially 13–27% aloins A and B (= barbaloin, aloin, 10-*C*-β-D-glucosyl diastereoisomers of aloe-emodin anthrone). In addition, the aloinosides A and B (= 11-*O*-α-L-rhamnosides of the aloins) in varying proportions or absent, depending on the source of the drug; 5-hydroxyaloin A, which is characteristic of Cape aloes; further, small amounts of aloe-emodin and chrysophanol; no compounds of the 7-hydroxyaloin type (cf. Barbados aloes). 1-Methyltetralins: feroxidin and two *O*-glucosylated derivatives, feroxins A and B [8]. Chromone derivatives: the main components (25–40%) are the 8-*C*-glucosylchromones aloeresins A and B and smaller amounts of aloeresin C (= 7-*O*-glucoside of aloeresin A) and iso-aloeresin A (in which the *p*-coumaroyl residue has the 2-*O*-*Z*-configuration [9]); the so-called aloeresin D (= 7-*O*-methyl derivative of aloeresin A, with the acetonyl side-chain reduced to an isopropoxy group) is found only in Kenya aloes (which is almost unobtainable on the Continent). 6-Phenyl-2-pyrone derivatives: the glycoside of the bitter substance aloenin B, which is made up of aloenin A (formerly aloenin) and *p*-coumaroyl-glucose is also present in Kenya aloes. The parent substance aloenin A, a 6-phenyl-2-pyrone *O*-glucoside (and not a chromenol glucoside [cf. 1]), in contrast with the data given in more recent textbooks, has not yet been detected in the official drugs and has only been isolated from *A. arborescens* MILLER, which is used in folk medicine. *p*-Coumaric acid methyl ester also occurs. (This summary of the constituents is taken from [1–3].)

Indications: see, Aloe barbadensis.

Making the tea: Not applicable. Nowadays, the drug is a component of the so-called "Swedish bitters", which originated in Sweden but which has become popular in Germany and elsewhere. The mixture includes: Aloes, Aurantii pericarpium, Croci stigma, Galangae rhizoma, Myrrha, Rhei radix, Sennae folium, and Sennae fructus; these are made into a tincture with alcohol and taken dropwise for indigestion and as a laxative. The mixture has been thought of, unjustifiably, as a panacea.

Phytomedicines: see, Aloe barbadensis.

Regulatory status (UK): General Sales List – Schedule 1, Table A; maximum single dose, 100 mg.

Authentication: Macro- (see: Description) and microscopically, following the Ph. Eur. 2 (BP 1988). For its differentiation by TLC from Aloe barbadensis, see there.

Quantitative standards: Ph. Eur. 2, etc.: *Hydroxyanthracene derivatives*, not less than 18.0% calculated as anhydrous aloin (M_r 418.4). *Loss on drying*, not more than 10.0%. BHP 1/1990: The material complies with the requirements of the appropriate monographs in the Ph. Eur. 2 or BP 1988.

Adulteration: see, Aloe barbadensis.
According to Conner et al. [12], screening for nataloin, i.e. nataloe-emodin (= 1,2,8-trihydroxy- 6-methylanthraquinone) 10-*C*-b-D-glucopyranoside, which is present in commercial Natal aloes, has failed to reveal its presence in the *Aloe* species supposedly contributing to the product.

Literature:
See: Aloe barbadensis.

Althaeae folium
Marshmallow leaf, Althaea leaf (BHP 1983)

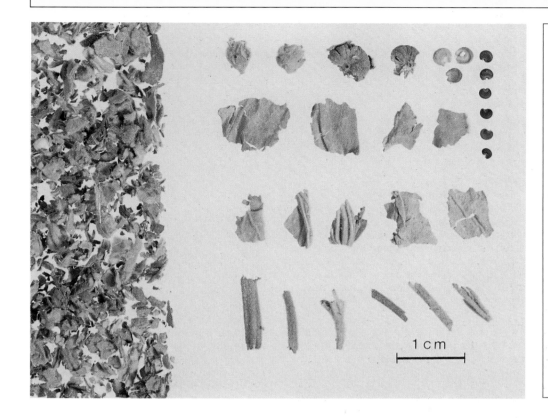

Fig. 1: Marshmallow leaf

<u>Description:</u> The finely tomentose to velvety pubescent pieces of leaf (pubescence on the upper surface – 2nd row – as well as on the lower surface – 3rd row) include fragments showing the characteristic palmate nervature. In the drug, there are always pubescent fragments of petiole and occasionally pieces of the inflorescence, as well as mericarps and seeds (1st row).

<u>Taste:</u> Mucilaginous.

Fig. 2: *Althaea officinalis* L.

Perennial, pubescent plant, up to 150 cm in height. Leaves 3- to 5-lobed, velvety, with palmate nervature; flowers white to pink, with 6–9 outer sepals fused at the bottom.

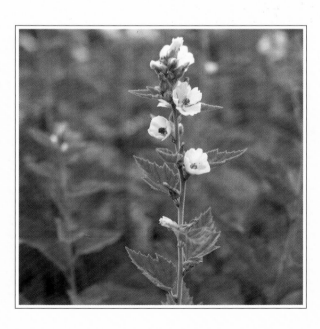

DAC 1986: Eibischblätter
ÖAB: Folium Althaeae
St.Zul. 1469.99.99

Plant source: *Althaea officinalis* L., marshmallow (Malvaceae).

Synonyms: Herba Malvae visci (Lat.), Eibischblätter, Altheeblätter (Ger.), Feuilles de guimauve (Fr.).

Origin: Marshmallow is distributed throughout Europe and western Asia and is also cultivated for drug purposes; it has become naturalized in the USA. The leaf drug is imported from eastern European countries.

Constituents: 6–9% mucilage (highest content in the leaves, which are harvested shortly before flowering), consisting essentially of arabinogalactans and galacturonorhamnans [1]. There are also traces of an essential oil of unknown composition. Flavonoids: the main one is 8-hydroxyluteolin 8-β-gentiobioside; the corresponding 8-glucoside is also present [2].

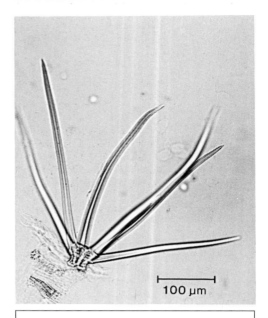

Fig. 3: Stellate trichome made up of six thick-walled, pointed cells; the base is pitted

Extract from the German Commission E monograph (BAnz no. 43, dated 02.03.1989)

Uses

For alleviating irritation of the mucous membranes of the mouth and throat and the associated dry cough.

Contraindications

None known.

Side effects

None known.

Interactions with other remedies

None known.

Warning: the absorption of other drugs being taken at the same time may be delayed.

Dosage

Unless otherwise prescribed: daily dose, 5 g drug; preparations correspondingly.

Mode of administration

Chopped drug for aqueous infusions and other galenical preparations for internal use.

Effect

Demulcent.

Wording of the package insert, from the German Standard Licence:

6.1. **Uses**

To alleviate irritation of the mucous membranes of the mouth and throat, as well as of the gastrointestinal tract; to ease irritation of the throat in bronchial catarrh.

6.2 **Dosage and Mode of administration**

Hot water (ca. 150 ml) is poured over 1 teaspoonful (1–2 g) of **Marshmallow leaf** and after 10 min. passed through a tea strainer. The tea can also be prepared by adding cold water and allowing it to draw for about an hour with occasional stirring.
Unless otherwise prescribed, a cup of the freshly prepared tea is drunk several times a day.

6.3 **Note**

Protect from light and humidity.

Indications: Particularly as an antitussive (demulcent, expectorant) in irritable coughs and catarrhal inflammation of the mouth and throat; it is also used for inflammation of the mucous membranes of the gastrointestinal tract. See further the BHP 1983. In *folk medicine,* it is recommended covering insect bites with the freshly bruised leaves.

Making the tea: Cold water is added to ca. 2 g (a heaped teaspoon) of the finely chopped drug, allowed to stand with frequent stirring, and strained after 1–2 hours; a cupful, slightly warmed, is drunk several times a day. The cold-water extract (cf. the Standard Licence) is to be preferred to the hot-water infusion.
1 Teaspoon = ca. 1.4 g.

Phytomedicines: Exclusively marshmallow root, rather than leaves, is used for the purpose.

Authentication: Macro- (see: Description) and microscopically, following the DAC 1986; see also the BHP 1983. The numerous stellate trichomes, comprising 2–8 (but mostly 6) thick-walled, pointed cells are characteristic (Fig. 3). In addition, there are tiered glandular trichomes, cluster crystals of calcium oxalate, and in the mesophyll mucilage cells.

Quantitative standards: DAC 1986: *Swelling index,* not less than 12; the drug is pre-moistened with 4.0 ml ethanol – a deviation from the standard method necessitated by the abundant pubescence. *Foreign matter,* not more than 8% of buds, flowers, fruits, and shoots; not more than 2% other foreign matter, including leaves attacked by rust – recognized by brown spots and the presence of teleutospores of *Puccinia malvacearum* (cf. Malvae folium, Fig. 5); leaves of other Malvaceae, especially *Lavatera thuringiaca* L. (teeth of the lamina twice as wide as long; structure of the basal part of the stellate trichomes which are on a hemispherical or columnar pulvinus), must be absent. *Loss on drying,* not more than 12%. *Ash,* not more than 18%. *Acid-insoluble ash,* not more than 2.0%.
ÖAB: *Swelling index,* not less than 12. *Foreign matter,* not more than 3%; spores of *Puccinia malvacearum* must not be present. *Ash,* not more than 15.0%. *Acid-insoluble ash,* not more than 2.0%.

Adulteration: Very rare, e.g. with leaves of other Malvaceae; see above.

Literature:
[1] M.S. Karawya, S.I. Balbaa, and M.S.A. Afifi, Planta Med. **20**, 14 (1971).
[2] J. Gudej, Acta Pol. Pharm. **44**, 369 (1987).

Althaeae radix (DAB 10), Marshmallow root (BHP 1/1990)

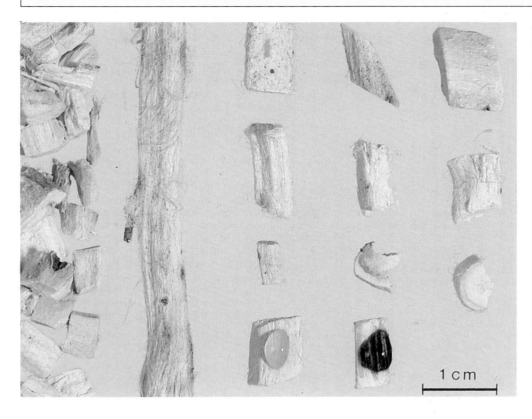

Fig. 1: Marshmallow root

<u>Description</u>: The drug consists of pieces of root, the outer bark layers of which have mostly been removed by peeling or scraping. They are yellowish white, almost cylindrical, and on the outside have dark scars originating from lateral roots, as well as small detaching groups of bark fibres. The fracture is fibrous in the outer part and short in the inner part, and shows a dark sinuate cambium line. With a hand lens, the concentric layers of the cortex can be easily recognized, especially after soaking in water.
The drug becomes yellow with ammonia solution (bottom row, left) and blue with iodine solution (bottom row, right).

<u>Odour</u>: Faint, characteristic, and somewhat mealy.

<u>Taste</u>: Mucilaginous and sweetish.

1 cm

For an illustration of *Althaea officinalis* L., see: Althaeae folium.

DAB 10: Eibischwurzel
ÖAB: Radix Althaeae
Ph. Helv. VII: Althaeae radix
St.Zul. 8899.99.99

Plant origin: *Althaea officinalis* L., marshmallow (Malvaceae).

Synonyms: Althaea root, Guimauve (Engl.), Eibischwurzel, Schleimwurzel (Ger.), Racine d'althée, Racine de guimauve (Fr.).

Origin: Native in Europe and western Asia. The drug comes from cultivated plants (at least two years old) grown in Bulgaria, former Yugoslavia, the former USSR, Hungary, and Belgium; production in Germany no longer covers its costs.

Constituents: 5–10% mucilage (depending greatly on the time of harvesting and on the further processing): a mixture mainly of acidic polysaccharides comprising an arabinan, glucans, and a rhamnogalacturonan [1–3]. Pectin, sugars, asparagine, and small amounts of sterols are also present.

Indications: As an antitussive, especially for irritable coughs and catarrhal inflammation of the throat, but **not** as expectorant; the total extract and the polysaccharide fraction have both been shown to produce a statistically significant cough-suppressant effect [3]. A less frequent use is for gastroenteritis, and occasionally as a poultice for skin inflammations or burns. A 2–3% macerate is also given as an enema in cases of proctitis (inflammation of the rectum).
In *folk medicine*, the drug is sometimes employed for diarrhoea, cystitis, and fluor albus, but in each case without proper justification.

Making the tea: Cold water is added to 3–10 g of the finely cut drug and macerated at room temperature for 30 min. with frequent stirring; it is then passed through a tea strainer or a piece of fine cloth. Marshmallow syrup is also a common preparation, e.g. Sirupus Althaeae ÖAB.
1 Teaspoon = ca. 3 g.

Herbal preparations: A few ready-prepared cough teas contain extracts of marshmallow root, e.g. Bronchostad®, Solubifix®, Broncholind®, Bronchialtee 400, etc.

Phytomedicines: Many prepared remedies which contain the finely powdered drug or extracts, e.g. Risinetten® (pastilles), etc.
In the UK, the drug is a component of Gerard House Golden Seal Tablets, Potter's Herbheal Ointment, etc.

Authentication: Macro- (see: Description) and microscopically, following the DAB 10; see also the BHP 1/1990. The microscopy of the powdered drug is described in [4].
The BHP 1/1990 TLC identification procedure, which is closely modelled on the method described in [5] for flavonoid drugs, provides a fingerprint chromatogram:

Test solution: 1 g powdered drug extracted for 10–15 min. with 10 ml methanol on the water-bath.

Reference solution: 2.5 mg rutin dissolved in 10 ml methanol.

Loadings: 20 μl of each solution, as 2-cm bands on silica gel.

Extract from the German Commission E monograph (BAnz no. 43, dated 02.03.1989)

Uses

Inflammation of the mucous membranes of the mouth and throat and the associated irritable dry cough.
Mild inflammation of the gastric mucosa.

Contraindications

None known.

Side effects

None known.

Interactions with other remedies

None known.
Warning: The absorption of other drugs being taken at the same time may be delayed.

Dosage

Unless otherwise prescribed: daily dose, 6 g drug; preparations correspondingly.
Marshmallow syrup, single dose 10 g.

Mode of administration

Pulverized drug for aqueous infusions and other galenical preparations for internal use.
As marshmallow syrup, only to be used for inflammation of the mucous membranes of the mouth and throat.
Note: Marshmallow syrup: diabetic patients must take into account the sugar content, ... % (stated by the manufacturer), equivalent to ... bread units.

Effects

Soothes, inhibits mucociliary activity, stimulates phagocytosis.

Mobile phase: ethyl acetate + anhydrous formic acid + glacial acetic acid + water (100 + 11 + 11 + 27), 15 cm run.

Detection: sprayed with 1% methanolic diphenylboryloxyethylamine and over-sprayed with 5% ethanolic polyethylene glycol 4000.

Wording of the package insert, from the German Standard Licence:

5.1 Uses

To soothe irritation arising from inflammation of the mucous membranes of the mouth and throat, upper respiratory tract, and gastrointestinal tract.

5.2 Dosage and Mode of administration

Cold water (ca. 150 ml) is poured over a tablespoonful (15 g) of **Marshmallow root**, allowed to stand with frequent stirring for $^1/_2$ hours, and then strained. Unless otherwise prescribed, a cup of the tea is drunk several times a day. The tea can be gently warmed before drinking and should be freshly prepared each time.

5.3 Note

Store away from light and moisture.

Evaluation: in UV 366 nm light. Test solution: relative to the reference rutin band, fluorescent bands at Rx 2.55 (narrow, blue), 2.5 (blue), 2.4 (blue), 0.9 (blue), 0.65 (blue).

Quantitative standards: DAB 10: *Swelling index*, not less than 10. *Foreign matter*, not more than 2% fragments with a brownish discoloration or not complying with the description of the microscopy; with the peeled drug, not more than 2% pieces with a cork layer should be present. *Loss on drying*, not more than 10.0%. *Ash*, not more than 6.0% for the peeled drug and not more than 8.0% for the unpeeled drug.
ÖAB: *Swelling index*, not less than 10. *Condition*, the drug must not be discoloured or smell musty; it should give an almost colourless mucilage which is neutral to litmus and smells neither sourish nor ammoniacal. *Ash*, not more than 6.0%.
Ph. Helv. VII: *Swelling index*, not less than 15. *Foreign matter*, not more than 2% woody roots and other foreign matter; no

brown fragments should be present. *Sulphated ash*, not more than 7.5%.
BHP 1/1990: *Swelling index*, not less than 10. *Water-soluble extractive*, not less than 22%. *Foreign matter*, not more than 2%. *Loss on drying*, not more than 12%. *Total ash*, not more than 8%. *HCl-insoluble ash*, not more than 3%.

Adulteration: Roots of *Althaea rosea* (L.) CAV., hollyhock, are occasionally encountered; they are coarsely fibrous, very woody, and the transverse surface is distinctly yellow. The adulteration with *Atropa belladonna* L., described in the literature (and for which the Ph. Helv. VII requires microscopical examination), does not occur in practice; it would be easily recognized by the presence of cells with calcium oxalate crystal sand (instead of clusters); cf. Bardanae radix. The Ph. Helv. VII includes the following test for bleaching agents (detection of SO_3^{2-}): 5 g drug and 30 ml water are put into a 250 ml wide-necked flask; 5 ml 25% phosphoric acid is then added and a moistened starch/iodide paper positioned in the neck of the flask which is carefully warmed with shaking on the waterbath at 30–35 °C. No (permanent or transient) blue colour should develop in the following 15 min.

Literature:
[1] Kommentar DAB 10.
[2] A. Madaus, W. Blaschek, and G. Franz, Pharm. Weekbl. (Sci. ed.) **9**, 239 (1987).
[3] G. Nosál'ova et al., Pharmazie **47**, 224 (1992).
[4] B.P. Jackson and D. W. Snowdon, Atlas of microscopy of medicinal plants, culinary herbs and spices, Belhaven Press, London, 1990, p. 158.
[5] H. Wagner, S. Bladt, and E.M. Zgainski, Plant drug analysis, Springer-Verlag, Berlin, Heidelberg, New York, Tokyo, 1984, pp. 163 et seq.

Ammeos visnagae fructus   (DAB 10), Ammi visnaga fruit

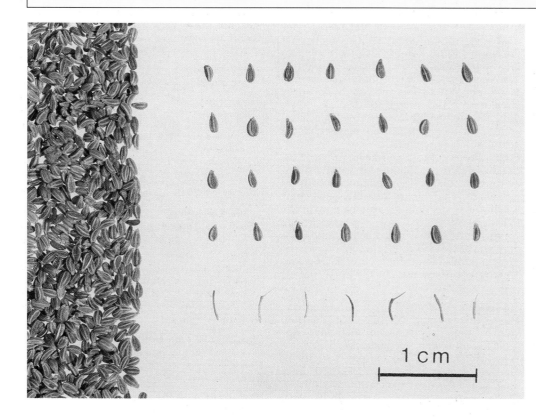

Fig. 1: Ammi visnaga fruit

<u>Description:</u> The small, greyish brown, ellipsoidal, broadly ovoid to pear-shaped double achenes are mostly split into the constituent mericarps; these are ca. 1.5–3 mm long and ca. 0.9 mm broad, ovoid and on the commisural surface somewhat flattened. They are glabrous, with five lighter coloured prominent ridges and at the upper end a brownish yellow stylopodium bearing the remains of the stigma (Fig. 3).

<u>Taste:</u> Somewhat bitter and aromatic.

Fig. 2: *Ammi visnaga* (L.) LAM.

An annual or biennial herb up to 1 m in height. Leaves repeatedly pinnatisect with linear segments. Umbrella-shaped compound umbels, the rays of which become woody and are used as toothpicks (hence the name).

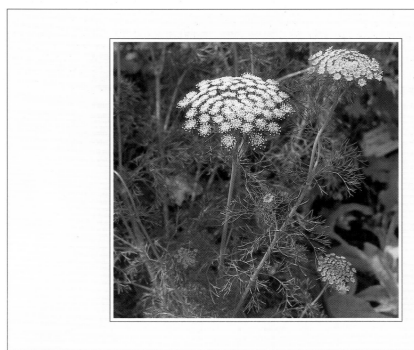

DAB 10: Ammi-visnaga-früchte

Plant source: *Ammi visnaga* (L.) LAM. (Apiaceae).

Synonyms: Fructus Ammi visnagae (Lat.), Visnaga fruit (Engl.), (Ammi-) Visnagafrüchte, Bischofskrautfrüchte (Ger.), Fruits de Khella (Fr.).

Origin: Indigenous in the Mediterranean region; cultivated in Argentina, Chile, Mexico, and North America. The major part of the drug comes from plantations in Morocco, Egypt, Tunisia, and more recently the former USSR.

Constituents: 2–4% furanochromones (γ-pyrones): 0.3–1.2% khellin (=visammin), 0.05–0.3% visnagin [1], 0.3–1% khellol and its glucoside khellenin, khellinol, ammiol and its glucoside, visammiol, khellinone, visnaginone. 0.2–0.5% pyranocoumarins (visnagans): visnadin, samidin, and dihydrosamidin. Traces only of the furanocoumarins xanthotoxin and ammidin [2, 5].

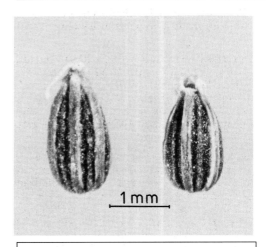

Fig. 3: Mericarps (achenes) of *Ammi visnaga*, with remains of the stigma

Flavonoids: quercetin and isorhamnetin and their 3-sulphates, kaempferol. 0.02–0.03% Essential oil, containing among other things camphor, carvone, α-terpineol, terpinen-4-ol, and linalool along with *cis*- and *trans*-linalool oxides. 12–18% Fixed oil. 12–14% Protein.

Indications: The drugs acts as a spasmolytic, especially on the musculature of the bronchi, gastrointestinal tract, biliary tract, urogenital system, and the coronary vessels, and also as a diuretic. The essential active principles are the furanochromones (khellin, visnagin). The coumarin derivatives (visnadin, samidin) are involved in the overall effect, especially through their spasmolytic, coronary-dilating action. The drug is indicated for whooping cough, cramp-like conditions of the gastrointestinal tract, biliary colic, painful menstruation, for the removal of small bladder and kidney stones, and in angina pectoris, and bronchial asthma. *It is rarely used as a tea. The preference is for ready-made preparations* with extracts containing the total active principles or the isolated pure substances khellin or visnadin.

Visnadin dilates the coronary vessels and brings about a distinct increase in coronary circulation. Its preparations, e.g. Carduben®, are therefore prescribed for heart conditions in which the circulation in the heart muscle is impaired.

Preparations containing khellin are used especially against asthmatic or spastic bronchitis, bronchial asthma, angina pectoris, as well as for renal, biliary, and intestinal colic. Khellin may also have a role to play in the treatment of vitiligo and psoriasis. Minor components – khellenin, khellol, ammiol – may have favourable effects on serum protein levels, total cholesterol levels, and atherosclerotic changes in the blood vessels [11].

Side effects: Prolonged use, or an overdose, may cause nausea, vertigo, constipation, lack of appetite, headache, allergic symptoms (itching), and sleeplessness.

When determining the chronic toxicity in the dog of *individual constituents* (10 times the therapeutic dose over 3 months!), toxic effects were observed particularly with samidin [3]. Weak phototoxic activity has also been demonstrated [4]. Experiments have shown that the natural accompanying substances in Ammi visnaga dry extract greatly increase the solubility and spontaneous dissolution of khellin [6].

Extract from the German Commission E monograph (BAnz no. 50, dated 13.03.1986)

Uses
Mild anginal symptoms. In supportive treatment for mild obstruction of the respiratory tract.
In post-operative supportive treatment of conditions associated with the presence of urinary calculi.

Contraindications
None known.

Side effects
None known.

Interactions with other drugs
None known.

Dosage
Unless otherwise prescribed: average daily dose, equivalent to 20 mg γ-pyrones (calculated as khellin).

Mode of administration
The powdered drug, or other galenical preparations, for internal use.

Effects
Increases coronary and myocardial circulation; mild positive inotropic effect; spasmolytic effect on smooth muscle.

Making the tea: Boiling water is poured over 0.5g of the powdered fruit and after 10–15 min. passed through a tea strainer.
1 Teaspoon = ca. 2.5g.

Phytomedicines: Prepared remedies containing extracts of the drug (percolates, fluid extracts), mostly with a standardized khellin or visnadin content, e.g. Stenocrat®, or with pure visnadin, e.g. Carduben®, or containing khellin or khellin derivatives, are included in: cardiac remedies (14), bronchospas-

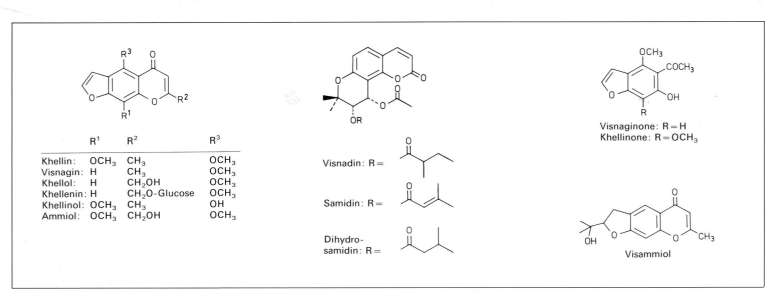

	R¹	R²	R³
Khellin:	OCH₃	CH₃	OCH₃
Visnagin:	H	CH₃	OCH₃
Khellol:	H	CH₂OH	OCH₃
Khellenin:	H	CH₂O-Glucose	OCH₃
Khellinol:	OCH₃	CH₃	OH
Ammiol:	OCH₃	CH₂OH	OCH₃

Visnadin: R =

Samidin: R =

Dihydro-samidin: R =

Visnaginone: R = H
Khellinone: R = OCH₃

Visammiol

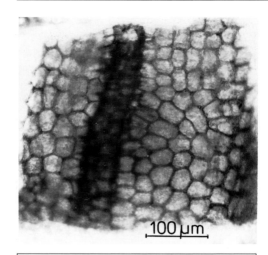

Fig. 4: Large-celled exocarp, with the dark brown secretory canal (oil duct, vitta) visible underneath

molytics (6), spasmolytics (3), urological remedies (4), and coronary remedies (3). It is also included in homoeopathic preparations.

Authentication: Macro- and microscopically, following the DAB 10. Among the diagnostic features are the large-celled and not, or only slightly, papillose exocarp with the secretory canals (vittae) visible underneath (Fig. 4) and the occurrence of large intercellular spaces in the ridges. For the detailed microscopy of the powdered drug, see [7]. The khellin and visnagin appear to be located in the secretory canals and endosperm, rather than in the endosperm [8].

The DAB 10 identification tests are as follows: 0.5 g powdered drug vigorously shaken for 1min. with 4 ml methanol, filtered, and 0.2 ml conc. sulphuric acid added to 0.2 ml of the filtrate, giving a pale lemon-yellow solution (formation of the oxonium salts of the γ-pyrone derivatives) and with *Ammi majus* furnishing a dark greenish brown colour (owing to the presence of furanocoumarins and the absence of γ-pyrones). This test is not satisfactory when the material is a mixture. The TLC test involves separation of the furanochromones [9]:

Test solution: 0.5 g powdered drug shaken for 30 min. with 10 ml 60% ethanol; filtrate reduced to 5 ml on the water-bath.

Reference solution: 5 mg khellin dissolved in 1.0 ml 60% ethanol.

Loadings: 20 µl test solution and 10 µl reference solution, as 2-cm bands on silica gel GF$_{254}$.

Solvent system: ethyl acetate, 10 cm run.

Evaluation: in UV 254 nm light. Reference solution: in the middle region, the khellin quenching zone and directly below it that of visnagin. Test solution: as for the reference solution; in the upper part of the chromatogram, no intense quenching zones close to each other (*Ammi majus*). In UV 365 nm light. Test solution: distinct greyish orange (khellin) and bright blue (visnagin) fluorescent zones; in the upper region, a further intense blue fluorescent zone; weak blue and greenish fluorescent zones possibly also present.

Between 5 and 19% admixture of *Ammi majus* fruits is indicated by strong quenching zones (belonging to xanthotoxin, bergapten, etc.) in the upper Rf region.

Spraying with 5% or 10% ethanolic potassium hydroxide intensifies the fluorescence.

20% Antimony(III) trichloride in chloroform can also be used as a detecting agent [10].

Quantitative standards: DAB 10: γ-*Pyrones*, not less than 1.0% calculated as khellin (M_r 260.2). *Foreign (vegetable and/or mineral) matter*, not more than 2%; fruit of *Ammi majus* must be absent (see below). *Loss on drying*, not more than 10.0%. *Ash*, not more than 10.0%.

Adulteration: Rare. Transverse sections of the macroscopically very similar fruits of *Ammi majus* L. (bullwort) can be recognized microscopically by the absence of large intercellular spaces in the ridges and the reticulate and ridge-like thickened cells in the ridges; in addition, the innermost mesocarp layer consists of large cells with unthickened brown walls; the outer cells of the epidermis of the fruit wall are smaller than those of *Ammi visnaga* and are often papillose.

Literature:
[1] P. Martelli et al., J. Chromatogr. **301**, 297 (1984).
[2] P.W. Le Quesne et al., J. Nat. Prod. **48**, 496 (1985).
[3] A. Kandil and E.E. Galal, J. Drug Res. **7**, 109 (1975).
[4] O. Schimmer, R. Beck and U. Dietz, Planta Med. **40**, 68 (1980).
[5] L.W. Tjarks, G.F. Spencer, and E. P. Seest, J. Nat. Prod. **52**, 655 (1989).
[6] K.H. Frömming, N. Eisenbach, and W. Mehnert, Pharmaz. Ind. **51**, 439 (1989).
[7] B.J. Jackson and D.W. Snowdon, Atlas of microscopy of medicinal plants, culinary herbs and spices, Belhaven Press, London, 1990, p. 240.
[8] G.G. Franchi, S. Ferri, L. Bovalini, and P. Martelli, Int. J. Crude Drug Res. **25**, 137 (1987).
[9] DAB 10.
[10] H. Wagner, S. Bladt, and E.M. Zgainski, Plant drug analysis, Springer-Verlag, Berlin, Heidelberg, New York, Tokyo, 1984, p. 160.
[11] R. Grünewald and H.-P. Stobernack, Z. Phytother. **11**, 65 (1990).

Angelicae radix   (DAB 10), Angelica root (BHP 1983)

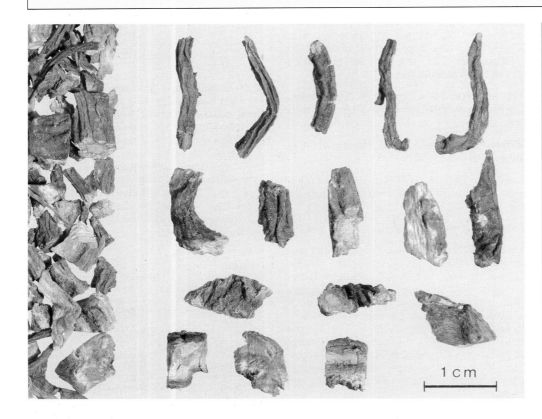

Fig. 1: Angelica root

Description: The grey, reddish, or dark brown longitudinally grooved, often thin, pieces of root have radially arranged secretory canals (diameter 100–200µm) in the bark and a radially striated yellow xylem. In addition, there are irregular fragments of rhizome, likewise with secretory canals.

Odour: Intensely spicy.

Taste: At first aromatic, then acrid, bitter, and lastingly pungent.

Fig. 2: *Angelica archangelica* L.

1–2.5 m tall, sturdy herbs having 2–3 times pinnately divided leaves with broad sheaths. Large compound umbels, without bracts, but with bracteoles about as long as the umbelets.

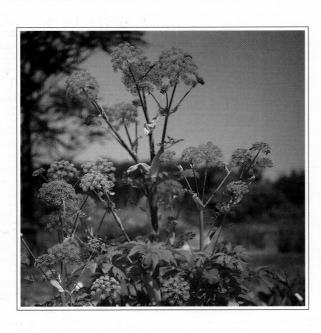

DAB 10: Angelikawurzel
ÖAB: Radix Angelicae
St.Zul. 1419.99.99

Plant source: *Angelica archangelica* L., garden angelica (Apiaceae = Umbelliferae).

Synonyms: Radix Archangelicae, Radix Angelicae sativae, Radix Syriacae (Lat.), The Root of the Holy Ghost (Engl.), Angelikawurzel, Heiligenwurzel (Ger.), Racine d'angélique (officinale) (Fr.).

Origin: In various subspecies and varieties, native throughout the temperate zones of Europe and Asia, especially in the northern regions. The drug comes almost exclusively from plants cultivated in Poland, the Netherlands, the eastern part of Germany, and less frequently from Belgium, Italy, or former Czechoslovakia.

Constituents: Ca. 0.35–1.9% essential oil comprising 80–90% monoterpene hydrocarbons, with β-phellandrene (13–28%), α-phellandrene (2–14%), and α-pinene (14–31%) as principal components [1, 10];

OR

Bergapten: R = CH₃

Isoimperatorin R =

Archangelicin

Xanthotoxin

Angelicin

Peucenin 7-methyl ether

HO

OH O

Archangelenone

$(CH_2)_n$ — CH_2

CH_2 — C

Macrocyclic lactones
n = 10, 12, 14

sesquiterpenes like β-bisabolene, bisabolol, β-caryophyllene, and the macrocyclic lactones tri-, penta-, heptadecanolide, and 12-methyltridecanolide. Over 20 furanocoumarins, including bergapten, isoimperatorin, xanthotoxin, angelicin, archangelicin (= kwannin), and the chromone peucenin 7-methyl ether [2, 3, 11]; coumarins: umbelliferone, osthol, etc. [10]; phenol-carboxylic acids; the flavanone archangelenone; sitosterol; fatty acids (C_{14}–C_{18}); tannins; saccharose.

Indications: Angelica root belongs to the group of bitters and aromatics (bitter substances and essential oil) which stimulate the gastric and pancreatic secretions. It is used to stimulate the appetite, as a stomachic in dyspepsia with insufficient gastric secretion, as well as a spasmolytic and antimicrobially active carminative. It forms a raw material for the production of spice extracts and for making bitters and liqueurs, such as Boonekamp, Bénédictine, Chartreuse, etc.
In *folk medicine* it is also sometimes used as an antiseptic expectorant, as a diuretic and emmenagogue, and in nervous insomnia (essential oil).
Besides the drug itself, the tincture, the essential oil (Oleum Angelicae), and Spiritus Angelicae compositus, are employed – often also externally as mild rubefacients in neuralgic and rheumatic complaints. The essential oil is toxic in large doses (in rats, 1.87 mg/kg) [4].

Note: The BHP 1983 also includes Angelica leaf, which is used in the USA as well. It has carminative and anti-inflammatory properties and is indicated in flatulent dyspepsia and pleurisy. The North American drug is derived from *Angelica atropurpurea* L., alexanders; its uses are very similar to those of the European plant.

Side effects: The furanocoumarins cause photodermatoses [5]. In combination with UV-A light, they are phototoxic, photomutagenic, and cancerogenic [6, 7]. Many of the coumarins also have strong calcium antagonist activity [11]. However, among other things, because of their slight solubility in water, no risks are likely from the tea [7].

Making the tea: 1.5 g of the finely cut or coarsely powdered drug is added to cold water and boiled for a short time or infused with boiling water in a covered vessel. A cupful, unsweetened, is taken half-an-hour before meals. 1 Teaspoonful = ca. 1.5 g.

Phytomedicines: Angelica root or extracts prepared from it are components especially of gastrointestinal remedies, e.g. Aciphyt®, Euvitan®, Ventrimarin®, Iberogast®, Legastol®, Carvomin®, Gastritol® „Dr. Klein", Stovalid®, Purgocit®, Dr. Klinger's-Bergischer-Kräutertee and Magentee, etc., as well as of roborants and tonics, spasmolytics, cholagogues and biliary remedies, and also hypnotics and sedatives.

Regulatory status (UK): General Sales List – Schedule 1, Table A.

Authentication: Macro- and microscopically, following the DAC 1986; see also the BHP 1983. TLC, however, offers greater certainty as a means of identification [8, 9]:

Test solution: 3.0 g powdered drug refluxed with 30 ml methanol for 30 min., cooled and filtered, and the filtrate taken to dryness under reduced pressure and the residue dissolved in 9 ml methanol.

Reference solution: 5 mg umbelliferone dissolved in 20 ml methanol.

Loading: 5 µl each of the test and reference solutions.

Solvent system: upper layer of diethyl ether + toluene (1 + 1), saturated with 12% aqueous acetic acid; 6 cm run.

Evaluation: in UV 366 nm light (Fig. 3). Test solution: immediately above the level of the umbelliferone zone, an intense blue fluorescent zone and above that three blue to yellowish fluorescent zone; directly below the umbelliferone zone, a bluish fluorescent zone and below that a yellowish brown fluorescent zone (much less intensely fluorescent in UV 254 nm light).
Deviating chromatograms point to adulteration by other Apiaceae (see: Fig. 3).

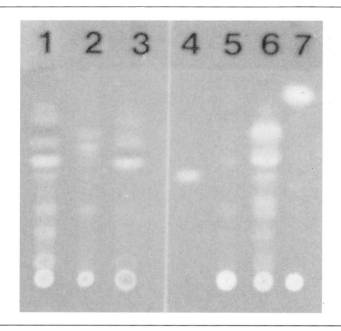

Fig. 3: TLC on 4 × 8 cm silica-gel foil Drugs from roots of various Apiaceae

1: Pimpinella peregrina (so-called "white" burnet saxifrage)
2: Pimpinella major/saxifraga ((greater) burnet saxifrage)
3: Heracleum sphondylium (hogweed)

4: Umbelliferone (reference substance)
5: Pastinaca sativa (wild parsnip)
6: Angelica archangelica (angelica)
7: Levisticum officinale (lovage)

For details, see the text

The DAC 1986 TLC method is similar, but the silica gel 60 F_{254} plate is evaluated in UV 365 nm light before and after spraying with 26% ammonia solution + methanol (20 + 80).

Quantitative standards: DAC 1986: *Volatile oil*, not less than 0.25%. *Extractive*, not less than 30.0%. *Foreign matter*, not more than 5% stem fragments and not more than 2% other foreign matter. *Loss on drying*, not more than 10%. *Ash*, not more than 10%. *Acid-insoluble ash*, not more than 2.0%. ÖAB: *Volatile oil*, not less than 0.3%. *Foreign matter*, not more than 5% stem fragments. *Ash*, not more than 10.0%. BHP 1983: *Total ash*, not more than 10%. *Acid-insoluble ash*, not more than 4%.

Adulteration: Possible, especially with the cut drug; roots of other Apiaceae may be involved, particularly *Levisticum officinale*, *Pimpinella* species, and *Heracleum sphon-*

dylium. For their TLC detection, see: Authentication.

Storage: Protected from light and in tightly closed containers (not made of plastic – essential oil).

Literature:

[1] I. Héthelyi et al., Herb. Hung. **24**, 149 (1985).
[2] S. Harkar, T.K. Radzan and E.S. Waight, Phytochemistry **23**, 419 (1984).
[3] H. Sun and J. Jakupovic, Pharmazie **41**, 888 (1986).
[4] G. Brownlee, Quart. J. Pharmacy **13**, 130 (1940).
[5] K.W. Glombitza, Dtsch. Apoth. Ztg. **112**, 1593 (1972).
[6] O. Schimmer, R. Beck and U. Dietz, Planta Med. **40**, 68 (1980).
[7] O. Schimmer, Planta Med. **47**, 79 (1983).
[8] O.B. Genius, Dtsch. Apoth. Ztg. **121**, 386 (1981).
[9] P. Rohdewald, G. Rücker and K.W. Glombitza, Apothekengerechte Prüfvorschriften, S. 619, Dtsch. Apoth. Verlag Stuttgart 1986.
[10] P. Gautier et al., Pharm. Weekbl. (Sci. ed.) **9**, 234 (1987).
[11] P. Härmälä et al., Phytochem. Anal. **3**, 42 (1992).

Anisi fructus   (DAB 10), Aniseed (Ph. Eur. 2, BP 1988)

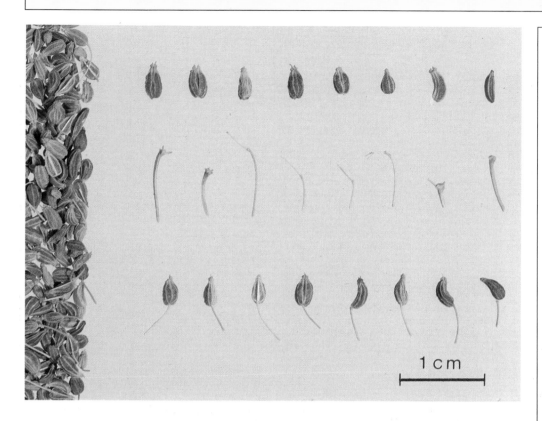

Fig. 1: Aniseed (middle row, parts of the stem and remains of the carpophore)

Description: The drug consists of the ca. 2 mm long, greyish green to greyish brown, finely ridged and finely pubescent (Fig. 4), obpyriform and laterally somewhat compressed, stalked cremocarps (double achene). The mericarps have five more or less straight ridges.

Odour: Reminiscent of anethole.

Taste: Sweetish, aromatic (aniseed-like).

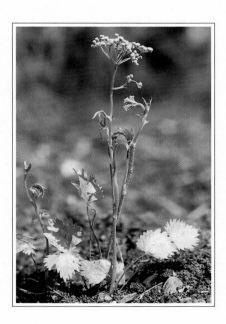

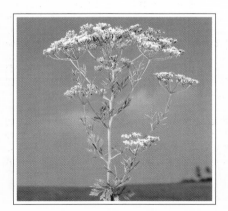

Figs. 2 and 3: *Pimpinella anisum* L.

Herbaceous plants, 30–60 cm tall, with basal leaves undivided and leaves towards the top increasingly pinnatisect. Compound umbels with 7–15 rays and mostly without bracts.

trans-Anethole   Methylchavicol   Anisaldehyde

2-Methylbutyricacidester of 4-Methoxy-2-(1-propenyl)-phenol

DAB 10: Anis
Ph. Helv. VII: Anisi fructus
ÖAB: Fructus Anisi
St.Zul.: 8099.99.99

Plant source: *Pimpinella anisum* L. (Apiaceae).

Synonyms: Semen Anisi, Semen Absinthii dulcis (Lat.), Pimpinella, Anise (Engl.), Anis, Kleiner Anis, Süßer Kümmel (Ger.), Anis vert, Fruit d'anis (Fr.).

Origin: Presumed to be native in the eastern Mediterranean region and western Asia; cultivated in southern Europe, the Mediterranean region, the Middle East, India, the former USSR, and in Mexico and Chile; imports come from Turkey, Egypt, and Spain.

Constituents: Main constituent: 1.5–5% essential oil, with *trans*-anethole (80–90% of the oil) chiefly responsible for the taste and smell. Also, the isomeric methylchavicol (estragole) (1–2%), which, although smelling like anise, does not taste sweet, and anisaldehyde (<1%); further, sesquiterpene hydrocarbons (especially γ-himachalene, ca. 2% [2]) and less than 1% monoterpene hydrocarbons (difference with the oil from *Illicium verum* HOOK. f.) [1–3]. The dimers of anethole (dianethole) and anisaldehyde (dianisoin) repeatedly mentioned in the litera-

ture and supposedly responsible for the oestrogenic activity in old drugs, could not be found after thorough investigation [4]. Characteristic of *genuine* aniseed oil is the presence of up to 5% of the 2-methylbutyryl ester of 4-methoxy-2-(1-propenyl)-phenol (= pseudoisoeugenyl 2-methylbutyrate) [2, 3]. In addition, aniseed contains fat and coumarins [5].

Indications: As an expectorant and carminative, on account of the secretolytic, spasmolytic, and secretomotor effects of its essential oil; like fennel, it is often used in paediatric practice [1, 6, 7]. In high doses, as an antispastic and antiseptic.
In *folk medicine* also as an emmenagogue, lactagogue (oestrogenic action?), and aphrodisiac. The essential oil is used externally (in a fatty-oil or ointment vehicle) as a stimulating liniment and against vermin. Aniseed and aniseed oil are also employed in the food and drink industry as flavour enhancers, e.g. in ouzo (Greek aniseed spirits), pastis, anisette (French aniseed drinks), and as an ingredient of Bénédictine, Boonekamp, Danziger Goldwasser, etc.

Making the tea: 1–5 g of the seeds, pounded or coarsely powdered immediately before use, is covered with boiling water and allowed to draw in a closed vessel for 10–15min.
1 Teaspoon = ca. 3.5g.

Herbal preparations: Several instant teas as powders containing aqueous extracts of aniseed, or as a tea paste, some preparations with micro-encapsulated aniseed oil.

Phytomedicines: As a constituent of numerous cough remedies (antitussives, expectorants), stomach and bowel remedies (carminatives, laxatives), especially in paediatric practice, in the form of teas, tea extracts, dragees, and sweets; often together with other essential-oil drugs, such as fennel.

Regulatory status (UK): General Sales List – Schedule 1, Table A (anise oil).

Authentication: Macro- (see: Description) and microscopically, following the DAB 10; see: Fig. 5. The diagnostic features of the powdered drug are described in [10].
The Ph. Eur. 2 (BP 1988, etc.) monograph includes the following TLC test of identity:

Test solution: 0.1g powdered drug shaken for 15min. with 2 ml dichloromethane, filtered, solvent carefully evaporated at ca. 60 °C, and the residue dissolved in 0.5 ml toluene.

Reference solution: 3 µl anethole and 40 µl olive oil dissolved in 1 ml toluene.

Loadings: 2 µl and 3 µl of the test solution and 1 µl, 2 µl, and 3 µl of the reference solution, at 2-cm intervals on silica gel GF_{254}.

Solvent system: toluene, 10 cm run.

Detection and Evaluation: in UV 254 nm light. Reference and Test solutions: dark spots in the centre part corresponding to anethole.
Sprayed with 20% phosphomolybdic acid in 96% ethanol, followed by heating at 120 °C for 5 min. Test solution: with the 2 µl loading of the test solution: anethole, a blue zone against a yellow background intermediate in size between the 1 µl and 3 µl zones of the reference solution; a blue zone, due to triglycerides, in the lower third of the chromatogram at about the same Rf as the blue zone of the olive-oil triglycerides.
The TLC can also be carried out according to the methods in [1, 8].

Quantitative standards: Ph. Eur. 2: *Volatile oil*, not less than 2.0%. *Foreign matter*, not more than 2%. *Water*, not more than 7.0%. *Acid-insoluble ash*, not more than 2.5%. *Sulphated ash*, not more than 12.0%.
BHP 1983: *Volatile oil*, not less than 2.0%. *Foreign organic matter*, not more than 2%; other fruits and seeds, not more than 2%. *Total ash*, not more than 10%. *Acid-insoluble ash*, not more than 2.5%.

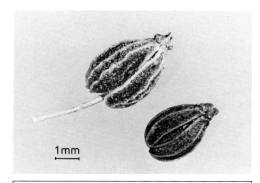

Fig. 4: Pubescent fruit of *Pimpinella anisum* (left) and smaller glabrous fruit of *Petroselinum crispum*, a possible contaminant (right)

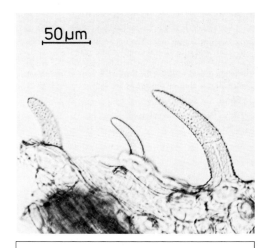

Fig. 5: 1- to 2-celled, thick-walled, curved trichomes with warty cuticle from *Pimpinella anisum*

Wording of the package insert, from the German Standard Licence:

6.1 Uses

For promoting the dissolution of phlegm in catarrh of the respiratory tract; flatulence and colicky symptoms in the gastrointestinal tract, especially in nursing babies and infants.

6.2 Contraindications

Allergy to aniseed and anethole.

6.3 Side effects

Occasional allergic reactions by the skin, respiratory tract, and the gastrointestinal tract.

6.4 Dosage and Mode of administration

Boiling water (150ml) is poured over 1–2 teaspoonfuls of crushed of **Aniseed** and after 10–15min. passed through a tea strainer.

Unless otherwise prescribed, to promote the dissolution of phlegm, a cup of the freshly prepared tea is taken in the morning and/or at night before going to bed. For gastrointestinal complaints, a tablespoonful of the tea is taken several times a day. Nursing babies and infants may be given a teaspoonful, if need be in their bottle.

6.5 Note

Store protected from light and moisture.

Adulteration: See [1]. Occasionally (in former times more often, nowadays very rarely), the highly toxic coniine-containing fruit of *Conium maculatum* L., hemlock, are encountered in individual lots of aniseed [9]. Morphologically, hemlock fruit can be recognized by the undulate (especially in the upper part of the fruit) ridges. On moistening the powdered fruit with potassium hydroxide solution, they should not smell like mouse urine (coniine). Adulteration with parsley fruit is readily detected because of their small size and lack of pubescence (Fig. 4).

Currently, almost all lots of aniseed are contaminated with up to 1% coriander fruit.

About pharmacopoeial anise oil, see: Anisi stellati fructus. Nowadays, commercial anise oils consist either of star-anise oil or (frequently) of natural, or technical grade, *trans*-anethole.

Adulteration of powdered aniseed or anise oil can be rapidly and reliably determined by direct mass spectroscopy via the "marker" compound pseudoisoeugenyl 2-methylbutyrate which only occurs in genuine "anise oil"; as little as 0.2–1.4% can be detected in the presence of 94% anethole, without the necessity of its having to be separated or the sample specially prepared [11].

Storage: Protected from moisture and light in glass or tin, but not plastic, containers (essential oil!).

Literature:

[1] Kommentar DAB 10.
[2] K.-H. Kubeczka, Acta Horticulturae **73**, 85 (1978). V. Formácek and K.-H. Kubeczka, Essential oil analysis by capillary gas chromatography and carbon-13 NMR spectroscopy, Wiley, Chichester, 1982.
[3] K.-H. Kubeczka, F. von Massow, V. Formácek, and M. A. R. Smith, Z. Naturforsch. **31b**, 283 (1976).
[4] A. Kraus and F.J. Hammerschmidt, Dragoco Report **27**, 31 (1980).
[5] Th. Kartnig and H. Scholz, Fette, Seifen **71**, 276 (1969).
[6] H. Braun and D. Frohne, Heilpflanzenlexikon für Ärzte und Apotheker, G. Fischer, Stuttgart – New York, 1987.
[7] E.M. Boyd, Pharmacol. Rev. **6**, 521 (1954).
[8] P. Pachaly, Dünnschichtchromatographie in der Apotheke, Wissenschaftliche Verlagsgesellschaft m.b.H., Stuttgart, 1983.
[9] W. Schier and W. Schultze, Dtsch. Apoth. Ztg. **127**, 2717 (1987).
[10] B.J. Jackson and D.W. Snowdon, Atlas of microscopy of medicinal plants, culinary herbs and spices, Belhaven Press, London, 1990, p. 8.
[11] W. Schultze, G. Lange, and K.-H. Kubeczka, Dtsch. Apoth. Ztg. **127**, 372 (1987).

Anisi stellati fructus   (DAB 10), Star anise fruit

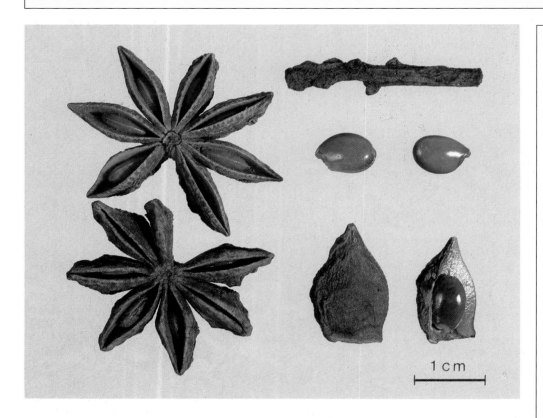

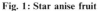

Fig. 1: Star anise fruit

<u>Description:</u> The cut drug consists of the hard pieces of the fruit wall, which are greyish brown on the outside and much wrinkled or roughly nodular and reddish brown, smooth, and shiny on the inside, together with the whole or fragmentary, very shiny chestnut-brown seeds.

The reddish brown, corky and woody, dehiscent syncarp comprises 6–11 (mostly 8) mostly unevenly developed mericarps (follicles), arranged stellately round a 6 mm high columella, which are boat-shaped and 12–20 mm long and 6–11 mm deep. The individual follicles, which are drawn out into a blunt point, are greyish brown and coarsely wrinkled on the outside and shiny reddish brown and smooth on the inside. When ripe, they spring open along the suture, exposing shiny chestnut-brown coloured, ovoid, compressed seeds, up to 8 mm long. The upper end of the columella is flat and sunken and usually ends at the level of the edges of the carpels; at its bottom end, the columella is often joined to the pedicel which is curved and thickened like a club at the top (Fig. 4).

<u>Odour:</u> Of anise.

<u>Taste:</u> Pungent and spicy.

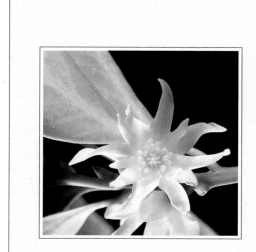

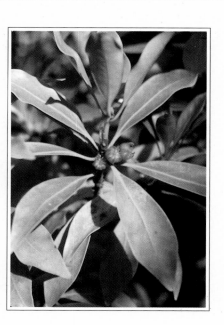

Figs. 2 and 3: *Illicium verum* HOOK.f.

A small evergreen tree with oblong, acuminate, entire leaves and spherical flowers comprising 10 strongly curved reddish perianth parts, 10 stamens, and generally 8 carpels forming when ripe a star-shaped syncarp with each follicle containing one seed.

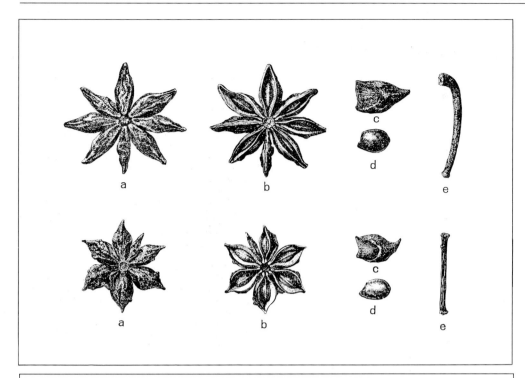

Fig. 4: **Star anise and Japanese star anise (shikimi) fruit (fruit, seeds, and pedicels). Top row:** *Illicium verum.* **Bottom row:** *Illicium anisatum.* **(a) Fruit seen from underneath. (b) Fruit seen from the top. (c) Single follicle seen from the side. (d) Seed removed from the fruit. (e) Pedicel of the fruit. Natural size. (From: G. Gassner,** *Mikroskopische Untersuchung pflanzlicher Lebensmittel,* **4th ed., G. Fischer Verlag, Stuttgart, 1973)**

DAB 10: Sternanis
ÖAB: Fructus Anisi stellati

Plant source: *Illicium verum* HOOK. f. (Illiciaceae; formerly, Magnoliaceae).

Origin: Said originally to have been native in southern China and northern Vietnam; not now known in the wild; cultivated in the tropics, including China, Indochina, Japan, Philippines. The drug is imported from China and Vietnam.

Synonyms: Chinese star anise (Engl.), Sternanis, Chinesischer Sternanis (Ger.), Fruit de badianier de Chine, Fruit d'anis étoilé (Fr.).

Constituents: 5–8% essential oil localized mainly in the pericarp; it comprises up to 80–90% *trans*-anethole and ca. 5% monoterpenoid hydrocarbons, including limonene and α-pinene, and linalool, which are almost completely absent from genuine anise oil (from Anisi fructus, q.v.). In contrast to genuine anise oil, the 2-methylbutyric acid ester of 4-methoxy-2-(1-propenyl)-phenol (= 5-methoxy-2-(2-methylbutyryloxy)-1-propenylbenzene = pseudoisoeugenyl 2-methylbutyrate) is also absent [1]. The drug also contains fixed oil (especially in the seed) and tannins.

Indications: Star anise is used principally as an aromatic and spice, and less often like

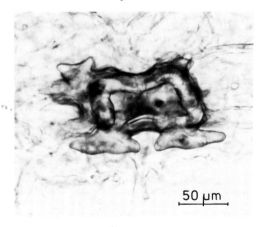

Fig. 5: **Gnarled, irregular sclereid from the pedicel of the fruit**

anise as a stomachic and expectorant [2]. Star anise oil is employed in pharmacy practice and in the food industry in the same way as the very expensive genuine anise oil (which has not been available in sufficient quantity for many years), as a component of alcoholic drinks, liqueurs, toothpastes, sweets, pharmaceutical preparations, and occasionally also as a perfume in soap.

Making the tea: Not often done. 0.5–1.0 g drug is coarsely powdered immediately before use and boiling water poured over it and after 10 min. strained.
1 Teaspoon = ca. 3.2 g.

Herbal preparations: Star anise is a component of herbal mixtures which are intended for making mulled wine.

Phytomedicines: Fewer than for anise, as a component of prepared antitussives and gastrointestinal remedies.

Regulatory status (UK): Anise oil: General Sales List – Schedule 1, Table A.

Authentication: Macro- (see: Description) and microscopically, following the DAB 10. The scattered, very irregular, ca. 0.4 mm sclereids that occur in the columella and fruit pedicel are particularly diagnostic: they are 91-220-440 µm long and up to 150 µm wide, and they vary greatly in shape – from gnarled to highly branched (Fig. 5). The testa of the seed consists of palisade-like stone cells with yellowish, strongly thickened, lignified, and extensively pitted walls; they are up to 200 µm high and 50 µm wide [8].

A detailed account of the microscopy of the powdered drug is given in [7].

For the TLC detection of anethole in star-anise oil, see: Anisi fructus. It is no longer necessary to differentiate between star-anise oil and "genuine" anise oil from *Pimpinella anisum*, since Anisi aetheroleum (anise oil) may now be obtained from both plants. The TLC differentiation can be based on the 5-methoxy-2-(2-methylbutyryl-oxy)-1-propenylbenzene quenching band in the chromatogram of "genuine" anise oil [4]. The foeniculin band [5, 6], which occurs only in the chromatogram of star-anise oil, is absent from that of "genuine" anise oil, but, unfortunately, this is not an adequate criterion, as the compound is present only in traces in some star-anise oils and cannot then be detected with certainty by TLC [6]. The DAB 10 TLC identity test is as follows:

Test solution: 0.20 g freshly powdered drug shaken for 15 min. with 2.0 ml toluene and filtered.

Reference solution: 3 µl anethole and 20 µl olive oil dissolved in 1.0 ml toluene.

Loadings: 20 µl each of the test and reference solutions, as 2-cm bands on silica gel GF$_{254}$.

Solvent system: toluene, 10 cm run.

Detection and Evaluation: In UV 254 nm light. Reference and Test solutions: in the middle on a light background, a quenching zone corresponding to anethole.

Sprayed with anisaldehyde reagent, followed by heating at 120 °C for 5 min. and examination in daylight. Test solution: anethole zone, a yellow to greenish yellow zone approximately equal in size and intensity to that corresponding zone of the reference solution; in the lower third, a red zone at the level of the olive-oil triglyceride zone in the reference chromatogram.

Quantitative standards: DAB 10: *Volatile oil*, not less than 7.0%. *Foreign (plant and inorganic) matter*, not more than 2%. *Water*, not more than 7%. *Ash*, not more than 5%.
ÖAB: *Volatile oil*, not less than 5.0%. *Foreign matter*, not more than 1%; fruit of *Illicium religiosum*, shikimi fruit, must be absent. *Ash*, not more than 5.0%.

Adulteration: Shikimi fruit, derived from *Illicium anisatum* L. (syn. *I. religiosum* SIEB. et ZUCC.), Japanese anise or Bastard star anise, is a possible adulterant. They are toxic because of their content of the sesquiterpene anisatin. However, in practice they are very rarely encountered.

Star anise and shikimi fruit have a "mosaic" of morphological and anatomical features which, according to the literature, supposedly belong **either** to star anise fruit **or** to shikimi fruit and which may suggest that a particular fruit is a "typical" star anise or shikimi fruit; there are also many transition forms [8].

In general, shikimi fruit are smaller, more yellowish brown, plumper, and more broadly dehiscent; in side view, the follicles are sharply beaked and their tips have a distinct upward bend. The sclereids of the columella are smaller (58-103-300 µm), roundish and unbranched, with only slight protuberances. In shikimi fruit the columella stops short, thus forming a depression, while in star anise it continues through to the top. The fruit pedicel is straight and not clavately thickened. The place where the fruit pedicel is attached in shikimi fruit often has a ring of cork, which is absent in star anise fruit (Fig. 4) [8].

Shikimi fruit do not have the pungent taste of anise, but are only slightly bitter and aromatic, sourish and resinous, and sometimes like camphor [8].

It is practically impossible to detect fragments of shikimi fruit in *powdered* star anise fruit, but the following TLC procedure, which will detect 5% admixture, depends on the detection of the phenylpropane myristicin (only present in shikimi fruit) at Rf ca. 0.19 (still well away from the enormous anethole zone, despite the necessary overloading) [9]: silica gel 60 F$_{254}$; hexane + toluene (1 + 1), 15 cm run; UV 254 nm light, then spraying with 10% ethanolic phosphomolybdic acid and heating at ca. 120 °C for a few min.

Nevertheless, the use of myristicin as a marker still has an element of uncertainty, since there are other toxic *Illicium* species and nothing is known of their myristicin content [9].

Direct mass-spectrometric analysis offers a rapid and highly effective, but sophisticated, means establishing such admixture [9].

Storage: Only as the whole drug, protected from light in tightly closed containers (not made of plastic).

Literature:

[1] V. Formácek and K.-H. Kubeczka, Essential oil analysis by capillary gas chromatography and carbon-13 NMR spectroscopy, Wiley, Chichester, 1982 (see: Anisi fructus).

[2] Kommentar DAB 10.

[3] Hager, vol. **5**, p. 228 (1976).

[4] K.-H. Kubeczka, Dtsch. Apoth. Ztg. **122**, 2309 (1982).

[5] V. Seger, H. Miething, and R. Hänsel, Pharm. Ztg. **132**, 2747 (1987).

[6] W. Schultze, A. Linde, and A. Zänglein, unpublished work (1987).

[7] B.P. Jackson and D.W. Snowdon, Atlas of microscopy of medicinal plants, culinary herbs and spices, Belhaven Press, London, 1990, p. 222.

[8] A. Zänglein, W. Schultze, and K.-H. Kubezcka, Dtsch. Apoth. Ztg. **129**, 2819 (1989).

[9] W. Schultze, A. Zänglein, G. Lange, and K.-H. Kubeczka, Dtsch. Apoth. Ztg. **139**, 1194 (1990).

Anserinae herba   Silverweed

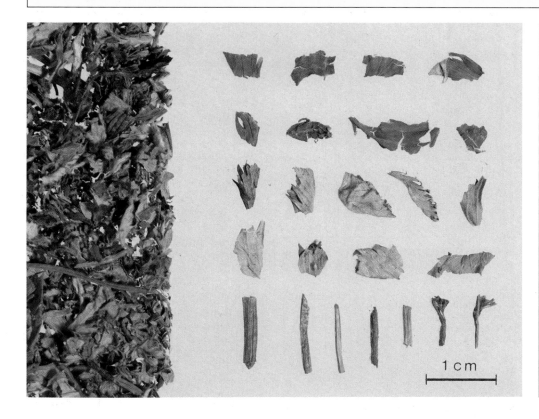

Fig. 1: Silverweed

Description: The 1–3 cm long leaflets have a serrate to pinnatifid margin. The leaf fragments are densely tomentous on the whitish (silvery) lower surface (Fig. 3) and have sparse hairs on the green upper surface. Pubescent pieces of stem and, occasionally, yellow petals or entire flowers are present.

Taste: Very faintly astringent.

1 cm

Fig. 2: *Potentilla anserina* L.

A perennial low herb with long, self-rooting runners. Leaves pinnate, the leaflets having a coarsely serrate margin. Flowers with five yellow petals and with long stalks.

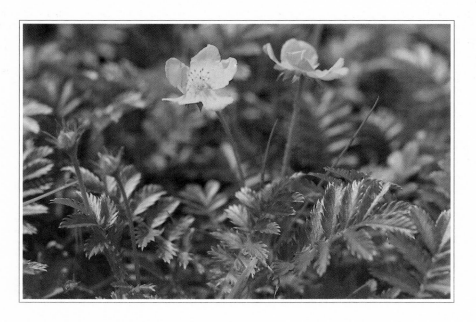

DAC 1986: Gänsefingerkraut
St.Zul. 9599.99.99

Plant source: *Potentilla anserina* L., silverweed (Rosaceae).

Synonyms: Herba Potentillae argentinae (Lat.), Gänsefingerkraut, Silberkraut, Gänserich (Ger.), Herbe d'ansérine (Fr.).

Origin: Widely distributed in the temperate zones. Drug imports come from Hungary, former Yugoslavia, and Poland.

Constituents: 6–10% tannins, no doubt mainly of the ellagic-acid type [1–3]; recently, monomeric and dimeric ellagitannins have been detected [4]. Flavonoids (quercetin and myricetin glycosides) and leucoanthocyanidins, as well as choline [5, 6] and compounds of unknown structure with spasmolytic activity (?) [7], are also present.

Indications: On the basis of the tannin content, the drug can be used as an astringent (both internally and externally).

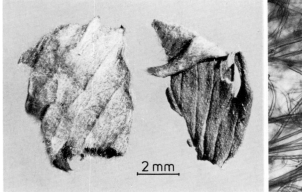 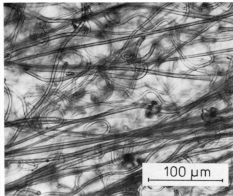

Fig. 3: *Potentilla anserina* **leaf fragments, showing the densely tomentous lower surface (left) and the darker, sparsely pubescent upper surface (right)**

Fig. 4: Dense tomentum of the lower leaf surface, consisting of straight stiff trichomes and underneath of long, tortuous, intertwined trichomes

Several publications deal with the reported spasmolytic action of silverweed; the findings are controversial [7–9]. According to medical experience, the drug is particularly useful in treating dysmenorrhoea of spastic origin [10].

Making the tea: Boiling water is poured over 2 g of the finely chopped drug and strained after 10 min.
1 Teaspoon = ca. 0.7g.

Herbal preparations: Silverweed is a component of prepared herbal mixtures (for the most varied indications) and instant teas.

Phytomedicines: Silverweed or extracts made from it are components of various prepared remedies with different indications, e.g. for the male climacteric and psychosexual problems; for nausea; Esberi-Nervin® (drops) for nervous restlessness.

Authentication: Macro- and microscopically, following the DAC 1986. The dense to-

mentum of the lower leaf surface is very characteristic – above the dense mat of unicellular thin-walled, tortuous trichomes is a layer of thicker-walled stiff trichomes (Fig. 4).
TLC of the flavonoids can be carried out according to [11]; for details of the system, see: Althaeae radix.

Evaluation: in UV 366 nm light. Test solution: up to eight orange fluorescent zones in the range Rf 0.3–0.9, with quercetin and myricetin monoglycosides at Rf ca. 0.6–0.7 and their diglycosides around Rf ca. 0.35.

Quantitative standards: DAC 1986: *Tannins precipitable with hide powder*, not less than 5.0%. *Foreign matter*, not more than 5%. *Loss on drying*, not more than 10%. *Ash*, not more than 13%. *Acid-insoluble ash*, not more than 2.0%.

Adulteration: Scarcely ever occurs.

Literature:
[1] E.C. Bate-Smith, J. Linn. Soc. (Bot.) **58**, 39 (1961).
[2] E. Eisenreichova, A. Buckowa, J. Leifertova and M. Babinska, Česk. Farm. **23**, 82 (1974).
[3] K. Herrmann, Pharm. Zentralh. **88**, 303 (1949).
[4] K. Lund, Dissertation Freiburg i. Br. 1986.
[5] W. Rodewald, Pharmazie **5**, 538 (1950).
[6] P. Tunmann and R. Janka, Arzneim.-Forsch. **5**, 20 (1955).
[7] W. Smetana and R. Fischer, Pharm. Zentralh. **102**, 624 (1963).
[8] G. Harnischfeger and H. Stolze, Bewährte Pflanzendrogen in Wissenschaft und Medizin, notamed.-Verl., Melsungen (1983).
[9] H.W. Younken et al., J. Am. Pharm. Assoc. **38**, 448 (1949).
[10] A.R. Bliss et al., J. Am. Pharm. Assoc. **29**, 299 (1940).
[11] H. Wagner, S. Bladt, and E.M. Zgainski, Plant drug analysis, Springer-Verlag, Berlin, Heidelberg, New York, Tokyo, 1984, pp. 168, 186.

Apii fructus   Celery seed (BHP 1/1990)

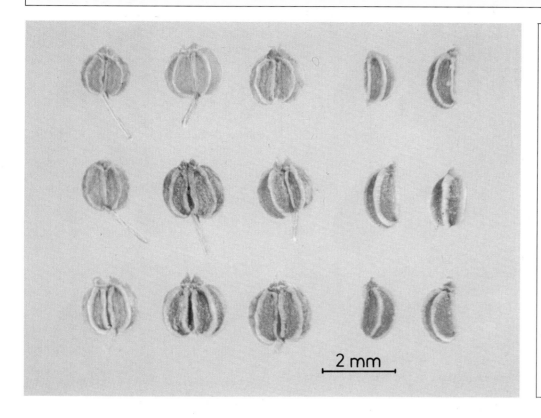

2 mm

Fig. 1: Celery seed

<u>Description:</u> The greyish green to brownish, oval cremocarps (double achenes) are only 0.8–1.5 mm long and they have a conical stylopod and the remains of two short styles. On the outer surface, there are five narrow, pale to whitish, prominent ridges. The cremocarps are to some extent split into the individual mericarps. Short pedicels may also be present.

<u>Odour:</u> Characteristic, spicy.

<u>Taste:</u> Spicy and somewhat bitter.

Figs. 2 and 3: *Apium graveolens* L.

A long cultivated, erect biennial, up to ca. 60 cm in height, with firm, 1–2 times pinnately divided leaves; the leaflets rhombic and frequently ternate. Small whitish flowers and spicy fruits on robust stems in compound umbels, without bracts and bracteoles.

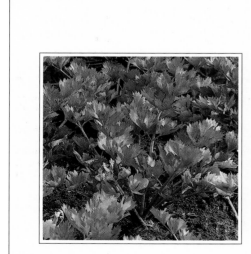

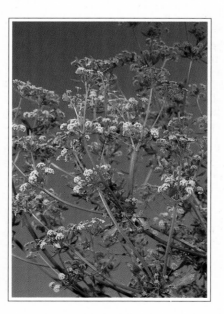

Plant source: *Apium graveolens* L., wild celery (Apiaceae = Umbelliferae).

Synonyms: Apium, Celery fruit (Engl.), Selleriefrüchte, Selleriesamen (Ger.), Ache des marais, Fruit de céleri (Fr.).

Origin: Native throughout Europe, western Asia to India, North and South Africa. On saline soils, almost cosmopolitan. Cultivated in various forms, as a useful plant. The drug comes only from cultivated plants and is imported from India and China, as well as certain parts of Europe.

Constituents: Ca. 2–3% essential oil, with limonene (60%) and selinene (10%) as the main components; further, *p*-cymene, *β*-terpineol, *β*-pinene, *β*-caryophyllene, *α*-santalol, and dihydrocarvone, and the butylphthalides sedanolide (2.5–3%), sedaenolide, and *n*-butylphthalide and sedanonic acid (ca. 0.5%) as aroma constituents; *C*-prenylcoumarins: osthenol, apigravin, celerin; furocoumarins and furocoumarin glucosides: apiumetin, rutaretin, nodakenetin, celereoin, etc. [1, 2]; flavonoids: apigenin,

Sedanolide

Osthenol: R = -H
Apigravin: R = -OCH₃

Apiumetin

isoquercitrin, etc.; alkaloids have been detected but not yet identified.

Indications: Celery seed is now only occasionally used in *folk medicine*, chiefly as a diuretic in bladder and kidney complaints, and an adjuvant in arthritic and rheumatic conditions. The effect is ascribed primarily to the essential oil. Use as a nervine for "nervous restlessness", and as a stomachic and carminative, has also been reported. The essential oil and various fractions from it have been described as having sedative activity [3, 4]. Various methylphthalides are spasmolytic and sedative [5]. *n*-Butylphthalide and *n*-butyl-4,5-dihydrophthalide have been shown to have anticonvulsant activity in rats and mice [6, 7]. Extensive animal experiments have demonstrated that the at most very slightly toxic alkaloid fraction has depressant, tranquillizing effects on the CNS [8]. Some coumarins also have central sedative and bactericidal properties.

Side effects: The drug is contraindicated in inflammation of the kidneys, since the essential oil (like other apiaceous oils) may increase the inflammation as a result of epithelial irritation. The furanocoumarins of the fruit, in combination with UV-A light, are toxic and bring about photodermatoses known variously as phyto(photo)dermatitis, phototoxic dermatitis, or Apium allergic contact dermatitis [9–12].

Making the tea: Not usual. Boiling water is poured over 1 g of the drug which has been crushed just before use and after 5–10 min. strained.
1 Teaspoon = ca. 1.5 g.

Phytomedicines: In the UK, celery seed is a component of almost 60 anti-inflammatory preparations [13], including Heath & Heather Celery Seed Tablets, Gerard House Celery Tablets, etc.

Regulatory status (UK): General Sales List – Schedule 1, Table A; likewise, celery oil.

Authentication: Macro- (see: Description) and microscopically. The transverse section shows the typical structure of an apiaceous fruit. There are two or three vittae in each of the slightly arcuate grooves and two vittae on the commisural surface. In surface view, the cells of the epicarp are sinuate, with a finely striated, and in places also warty, cuticle. The detailed microscopy of the seed and powdered seed is to be found in the BHP 1/1990 and [14].

The BHP 1/1990 TLC identification procedure is the same as that described under Althaeae radix (q.v.):

Evaluation: in UV 366 nm light. Test solution: relative to the rutin reference band, fluorescent bands at Rx ca. 1.05 (broad and orange) and Rx ca. 1.7 (orange).

Quantitative standards: BHP 1/1990: *Volatile oil*, not less than 1.5%. *Water-soluble extractive*, not less than 15%. *Foreign matter*, not more than 2%. *Total ash*, not more than 10%. *HCl-insoluble ash*, not more than 2%.

Adulteration: Scarcely known in practice. Confusion with the likewise rather small fruits of Petroselini fructus (parsley, q.v.) or with those of Ammeos visnagae fructus (*Ammi visnaga*, q.v.) can be recognized microscopically.

Storage: Protected from light and moisture, but not in plastic containers.

Literature:
[1] V.K. Ahluwalia et al., Phytochemistry **27**, 1181 (1988).
[2] A.K. Jain et al., Planta Med. **52**, 246 (1986).
[3] A. Osol and G.E. Farrer, The Dispensatory of the United States of America. 5th ed. **2**, 1620 (1955).
[4] R.P. Kohli, P.R. Dua, K. Shanker and R.C. Saxena, Indian J. Med. Res. **55**, 1099 (1967).
[5] M.J.M. Gijbels, J.J.C. Scheffer and A. Baerheim Svendsen, Rivista Italiana E.P.P.O.S. **61**, 335 (1979).
[6] Sh. Yu and Sh. You, Yaoxue Xuebao **19**, 566 (1984); C. A. **101**, 222522 (1984).
[7] J. Yang and Y. Chen, Yaoxue Tangbao **19**, 670 (1984); C. A. **103**, 92687 (1984).
[8] V.K. Kulshrestha, N. Singh, R.L. Saxena and R.P. Kohli, Indian J. Med. Res. **58**, 99 (1970).
[9] O. Schimmer, Planta Med. **47**, 79 (1983).
[10] K.W. Glombitza, Dtsch. Apoth. Ztg. **112**, 1593 (1972).
[11] J. Mitchell and A. Rook, Botanical dermatology. Plants and plant products injurious to the skin. H. Kimpton, Vancouver, 1979, pp. 787.
[12] C. Benezra, G. Ducombs, Y. Sell, and J. Foussereau, Plant contact dermatitis. Decker, Toronto – Philadelphia; Mosby, Saint Louis – Toronto – London, 1985, pp. 353.
[13] J.D. Phillipson and L.A. Anderson, Pharm. J. **233**, 80, 111 (1984).
[14] B.P. Jackson and D.W. Snowdon, Atlas of microscopy of medicinal plants, culinary herbs and spices, Belhaven Press, London, 1990, p. 52.

Arnicae flos   (DAB 10), Arnica (BHP)

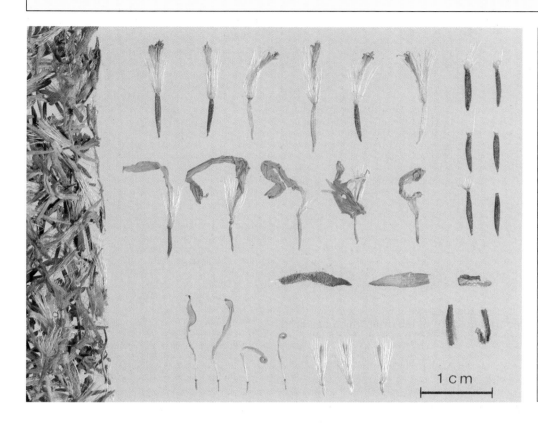

Fig. 1: Arnica (the bottom row shows ligulate and tubular florets of the adulterant "Mexican Arnica", *Heterotheca inuloides* Cass.)

<u>Description:</u> The drug consists of the dried, whole, but mostly fallen, flower-heads (capitula) or of individual ligulate and tubular florets which have come loose from the involucre and receptacle (Flores Arnicae sine calycibus or receptaculis; see the ÖAB). The greyish white, bristly pappus hairs which form a wreath at the upper end of the long, slender, brown ovary (the later achenes) of the ligulate and tubular florets are characteristic and are responsible for the greyish white appearance of the drug. The golden-yellow crown of ligulate florets surrounded by the pappus is much shrivelled, that surrounding the tubular florets is inconspicuous. There are also a few slightly convex receptacles with involucral bracts but without florets.

<u>Odour:</u> Faintly aromatic.

<u>Taste:</u> Slightly bitter, somewhat pungent and spicy.

Figs. 2 and 3: *Arnica montana* L.

A 20–30 cm tall perennial herb with opposite leaves. 1–3 (rarely 5) flower-heads, one terminal and the others arising from the axils of the leaves. Receptacles 5–8 cm broad, with 15–25 ligulate florets.

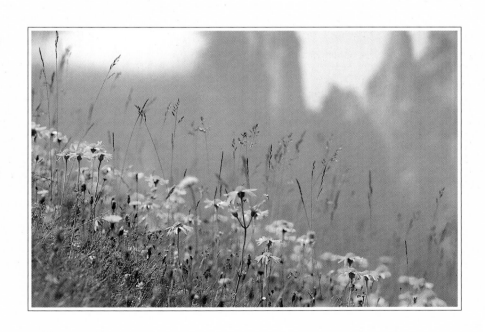

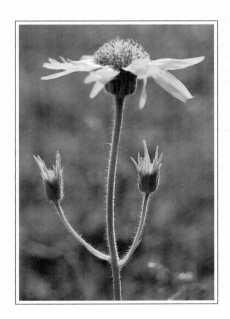

DAB 10: **Arnikablüten**
Ph. Helv. VII: **Arnicae Flos**
ÖAB: **Flos Arnicae**
St.Zul.: **8199.99.99**

Plant sources: *Arnica montana* L. (Asteraceae). This is a protected species in Germany and hence the DAB 10 also permits *A. chamissonis* LESS. subsp. *foliosa* (NUTT.) MAGUIRE (North American meadow arnica). The BHP 1983 only allows *A. montana*. The sources of the American drug are *A. fulgens* PURSH, *A. sororia* GREENE, and *A. cordifolia* HOOK. [40].

Synonyms: Arnica flowers, Leopard's or Wolf's bane, Mountain tobacco (Engl.), Arnikablüten, Bergwohlverleih, Wundkraut, Kraftwurz (Ger.), Fleurs d'arnica (Fr.).

Origin: From wild plants growing in Europe to southern Russia. At present, the main suppliers are former Yugoslavia, Spain, Italy, and Switzerland. *A. chamissonis* is being cultivated in Russia and the eastern part of Germany, and a start has been made with the cultivation of the subsp. *foliosa* in the western part of Germany.

Constituents [41, 42]: Pseudoguaianolide-type sesquiterpene lactones: *A. montana*

Helenalins

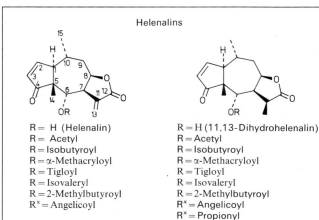

R = H (Helenalin)
R = Acetyl
R = Isobutyroyl
R = α-Methacryloyl
R = Tigloyl
R = Isovaleryl
R = 2-Methylbutyroyl
Rˣ = Angelicoyl

R = H (11,13-Dihydrohelenalin)
R = Acetyl
R = Isobutyroyl
R = α-Methacryloyl
R = Tigloyl
R = Isovaleryl
R = 2-Methylbutyroyl
Rˣ = Angelicoyl
Rˣ = Propionyl

* Only in A. chamissonis flowers

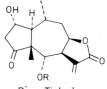

R* = Tigloyl
R* = Angelicoyl
R* = Senecioyl

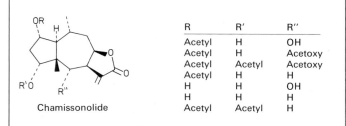

Chamissonolide

R	R′	R″
Acetyl	H	OH
Acetyl	H	Acetoxy
Acetyl	Acetyl	Acetoxy
Acetyl	H	H
H	H	OH
H	H	H
Acetyl	Acetyl	H

R* = Tigloyl
R* = Angelicoyl
R* = Senecioyl
Rˣ = Isovaleryl

* Only in A.chamissonis flowers

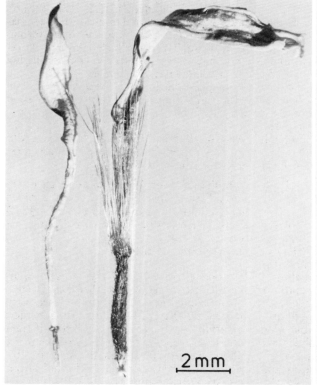

2 mm

Fig. 4

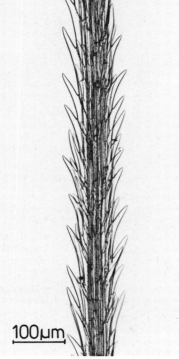

100 μm

Fig. 5

Fig. 4: Ligulate florets of *Heterotheca inuloides* (left) and *Arnica montana* (right)

Fig. 5: Pappus bristle from *Arnica montana*

flowers 0.2–0.8%; *A. chamissonis* subsp. *foliosa* flowers 0.2–1.5%. In *A. montana* flowers, esters of helenalin and 11α,13-dihydrohelenalin with lower fatty acids (acetic, isobutyric, 2-methylbutyric, isovaleric, metha-crylic, and tiglic acids) [1]. Central European flowers contain principally helenalin esters; in Spanish flowers, dihydrohelenalin methacrylate, tiglate, and isobutyrate are predominant, with only small amounts of helenalin esters [2]. *A. chamissonis* subsp. *foliosa* flowers have, in addition to helenalin and 11,13-dihydrohelenalin esters (= helenalins), their 2,3-dihydro-2α-hydroxy derivatives (= arnifolins) and 2,3-dihydro-2α,4α-dihydroxy derivatives (= chamissonolides) [3–7]; there is considerable variation, depending on the origin of the plant material. There are sources in which the 11,13-dihydrohelenalin esters (>80%) or helenalin and dihydrohelenalin esters (>70%) dominate, and are thus similar to *A. montana* flowers, as well as sources in which the helenalins, arnifolins, and chammisonolides occur in more or less equal proportions or in which the arnifolins predominate [6]. Flowers of the subsp. *chamissonis* (subsp. *genuina*) contain almost entirely chamissonolides, but traces of the eudesmanolide ivalin are also present [8]. Flavonoids (0.4–0.6%): numerous flavonoid aglycones [9–11] and glycosides (17 from the flowers of *A. montana*, 27 from those of *A. chamissonis* subsp. *foliosa* [12–15]; in both species, the flavonols mostly have the sugar at the 3-position and the flavones mostly at the 7-position; the two species are distinguished by the presence only in *A. chamissonis* of acylated glycosides, the flavonol glucosides being esterified with acetic acid and the flavone glucosides with 2- methylbutyric acid [43]).
0.2–0.35% essential oil of a buttery consistency, with ca. 40–50% fatty acids and ca. 9% *n*-alkanes (C_{19}–C_{30}) [16], thymol derivatives, and mono- and sesquiterpenes (including α- phellandrene, myrcene, humulene, δ-cadinene, caryophyllene oxide) [17,18]; cinnamic acid and derivatives (among them chlorogenic acid, cynarin, caffeic acid); coumarins (umbelliferone, scopoletin); polyacetylenes; 0.1% choline; xanthophylls.

Indications: For wound healing, and as a wound antiseptic, antiphlogistic, antirheumatic, and antineuralgic. Used for injuries and accidents (sprains, dislocations, bruising, haematomas, oedema associated with fractures), in phlebitis and thrombosis, in arthralgia and rheumatic pains in the joints, for furuncles and inflamed insect bites, in inflammation of the mucous membranes especially of the mouth. For use as a cardiotonic and analeptic, see: Side effects.

The essential active principles are the helenalin and dihydrohelenalin esters, which have been shown to have strong antimicrobial [18, 19], antiphlogistic, antirheumatic, anti-arthritic [21, 22], antihyperlipidaemic [22], and respiratory analeptic [23, 24] properties. They also affect the heart and circulation [23–27]. Flavonoids, essential oil, xanthophylls, and polyacetylenes may also be involved in some of the effects. See further [42].
In addition, cholagogic and diuretic effects (sesquiterpene lactones, flavonoids, chlorogenic acid, cynarin, caffeic acid), as well as reflex-modulating effects on the central nervous system, have been described.
The most frequently used form of the drug is the tincture (Arnicae tinctura) prepared from 1 part drug and 10 parts 70% ethanol, as described in the DAB 10.
In *folk medicine,* the drug has often been used as an abortifacient, which can be explained on the basis of the proved oxytocic activity of its sesquiterpene lactones.

Side effects: Owing to the toxicity of the sesquiterpene lactones, oral use must be very carefully controlled or avoided altogether, since investigation of the pharmacokinetics and therapeutic spectrum of these highly active substances is almost entirely lacking. With too high doses, gastroenteritis intervenes [28–30]; and with very high doses, death through cardiac arrest following dyspnoea may occur. The helenolides are known to have damaging effects on the heart [27]. Helenalin shows a concentration-dependent inotropic effect (EC_{50} 1.4×10^5) on the guinea-pig auricle and on the isolated

cat papillary muscle, which arises from an indirect sympathomimetic action [26, 27, 31, 32]. At higher concentrations, or after a longer period of action, the time of contraction is reduced and the rate of relaxation is decreased. Helenalin slows down the recovery kinetics of calcium, probably via a membrane-stabilizing action, which is responsible for the toxic effects [31]. With longer and more frequent external application, oedematous dermatitis may occur, with the formation of small vesicles. Helenalin and its esters have been shown to be sensitizing agents and to act as allergens [33–35].
Biological effects of the sesquiterpene lactones present in *Arnica* species are reviewed in [44].

Making the tea: 2.0 g arnica is brewed with boiling water, which is poured through a tea strainer after 5–10 min.

Warning: Not for prolonged application; internal use problematic and to be avoided (see: Standard Licence). Beware of side effects! Externally, as the infusion (2%) or the (diluted) tincture.
1 Teaspoon = ca. 0.5 g.

Phytomedicines: With 271 preparations, arnica heads the list of phytotherapeutic remedies [36]. In the "Rote Liste"® (Red List) there are 200 specialities containing extracts of arnica which cover twenty-six different areas of use; more than half of them are allopathic products, and the rest are homoeopathic remedies. The main indications are as cardiac remedies (33), analgesics and antirheumatics (31), and phlebitis and vari-

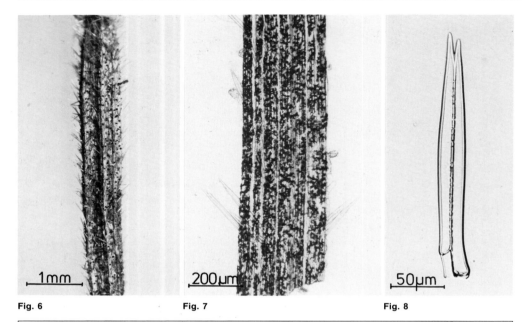

Fig. 6   Fig. 7   Fig. 8

Fig. 6: Ovary with paired trichomes and peltate glandular trichomes (dark spots)

Fig. 7: Phytomelan deposits in the fruit wall

Fig. 8: Paired trichomes

---

be brownish grey to dark brown (sesquiterpene lactones). If flowers of *A. chamissonis* subsp. *chamissonis*, *Heterotheca* (Mexican "Arnica"), or *Calendula* are present, the lower phase takes on a faint reddish colour.

The Zimmermann reaction can also be used for the photometric quantitative determination [37] or by HPLC or GC of the sesquiterpene lactones [7]. But, TLC of the sesquiterpene lactones is a more convenient proof of identity [38]. Checking the purity according to the DAB 10 method, by TLC of the flavonoids, enables the most important adulterants to be recognized through the occurrence of rutin, which is not present in arnica flowers:

Test solution: 1.0 g powdered drug shaken for 5 min. with 10 ml methanol on the water-bath at 65 °C, filtered and cooled.

Reference solution: 1.0 mg each of chlorogenic and caffeic acids and 2.5 mg hyperoside and rutin dissolved in 10 ml methanol.

Loadings: 30 µl test solution and 10 µl reference solution, as 2-cm bands on silica gel G.

Solvent system: anhydrous formic acid + water + ethyl methyl ketone + ethyl acetate (10 + 10 + 30 + 50), 15 cm run.

Detection: dried at 100–105 °C and while warm sprayed with 1% methanolic diphenylboryloxyethylamine and then with 5% methanolic Macrogol 400.

Evaluation: after 30 min. in UV 365 nm light. Test solution: at about the middle, the intense bright blue fluorescent chlorogenic acid zone (also in the chromatogram of the reference solution); above it, three yellowish brown to orange zones, the middle one being sometimes very faint and the upper one being assigned to isoquecetrin and luteolin 7-glucoside; above the group of three, the greenish fluorescent astragalin zone (with *A. chamissonis* subsp. *foliosa*, only in traces and between the hyperoside and caffeic acid zones a yellowish brown to orange fluorescent zone); slightly below the caffeic acid zone, two intense turquoise fluorescent zones, the lower one being distinctly larger. There must be **no** greenish yellow or yellowish brown fluorescent zones at the same level as, or below, the rutin zone (*Calendula* and/or *Heterotheca* flowers).

Diagrams of the flavonoid-glycoside chromatograms from *A. montana*, *A. chamissonis* subsp. *foliosa*, and *Heterotheca* flowers, with the assignments of the bands, are to be found in [45].

Quantitative standards: DAB 10: *Foreign matter*, absence of *Calendula* and *Heterotherca* flowers tested by TLC as above.

---

cosis remedies (30). About half the preparations are for external use.

Authentication: Macro- and microscopically, following the DAB 10; see also the BHP 1983. Among the important diagnostic features are the pappus bristles (see: Adulteration) on both ligulate and tubular florets (Figs. 4 and 5). The ovary in genuine arnica flowers is long and slender, and phytomelan deposits (Fig. 7), paired trichomes (Figs. 6 and 8), and glandular trichomes (Fig. 6) can be recognized. The tips of the involucral bracts in *A. montana* have numerous glandular trichomes, those of *A. chamissonis* tufts mostly of unicellular trichomes.

The DAB 10 identity test is based on the Zimmermann reaction:
1.0 g powdered drug shaken for 5 min. with 15 ml hexane and the extract then filtered through anhydrous sodium sulphate, rinsed with a further 3 ml hexane, and carefully concentrated to 3 ml on the water-bath; 1.0 ml 5% 1,3-dinitrobenzene in toluene and 2.0 ml methanolic sodium hydroxide solution (0.6 g NaOH dissolved in 2.5 ml water and 4.5 ml methanol added), and shaken for 3 min. After 30 min., the lower layer should

---

Wording of the package insert, from the German Standard Licence:

5.1 Uses

In supportive treatment for dislocations, sprains, muscle and joint pains, swelling resulting from injury and bruising; promoting wound healing and the absorption of extravasated blood.
Warning: not for internal use.

5.2 Contraindications

Known hypersensitivity to members of the daisy family, such as arnica, chamomile, marigolds, or yarrow.

5.3 Side effects

In using preparations of arnica, hypersensitivity (allergy) may occur in the form of painful, itching and inflammatory changes in the skin. The treatment should then be stopped and a doctor consulted.

5.4 Dosage and Mode of administration

About 1–2 teaspoonfuls (2–3 g) **Arnica** are covered with hot water (ca. 150 ml) and after 10 min. passed through a tea strainer. Unless otherwise prescribed, linen or cellulose wadding or a similar material is soaked in the infusion and then placed on the affected part of the body. The poultice is changed several times a day.

5.5 Note

Store protected from light and moisture.

Loss on drying, not more than 9.0%. *Ash*, not more than 10.0%.
ÖAB: *Foreign matter*, not more than 1%. *Ash*, not more than 8.0%.
Ph. Helv. VII: *Water-soluble extractive*, not less than 17.0%. *Foreign matter*, not more than 1% stem fragments; capitula of other Asteraceae absent. *Sulphated ash*, not more than 13%.
BHP 1983: 45% *Alcohol-soluble extractive*, not less than 15%. *Foreign organic matter*, not more than 2%; receptacles with attached involucre, not more than 25–33%. *Total ash*, not more than 8%.

Adulteration: Relatively frequent, since in many countries *Arnica montana* is a protected species and, as a result, the genuine drug is not always available in sufficient quantity. The adulterant most often encountered is "Mexican Arnica", the flower-heads of *Heterotheca inuloides* CASS. (Asteraceae) [45]. They can be recognized by the following features: ligulate florets without a pappus, tubular florets with a double pappus (the outer ring being shorter), V-shaped stigma (style not bent as in *A. montana*); fruit short and ovoid, without phytomelan (in *A. montana* very long and slender, with phytomelan); paired trichomes on the ovary very long and slender; sesquiterpene lactones absent. A detailed description can be found in [39].
Other forms of adulteration, e.g. with the flowers of *Calendula officinalis* (see: Calendulae flos) or with *Doronicum* species, are seldom met with [45] and are easily recognized microscopically.

Literature:
[1] G. Willuhn, P.-M. Röttger, and U. Matthiesen, Planta Med. **49**, 226 (1983).
[2] C. Luley and G. Willuhn, Acta Agron. Hungar. **34** (Suppl.), 75 (1985).
[3] G. Willuhn, J. Kresken, and D. Wendisch, Planta Med. **47**, 157 (1983).
[4] G. Willuhn and J. Kresken, Planta Med. **45**, 132 (1982).
[5] J. Kresken, Thesis, Univ. Düsseldorf, 1984.
[6] W. Leven, Thesis, Univ. Düsseldorf 1988.
[7] W. Leven and G. Willuhn, J. Chromatogr. **410**, 329 (1987).
[8] G. Willuhn et al., Planta Med. **51**, 398 (1985).
[9] I. Merfort, Planta Med. **50**, 107 (1984).
[10] I. Merfort, Planta Med. **51**, 136 (1985).
[11] I. Merfort, C. Marcinek, and A. Eggert, Phytochemistry **25**, 2901 (1986).
[12] I. Merfort and D. Wendisch, Planta Med. **53**, 434 (1987).
[13] I. Merfort, Pharm. Weekbl. **9**, 240 (1987).
[14] I. Merfort and D. Wendisch, Planta Med. **54**, 247 (1988).
[15] I. Merfort, Phytochemistry **27**, 3281 (1988).
[16] H. Kating, W. Rinn, and G. Willuhn, Planta Med. **18**, 130 (1970).
[17] G. Willuhn, R. Schneider, and U. Matthiesen, Dtsch. Apoth. Ztg. **125**, 1941 (1985).
[18] K.H. Lee, T. Ikuba, R.Y. Wu, and T.A. Geissmann, Phytochemistry **16**, 1177 (1977).
[19] G. Willuhn, P.-M. Röttger, and W. Quack, Pharm. Ztg. **127**, 2183 (1982).
[20] I.H. Hall et al., J. Pharm. Sci. **68**, 537 (1979).
[21] I.H. Hall, C. O. Sturnes, K.H. Lee, and T.G. Waddell, J. Pharm. Sci. **69**, 537 (1980).
[22] I.H. Hall et al., J. Pharm. Sci. **69**, 694 (1980).
[23] P.H. List and B. Friebel, Arzneimitt.-Forsch. **24**, 148 (1974).
[24] G. Willuhn, Pharmazie in unserer Zeit **10**, 1 (1981).
[25] G. Willuhn and P.-M. Röttger, Planta Med. **45**, 131 (1982).
[26] K. Takeya, M. Itoigawa, and H. Furukawa, Chem. Pharm. Bull. **31**, 1719 (1983).
[27] G. Willuhn. Dtsch. Apoth. Ztg. **127**, 2511 (1987).
[28] H. Schulz, Wirkung und Anwendung der Deutschen Arzneipflanzen, 2nd ed., Leipzig, 1929.
[29] K. Stuhlfauth, Hippokrates (D) **9**, 1131 (1938).
[30] Arzneimittelkommission der Deutschen Apotheker, Pharm. Ztg. **126**, 2082 (1981).
[31] A. Konder et al., Farm. Tijdschr. Belg. **61e**, 240 (1984).
[32] M. Itoigawa, K. Takeya, H. Furukawa, and K. Ito, Cardiovascular Pharmacol. **9**, 193 (1987).
[33] H.-D. Herrmann, G. Willuhn, and B.M. Hausen, Planta Med. **34**, 299 (1978).
[34] B.M. Hausen, H.-D. Herrmann, and G. Willuhn, Contact Dermatitis **4**, 3 (1978).
[35] B.M. Hausen, Hautarzt **31**, 10 (1980).
[36] Statistik, Verbrauchzahlen für Drogen im Jahr 1982, Dtsch. Apoth. Ztg. **123**, 1653 (1983).
[37] W. Leven and G. Willuhn, Planta Med. **52**, 537 (1986).
[38] G. Willuhn, J. Kresken, and I. Merfort, Dtsch. Apoth. Ztg. **123**, 2431 (1983).
[39] J. Saukel, Sci. Pharm. **52**, 35 (1984).
[40] V.E. Tyler, The new honest herbal, 2nd ed., G.F. Stickley Co., Philadelphia, 1980, p. 26.
[41] T.M. Pinchon and M. Pinkas, Pl. Méd. Phytothérap. **22**, 124 (1988).
[42] G. Willuhn, Pharm. Ztg. **136**, 2453 (1991).
[43] I. Merfort and D. Wendisch, Pl. Med. **58**, 355 (1992).
[44] B.M. Hausen, in: P.A.G.M. de Smet, K. Keller, R. Hänsel, and R.F. Chandler, Adverse effects of herbal drugs, Springer, Berlin – Heidelberg – New York, 1992, vol. **1**, p. 237.
[45] I. Merfort, G. Willuhn, and C. Jerga, Dtsch. Apoth. Ztg. **130**, 980 (1990).

Artemisiae herba   Mugwort, Artemisia vulgaris (BHP 1983)

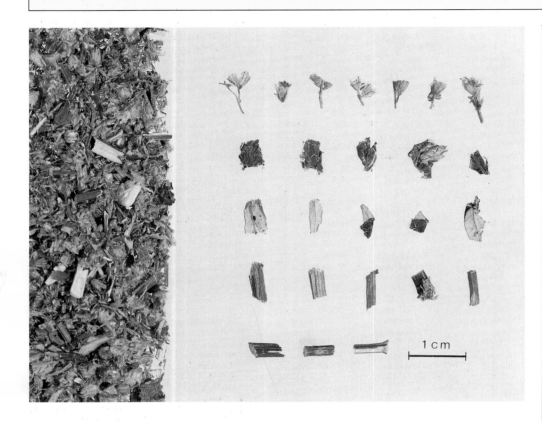

Fig. 1: Mugwort

Description: The drug consists of the 60–70 cm long flowering tops. In the cut drug, there are the leaf tips which are often lanceolate and mostly with an entire or serrate margin tip, derived from the pinnate or bipinnate leaves. The leaf fragments are glabrous on the upper surface and dark to very dark green; they have a silvery grey, woolly indumentum on the lower surface (distinction from Absinthii herba). The many T-shaped trichomes (Fig. 4) cause the drug to more or less clump together. There are numerous ovoid flower receptacles with greyish white, woolly, imbricate sepals and yellowish or reddish flowers, often present as broken panicles (Fig. 1, top row). The receptacle is glabrous (in contrast with Absinthii herba). Longitudinally ridged pieces of stem with a pith, which are green or which usually have a reddish violet flush on the outside, also occur.

Odour: Pleasantly aromatic.

Taste: Spicy and somewhat bitter.

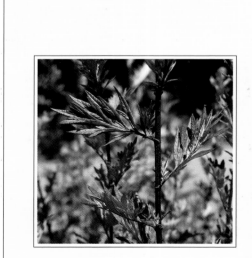

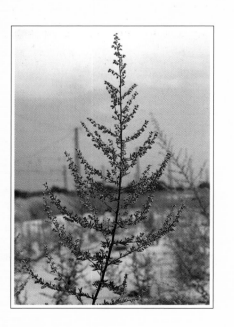

Figs. 2 and 3: *Artemisia vulgaris* L.

50–150 cm tall herbs with bipinnate leaves having an indumentum only on the lower surface. Small, yellow to red-brown flower-heads arranged in panicles.

Erg. B. 6: Herba Artemisiae

Plant origin: *Artemisia vulgaris* L., mugwort (Asteraceae).

Synonyms: Summitates Artemisiae (vulgaris) (Lat.), Felon herb, Wild wormwood, St. John's plant (Engl.), Beifußkraut, Wilder Wermut (Ger.), Feuilles d'armoise commune (Fr.).

Origin: Distributed throughout Europe, Asia, and North America, especially in fields lying fallow, hedges, cuttings, and on rubbish tips and river banks. The drug comes from collections made in the wild in eastern Europe.

Constituents: Essential oil (0.03–0.3%) with over 100 identified components and a composition varying both qualitatively and quantitatively [1–6]. Depending on the origin, 1,8-cineole, camphor, linalool, or thujone may be the main component, along with 4-terpineol, borneol, α-cadinol, spathulenol, and 21 irregularly built monoterpenes [7]; sesquiterpenes, including small amounts of eudesmane derivatives [21], and sesquiterpene lactones, among them the eudesmane derivative vulgarin (=tauremisin), and psilostachyin and psilostachyin C [8]; the flavonol glycosides quercetin 3-*O*-glucoside and 3-*O*-rhamnosidoglucoside (rutin), as well as isorhamnetin 3-*O*-glucoside and 3-*O*-rhamnosidoglucoside [9]; coumarins (1.9%), including aesculetin, aesculin, umbelliferone, scopoletin, coumarin, and 6-methoxy-7,8-methylene-dioxycoumarin [10,11]; polyacetylenes [12, 22]; pentacyclic triterpenes [13–15], sitosterol, stigmasterol [14]; carotenoids [16].

Indications: Nowadays, the drug is only rarely used as a bitter aromatic to stimulate secretion of the gastric juices in lack of appetite or anacid or sub-acid gastritis, as well as against flatulence and a feeling of distension. The uses correspond to those of wormwood, but the action is weaker. In *folk medicine*, mugwort is also employed as a choleretic and formerly as an anthelmintic, as well as for amenorrhoea and dysmenorrhoea. The essential oil has been shown to have considerable repellent activity and to be antibacterial and antifungal [18].

Side effects: In therapeutic doses, none. A case of contact dermatitis has been described in the literature [19].

Extract from the German Commission E monograph
(BAnz no. 122, dated 06.07.1988)

Uses

Mugwort is used in complaints and problems involving the gastrointestinal tract, such as colic, diarrhoea, constipation, cramps, weak digestion, to stimulate secretion of gastric juice and bile, as a laxative in cases of obesity and "for the liver", also against worm infestations, and for hysteria, epilepsy, persistent vomiting, convulsions in children, menstrual problems and irregular periods, to promote the circulation and to act as a sedative.

The root is used in asthenic states as a tonic, and in combination with other remedies also for psychoneuroses, neurasthenia, depression, hypochondria, autonomic neuroses, general irritability and restlessness, insomnia, and anxiety states.

The efficacy of mugwort preparations in the conditions indicated has not so far been substantiated.

Risks

An abortifacient action has been described. Allergic reactions may be elicited in previously sensitized subjects.

Evaluation

As the efficacy of the drug in the various indications claimed has not been substantiated, its therapeutic use cannot be endorsed.

Making the tea: Boiling water (150 ml) is poured over a teaspoonful of the drug, allowed to draw for 5 min. in a covered vessel, and then strained. To stimulate the appetite, two or three cups a day are drunk before meals.
1 Teaspoon = ca. 1.2 g.

Phytomedicines: Mugwort extracts are included in Famitra-Diät-Tabletten (diet tablets), Famitra-Kräuter-Extrakt-Tabletten (herb extract tablets). The drug is a constituent of Famitra Kräuterkur 23 Komplex Magentee (stomach tea).

Authentication: Macro- (see: Description) and microscopically. The T-shaped trichomes, with horizontal cells which are up to 1 mm in length, thin, or variably thickened, and often twisted (Fig. 5), are characteristic. The leaves have stomata only on the lower epidermis and mostly only one palisade layer. Rounded, smooth pollen grains with three apertures and peltate glandular trichomes are also present [20] (Fig. 6). For a more detailed description of the macro- and microscopy, see the BHP 1983.

Quantitative standard: Erg. B. 6: *Ash*, not more than 9%.

Adulteration: Only occasionally. Wormwood has an indumentum on both leaf surfaces and a pubescent receptacle.

Storage: Protected from light. Not to be kept in plastic containers.

Literature
[1] G.M. Nano, C. Bicchi, C. Frattini and M. Gallino, Planta Med. **30**, 211 (1976).
[2] H. Jork and S.M.K. Juell, Arch. Pharm. (Weinheim) **312**, 540 (1979).
[3] M. Hurabielle, M. Malsot and M. Paris, Riv. Ital. EPPOS **63**, 296 (1981); C.A. **95**, 225461 (1981).
[4] K. Michaelis et al., Z. Naturforsch. C: Biosci. **37c**, 152 (1982).
[5] A.P. Carnat et al. Ann. Pharm. Fr. **43**, 397 (1986); C.A. **104**, 222004 (1986).

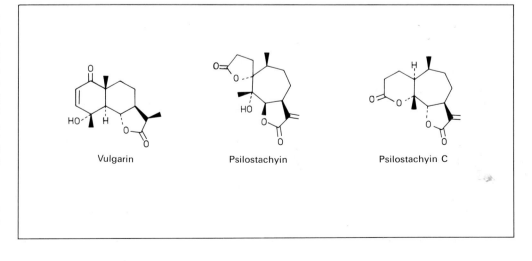

Vulgarin   Psilostachyin   Psilostachyin C

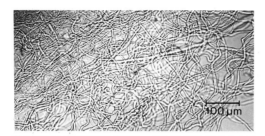

Fig. 4: Woolly indumentum on the lower surface of the leaf, made up of T-shaped trichomes (Fig. 5)

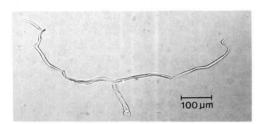

Fig. 5: A single T-shaped trichome from the lower epidermis

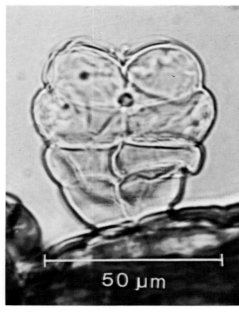

Fig. 6: Peltate glandular trichome

[6] L.N. Misra and S.P. Singh, J. Nat. Prod. **49**, 941 (1986).

[7] R. Naef-Mueller, W. Pickenhagen and B. Willhalm, Helv. Chim. Acta **64**, 1424 (1981).

[8] M. Stephanovic, A. Jokic and A. Behbud, Glas. Hem. Drus. (Beograd) **37**, 463 (1972); C.A. **80**, 80080 (1974).

[9] B. Hoffmann and K. Herrmann, Z. Lebensm. Unters. Forsch. **174**, 211 (1982).

[10] M.A. Ikasanova, T.R. Berezovskaya and E.A. Serykh, Khim. Prir. Soedin 110 (1986); C.A. **104**, 203928 (1986).

[11] R.D.H. Murray and M. Stephanovic, J. Nat. Prod. **49**, 550 (1986).

[12] D. Drake and J. Lam, Phytochemistry **13**, 455 (1974).

[13] S.K. Kundu, A. Chatterjee and A.S. Rao, Austr. J. Chem. **21**, 1931 (1968).

[14] S.K. Kundu, A. Chatterjee and A.S. Rao, J. Indian Chem. Soc. **46**, 584 (1969).

[15] M. Stephanovic, M. Dermanovic und M. Verencevic, Glas, Hem. Drus. (Beograd) **47**, 7 (1982); C.A. **96**, 177968 (1982).

[16] T. Shimizu et al., Sagami Joshi Daigaku Kiyu **45**, 5 (1981); C.A. **97**, 125913 (1982).

[17] Y.S. Hwang et al., J. Chem. Ecol. **11**, 1297 (1985); C.A. **103**, 175478 (1985).

[18] V.K. Kaul, S.S. Nigam and K.L. Dhar, Indian J. Pharm. **38**, 21 (1976).

[19] G. Kurz and M.J. Rapaport, Contact Dermatitis **5**, 407 (1979).

[20] P. Rohdewald, G. Rücker and K.-W. Glombitza, Apothekengerechte Prüfvorschriften, S. 645, Deutscher Apotheker Verlag, Stuttgart 1986.

[21] J.A. Marco, J.F. Sanz, and P. del Hierro, Phytochemistry **30**, 2403 (1991).

[22] B. Wallnöfer, O. Hofer, and H. Greger, Phytochemistry **28**, 2687 (1989).

Aurantii flos   Orange flowers

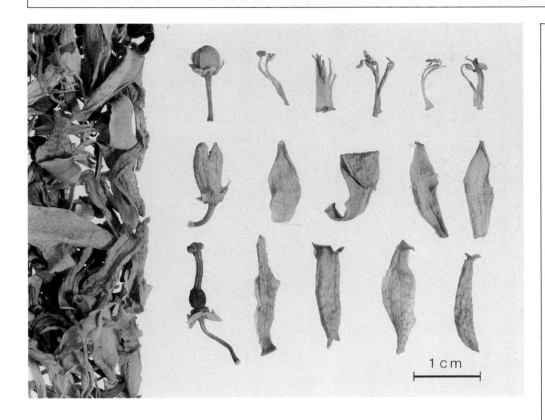

1 cm

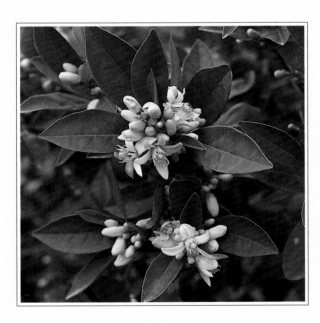

Fig. 1: Orange flowers

<u>Description</u>: The drug consists of the light brownish yellow, 1–2 cm long, stalked and still closed, dried flower buds. They are gamopetalous and have an obscurely five-toothed calyx with short stout spreading tips. The five glabrous petals are covered with distinct brownish dots (secretory glands with essential oil) and form a dome which broadens from the bottom. In cross-section, or in fragments, numerous (20–35) filaments are visible, which at the bottom are fused into bands. The superior, brownish black ovary is spherical and has a thick pistil with capitate stigma.

<u>Odour</u>: Faint, but characteristically aromatic.

<u>Taste</u>: Spicy and aromatic, and very slightly bitter.

Fig. 2: *Citrus aurantium* L.

A small, ca. 5 m tall tree with broadly elliptic, evergreen, entire leaves on petioles distinctly winged in the upper part (in contrast, petioles of *Citrus limon*, the lemon, only slightly winged). Scented, actinomorphic, white flowers having 5(–8) punctate petals (oil glands) and numerous stamens with filaments fused together at the base to form broad bands. Fruit a multilocular berry.

ÖAB: Flos Aurantii
Ph. Helv. VII: Aurantii flos
Erg. B. 6: Flores Aurantii

Plant sources: *Citrus aurantium* L. subsp. *aurantium* (= subsp. *amara* (L.) ENGL.), bitter orange (Rutaceae); the Ph. Helv. VII also permits *Citrus sinensis* (L.) OSBECK, sweet orange.

Synonyms: Flores Naphae (Lat.), Bitter orange or Seville orange or Bigarade or Neroli flowers (Engl.), Orangen-, Bigarade-, or Neroliblüten (Ger.), Fleurs de bigaradier, Fleurs d'oranger amer (Fr.).

Origin: Cultivated in southern Europe and in regions with a subtropical climate. The drug is imported from Spain and Mexico.

Constituents: Ca. 0.2–0.5% essential oil, consisting mainly of monoterpenes, e.g. linalyl acetate, α-pinene, limonene, linalool, nerol, geraniol, etc.; methyl anthranilate is a characteristic constituent. Bitter substances and flavonoids are also present.

Indications: Exclusively in *folk medicine,* as a mild sedative for nervousness and disturbed sleep. For the rest, it is used as an aromatic.

The neroli oil obtained from fresh orange flowers by steam distillation is extensively used in perfumery, e.g. for eau de cologne, etc.

Making the tea: Boiling water is poured over 1–2 g of the drug and after 5 min. passed through a tea strainer. As a mild sedative, one or two cups of the tea are drunk in the evening.
1 Teapoon = ca. 1 g.

Herbal preparations: The drug is also available in tea bags (1.2 g).

Phytomedicines: The drug is present in some prepared remedies for a range of very different indications, in most cases doubtless simply as an aromatic.

Authentication: Macro- (see: Description) and microscopically. In the mesophyll of the sepals there are large clusters of calcium oxalate crystals and on the epidermis unicellular trichomes. The epidermal cells of the petals show a distinctly striated cuticle and the schizolysigenous oil glands are ca. 100 mm in diameter. The pollen grains are spherical, with a delicately punctate exine. The essential oil (neroli oil) can be examined by TLC as follows [1]:

Reference solution: citral 1:30 in toluene.

Loadings: 5 µl of a 1:10 dilution of the oil and 3 µl reference solution, as 2-cm bands on silica gel 60F$_{254}$.

Solvent system: toluene + ethyl acetate (93 + 7), 15 cm run.

Detection: sprayed with 5% ethanolic sulphuric acid and oversprayed with 1% ethanolic vanillin, followed by heating at 110° for 5–10 min.

Evaluation: in daylight. Test solution: major blue spots at Rf ca. 0.6 (linalyl acetate) and 0.25 (linalool); other terpene alcohols below the linalool band.

Quantitative standards: Erg. B. 6: *Volatile oil,* not less than 0.2%. *Ash,* not more than 7%.
ÖAB: *Volatile oil,* not less than 0.2%.
Ph. Helv. VII: *Volatile oil,* not less than 0.18%. *Foreign matter,* not more than 20% discoloured and fully open flowers. *Sulphated ash,* not more than 10%.

Adulteration: In practice rare.

Literature:
[1] H. Wagner, S. Bladt, and E. M. Zgainski, Plant drug analysis, Springer-Verlag, Berlin, Heidelberg, New York, Tokyo, 1984, pp. 15, 44.

Aurantii fructus immaturi   Unripe orange

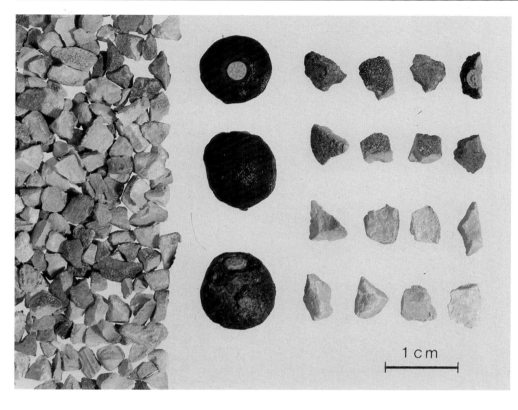

1 cm

Fig. 1: Unripe orange

Description: Unripe orange consists of almost spherical, very hard fruit, 0.5–2 cm in diameter, which on the outside are dark green to brownish grey and knobbly or wrinkled with numerous punctate depressions (oil glands). Examination of the cross-section (Fig. 2) with a hand lens reveals the oil glands lying just underneath the surface; the locules of the ovary, which are in the centre, can also be recognized.

Odour: Spicy and aromatic.

Taste: Spicy and bitter.

For the description and illustrations of the plant source, see: **Aurantii pericarpium.**

Plant source: See, Aurantii pericarpium.

Synonyms: Orange peas (Engl.), Unreife Pomeranzen, Grüne Orange, Orangetten (Ger.), Fruits d'oranger amer verts (Fr.).

Origin: See, Aurantii pericarpium.

Constituents: See, Aurantii pericarpium. In addition, there are limonin-type triterpenoid bitter substances in the seeds.

Indications: As for Aurantii pericarpium (q.v.).

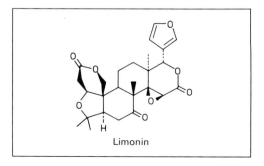

Limonin

Making the tea: As for Aurantii pericarpium (q.v.).

Authentication: Macro- (see: Description) and microscopically. In the small-celled epidermis, there are very large stomata. The

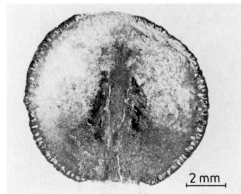

Fig. 2: Transverse section through the unripe fruit, showing the many large secretory glands below the epidermis

parenchyma of the fruit wall contains a few calcium oxalate crystals. Hesperidin occurs in the parenchyma as amorphous masses; it is insoluble in water, but dissolves in potassium hydroxide solution to yield an intense yellow solution and in conc. sulphuric acid to give an orange-yellow colour which on gentle warming changes to red.

Quantitative standard: *Bitterness value,* should be not less than 1000.

Adulteration: Rare. Unripe lemons are oblong and at the top they have a teat-like projection; they taste only slightly bitter.

Storage: As for Aurantii pericarpium (q.v.).

Aurantii pericarpium   (DAB 10), Dried bitter-orange peel (*BAN*; BP 1988)

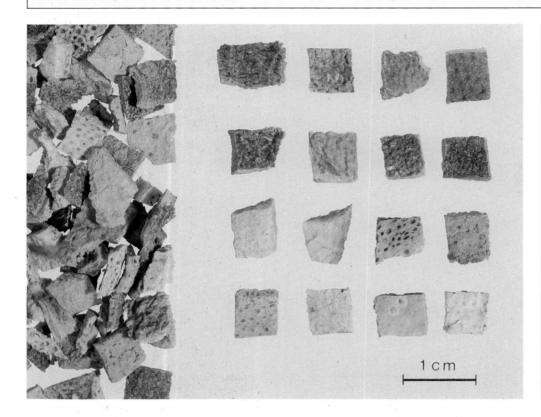

Fig. 1: Bitter-orange peel

Description: The drug consists of the outer layer (flavedo) of the fruit wall obtained by peeling ripe bitter oranges and making sure that the spongy white parenchyma (albedo) is largely removed. The coarsely knobbly strips or pieces are up to ca. 2 mm thick and twisted or curved. On the outside, they are yellowish to reddish brown and on the inside whitish yellow to light ochre; they appear punctate because of the oil glands that shine through (Fig. 4).

Odour: Spicy and aromatic.

Taste: Spicy and bitter.

Figs. 2 and 3: *Citrus aurantium* L.
A small ca. 5 m tall tree bearing broadly elliptic, evergreen, entire leaves, on petioles with a distinctly winged upper part (in contrast, in *Citrus limon*, the lemon, the petioles only slightly winged). Scented, actinomorphic, white flowers with 5(-8) punctate petals (oil glands) and numerous stamens, the lower parts of the filaments being fused together to form broad bands. Fruit a multilocular berry.

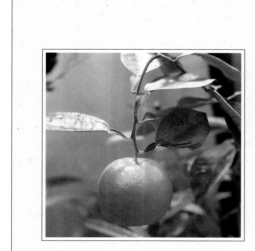

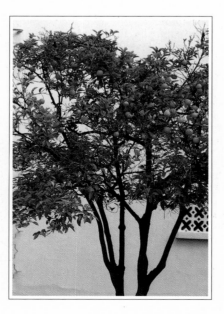

DAB 10: Pomeranzenschale
ÖAB: Pericarpium Aurantii amari
Ph. Helv. VII: Aurantii amari flavedo
St.Zul. 1629.99.99

Plant source: *Citrus aurantium* L. subsp. *aurantium* (syn. *C. aurantium* subsp. *amara* (L.) ENGLER) (Rutaceae).

Synonyms: Aurantii amari cortex, Aurantii cortex siccatus, Flavedo aurantii amari (Lat.), Pomeranzenschale, Bitterorangenschale, Bigaradeschale (Ger.), Écorce de fruit d'orange amer (Fr.).

Origin: Cultivated in southern Europe and other subtropical regions. Imports of the drug come from Spain, Portugal, Israel, and the West Indies.

Constituents: Bitter-tasting flavonoid glycosides such as neohesperidin and naringin, the sugar component of which, neohesperidose (2-*O*-α-L-rhamnopyranosyl-β-D-glucopyranose, isomeric with rutinose = 6-rhamnosylglucose) is responsible for the bitter taste; non-bitter flavonoids, such as hes-

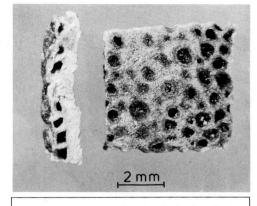

Naringin: R^1 = R^2 = H
Neohesperidin: R^1 = CH$_3$, R^2 = OH

(+)-Limonene

Fig. 4: Pitted fruit wall with oil glands, side-view (left) and top plan view (right)

peridin, rutoside, and more highly methoxylated lipophilic flavonoids like sinensetin, nobiletin, tangeretin; 1% up to more than 2% essential oil, with limonene as the main component; considerable amounts of pectin; furanocoumarins (photosensitizing, see the German Commission E monograph).

Indications: As a bitter aromatic to stimulate secretion of gastric juice and the appetite, in gastric hypo-acidity. It is often used as a flavour enhancer.

Making the tea: Not very usual. The drug is more often used as a tincture or syrup (1 g Aurantii tinctura (1 part drug percolated with 5 parts 70% ethanol) = 25 drops or 6 g Sirupus Aurantii amari = 1 teaspoon), diluted with water or tea. The drug is a frequent component of so-called "Swedish bitters" (see note under: Aloe capensis) and the "Elixir ad longam vitam" (also known as Tinctura Aloes composita – see: DAB 6).

Phytomedicines: Bitter-orange peel extract, tincture, or the powdered drug is present in numerous prepared gastrointestinal remedies, tonics, and roborants and cholagogues, e.g. Carminativum Hetterich®, etc.

Authentication: Following the DAB 10. Microscopical examination has little point. On the other hand, the DAB 10 TLC examination for flavonoids and coumarins can be used for determining the identity and purity; the method is described under Arnica flos (q.v.):

Evaluation: Test solution: a distinct yellowish brown fluorescent rutin zone, with slightly above it the conspicuous red fluores-

Extract from the German Commission E monograph
(BAnz no. 193, dated 15.10.1987)

Uses
Loss of appetite; dyspeptic complaints.

Contraindications
None known.

Side effects
Photosensitization may occur, especially in people with a fair skin.

Interactions with other remedies
None known.

Dosage
Daily dose, 4–6 g drug.
Tincture (DAB 7): 2–3 g.
Extract (Erg. B. 6): 1–2 g.

Mode of administration
Crushed drug for infusions; other bitter-tasting galenical preparations for internal use.

cent eriocitrin zone; in ascending order, the greenish fluorescent hesperidin zone and next to it the greenish fluorescent naringin zone – the latter being slightly below the level of the reference chlorogenic acid zone; at an Rf value in between those of the reference chlorogenic and hyperoside zones, a distinct dark blue fluorescent zone; near the solvent front four clear-cut blue fluorescent zones, the uppermost one being at about the same Rf as the reference caffeic acid zone; other, fainter brownish yellow to greenish and blue fluorescent zones present.
Relevant illustrations are given in [1].

Quantitative standards: BP 1988: *Volatile oil*, not less than 2.5%.
DAB 10: *Bitterness value*, not less than 600. *Volatile oil*, not less than 1.0%. *Foreign (vegetable and/or mineral) matter*, not more than 2%. *Loss on drying*, not more than 10.0%. *Ash*, not more than 7.0%.
ÖAB: *Bitterness value*, not less than 600. *Volatile oil*, not less than 3.0%.
Ph. Helv. VII: *Bitterness value*, not less than 15 Ph. Helv. units. *Volatile oil*, not less than 3.0%. *Foreign matter*, not more than 2%. *Sulphated ash*, not more than 10%.

Adulteration: Hardly ever occurs in practice. Peel from other *Citrus* species with a yellowish or yellowish green outer skin has a much smaller bitterness value and can be recognized by deviating chromatograms.

Storage: Protected from light, in well-closed containers not made of plastic.

Literature:
[1] H. Wagner, S. Bladt and K. Münzing-Vasirian, Pharm. Ztg. **120**, 1262 (1975).

Wording of the package insert, from the German Standard Licence:

6.1. Uses
As a supportive measure in treating stomach complaints, e.g. insufficient formation of gastric juice; to stimulate the appetite.

6.2 Contraindications
Stomach or intestinal ulcers.

6.3 **Dosage and Mode of administration**
Hot water (ca. 150 ml) is poured over one teaspoonful (2–3 g) of well comminuted **Bitter-orange peel** and after

10–15 min. passed through a tea strainer. The tea can also be prepared by adding the drug to cold water and allowing it to soak for 6–8 hours, with occasional stirring.

Unless otherwise prescribed, a cup of the tea is drunk cold or moderately hot several times a day half-an-hour before meals.

Note
Store away protected from light and moisture.

Avenae herba (recens)   Oats (green tops)

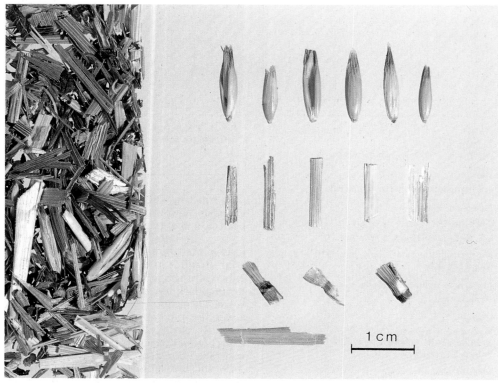

Fig. 1: Oats (green tops)

<u>Description:</u> For drug purposes, the green or rapidly dried (fresh) aerial parts of the plant harvested just before it is in full flower are used. The dried, chopped cut drug consists of the mostly longitudinally cut pieces of stem, longitudinally curled-up fragments of the leaf sheaths, and flat pieces of the leaf blades. In addition, there are some whole or fragmentary husks [8].

1 cm

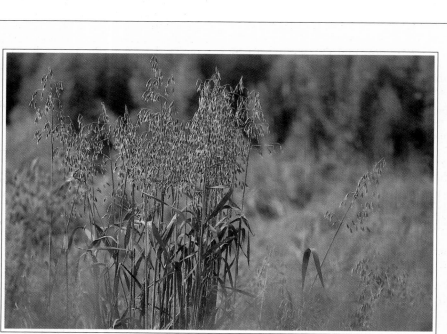

Fig. 2: *Avena sativa* L.

A 0.6–1 m tall, erect, cultivated cereal plant, with narrow, linear leaves. Spikelets with 2–3 florets in loose panicles.

Plant origin: *Avena sativa* L., oat (Poaceae = Gramineae).

Synonyms: Green oats (Engl.), Grüner Hafer (Ger.), Herbe d'avoine (Fr.).

Origin: The oat, which derives from wild grasses such as *Avena fatua* L., *A. sterilis* L., and *A. barbata* Pott, was, to begin with, an accidentally cultivated plant, which first occurred as an undesired accompaniment to other cereal plants. It proved to be very tolerant of climate and locality and was therefore able to continue its expansion during climatic deterioration. Since 100 BC, the oat has been cultivated mainly in northern latitudes, nowadays in many varieties [1].

Constituents: In the ash, up to 55–70% SiO_2, of which up to 2% occurs in the dried, green leaves (and in the straw) in soluble form, e.g. as esters of silicic acid with polyphenols and mono- and oligosaccharides [2]. In comparison with other cereals, the content of iron (39 mg/kg dry weight), manganese (8.5 mg), and zinc (19.2 mg) is very high (according to [2]). The inflorescence is particularly rich in flavones [4]; the leaves contain triterpenoid saponins of the furostanol type (avenacosides; ca. 1–3 mg/g fresh weight) with strong *in-vitro* fungicidal activity [5]; carotenoids and chlorophyll derivatives are also present.

Indications: In *folk medicine*, oat-herb tea (like the homoeopathic mother tincture obtained from fresh flowering plants) is used as

---

Extract from the German Commission E monograph (BAnz no. 193, dated 15.10.1987)

Uses

Preparations of oats (green tops) are used in acute and chronic anxiety, stress, and excitatory states, neurasthenic and pseudo-neurasthenic syndromes, skin conditions, weakness of the connective tissue and of the bladder, as well as a tonic and restorative.

In combination with other drugs, preparations are used for disorders and complaints of the cardiovascular and respiratory systems, in metabolic and geriatric disorders, various forms of anaemia, hyperthyroidism, neuralgia, and neuritis, as well as for treating loss of blood, pulled muscles, sexual disorders, tobacco abuse, cramps, and as a lactagogue and to improve physical endurance.
The efficacy of the drug in the various indications listed has not been substantiated.

Risks

None known.

Evaluation

Because the effects of preparations of oats (green tops) have not been substantiated, their therapeutic use cannot be endorsed.

---

a sedative in nervous exhaustion, sleeplessness, and so-called "weakness of the nerves". A scientifically-based association of these indications with particular constituents has not yet been possible. Tea from oats (green tops) is said to lower the blood uric-acid level, and the drug therefore finds use in the Kneipp therapy as an adjuvant in rheumatism and arthritis. The tea is also considered to be a suitable diuretic in irrigation therapy (water diuresis). Further details about the possible effects of the different organs of the oat and their constituents are given in [2]. Be that as it may, activity against these indications has not been proved medically. Thus, use of a tincture of oats (green tops) against tobacco abuse, which was proposed at one time [6], has not received any clinical confirmation [7]. The above-mentioned (and other) areas of use have no doubt come from the homoeopathic application of oats (green tops) in phytotherapy.

Note: In *folk medicine*, baths are prepared from oat straw (Stramentum Avenae) for use against arthritis, rheumatism, paralysis, and liver and skin disorders. These baths are also said to give good results as a sedative in hypertonia. The grain (Avenae fructus), in the form of rolled oats, porridge, or oatmeal, is prescribed as a diuretic and roborant during convalescence. A skin cream against sunburn produced in the UK is said to contain oat mucilage [2].

Side effects: In therapeutic doses, none known.

Making the tea: A heaped tablespoonful of the drug (ca. 3 g) is brewed up with $^1/_4$ litre boiling water, which is allowed to cool to room temperature, and the drug is then removed with a tea strainer. A cup of the tea is drunk unsweetened, or only slightly sweetened, several times a day or shortly before going to bed.

Phytomedicines: Oats (green tops) as a tea, e.g. Vollmer's prepared oats (green tops) tea. As the homoeopathic mother tincture (and dilutions) or as an extract, the drug is a component of allopathic preparations mostly categorized as plant sedatives, e.g. Esberi-Nervin®, Vivinox®-Beruhigungsdragees (sedative dragees).

Regulatory status (UK): General Sales List – Schedule 1, Table A (oats).

Authentication: Macroscopically (see: Description). W. Schier [8] has provided the following description of the anatomy and microscopy of the drug:
Stem: (a) Epidermis in surface view: "long", straight-walled, sometimes slightly wavy, thick-walled, heavily pitted cells which alternate with "short", thick-walled, and heavily pitted cells. Paracytic graminaceous stomata. (b) Transverse section: typical of a monocot stem. Cuticle thin; epidermis of cells strongly thickened particularly on the outside. Underneath, generally a two- cell thick hypodermis consisting of thick-walled cells, interrupted by regions of thin-walled assimilating cells, these including occasional small groups (mostly 3) of fibres sometimes reaching as far as the epidermis and towards the inside surrounding a continuous collateral vascular bundle. Following a closed ring of fibres, large-celled parenchymatous tissue with triangular intercellular spaces with scattered continuous collateral vascular bundles surrounded by a sheath of sclerenchyma.
Leaf sheath: (a) Outer surface: a thin, mostly smooth cuticle, as well as thick- and very wavy-walled epidermal cells. Stomata frequent. (b) Inner surface: thin- and straight-walled epidermal cells, together with only a few stomata.
Lamina: (a) Upper surface – surface view: epidermal cells elongated, straight-walled, and pitted. Graminaceous paracytic stomata (Fig. 3). At the margin, short, curved and pointed trichomes with a very broad base. In the mesophyll, various-sized crystals (small needles, prisms, occasional sphaerocrystals). (b) Lower surface – surface view: cuticle somewhat warty, elongated and straight-walled epidermal cells. Stomata frequent. Over the nerves, rows of slightly curved trichomes with a broad, thick-walled, pitted base (Fig. 4). In between, thicker and wavy-walled cells. Crystals like those of the upper surface. In the mesophyll, palisade-like cells with a round transverse section.
Glume: Outer epidermis comprising long and short cells (Fig. 5) – the long cells with markedly sinuous walls and thickened at the ends of each sinus, the short cells single or in pairs (twinned) with one roundish and one halfmoon-shaped cell. Inner epidermis comprising long, thin-walled cells with occasional stomata.
Palea: Structurally similar to the glume, but with the various types of cells thinner-walled and more delicate. Outer epidermis with stomata and at the margin trichomes like those described above.
See also [9] for a description and illustrations of the microscopy of the powdered drug.
The following TLC method can be used to detect the saponins [10]:

Test solution: 2 g powdered drug refluxed with 10 ml 70% ethanol for 10 min., then filtered and the filtrate concentrated to 5 ml. Alternative extractant: *n*-butanol.

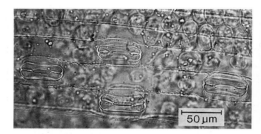

Fig. 3: Graminaceous stomata with dumb-bell-shaped guard cells, from the upper surface of the leaf

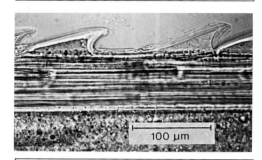

Fig. 4: Pointed, unicellular trichomes with a broad base, from the lower surface of the leaf

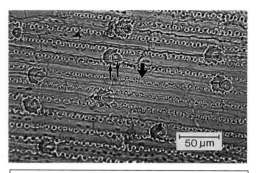

Fig. 5: Outer epidermis of the glume with long (thick arrow) and short (thin arrows) cells

Reference solution: 10 mg vanillin and/or avenacoside B in 10 ml methanol.

Loadings: 25–40 μl test solution and 10 μ reference solution, as 2-cm bands on silica gel $F60_{254}$.

Solvent system: chloroform + methanol + water (64 + 50 + 10), the composition to be followed exactly using analytical grade chloroform.

Detection; sprayed with 5% ethanolic sulphuric acid, oversprayed with 1% ethanolic vanillin; plate heated at 110 °C for 5–10 min.

Evaluation: in daylight. Reference solution: vanillin zone at Rf ca. 0.55 and avenacoside B zone at Rf ca. 0.2. Methanol extract: about 16 mostly grey to reddish violet bands over the whole Rf range; with longer heating, bands clearer but uniformly red-brown. Butanol extract: saponin bands more conspicuous.

Adulteration: Practically never occurs.

Storage: Protected from light and moisture.

Literature:
[1] H. D. Belitz and W. Grosch, Lehrbuch der Lebensmittelchemie, Berlin, 1982.
[2] E. Schneider, Z. Phytotherap. **6**, 165 (1985).
[3] S.W. Souci, W. Fachmann, and H. Kraut, Zusammensetzung der Lebensmittel, Stuttgart, 1981.
[4] G. Popovici et al., Z. Pflanzenphysiol. **85**, 103 (1977).
[5] B. Wolters, Dtsch. Apoth. Ztg. **106**, 1729 (1966).
[6] C.L. Anand, Nature (London) **233**, 496 (1971).
[7] K. Geckleiter et al., Münch. Med. Wochenschr. **116**, 581 (1974).
[8] W. Schier, unpublished observations (1987).
[9] B.P. Jackson and D.W. Snowdon, Atlas of microscopy of medicinal plants, culinary herbs and spices, Belhaven Press, London, 1990, p. 112.
[10] H. Wagner, S. Bladt, and E.M. Zgainski, Plant drug analysis, Springer, Berlin – Heidelberg – New York – Tokyo, 1984, p. 242.

Bardanae radix Burdock root (BHP 1/1990)

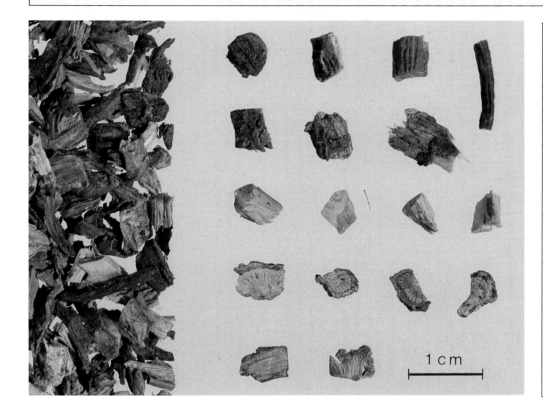

1 cm

Fig. 1: Burdock root

<u>Description</u>: **The very hard, horny, scarcely fibrous pieces of root have a greyish brown to brownish black, longitudinally wrinkled, external surface (cork). The transverse section shows a whitish to light brown cortex, a darkish cambial zone, a radially striated yellowish brown xylem, and a spongy, frequently torn pith (Fig. 3). In older pieces of root, the gaps often extend as far as the cortex. With a hand lens, in pieces of young root, a ring of brown secretory glands (resin canals) can be recognized.**

<u>Taste</u>: **The drug becomes soft on chewing and tastes sweetish and mucilaginous; later on, it becomes bitter.**

Fig. 2: *Arctium lappa* L.

A member of the Asteraceae, about 1 m in height, with large ovate, acuminate leaves. Ca. 4 cm broad flowerheads, consisting only of reddish violet tubular florets, surrounded by numerous involucral bracts ending in a stiff spiny or hooked tip.

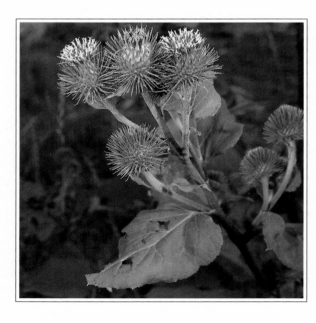

Erg. B. 6: Radix Bardanae

Plant sources: *Arctium lappa* L. (= *A. majus* BERNH.), great burdock, as well as *A. minus* BERNH. s.l., lesser burdock, and *A. tomentosum* MILL., woolly burdock (Asteraceae). Only the first two plants are a source of burdock root in the UK; cf. the BHP 1/1990.

Synonyms: Radix Arctii or Lappae or Personatae (Lat.), Lappa root, Bardane root (Engl.), Klettenwurzel, Dollenkrautwurzel, Kleberwurzel (Ger.), Racine de bardane (Fr.).

Origin: Native in Europe, northern Asia, and North America. The drug (*A.lappa*) comes from plants cultivated especially in Bulgaria, former Yugoslavia, Poland, and Hungary.

Constituents: Ca. 27–45% inulin, mucilage (carbohydrates, altogether ca. 69%); 0.06–0.18% essential oil with so far 66 identified components, among them phenylacetalde-

R = CH₂OH: Arctinone
R = CHOH-CH₂OH: Arctinol
R = CHO: Arctinal
R = COOH: Aretic acid

$H_3C-CH=CH-(C\equiv C)_4-CH=CH_2$

Trideca-1,11-diene-3,5,7,9-tetrayne

Arctiin

Dehydrocostuslactone

Costus acid

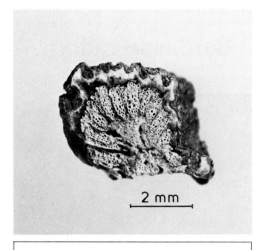

Fig. 3: A wrinkled piece of root, showing the darker cambial region and the radially striated and fissured xylem

hyde, benzaldehyde, and 2-alkyl(C_3 to C_5)-3-methoxypyrazines and 2-methoxy-3-methylpyrazine, and also 32 acids as important aroma substances in the root [1]; 14 polyacetylenes, the principal components being trideca-1,11-diene-3,5,7,9-tetrayne (0.0002%) and 10 sulphur-containing acetylenic compounds, such as aretic acid, arctinone, arctinol, arctinal, etc.; the costus acids and, as bitter substances, the guaianolides dehydrocostuslactone and 11,13-dihydrodehydrocostuslactone [1]. 1.9–3.65% polyphenols, including caffeic acid, chlorogenic acid, isochlorogenic acid, and other caffeic acid derivatives; probably, the lignan-olide arctiin. Sitosterol and stigmasterol, as well as γ-guanidino-n-butyric acid, are also present.

Indications: Burdock root is more or less obsolete as a herbal drug (but cf. the note under: Authentication). Nevertheless, extracts still find use as adjuvants in various prepared remedies, especially homoeopathic ones.
In *folk medicine,* it is used as a diuretic ("for purifying the blood"), as a laxative, for renal or urinary calculi, in rheumatic complaints, as well as externally against eczema and poorly healing wounds. Root extracts have antibiotic activity. Stimulation of liver and bile function has been demonstrated in older investigations. The active substances may be podophyllin-type lignan derivatives and guaianolide-type sesquiterpene lactones. Root extracts reduce blood-sugar levels in rats and raise carbohydrate tolerance [3] (guanidinobutyric acid ?).

Externally, burdock-root oil (extract with olive or peanut oil) is applied against dry seborrhoea of the scalp. There is **no** evidence for the supposed stimulation of hair growth (the reason why it is included in many hair preparations); this use may derive from the doctrine of signatures, according to which the powers responsible for the dense hairiness of the plant would have the same effect in human beings.

Making the tea: 2.5 g of the finely chopped or coarsely powdered drug is put into cold water (and may be left for several hours), then boiled for up to an hour, and finally passed through a strainer.
1 Teaspoon = ca. 2 g.

Phytomedicines: Prepared (usually homoeopathic) remedies with burdock-root extracts as adjuvants belong to the following groups, among others: cholagogues and biliary remedies, analgesics and antirheumatics, gastrointestinal remedies, coronary remedies, preparations for oral and pharyngeal hygiene, alteratives, liver remedies, urological remedies.
Burdock root is a component of the following UK preparations, among others: Seven Seas Rheumatic Pain Tablets, and Potter's Rheumatic Pain Tablets, Tabritis Tablets, Catarrh Mixture (oral liquid), and Skin Eruptions Mixture (oral liquid); extracts of burdock are present in Potter's G. B. Tablets and Gerard House Blue Flag Root Compound Tablets.

Regulatory status (UK): General Sales List – Schedule 1, Table A (as: Lappa).

Authentication: Macro- (see: Description) and microscopically, following [4]; see also the descriptions in the BHP 1/1990. The root does not contain starch, i.e. transverse sections do not give a blue colour with iodine solution, but because of the inulin content they do give a strong red-violet colour with α-naphthol/sulphuric acid reagent. Oxalate is absent. In fragments of young root (with both epi- and endodermis), brown secretory glands (resin canals) can be seen in the cortex; in older roots (cork), there are groups of yellow phloem fibres.
The TLC method of identification prescribed by the BHP 1/1990 is the same as for Althaeae radix (q.v.):

Evaluation: in UV 366 nm light. <u>Test solution</u>: relative to rutin, major fluorescent bands at about Rx 2.35 (narrow and intense blue), 2.1 (whitish blue), 1.75 and 1.4 (both pale blue).

Quantitative standards: <u>Erg. B. 6</u>: *Ash*, not more than 6%.
<u>BHP 1/1990</u>: *Water-soluble extractive*, not less than 24%. *Foreign matter*, not more than 2%. *Loss on drying*, not more than 15%. *Total ash*, not more than 12%. *HCl-insoluble ash*, not more than 3%.

Note: The BHP 1/1990 also has a monograph on Burdock leaf (Bardanae folium, Lappa herb), the uses of which are similar to those of Burdock root; in the UK, lappa herb is a component of more than 30 anti-inflammatory preparations [5].

Adulteration: Confusion is possible with the externally very similar roots of *Atropa belladonna* L., deadly nightshade; they contain over 20 alkaloids, comprising tropanes, tropine esters, and *N*-oxides [6], many of which are highly active physiologically. Belladonna roots can be distinguished microscopically, since they have starch and cells with microsphenoidal ("sandy") crystals of calcium oxalate. TLC can be used to detect small amounts:

Test solution: 1 g powdered drug boiled with 10 ml methanol and filtered.

Loading: 40 µl of the filtrate, as a 1.5-cm band on silica gel.

Solvent system: chloroform + ethanol (98 + 2), 10 cm run.

Detection: sprayed with 10% methanolic potassium hydroxide.

Evaluation: in UV 365 nm light. **No** bluish green fluorescent band at Rf ca. 0.2.
This procedure allows the detection of 0.5% admixture of belladonna root.

Literature:
[1] T. Washino et al., Nippon Nogei Kagaku Kaishi **59**, 389 (1985); C. A. **103**, 52880 (1985).
[2] T. Washino, M. Yoshikura and S. Obata, Agric. Biol. Chem. **50**, 263 (1986); C. A. **104**, 203839 (1986).
[3] O. Lapinina and T.F. Sisoeva, Farmatsevt. Zh. (Kiew) **19**, 52 (1964); C. A. **66**, 140, 1451 (1967).
[4] P. Rohdewald, G. Rücker and K.-W. Glombitza, Apothekengerechte Prüfvorschriften, S. 827, Deutscher Apotheker Verlag, Stuttgart 1986.
[5] J.D. Phillipson and L.A. Anderson, Pharm. J. **233**, 80, 111 (1984).
[6] F. Oprach, T. Hartmann, L. Witte, and G. Toppel, Planta Med. **52**, 513 (1986).

Barosmae folium   Buchu (BHP 1/1990)

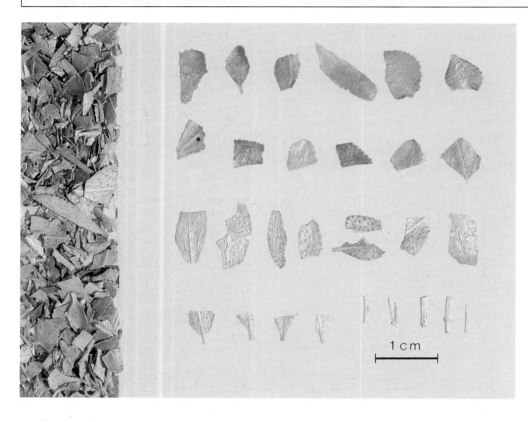

1 cm

Erg. B. 6: Folia Bucco

Plant source: *Agathosma betulina* (BERGIUS) PILLANS (syn. *Barosma betulina* (BERGIUS) BARTL. et H.L. WENDL.), the round or short buchu of English commerce (Rutaceae).

Synonyms: Folia Bucco, Folia Buchu, Folia Diosmeae (Lat.), Agathosma (BHP 1983), Round or Short buchu (Engl.), Buccoblätter (Ger.), Feuilles de buchu (Fr.).

Origin: *Agathosma* species are native to the Cape region of South Africa, from where the drug is imported.

Constituents: Ca. 2% essential oil in schizolysigenous oil glands. The main component in the distilled oil is the monoterpene diosphenol which at room temperature separates in crystalline form (buchu camphor); it is presumably derived (through the effect of the plant acids present?) from the genuine constituent piperitone epoxide. Other components of the essential oil are limonene, (−)-isomenthone, (+)-menthone, (−)-pulegone, terpinen-4-ol, and *p*-men-

than-3-on-8-thiol which is chiefly responsible for the odour [1–3, 5]. Besides mucilage and resins, there are flavonoids, which, together with the main constituent diosmin, play a significant part in the activity of the drug.

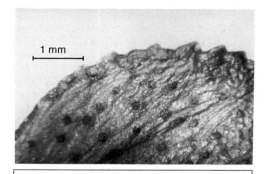

Fig. 2: Leaf fragment showing the crenulate-serrulate margin and translucent oil glands (hand lens)

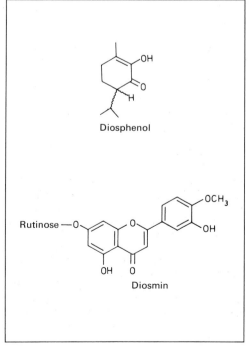

Diosphenol

Diosmin

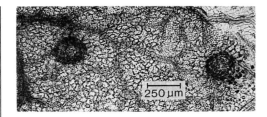

Fig. 4: Spherical oil glands in the mesophyll of buchu

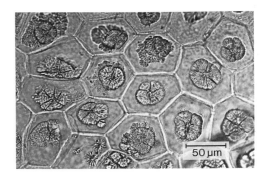

Fig. 3: Upper epidermis, showing sphaerocrystalline masses of diosmin

Indications: Buchu can be used as a disinfectant and diuretic in cases of mild inflammation of the urinary tract. Diosphenol is considered to be responsible for the antibacterial effect; it is a phenol which is excreted mainly as the glucuronic acid conjugate, so that perhaps just as with bearberry leaves an antibacterial effect can be expected. The diuretic activity may come from the flavonoids and also terpinen-4-ol (components which are also present in the essential oil of juniper berries – Juniperi fructus – for example).

Side effects: Not expected at therapeutic dose levels.

Making the tea: Boiling water is poured over ca. 1 g of the drug, covered and allowed to stand for 10 min. before being strained. A cup of the infusion is drunk several times a day as a diuretic.
1 Teaspoon = ca. 1.0 g.

Herbal preparations: The drug is a component of about 10 prepared herbal teas, including Buccotean® Tee (also available as an instant tea), Buccosperin® Tee, and Uron-Tee tea bags.
Buchu is a constituent of the UK product Potter's Kas-bah Herb.

Phytomedicines: There are no monovalent preparations, but about a dozen combinations, chiefly urological remedies; the drug is also present in prostate remedies.
Among the preparations containing buchu available in the UK are: Potter's Diuretabs, Antitis Tablets and Backache Tablets, and Stomach Mixture (oral liquid); Gerard House Herbal Powder No. 8 and Buchu Compound Tablets, this latter containing an extract.

Regulatory status (UK): General Sales List – Schedule 1, Table A.

Authentication: Macroscopy (see: Description), Microscopical diagnostic features include a thick cuticle, mucilage-containing epidermal cells, and diosmin crystals in the upper epidermis (Fig. 3). The leaf has a bilateral structure with a single palisade layer, and in the mesophyll there are calcium oxalate clusters and large spherical oil glands (Fig. 4). The detailed microscopy of the powdered drug is presented in [6].
The BHP 1/1990 TLC identification test is carried out as for Althaeae radix (q.v.):

Evaluation: in UV 366 nm light. Test solution: relative to the rutin reference band, major fluorescent bands at Rx 2.4, 2.3, and 1.3 (all blue), and 1.0 (orange).

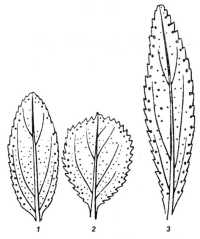

1 B. crenulata; *2* B. betulina; *3* B. serratifolia

Quantitative standards: Erg. B. 6: *Volatile oil*, not less than 0.8%. *Ash*, not more than 5%.
BHP 1/1990: *Volatile oil*, not less than 1.3%. *Water-soluble extractive*, not less than 14%. *Stems*, not more than 5%. *Foreign matter*, not more than 1%. *Total ash*, not more than 5%. *HCl-insoluble ash*, not more than 1.5%.

Adulteration: Unlike the round, serrulate leaves of *Agathosma betulina*, the leaves of other *Agathosma* species usually contain little or no diosphenol. The ovate leaves of *A. crenulata* (L.) Pillans p.p., oval buchu, and the lanceolate leaves of *A. serratifolia* (Curtis) Spreeth, long buchu, are encountered [5], and possibly also leaves from *A. ericifolia* Andr. or of *Adenandra fragrans* (Sims) Roem. et Schult.

	length/width [5]
1. A. crenulata;	2.34
2. A. betulina;	1.95
3. A. serratifolia	5.35

Leaves of hybrids between *A. betulina* and *A. crenulata* are not readily differentiated morphologically from those of *A. betulina*; however, they have a lower diosphenol content [1].
TLC and/or GLC can be used to distinguish between the leaves of *A. betulina* and *A. crenulata*, the diosphenol zone or peak being absent with the latter species [4, 5].

Literature:
[1] K.L.M. Blommaert and E. Bartel, J. S. Afr. Bot. **42**, 121 (1976).
[2] D. Lamparsky and P. Schudel, Tetrahedron Lett. **36**, 3323 (1971).
[3] R. Kaiser, D. Lamparsky, and P. Schudel, J. Agric. Food Chem. **23**, 943 (1975).
[4] S.M. Doran, I. Havlik, and D.W. Oliver, Planta Med. **54**, in press (1988).
[5] A.D. Spreeth, J.S. Afr. Bot. **42**, 109 (1976).
[6] B.P. Jackson and D.W. Snowdon, Atlas of microscopy of medicinal plants, culinary herbs and spices, Belhaven Press, London, 1990, p. 26.

Basilici herba   Basil

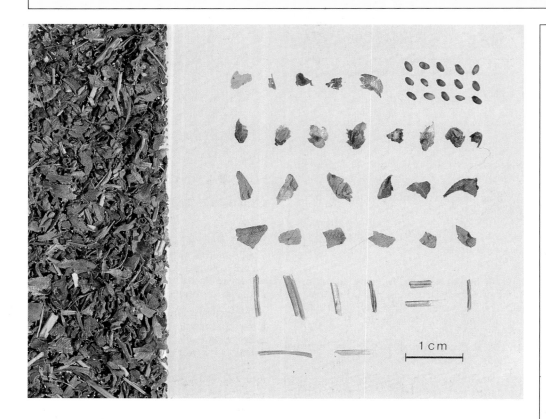

1 cm

Fig. 1: Basil

Description: Basil consists of the aerial parts collected at the time of flowering. The whole drug has 4-angled stems which are almost glabrous at the bottom and covered with soft hairs towards the top. The leaves are opposite and petiolate, up to 2 cm long and about 12 mm wide, ovate or oblong-ovate, and blunt or acute at the tip. The main nerve and curved lateral nerves are a prominent feature of the glabrous lamina; the margin may be serrate or entire and ciliate. The flowers are white, purple, or multi-coloured and are borne in axillary pseudo-umbels on the upper parts of the stem or at the ends of the branches. The campanulate, two-lipped calyx is 5-toothed, and the upper tooth is flat, almost orbicular, and very large. The two-lipped corolla has a 4-part upper lip and a divided bottom lip. The fruit contains four, very small, ovoid, brown to black, glabrous seeds.

The cut drug consists of leaf fragments with a serrate or entire margin (Fig. 1, third and fourth rows from the top) and numerous glandular trichomes (hand lens); pieces of glabrous 4-angled stem (Fig. 1. bottom row); white, purple, or multi-coloured flower parts (Fig. 1, top left); brown, ovoid seeds (Fig. 1, top right); and calyx remains with fruits (Fig. 1, second row from the top).

Odour: Pleasantly aromatic.

Taste: Spicy and slightly salty.

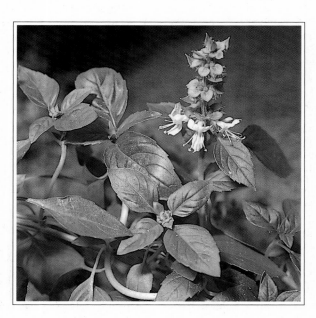

Fig. 2: *Ocimum basilicum* L.

A 20–50 cm tall annual with ovate, acuminate leaves. Flowers zygomorphic, yellowish white to red, and mostly in whorls of six.

St.Zul.: 1429.99.99

Plant source: Various races (subspecies?; chemotypes?) of *Ocimum basilicum* L. (Lamiaceae = Labiatae).

Synonyms: Sweet or Garden basil (Engl.), Basilikumkraut (Ger.), Herbe de grand basilic (Fr.).

Origin: Its place of origin is uncertain (South Asia ?); nowadays, it is cultivated in the subtropics, especially throughout the Mediterranean region, in various races and varieties differing not only in their constituents but also to a considerable degree in their morphology; it often runs wild. Imports come from plantations in France, Morocco, Italy, as well as Egypt, Bulgaria, and Hungary.

Constituents: Depending on the variety and chemotype, on the origin, and when collected, the essential-oil content varies from 0.04 to 0.70%. The main components of the oil are linalool (some chemotypes, up to 75% of the oil), methylchavicol (= estragole; up to 87%), and eugenol (up to 20%); there are other monoterpenes (among them, ocimene and cineole), as well as sesquiterpenes and phenylpropanes (including methyl cinnamate) [1–3]. The drug also contains tannins, flavonoids (quercetin and kaempferol glycosides, etc.), caffeic acid, and aesculoside [4, 5], and possibly saponins.

Indications: Basil is widely used in the fresh and dried state as a spice (for salads, soups, soft cheeses, fish dishes, etc.). In folk medicine, especially in Mediterranean countries, the drug is employed as a stomachic in lack of appetite, as a carminative against flatulence and a feeling of distension, occasionally as a diuretic, galactagogue, and externally as a gargle and astringent for inflammation of the throat. Alcoholic extracts of the drug are included in ointments for treating poorly healing wounds. Water and methanol extracts of basil leaves are reported to have anti-ulcerogenic activity in rats, perhaps due in part to the flavonoids present [13]. The essential oil has anthelmintic activity [6] and it is also widely employed in the perfumery and cosmetic industry. The herb finds use in the fish preservation industry.

Side effects: None in therapeutic doses. Nevertheless, it should be noted that methylchavicol (estragole) is a known hepatocarcinogen in animals [9]; basil oil is reputedly non-toxic [10].

Making the tea: Boiling water (ca. 150 ml) is poured over 1–2 heaped teaspoonfuls (2–4 g)

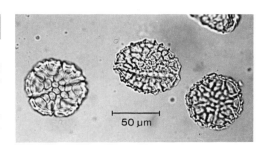

Fig. 3: Lenticular, hexacolpate pollen grains with a reticulate exine

of the herb, allowed to draw for 10–15 min., strained, and drunk unsweetened as required. For chronic flatulence, a cup of the tea is drunk two to three times a day between meals; after eight days, the treatment is stopped for 14 days, and then resumed for a further eight days [7, 8].
1 Teaspoon = ca. 1.5 g.

Phytomedicines: Ethanolic extracts of the drug – together with extracts of caraway, fennel, chamomile, peppermint, etc. – are included in a number of carminatives and stomachics, e.g. Gastrol®-Tropfen (drops).

Authentication: Macro- (see: Description) and microscopically. Besides the yellowish brown peltate glandular trichomes and the fewer and smaller capitate trichomes, there are 2–3-celled, stout-walled covering trichomes with a club-shaped basal cell. The relatively large (mostly > 50 μm), more or less lenticular pollen grains with a reticulate exine are particularly characteristic (Fig. 3). A detailed account of the microscopy of the powder is presented in [11].
The St.Zul. TLC identification test is as follows:

Test solution: 0.5 ml of the oil from the essential-oil determination dissolved in 10 ml toluene.

Reference solution: 10 μl each of eugenol and linalool dissolved in 10 ml toluene.

Loadings: 20 μl each of the test and reference solutions, as 2-cm bands on silica gel GF$_{254}$.

Solvent system: toluene + ethyl acetate (90 + 10), 15 cm run.

Detection and Evaluation: in UV 254 nm light. Reference solution: at Rf 0.5, eugenol as a quenching zone. Test solution: at about the same Rf, a quenching zone (sometimes weak); at Rf 0.6–0.7, possibly other quenching zones.

Wording of the package insert, from the German Standard Licence:

7.1 Uses
In supportive treatment for a feeling of distension and flatulence.

7.2 Dosage and Mode of administration
Ca. 150 ml boiling water is poured over two teaspoonfuls (ca. 4 g) of **Basil** and after 10–15 mins. passed through a tea strainer.
Unless otherwise prescribed, a cup of the freshly prepared tea is drunk two to three times a day between meals.

7.3 Note
Store away from light and moisture.

Sprayed with anisaldehyde reagent, followed by heating at 100–110 °C for ca. 10 min. In UV 365 nm light. Reference and Test solutions: eugenol as a yellow fluorescent zone. In daylight. Reference solution: eugenol as a brownish violet zone; at Rf ca. 0.4, linalool as a dark violet zone. Test solution: likewise; in ascending order at Rf 0.5–0.6, a grey and a pinkish red zone and directly below the solvent front a violet zone; other grey to brown zones possibly present.

Note: methylchavicol has the same Rf value as eugenol in this system.
Another suitable TLC method is given in [12].

Quantitative standards: St.Zul. 1429.99.99: *Volatile oil*, not less than 0.4%. *Foreign matter*, not more than 2%. *Loss on drying*, not more than 10%. *Ash*, not more than 15.0%.

Adulteration: Rarely occurs.

Storage: Protected from light and moisture in glass or metal (not plastic) containers.

Literature:
[1] H.H. Peter and M. Remy, Parfums, Cosmétiques, Arômes **21**, 61 (1978).
[2] G. Vernin et al., Perfum. Flavor. **9**, 71 (1984).
[3] Th. Kartnig and B. Simon, Gartenbauwissenschaft **51**, 223 (1986).
[4] Th. Kartnig and A. Gruber, personal communication (1987).
[5] M.O. Fatope and Y. Takeda, Planta Med. **54**, 190 (1988).
[6] M.L. Jain and S.R. Jain, Planta Med. **22**, 66 (1972); *ibid.*, **24**, 286 (1973).
[7] M. Pahlow, Das große Buch der Heilpflanzen, Gräfer und Unzer, Munich, 1985.
[8] Hager, vol. **6**, p. 288 (1977).
[9] D.L.J. Opdyke, Food, Cosmet. Toxicol. **11**, 867 (1973).
[10] E. C. Miller et al., Cancer Res. **43**, 1124 (1983).
[11] B.P. Jackson and D. W. Snowdon, Atlas of microscopy of medicinal plants, culinary herbs and spices, Belhaven Press, London, 1990, p. 12.
[12] H. Wagner, S. Bladt, and E.M. Zgainski, Plant drug analysis, Springer-Verlag, Berlin, Heidelberg, New York, Tokyo, 1984, p. 26.
[13] M.S. Akhtar, A.H. Akhtar, and M.A. Khan, Internat. J. Pharmacog. **30**, 97 (1992).

Betulae folium   (DAB 10), Birch

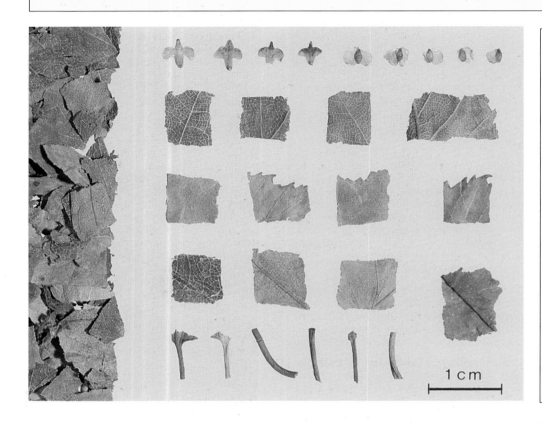

Fig. 1: Birch leaf, uppermost row: fruit scales and fruits

Description: The leaves of *Betula pendula* are ca. 3–7 cm long and ca. 2–4 cm wide, triangular to rhombic and acuminate, with a doubly serrate margin, glabrous, and densely punctate with glands on both surfaces. The leaves of *Betula pubescens* are ca. 2.5–5 cm long and ca. 1.8–4 cm wide, ovate to rounded triangular, with a coarsely serrate margin, slightly pubescent on both surfaces, and with only a few glands on both surfaces; on the lower surface, in the angles of the nerves, there are small yellowish grey tufts of hairs. The upper surface of the leaves is dark green; the lower surface is lighter and on it the pale coloured nerves are particularly prominent. Often, 3-lobed fruit scales and winged fruits (see: Fig. 4) can be found among the leaves.

Odour: Faintly aromatic.

Taste: Somewhat bitter.

Fig. 2: *Betula pendula* ROTH

A tree up to 25 m in height, the trunk silvery white when young, becoming dark later (difference with *B. pubescens* EHRH.). Branches pendent.

Fig. 3: Leaves and inflorescences (catkins) of *Betula pendula* ROTH

Leaves triangular to rhombic, with a sharply doubly serrate margin.

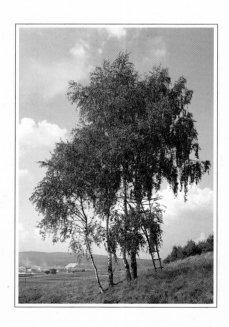

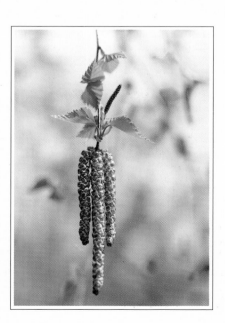

DAB 10: Birkenblätter
ÖAB: Folium Betulae
Ph. Helv. VII: Betulae folium
St.Zul. 8399.99.99

Plant sources: *Betula pendula* ROTH (syn. *B. verrucosa* EHRH.), silver birch, and *B. pubescens* EHRH., birch or downy birch (Betulaceae); also hybrids of these two species (Ph. Helv. VII).

Synonyms: Birch leaf (Engl.). Birkenblätter, *B. pendula*: Rauhbirke, Weißbirke; *B. pubescens*: Behaarte Birke, Besenbirke (Ger.); Feuilles de bouleau (Fr.).

Origin: Indigenous in temperate Europe. The drug is imported from China, the former USSR, and various eastern European countries.

Constituents: Up to 3% flavonoids (especially hyperoside, quercitrin, myricetin galactoside, and other kaempferol, myricetin, and quercetin glycosides; in the buds, also lipophilic flavone methyl ethers); further, among other things, up to 0.1% essential oil

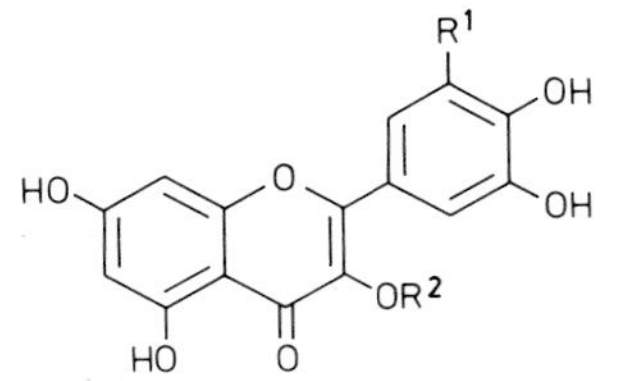

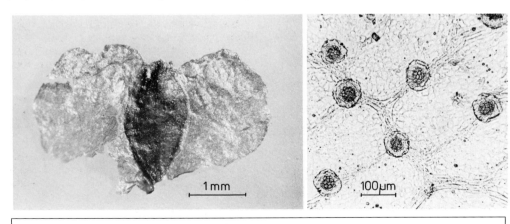

Quercetin: $R^1 = H$, $R^2 = H$
Hyperoside: $R^1 = H$, $R^2 =$ Galactosyl
Quercitrin: $R^1 = H$, $R^2 =$ Rhamnosyl
Myricetin-digalactoside: $R^1 = OH$, $R^2 =$ Digalactosyl

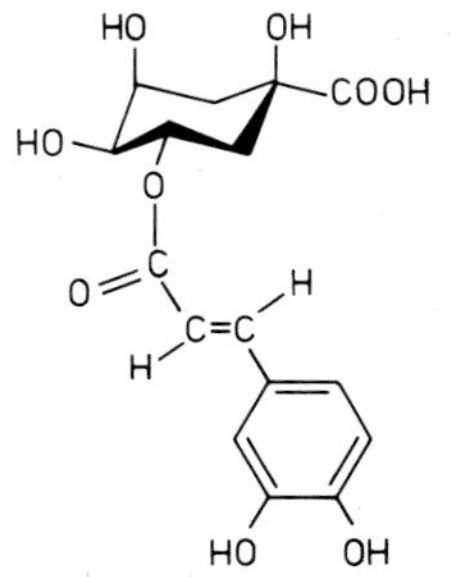

Chlorogenic acid

(containing sesquiterpene oxides, etc.); (+)-catechin and its 7-*O*-β-D-xylopyranoside and (−)-epicatechin, and a range of bi- and triflavonoid procyanidins; up to 0.5% ascorbic acid, phenol-carboxylic acids (among them, chlorogenic and caffeic acids), resins of unknown composition, triterpene alcohols (dammarane type), and questionably, haemolytically active substances (saponins) [1–3, 10–13].

Indications: As a *diuretic* to bring about water diuresis. It is used in irrigation therapy of the urinary tract against bacterial, inflammatory, and cramp-like disorders, e.g. pyelonephritis, ureteritis, cystitis, and urethritis. Whether the phytotherapy on its own is sufficient, or whether combination with chemotherapy is required, depends on the bacterial count as well as the on nature of the infecting bacteria [4]. The diuretic and saluretic (?) actions of the drug [5], which have been confirmed in animal experiments, is doubtless to be ascribed particularly to the flavonoids present [6, 7]; this effect may perhaps be enhanced by the relatively high vitamin C content [2]. The increased diuresis prevents the formation of urinary and renal calculi.
In *folk medicine,* birch is in use against arthritis and rheumatism and against loss of hair and skin rashes; it is also included in "spring cures" for "purifying the blood" [cf. 3].

Making the tea: Boiling water is poured over 2–3 g of the finely cut drug and after 10–15 mins. passed through a tea strainer.
1 Teaspoon = ca. 1 g, 1 tablespoon = ca. 2 g.

Note the divergent details given in the Standard Licence.

Herbal preparations: The drug is also available in tea bags (mostly 1.8 g).
Aqueous extracts are components of instant teas, e.g. Solubitrat®, Uroflux®, Solvefort®, Nieron®, NB-tee Siegfried, Harntee 400®, etc.

Phytomedicines: As diuretics and urological remedies, together with other drugs, such as Orthosiphonis folium, Equiseti herba, Juniperi fructus, Petroselini radix, in the form of mixed herbal teas, extracts, drops, capsules, and dragees.

Authentication: Macro- (see: Description) and microscopically, following the DAB 10. The diagnostic features include: peltate glandular trichomes, occurring on both leaf surfaces – numerous in the case of *Betula pendula* and scattered in the case of *B. pubescens* – which are up to 100 µm in diameter (Fig. 5) and whose innermost small suberized cells are covered by a flat shield consisting of large, thin-walled cells. *B. pubescens* also has a few, thick-walled, pointed covering trichomes that are often curved near the base; they range in length from ca. 80 to 600 µm, but are mostly ca. 100 to 200 µm, though in the angles of the nerves they can be up to ca. 1000 µm, and occasionally the wall is spirally thickened.
The DAB 10 test of identity [cf. 6] is as follows:

Test solution: 0.5 g powdered drug shaken for 5 min. with 10 ml methanol on the water-bath, cooled, and filtered.

Reference solution: 1.0 mg caffeic acid and 2.0 mg rutin dissolved in 10 ml methanol.

Extract from the German Commission E monograph
(BAnz no. 50, dated 3.03.1986)

Uses

For irrigation therapy in bacterial and inflammatory conditions of the lower urinary tract and renal gravel; as supportive treatment in rheumatic complaints.

Contraindications

None known.

Warning: No irrigation therapy in patients with oedema arising from impaired cardiac or renal function.

Interactions with other drugs

None known.

Dosage

Unless otherwise prescribed: average daily dose, 2.0–3.0 g drug several times a day; preparations correspondingly.

Mode of administration

Powdered drug or dry extracts for infusions and other galenical preparations and freshly pressed plant juice, for internal consumption.

Warning: During irrigation therapy, care must be taken to ensure a generous fluid intake.

Effect

Diuretic.

Fig. 4: Yellowish brown, winged achenes

Fig. 5: Brown, multicellular glandular trichomes on the lower surface of *Betula pendula* leaves

Loadings: 10 µl each of the test and reference solutions, as 2-cm bands on silica gel G.

Solvent system: water + 98% acetic acid + butan-1-ol (17 + 17 + 66), 10 cm run.

Detection: after drying at 100–105 °C, while still warm sprayed with 1% methanolic diphenylboryloxyethylamine, followed by 5% methanolic Macrogol 400.

Evaluation: after 30 min., in UV 365 nm light. Reference solution: bright blue fluorescent caffeic acid zone and yellowish brown fluorescent rutin zone. Test solution: uppermost zone, red fluorescent (chlorophyll); slightly below it and above the level of the reference caffeic acid zone, a yellowish brown fluorescent zone (quercitrin); above

the level of the reference rutin zone, several brownish yellow fluorescent zones, the most intense corresponding to hyperoside; usually, also a faint rutin zone; other brownish yellow and bluish fluorescent zones present. Quantitative determination of the total flavonoids (calculated as hyperoside) can be carried out according to the DAB 10 or by HPLC or OPLC [9, cf. 12].

Quantitative standards: DAB 10: *Flavonoids*, not less than 1.5% calculated as hyperoside (M_r 464.4). *Foreign matter*, not more than 3% pieces of branches and female catkins, and not more than 3% other foreign matter. *Loss on drying*, not more than 10.0%. *Ash*, not more than 5.0%.

ÖAB: *Flavonoids*, not less than 1.5% calculated as hyperoside. *Foreign matter*, not

more than 3%. *Water content*, not more than 10%. *Sulphated ash*, not more than 5.0%.

Ph. Helv. VII: *Flavonoids*, not less than 1.5% calculated as hyperoside (M_r 464.4). *Foreign matter*, not more than 3% woody branches and fragments of female catkins. *Sulphated ash*, not more than 6.5%.

Adulteration: In practice, rare.

Literature:

[1] Kommentar DAB 10.
[2] R. Hänsel and H. Haas, Therapie mit Phytopharmaka. Springer, Berlin/New York 1983.
[3] G. Harnischfeger and H. Stolze, Bewährte Pflanzendrogen in Wissenschaft und Medizin. notamed. Bad Homburg/Melsungen 1983.
[4] H. Schilcher, Z. Phytother. **8**, 141 (1987).
[5] H. Schilcher, according to [2].
[6] H. Schilcher and R. Braun: Ref. in Abstracts zum Intern. Congr. for Research on Medicinal Plants, p. 72. München 1976.
[7] H. Schilcher, Dtsch. Apoth. Ztg. **124**, 2429 (1984).
[8] P. Pachaly, Dünnschichtchromatographie in der Apotheke. Wissenschaftl. Verlagsges. mbH., 2. Aufl., Stuttgart 1983.
[9] K. Dallenbach-Tölke, S. Nyiredy and O. Sticher, Dtsch. Apoth. Ztg. **127**, 1167 (1987).
[10] K. Dallenbach-Toelke, Sz. Nyiredy, G. A. Gross, and O. Sticher, J. Nat. Prod. **49**, 1155 (1986).
[11] H. Kolodziej, Phytochemistry **28**, 3487 (1989).
[12] K. Dallenbach-Toelke, S. Nyiredy, B. Meier, and O. Sticher, Planta Med. **53**, 189 (1987).
[13] B. Rickling and K.W. Glombitza, Planta Med. **59**, 76 (1993).

Boldo folium

Boldo, Peumus (BHP 1983)

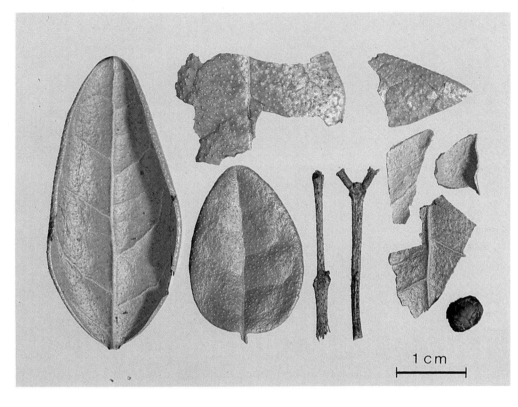

Fig. 1: Boldo leaf

Description: The stiff, leathery, and brittle, elliptic-ovate leaves have an entire margin that is usually slightly revolute. The small, pale protuberances on the upper surface are characteristic; the stout main nerve and the curved lateral nerves are prominent features of the lower surface. In the cut drug, there are occasional reddish brown pieces of twig with pale, linear lenticels and hard, brown, oval seeds (Fig. 1, bottom right).

Odour: Strongly spicy, characteristic.

Taste: Pungently spicy, somewhat bitter.

DAC 1986: Boldoblätter
Ph. Helv. VII: Boldo folium

Plant source: *Peumus boldus* MOLINA (Monimiaceae).

Synonyms: Boldo leaf (Engl.), Boldoblätter (Ger.), Feuilles de boldo (Fr.).

Origin: Chile. A shrub or small tree characteristic of arid vegetation. The drug is imported from Chile.

Constituents: 0.25–0.50% aporphine alkaloids, with boldine as the principal base; 2–3% essential oil, containing *p*-cymol, cineole, ascaridole, and other monoterpenes; small amounts of flavonoids.

Indications: Owing to its boldine content, mainly as a choleretic (but see below); boldo leaf and its preparations stimulate the production of bile, and its secretion from the gall bladder, and the secretion of gastric juice. Boldine has been shown to have mild diuretic, uric-acid excretory, and weak hypnotic effects [1].

In *folk medicine*, boldo is used as a diuretic, stomachic, and sedative. In Chile, the leaves are also employed as an anthelmintic, the activity arising from the ascaridole content of the essential oil [2].

Making the tea: Boiling water is poured over 1–2 g of the finely cut drug and after 10 min. passed through a tea strainer. As a choleretic, a cupful is drunk two or three times a day.
1 Teaspoon = ca. 1.5 g.

Boldine

Note: Detailed investigations have shown that, depending upon the extraction conditions (pH of the extractant, ethanol content, temperature), losses of up to more than 80% of the boldine may occur [3]. Standardized preparations are therefore to be preferred.
In this connection, it may be noted that pharmacological evaluation in rats of an aqueous alcoholic extract of the drug (Hepatran®) did not confirm the reputed choleretic activity of the drug, but did reveal significant hepato-protective activity, in which boldine appears to be implicated, and dose-dependent anti-inflammatory effects, which seem not to involve boldine [4].

Herbal teas: Some instant teas contain extracts of boldo, e.g. Solu-Hepar®, etc.
The drug is also a component of the UK product Potter's Sciargo Herb Mixture, which is put up in tea bags.

Phytomedicines: In several prepared cholagogues and biliary remedies, e.g. Losapan® (powder, granules), Pankreaticum, Gallemolan® (drops), Galenavowen® (dragees), etc.

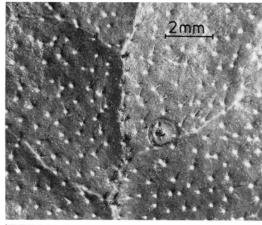
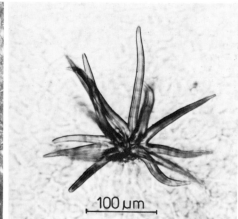

Fig. 2: Upper leaf surface of *Peumus boldus*, showing numerous white protuberances with trichomes

Fig. 3: Multicellular stellate trichome, from the lower leaf surface

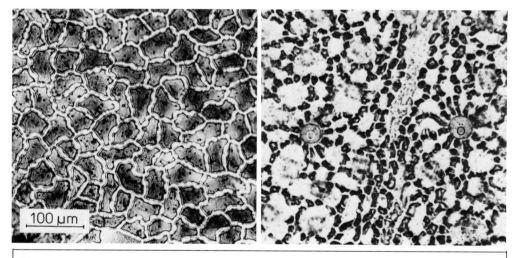

Fig. 4: Warty epidermis of the lower leaf surface

Fig. 5: Oil cells (Ö) in the intercellular spaces of the spongy parenchyma

Among the multi-ingredient UK products are: Opobyl® (tincture) and Potter's Boldo Tablets (aqueous extract), Boldo Aid to Slimming Tablets (standardized extract), and Sciargo (tablets).

Regulatory status (UK): General Sales List – Schedule 1, Table A; maximum single dose 1.5 g.

Authentication: Macro- (see: Description) and microscopically. Moderate magnification suffices to show the presence on the upper surface of numerous small white protuberances with trichomes (Fig. 2); increasing the magnification reveals the characteristic stellate nature of the trichomes, which also occur on the lower surface but without the protuberances on the epidermis (Fig. 3). The epidermal cells are thickened and warty (Fig. 4) and the cells of the hypodermis lying beneath also have thickened walls. In the mesophyll there are spherical secretory cells filled with essential oil (Fig. 5). See also the description in the BHP 1983.
The following TLC examination is for boldine (modified according to the DAC 1986):

Test solution: 1 g powdered drug shaken for 10 min. with 50 ml 1% hydrochloric acid and filtered; 1.5 ml dilute ammonia solution + 0.6 g sodium hydrogen carbonate added to 30 ml filtrate and the whole shaken with 3 × 50 ml chloroform + isopropanol (3 + 1); the combined organic phases dried with 10 g anhydrous sodium sulphate, taken to dryness under reduced pressure, and the residue dissolved in 1.0 ml methanol.

Reference solution: 1 mg boldine in 1.0 ml methanol.

Loadings: 40 µl each of test and reference solutions, as 2-cm bands on silica gel.

Solvent system: toluene + methanol + diethylamine (10 + 1 + 1), 12 cm run.

Detection: after drying, sprayed with iodine solution or Dragendorff reagent.

Evaluation: in daylight. Reference solution: boldine zone in the lower third. Test solution: a corresponding boldine zone.

Quantitative standards: DAC 1986: *Total alkaloid*, not less than 0.1% calculated as boldine (M_r 327.4). *Foreign matter*, not more than 2% leaves of *Cryptocarya peumus* NEES (Lauraceae) and not more than 2% other foreign organic matter. *Loss on drying*, not more than 12.0%. *Ash*, not more than 13.0%.

Ph. Helv. VII: *Volatile oil*, not less than 2%. *Total alkaloid*, not less than 0.1% calculated as boldine (M_r 327.4). *Foreign matter*, not more than 5% woody stems. *Sulphated ash*, not more than 4%.

BHP 1983: *Total ash*, not more than 12%. *Acid-insoluble ash*, not more than 6%.

Adulteration: Especially with the very similar smelling leaves of *Cryptocarya peumus* NEES (Lauraceae), a tree with the same distribution as *Peumus boldus*. These leaves are somewhat larger and the undulate margin is only slightly revolute. Protuberances and stellate trichomes are absent, but secretory cells with essential oil are present as with boldo.

Storage: Protected from light in closed containers (not made of plastic) and kept cool.

Literature:
[1] H. Schindler, Arzneimittel.Forsch. **7**, 747 (1957).
[2] Hager, vol. **6A**, 555 (1977).
[3] C. van Hulle et al., J. Pharm. Belg. **38**, 97 (1983).
[4] M.C. Lanhers et al., Planta Med. **57**, 110 (1991).

Bursae pastoris herba   Shepherd's purse, Capsella (BHP 1983)

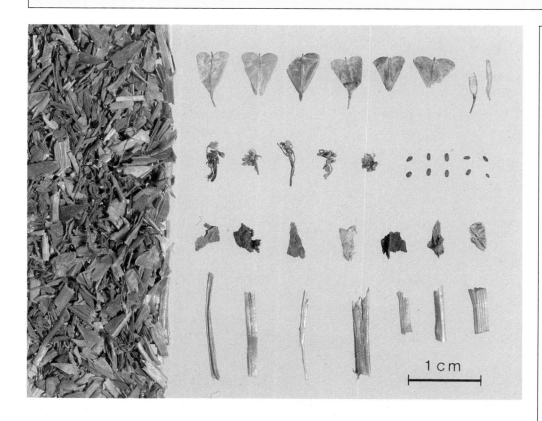

Fig. 1: Shepherd's purse (top row: fruits)

<u>Description:</u> A notable feature of the cut drug is the entire or fragmentary triangular obcordate, flattened, green to light yellow long-pedicellate pods, which are septate at the narrowest point and have keeled valves. There are also numerous brownish red seeds; small clumps of greenish white, much shrivelled inflorescences; light green, round or angular pieces of stem with fine longitudinal striations; and fragments of leaves.

<u>Odour:</u> Faint and unpleasant.

<u>Taste:</u> Somewhat acrid and bitter.

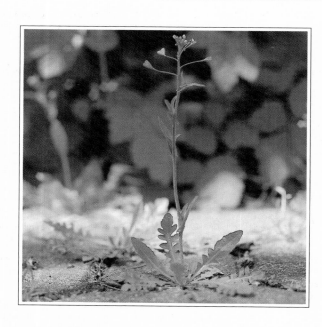

Fig. 2: *Capsella bursa-pastoris* (L.) MEDIKUS

An annual or biennial plant, up to 80 cm in height, growing on waste ground. Rosette of basal entire to deeply pinnatifid leaves; stem leaves broadly winged and embracing the stem. Flowers white, small, on long pedicels. Pods triangular, obcordate.

St.Zul.: 1539.99.99

Plant source: *Capsella bursa-pastoris* (L.) MEDIKUS, shepherd's-purse (Brassicaceae).

Synonyms: Herba Sanguinariae (no doubt because of the styptic effect) (Lat.), Hirtentäschelkraut (Ger.), Herbe de bourse à pasteur (Fr.).

Origin: Cosmopolitan; the drug comes from collections in the wild in Europe (the former USSR, former Yugoslavia, Hungary, and Bulgaria).

Constituents: Much old information about certain compounds needs to be re-examined. Thus, Japanese workers have doubted the earlier supposed detection of biogenetic amines (up to 1% choline, acetylcholine, tyramine) [1]. The presence of saponins (triterpenes?) also requires further study. The drug contains flavonoids, including luteolin and quercetin 7-rutinosides and luteolin 7-galactoside; sinigrin and other glucosinolates are present; and largish amounts of potassium salts and vitamin C have been found [2].

Extract from the German Commission E monograph (BAnz no. 173, dated 18.09.1986)

Uses

Internally: symptomatic treatment of mild menorrhagia and metrorrhagia; for topical application in nose bleeds.
Externally: superficial, bleeding injuries to the skin.

Contraindications

None known.

Side effects

None known.

Interactions with other remedies

None known.

Dosage

Unless otherwise prescribed: average daily dose, 10–15 g drug; preparations correspondingly.
Topical application: 3–5 g drug to a 150 ml infusion.

Fluid extract (according to Erg. B. 6): daily dose, 5–8 g.

Mode of administration

Chopped drug for infusions and other galenical preparations for internal and topical use.

Effects

Only on parenteral administration: muscarine-like effects with dose-dependent hypo- and hypertension, positive inotropic and chronotropic cardiac activity, and increased contraction of the uterus.

The occurrence of amino acids, including proline [3], and of a peptide with a haemostyptic action has been described [4].

Indications: Extracts of the drug have a haemostyptic action, which is said to be due to a peptide with *in-vitro* oxytocin-like activity [4]; here, the remarkable point is also mentioned that the maximum activity of shepherd's-purse preparations is supposedly reached three months after they have been made.
In *folk medicine,* the drug is still occasionally used as a styptic. The former common use as a substitute for ergot in uterine bleeding is obsolete and, because of the very inadequate activity, is not recommended. The drug is still used in *folk medicine* to treat dysmenorrhoea.

Making the tea: Boiling water is poured over 3–5 g of the finely chopped drug and after 10–15 min. passed through a tea strainer.
1 Teaspoon = ca. 1.5 g.

Phytomedicines: As the extract, in a few plant antidysmenorrhoeic remedies.
The herb is a component of the UK products Potter's Antitis Tablets and Seven Seas Backache Tablets.

Authentication: Macro- (see: Description) and microscopically. Diagnostic features of the light green drug powder are: (a) unicellular, flat, stellate trichomes with 3–5 radiating branches (Fig. 3) and a warty cuticle, and (b) up to 500 μm long, unicellular, tapering, thickened trichomes with a smooth cuticle [5, 6].
The following TLC test of identity can be used:

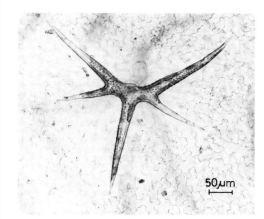

Fig. 3: Stellate trichome with warty cuticle, from the lower leaf surface of *Capsella bursa-pastoris*

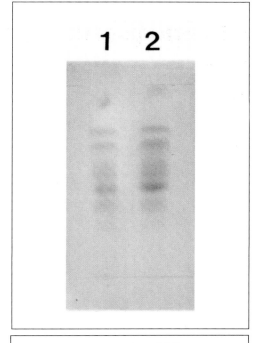

Fig. 4: TLC on 4 × 8 cm silica-gel foil
1: Shepherd's purse
2: Reference solution
For details, see the text.

Test solution: 1.0 g powdered drug refluxed for 20 min. with 20 ml 50% aqueous ethanol; the clear filtrate concentrated under reduced pressure to ca. 10 ml.

Reference solution: authentic drug similarly treated, or 10 mg leucine + 10 mg threonine dissolved together in 10 ml 50% aqueous ethanol.

Loadings: 5 μl each of the test and reference solutions, as bands.

Wording of the package insert, from the German Standard Licence:

6.1 **Uses**

As supportive treatment for nose bleeds and excessive menstruation.

6.2 **Dosage and Mode of administration**

Boiling water (ca. 150 ml) is poured over about 1–2 teaspoonfuls (2–4 g) of **Shepherd's purse** and after about 15 min. passed through a tea strainer.
Unless otherwise prescribed, a cup of the freshly prepared infusion is drunk warm two to four times a day between meals.
Note: If the bleeding persists, a doctor should be consulted.

6.3 **Note**

Store away from light and moisture.

Solvent system: butan-1-ol + acetone + glacial acetic acid + water (35 + 35 + 10 + 20), 6 cm run.

Detection: after drying in a current of warm air, sprayed with a solution of 30 mg ninhydrin in 10 ml butan-1-ol + 0.3 ml glacial acetic acid and heated at 100–105 °C for 10 min. while under observation.

Evaluation: in daylight. Reference solution: two pinkish red zones – the lower one threonine, the upper one leucine. Test solution: pink to pinkish red zones at the same Rf values, the more intense one at the same height as threonine; somewhat lower, an in-tense yellow spot (proline); above the leucine spot, 3–4 additional pinkish red spots (Fig. 4).

The St.Zul. procedure is similar, but makes use of silica gel GF_{254}, with proline as the reference substance; the chromatogram is also examined under UV 365 nm light.

Quantitative standards: St.Zul. 1539.99.99: *Water-soluble extractive*, not less than 18%. *Foreign (vegetable and/or mineral) matter*, not more than 2%. *Loss on drying*, not more than 10.0% *Ash*, not more than 10.0%. BHP 1983: *Total ash*, not more than 10%. *Acid-insoluble ash*, not more than 2.5%.

Adulteration: Has not been observed in the drug trade.

Literature:
[1] K. Kuroda and T. Kaku, Life Sci. **8**, 151 (1969); C. A. **70**, 76342 (1969).
[2] N.N. Sabri, T. Sarg, and A.A. Seif El-Din, Egypt. J. Pharm. Sci. **16**, 521 (1975).
[3] T. Perseca and Z. Curta, Stud. Univ. Babes-Bolyai [Ser.] Biol. **28**, 24 (1983); C.A. **99**, 181335 (1983).
[4] K. Kuroda and K. Takagi, Nature (London) **220**, 707 (1968).
[5] Berger, vol. **4**, 83 (1954).
[6] Hager, vol. **3**, 666 (1972); Vol. **4**, 655 (1992).

Calami rhizoma   Calamus, Acorus (BHP 1983)

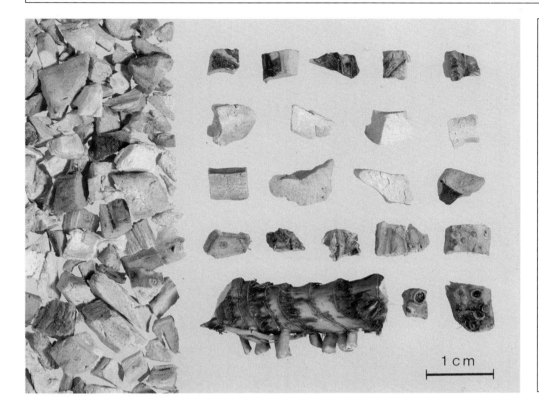

Fig. 1: Calamus rhizome

<u>Description</u>: The rhizome, freed from roots, leaf sheaths, and stems, is often split longitudinally and peeled; it exhibits triangular leaf and roundish root scars (Fig. 3). It is up to 2 cm thick, whitish with a reddish tinge, and soft (lacunose tissue, aerenchyma). The demarcation between the bark and the central stele can be recognized in the transverse section.

<u>Odour</u>: Characteristic and faintly aromatic.

<u>Taste</u>: Aromatic and bitter, somewhat spicy.

Fig. 2: *Acorus calamus* L.

A perennial, ca. 1 m tall marsh plant with distichous, linear leaves and a triangular stem. Densely crowded flowers in a club-like spike.

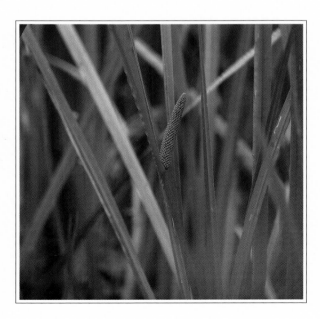

DAB 6: Rhizoma Calami
ÖAB: Radix Calami
Ph. Helv. VII: Calami rhizoma (Kalmus)

Plant source: *Acorus calamus* L., sweet flag, with different degrees of ploidy: var. *americanus* WULFF (diploid), var. *calamus* (triploid), var. *angustatus* ENGL. (tetraploid) (Araceae) [1].

Synonyms: Acorus or Sweet flag root (Engl.), Kalmuswurzelstock, Gewürzkalmus, Deutscher Ingwer (Ger.), Rhizome d'acore vrai (Fr.).

Origin: The drug is collected mostly from wild plants. Imports come from the former USSR, former Yugoslavia, and India.

Constituents: 2–6 (and up to as much as 9)% essential oil (in oil cells), consisting of sesquiterpenes and phenylpropanes. The composition of the oil (and also the oil content of the drug) varies greatly, depending on the degree of ploidy of the plants (see: Plant source). *Cis*-Isoasarone (β-asarone), often together with eugenol methyl ether, is the main component (up to 80%), but may be completely absent in the American drug [2–4]. Further constituents: bitter substances, among them acorone, a sesquiterpene diketone with a spiran structure, which is one of the volatile components present in the essential oil; in the oil of triploid plants, sesquiterpene ketones (shyobunones) predominate; in addition, tannins, mucilage, small starch grains.

Indications: On the basis of its constituents, the drug can be called a bitter aromatic; it is principally used as a stomachic and carminative. It is also employed externally as a rubefacient. The former common use in *folk medicine* as a "nervine" was perhaps connected with the tranquillizing property of *cis*-isoasarone.
In popular books on medicinal plants, the plant is praised as a "wonder drug".

Side effects: *Cis*-Isoasarone also has cancerogenic [5–7] and mutagenic [8] or chromosome-damaging [9] properties. Hence, to avoid any risk, the spasmolytically active American drug, which is free of *cis*-isoasarone, has to be employed. However, with a more pragmatic view of the situation, provided a limit is set on the *cis*-isoasarone content and prolonged use of the drug is avoided, the triploid European races poor in *cis*-isoasarone may be considered as acceptable [12].

Making the tea: Boiling water is poured over 1–1.5 g of the finely chopped or coarsely powdered drug, or cold water is added to the drug and boiled for a short time; after 3–5 min., it is strained. As an aromatic bitter, a cup of the tea is drunk at mealtimes. 1 Teaspoon = ca. 3 g.

Herbal preparations: Calamus is included in several prepared herbal mixtures (stomach teas, and also other indications).

Phytomedicines: Calamus-root extracts are present, usually in small amounts, in many multi-ingredient products, mostly gastrointestinal remedies and a few cholagogues, e.g. Carvomin®, Gastrol®, and many others. Calamus oil is also a component of remedies for external use.

Authentication: Macro- (see: Description) and microscopically. A particularly diagnostic feature is the lacunose tissue (aerenchyma) (Fig. 4) with secretory cells, some containing essential oil and some containing tannin inclusions that stain red with vanillin/hydrochloric acid. Closer examination of the parenchyma cells of this tissue also reveals small triangular air spaces and abundant small starch grains. The generally

scalariform vessels are in the vascular bundles, which are collateral outside the endodermis are and amphivasal (leptocentric) in the inner part of the rhizome. However, in the usual, more or less carefully peeled, drug, the endodermis is missing and the fibres and crystal sheath surrounding the outer vascular bundles are rare.
The detailed microscopy of the powdered drug is described and illustrated in [10].

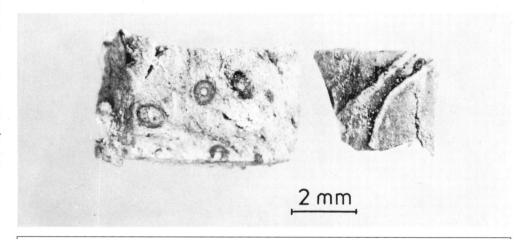

Fig. 3: **Pieces of the rhizome with roundish root (left) and elongated leaf (right) scars**

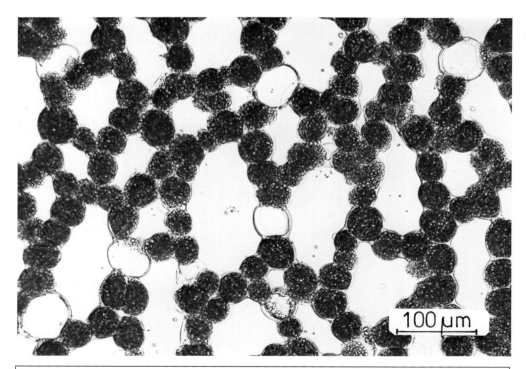

Fig. 4: **Starch-containing lacunose tissue (aerenchyma) with oil cells**

Cis-Isoasarone (β-Asarone)   Acorone   Shyobunone

The following TLC method can be used to establish the presence of *cis*-isoasarone (*β*-asarone) in calamus oil [11]:

Test solution: essential oil diluted 1 : 10 in toluene.

Reference solution: *cis*-isoasarone and eugenol, each diluted 1:30 in toluene.

Loadings: 5 μl of the test solution and 3 μl of the reference solutions, on silica gel 60F$_{254}$.

Solvent system: toluene + ethyl acetate (93 + 7) and/or (97 + 3).

Detection: sprayed with 5% ethanolic sulphuric acid, followed by 1% ethanolic vanillin, and then heated at 110 °C for 5–10 min. while under observation.

Evaluation: Reference solution: a reddish brown zone at Rf ca. 0.4 (*cis*-isoasarone); a reddish zone at Rf ca. 0.5 (eugenol). Test solution: a series of violet, blue, and brownish violet zones from about Rf 0.1 to the solvent front; size and intensity of the reddish brown *cis*-isoasarone zone at Rf ca. 0.4 depending on the origin and chemical race (illustrative chromatograms in [11]); only a faint zone present at the Rf ca. 0.5 (the level of eugenol), with above it several blue to bluish violet zones (sesquiterpenes).

Quantitative standards: DAB 6: *Volatile oil*, not less than 2.5%. *Ash*, not more than 6%. ÖAB: *Volatile oil*, not less than 2.0%. *Foreign matter*, in powdered Radix Calami starch grains with a diameter greater than 10 μm, stone cells, or considerable amounts of phloem fibres may not be present. *Ash*, not more than 6.0%.

Ph. Helv. VII: *Volatile oil*, not less than 2.0%. *Asarone content*, not more than 0.5%. *Foreign matter*, not more than 1%. *Sulphated ash*, not more than 7.0%.

BHP 1983: *Total ash*, not more than 6%. *Acid-insoluble ash*, not more than 1.0%.

Adulteration: In practice, rare.

Literature:
[1] L.C.M. Röst, Planta Med. **37**, 289 (1979).
[2] K. Keller and E. Stahl, Dtsch. Apoth. Ztg. **122**, 2463 (1982).
[3] K. Keller and E. Stahl, Planta Med. **47**, 71 (1983).
[4] E. Stahl and K. Keller, Planta Med. **43**, 128 (1981).
[5] J.M. Taylor, et al., Toxicol. Appl. Pharmacol. **10**, 405 (1967).
[6] M.A. Gross, et al., Proc. Am. Assoc. Cancer Res. **8**, 24 (1970).
[7] R.T. Habermann, Project P-153-70, Report of the Food and Drug Administration (1971).
[8] W. Göggelmann and O. Schimmer, Mutat. Res. **121**, 191 (1983).
[9] G. Abel, Planta Med. **53**, 251 (1987).
[10] B.P. Jackson and D.W. Snowdon, Atlas of microscopy of medicinal plants, culinary herbs and spices, Belhaven Press, London, 1990, p. 26.
[11] H. Wagner, S. Bladt, and E.M. Zgainski, Plant drug analysis, Springer-Verlag, Berlin, Heidelberg, New York, Tokyo, 1984, p. 24.
[12] K. Schneider and J. Jurenitsch, Pharmazie **47**, 79 (1992).

Calendulae flos   Marigold

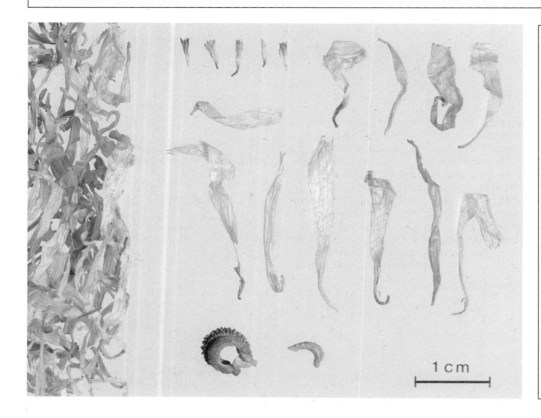

Fig. 1: Marigold

Description: The commercial drug consists of the entire or partly broken-up flower-heads (diameter 5–7 cm), especially of double varieties with numerous ligulate florets and few tubular florets, and of individual florets free of the receptacle and involucral bracts (Flores Calendulae sine calycibus). The yellowish red, shiny, female ligulate florets are characteristic; they are 20–30 mm long and 5–7 mm broad and they readily fade on keeping; at the top they are tridentate and they do not have a pappus.
The much smaller tubular florets occur less frequently (upper left).
There should be few or none of the curved, navicular fruits with short spines on the dorsal surface (bottom row).

Odour: Faint, but characteristic.

Taste: Somewhat bitter and salty.

Figs. 2 and 3: *Calendula officinalis* L.

An annual or biennial aromatic plant with broadly lanceolate leaves and flowering heads, 4–7 cm in diameter, comprising many orange-yellow ligulate and tubular florets.

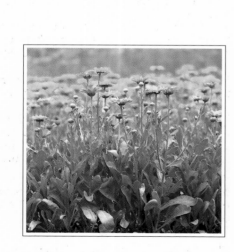
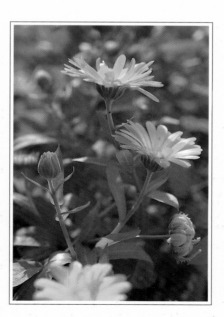

DAC 1986: Ringelblumenblüten
St.Zul.: 1209.99.99

Plant source: *Calendula officinalis* L., (pot) marigold (Asteraceae).

Synonyms: Calendula, Mary-bud, Goldbloom (Engl.), Ringelblumen, Goldblume (Ger.), Fleur de souci officinal, Fleur de tous les mois, Fleur de Calendule (Fr.).

Origin: Native in central, eastern, and southern Europe. It is cultivated in Mediterranean countries, in the Balkans, in eastern Europe, and to a small extent in Germany. Imports of the drug come from Egypt, Poland, and Hungary.

Constituents: Essential oil (ligulate florets up to 0.12%, receptacles of the inflorescence up to 0.4%), including menthone, isomenthone, γ-terpinene, α-muurolene, γ-and δ-cadinene, caryophyllene, pedunculatine, α- and β-ionone, β-ionone 5,6-epoxide, dihydro-actinidiolide, geranylacetone, carvone, caryophyllene ketone [1]. Sesquiterpene, al-

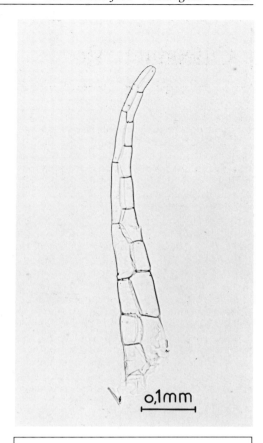

OCH₃ / Isorhamnetin structure

Isorhamnetin

Oleanolic acid-glycosides

R¹			R²
Glucose (1-4) Galactose (1-3)	Glucuronic acid		Glucose
Glucose (1-4) Galactose (1-3)	Glucuronic acid		H
Galactose (1-3)	— Glucuronic acid		Glucose
Galactose (1-4)	— Glucuronic acid		H
Glucose (1-4)	— Glucuronic acid		H
Glucuronic acid			H

Loliolide

loaromadendrol and epicubebol, glycosides active against vesicular stomatitis virus (VSV) [16]. Flavonol glycosides, chiefly the 2′-rhamnosylrutinoside, 3-*O*-rutinoside, and 3-*O*-neohesperidoside of isorhamnetin (together, 0.3-1.0-1.5%), and the corresponding quercetin derivatives, etc. [17, 18]. A mixture of several haemolytically active bisdesmosidic saponins (2–10% dry wt., depending on the variety and time of harvesting), with the basic unit oleanolic acid 3-*O*-β-D-glucuronide (mainly calendulosides A, C, and E, together with variable or minor amounts of B, D, and F) [19–21]. Triterpene alcohols, including α- and β-amyrin, taraxasterol, calenduladiol, arnidiol, faradiol, pentacyclic triterpene triols [2]. Free, esterified, and glucosidic sterols; carotenes and xanthophylls; polyacetylenes; phenol-carboxylic acids; bitter substances, but the sesquiterpene lactone calendin, mentioned in the literature, does not occur – it is identical with the xanthophyll degradation product loliolide [3]; tannins; immunostimulant polysaccharides

(a rhamnoarabino- galactan and two arabinogalactans) [22].

Indications: Preparations of the drug inhibit inflammation and promote the formation of granulation tissue. They are used in the same way as Arnicae flos: externally, in the form of infusions, tinctures, and ointments as a wound-healing remedy for inflammation of the skin and mucous membranes, for poorly healing wounds, bruises, boils, and rashes, e.g. pharyngitis, dermatitis, ulcus cruris (leg ulcers). The *internal use* as an antiphlogistic and spasmolytic in, e.g. cholecystitis, cholangitis, gastritis, cystitis, gastrointestinal spasms, is *largely obsolete*, although the drug is still a component of some prepared remedies. The actual active principle of the drug has not yet been clarified [4]; the essential oil and xanthophylls, as well as still unidentified bitter substances, have all been considered. The essential oil has been shown to have a trichomonacidal action [1]. More recent studies in rats have again demonstrated the antiphlogistic effect (on carrageenan- and prostaglandin E_1-induced inflammation) and inhibition of leucocyte infiltration [6, 7], as well as a uterotonic effect by aqueous extracts [8], an antiphlogistic and choleretic action of a flavonoid extract [9], and a bactericidal effect against *Staphylococcus aureus* [10].

Fig. 4: Biseriate trichome from the base of the (ligulate) floret of *Calendula officinalis*

In animal experiments (rats), isolated constituents, e.g. the calendulosides, have shown an anti-hyperlipidaemic effect and also a certain action on the central nervous system [11, 12].
A triterpene saponin-enriched extract of the flowers (and leaves and stems) has been shown both *in vivo* and *in vitro* to have cytotoxic and antitumoral activity [13].
Much of the drug is used to add to herbal mixtures in order to enhance their appearance.
In *folk medicine,* the drug is employed as a diaphoretic, diuretic, antispasmodic, anthelmintic, emmenagogue, and for liver complaints, but a scientific basis for these uses is lacking.

Making the tea: Boiling water is poured over 1 g of the drug and after 5–10 min. passed through a tea strainer.
1 Teaspoon = ca. 0.8 g.

Phytomedicines: Marigold flowers are a component of many herbal mixtures belonging to different groups, where it evidently fulfils the function of enhancing their appearance. Extracts of the drug are present in several prepared dermatological remedies, wound remedies (ointments, dusting powders), and cholagogues.

Authentication: Macro- (see: Description) and microscopically. At the base of the ligulate florets, there are long, biseriate trichomes (Fig. 4). Other parts of the drug are pubescent, especially with ordinary trichomes and shaggy glandular trichomes; characteristic asteraceous glandular trichomes are lacking. The detailed microscopy of the powdered drug is set out and illustrated in [23]. The TLC test of identity can be based on an examination of the flavonoids (characteristic isorhamnetin glycosides), using the method described under Arnicae flos (q.v.), where a reference to *Calendulae flos* is given. The very characteristic fingerprint chromatogram is evaluated as follows:

Evaluation: Test solution: greenish yellow or yellowish brown to orange fluorescent zones at about the same Rf value as the rutin zone, or a little lower, point to the presence of *Calendula* or *Heterotheca* flowers.

The St.Zul. solvent system is very similar: ethyl acetate + anhydrous formic acid + water (8 + 1 + 1); other chromatographic systems and illustrations to help in evaluating the chromatograms are to be found in [14, 15, 24]. A combined 2D-TLC and HPLC procedure for analysing the glycosides (flavonoids and saponins) is available [25]. Another HPLC method for the saponins is given in [21a].

Quantitative standards: St.Zul. 1209.99.99: *Foreign matter*, not more than 5% sepals and only occasional fruits. *Loss on drying*, not more than 10%. *Ash*, not more than 10%.

BHP 1983: *Water-soluble extractive*, not less than 20%. *Total ash*, not more than 9%. *Acid-insoluble ash*, not more than 2%.

Note: Calendulae flos is the subject of an ESCOP draft proposal for a harmonized European monograph.

Adulteration: Very rare.

Wording of the package insert, from the German Standard Licence:

6.1 Uses

Inflammation of the skin and mucous membranes; lacerated wounds, bruises, and burns.

6.2 Dosage and Mode of administration

Hot water (ca. 150 ml) is poured over between one and two teaspoonfuls (2–3 g) of **Marigold** and after 10 min. passed through a tea strainer.
Unless otherwise prescribed, for inflammation in the mouth or throat, the still-warm infusion is used as a rinse or gargle several times a day. For treating wounds, linen, or a similar material, is soaked in the infusion and placed on the wound; the dressing is changed several times a day.

6.3 Note

Store protected from light and moisture.

Literature:
[1] L. Gracza, Planta Med. **53**, 227 (1987).
[2] B. Wilkomirski, Phytochemistry **24**, 3066 (1985).
[3] G. Willuhn and R.-G. Westhaus, Planta Med. **53**, 304 (1987).
[4] J.J.C. Scheffer, Pharm. Weekbl. **114**, 1149 (1979).
[5] O. Gessner and G. Orzechowski, Gift- und Arzneipflanzen von Mitteleuropa, 3rd ed., C. Winter Universitätsverlag, Heidelberg, 1974.
[6] T. Shipochliew, A. Dimitrov, and E. Aleksandrova, Vet. Med. Nauki **18**, 87 (1981).
[7] J. Peyroux, P. Rossignol, and P. Delaveau, Plantes Méd. Phytothérap. **15**, 210 (1982).
[8] T. Shipochliew, Vet. Med. Nauki **18**, 94 (1981).
[9] T.J. Isakowa, Farmatsiya (Moscow) (5), 31 (1980).
[10] G. Dumenil et al., Ann. Pharm. Franç. **38**, 493 (1980).
[11] J. Lutomski, Pharmazie in unserer Zeit **12**, 149 (1983).
[12] L. Samochowiec, Herba Polon. **29**, 151 (1983).
[13] Y. Bochaud-Maitre, O. Algernon, and J. Raynaus, Pharmazie **43**, 220 (1988).
[14] P. Rohdewald, G. Rücker, and K.-W. Glombitza, Apothekengerechte Prüfvorschriften, Deutscher Apotheker Verlag, Stuttgart, 1986, p. 933.
[15] E. Stahl and S. Juell, Dtsch. Apoth. Ztg. **122**, 1951 (1982).
[16] N.D. Tommasi et al., J. Nat. Prod. **53**, 830 (1990).
[17] E. Vidall-Ollivier et al., Planta Med. **55**, 73 (1989).
[18] E. Vidall-Ollivier et al., Pharm. Acta Helv. **66**, 318 (1991).
[19] E. Vidall-Ollivier et al., Plantes Méd. Phytothérap. **22**, 235 (1989).
[20] E. Vidall-Ollivier et al., J. Nat. Prod. **52**, 1156 (1990).
[21] (a) E. Vidall-Ollivier et al., Pharm. Acta Helv. **64**, 156 (1989); (b) idem., *ibid.* **65**, 236 (1990).
[22] J. Varljen, A. Liptak, and H. Wagner, Phytochemistry **28**, 2379 (1989).
[23] B.P. Jackson and D.W. Snowdon, Atlas of microscopy of medicinal plants, culinary herbs and spices, Belhaven Press, London, 1990, p. 154.
[24] H. Wagner, S. Bladt, and E.M. Zgainski, Plant drug analysis, Springer-Verlag, Berlin – Heidelberg – New York – Tokyo, 1984, pp. 174, 176.
[25] W. Heisig and M. Wichtl, Dtsch. Apoth. Ztg. **130**, 2058 (1990).

Cardui mariae fructus   (DAB 10), Milk-thistle fruit

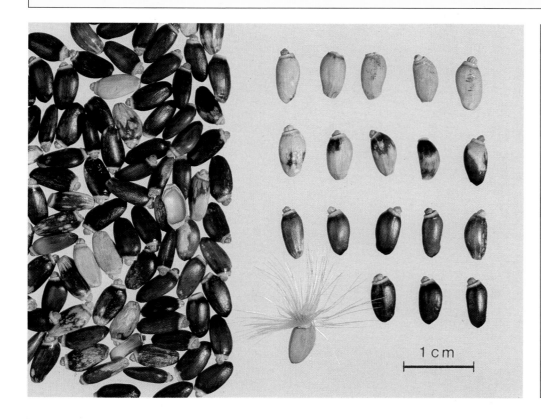

Fig. 1: Milk-thistle fruit

<u>Description:</u> The drug consists of the obliquely obovoid fruit (achenes) which are 6–7 mm long, up to 3 mm broad, and 1.5 mm thick. The testa is shiny brownish black or matt greyish brown, with dark or greyish white dots. At the tip, there is a yellowish projecting cartilaginous, swollen ring and at the bottom at the side a canaliculate hilum. The silvery pappus is absent from the drug (since it readily falls off). Commercial varieties are white, grey, and black.

<u>Odour:</u> Scarcely perceptible.

<u>Taste:</u> Oily (seeds) and bitter (testa).

Fig. 2: Fruit of *Silybum marianum* (L.) GAERTN. with pappus

For an illustration and description of the plant, see: Cardui mariae herba (Milk-thistle herb).

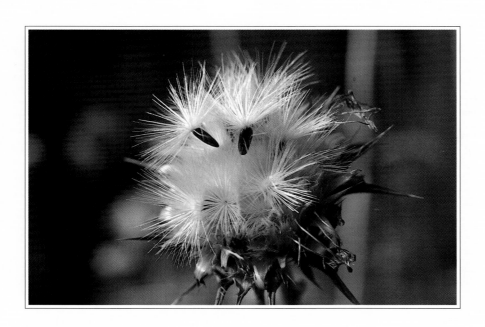

DAB 10: Mariendistelfrüchte
St.Zul. 1589.99.99

Plant source: *Silybum marianum* (L.) GAERTN. (syn. *Carduus marianus* L.), milk thistle (Asteraceae).

Synonyms: Fructus Silybi mariae (Lat.), Marian thistle (Engl.), Mariendistelfrüchte, Marienkörner, Frauendistelfrüchte (Ger.), Fruit de chardon Marie (Fr.).

Origin: Native in southern Europe, southern Russia, Asia Minor, and North Africa; naturalized in North and South America, South Australia, and Central Europe. The drug comes exclusively from cultivated plants: grown to a limited extent in northern Germany, but mainly imported from Argentina, China, Romania, and Hungary.

Constituents: 1.5–3% silymarin, a mixture of various flavanone derivatives (flavonolignans) present only in the fruit. The principal components are silybin (=silibinin), silychristin, and silydianin; in addition, the 3-desoxy-derivatives of silychristin and silydi-

Silybin

Silychristin

Silydianin

Taxifolin
2,3-Dihydroquercetin

anin (= silymonin), isosilychristin, isosily-bin and its 3-desoxy derivative silandrin, the 3-desoxy compounds silyhermin, neosily-hermin A and B, 2,3-dehydrosilybin, as well as tri- to pentamers of silybin (=silybino-mer); other constituents: taxifolin, querce-tin, dihydrokaempferol, kaempferol, apigen-in, naringin, eriodyctiol, chrysoeriol, and 5,7-dihydroxychromone; dehydrodiconifer-yl alcohol. Ca. 20–30% fixed oil with a high proportion of linoleic acid (ca. 60%), oleic acid (ca. 30%), and palmitic acid (ca. 9%) in the triglycerides; 0.038% tocopherol, 0.63% sterols: cholesterol, campesterol, stigmas-terol, sitosterol; ca. 25–30% protein; some mucilage.

Indications: For the prophylaxis and treat-ment of liver damage caused by metabolic toxins, e.g. alcohol, tissue poisons, in liver dysfunction and after hepatitis (post-hepati-tis syndrome), in chronic degenerative liver conditions, such as liver cirrhosis and fatty liver, and in latent hepatopathies.
Silymarin is the active antihepatotoxic com-plex; and there is an extensive literature dealing with its pharmacodynamic and ther-apeutic action [1, 2]. *In-vitro* and *in-vivo* ad-ministration of silymarin competitively sup-presses the action of hepatotoxic substances, e.g. carbon tetrachloride, thioacetamide, and the *Amanita* toxins phalloidin and α-amanitin, which lead to liver necrosis and cirrhosis. Prophylactic administration is more effective than therapeutic administra-tion after the liver damage has occurred. Thus, it was found that the most favourable time was 6 hours before giving the toxin; in the 30 mins. after giving the toxin (phalloid-in) the toxic effect was reduced, and subse-quently no further toxic effect could be ob-served. The demonstrated antihepatotoxic effect is explained by a "membrane-stabiliz-ing action", probably through antioxidant and radical-scavenging actions [3, 4]. The membrane-stabilizing effect of silymarin has also been established with nystatin-dam-aged yeast cells [5].
It has also been found, both *in vitro* and *in vivo*, that silybin increases the rate of synthe-sis of ribosomal ribonucleic acids through stimulation of the nucleolar polymerase I. This reinforces protein synthesis and accel-erates cell-regeneration processes, so that,

besides the prophylactic action, there may also be a curative effect [6, 7]. In a double blind study, it could be shown that silymarin (140 mg, 3 × daily) significantly reduced the mortality of patients with liver cirrhosis due to alcohol [8].
Even when administered in large doses (20.0 g/kg mouse, *per os*) silymarin is non-toxic. In man, it is excreted in the form of sulphate and glucuronidate conjugates pri-marily via the bile (ca. 20–40% within 24 hours; via the kidneys, ca. 3–7%) [9]. Cumu-lation does not occur. The concentration of silybin present in the bile after the adminis-tration of therapeutic doses is at a pharma-cologically effective level [10]; hence, in man the pharmacokinetic behaviour of silybin is in agreement with its therapeutic activity.
The components of silymarin are poorly sol-uble in water when pure. Clinical reports in the older literature, which also indicate cholagogic and spasmolytic effects [see: 11], relate solely to alcoholic extracts (tinctures). Teas are recommended only as supportive treatment in functional gall-bladder disor-ders. When teas are made, only a small pro-portion of the silymarin gets into the aqueous extract [12], so that pharmacologi-cally active doses are not attained and an antihepatotoxic effect is unlikely to be pro-duced.

Making the tea: Not very usual; taking a preparation with a standardized silymarin content is preferable. 3 g crushed fruits is put into cold water and boiled for a brief period, or brewed up with boiling water, and strained after 20–30 min.
1 Teaspoon = ca. 3.5 g.

Phytomedicines: Many prepared chola-gogues and biliary remedies and liver reme-dies, containing either the isolated active complex silymarin, e.g. Legalon®, Durasily-marin®, etc., or standardized extracts (more than 50 preparations), as well as gastrointes-tinal remedies and antiphlebitis remedies (10 preparations); inclusion in the latter type of remedy is doubtless based on the assumed effect that obstruction of the portal vein will have on venous reflux.

Authentication: Macro- and microscopical-ly, following the DAB 10. Microscopically, there are several diagnostic features. The pericarp epidermis is a colourless palisade layer of cells (ca. 75 μm × 8 μm) with a strongly thickened outside wall which re-duces the lumen in that part of the cell to a slit; the subepidermal layer comprises colourless thin-walled parenchyma cells or groups of cells alternating with a variable number of pigmented cells; the innermost layer is mostly collapsed and contains cigar-shaped or monoclinic prisms of calcium ox-

Uses

Crude drug: dyspeptic disorders.
Preparations: toxic liver damage; as supportive treatment in chronic inflammatory liver conditions and liver cirrhosis.

Contraindications

None known.

Side effects

None known.
Preparations: a mild laxative effect is occasionally observed.

Interactions with other remedies

None known.

Dosage

Unless otherwise prescribed: average daily dose of the crude drug, 12–15 g; preparations, equivalent to 200–400 mg silymarin, calculated as silibinin.

Mode of administration

Chopped drug for infusions and other galenical preparations for internal use.

Effects

Silymarin acts as an antagonist in many liver-damage models: phalloidin and α-amanitin (death-cap toxins), lanthanides, carbon tetrachloride, galactosamine, thioacetamide, and the hepatotoxic virus FV_3 of cold-blooded animals.
The therapeutic activity of silymarin is based on two sites or mechanisms of action: (a) it alters the structure of the outer cell membrane of the hepatocytes in such a way as to prevent penetration of the liver poison into the interior of the cell; (b) it stimulates the action of the nucleolar polymerase A, resulting in an increase in ribosomal protein synthesis, and thus stimulates the regenerative ability of the liver and the formation of new hepatocytes.

alate. The epidermis of the testa consists of large, lemon-yellow palisade-like, elongated (ca. 150 μm) cells with striated walls and a narrow lumen widening slightly at the ends; the subepidermal layers have lignified and pitted cells with closely arranged bands of thickening.

5.1 Uses

Mild digestive disorders.

5.2 Dosage and Mode of administration

Boiling water is poured over a heaped teaspoonful (3–5 g) of (freshly) crushed **Milk-thistle fruit** and after 10–15 min. passed through a tea strainer.
Unless otherwise prescribed, a cup of the freshly prepared infusion is drunk three or four times a day half- an-hour before meals.

5.3 Duration of use

To effect a cure, preparations of milk-thistle fruit need to be taken over an extended period of time.

5.4 Note

Store protected from light and moisture.

The DAB 10 TLC test of identity entails detection of silymarin and taxifolin:

Test solution: 1.0 g powdered drug shaken for 5 min. with 10 ml methanol on the water-bath at 65 °C, cooled, filtered, carefully taken to dryness, and the residue dissolved in 1.0 ml methanol.

Reference solution: 1.0 mg caffeic acid dissolved in 10 ml methanol.

Loadings: 30 µl test solution and 10 µl reference solution, as 2-cm bands on silica gel G.

Solvent system: anhydrous formic acid + acetone + chloroform (8.5 + 16.5 + 75), 2 × 10 cm run.

Detection: while still warm, sprayed with 1% methanolic diphenylboryloxyethylamine and then oversprayed with 5% methanolic Macrogol 400.

Evaluation: after 30 min. in UV 365 nm light. Reference solution: at about the middle, the bright blue fluorescent caffeic acid zone. Test solution: at the same height, the most intense zone, the yellowish green fluo-

rescent silybin zone; above the silybin zone, several fainter fluorescent zones and below it, as far as the starting line, further distinctly fluorescent zones (silydianin, silychristin, etc.) including the brownish yellow fluorescent taxifolin zone; the first zone below the silybin one may be stronger than the silybin zone.
A coloured illustration of the chromatogram is to be found in [13].

Quantitative standards: <u>DAB 10</u>: *Silymarin,* not less than 1.0% calculated as silybin (M_r 482.4). *Condition,* the drug must not smell or taste rancid. *Foreign (vegetable and/or mineral) matter,* not more than 2%. *Loss on drying,* not more than 8.0%. *Ash,* not more than 8.0%.

Adulteration: Practically never occurs.

Literature:
[1] R. Braatz and C.C. Schneider (Eds.), Symposium on the pharmacodynamics of silymarin, Köln 1974, Urban & Schwarzenberg, München, Berlin, Wien 1976.
[2] Experimentelle und klinische Hepatologie. III. Internationales Lebersymposium, Köln 1978. Hansisches Verlags-Kontor, Lübeck 1979.
[3] V. Valenzuela, R. Guerra and A. Garrido, Planta Med. **53**, 402 (1987).
[4] V. Valenzuela, R. Guerra and L.A. Videla, Planta Med **52**, 438 (1986).
[5] H.P. Koch, J. Bachner and E. Loeffler, Dtsch. Apoth. Ztg. **126**, 2050 (1986).
[6] H. Wagner, in: Natural Products as Medicinal Agents (Hrsg. J. Beal und E. Reinhard), Hippokrates, Stuttgart 1981, S. 217
[7] J. Sonnenbichler et al., Biochem. Pharmacol. **35**, 538 (1987).
[8] P. Ferenci et al., Heptaology **4**, 1093 (1984).
[9] P.J. Flory, G. Krug, D. Lorenz and W.H. Mennicke, Planta Med. **38**, 227 (1980).
[10] D. Lorenz, W.H. Mennicke and H. Berendt, Planta Med. **45**, 216 (1982).
[11] W. Spaich, Moderne Phytotherapie, Haug-Verlag, Heidelberg 1977.
[12] I. Merfort and G. Willuhn, Dtsch. Apoth. Ztg. **125**, 695 (1985).
[13] H. Wagner, S. Bladt, and E.M. Zgainski, Plant drug analysis, Springer-Verlag, Berlin, Heidelberg, New York, Tokyo, 1984, p. 190.

Cardui mariae herba   Milk-thistle herb

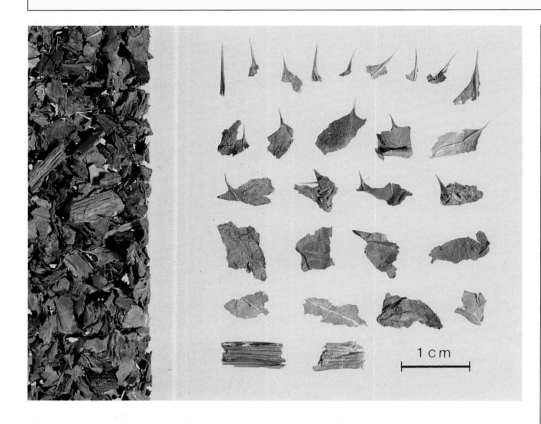

Fig. 1: Milk-thistle herb

<u>Description:</u> The drug comes from plants gathered before or during the flowering period, and it may therefore vary in appearance. There are deep green leaf fragments with white spots along the nerves and a sinuate-lobed margin that often bears stout yellow spines. Branching, somewhat brownish, slightly cottony pieces of stem are also present. Depending on the time of harvesting, there may also be flower-heads with purplish brown flowers and fruits are usually present as well (see: Milk-thistle fruit).

<u>Taste:</u> Distinctly bitter, sharp and unpleasantly salty.

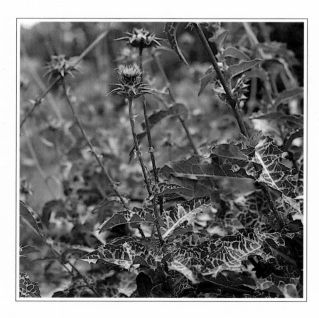

Fig. 2: *Silybum marianum* (L.) GAERTN.

A biennial thistle-like plant, up to 1.5 m in height (in cultivation even taller), with large and spiny, sinuate-lobed leaves, characteristically flecked with white especially along the nerves. Flower-heads, ca. 6 cm in diameter, comprising reddish violet tubular florets only, and with bracts ending in a stout recurved thorn. At the top of the fruit, a multiradiate white pappus.

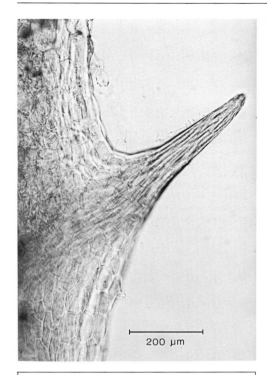

Fig. 3: Small spine at the leaf margin

Plant source: *Silybum marianum* (L.) GAERTN. (syn. *Carduus marianus* L.), milk thistle (Asteraceae).

Synonyms: Mariendistelkraut (Ger.).

Origin: see, Cardui mariae fructus (Milk-thistle fruit).

Constituents: Flavonoids: apigenin and its 7-*O*-glucoside, 7-*O*-glucuronide, and 4,7′-diglucoside, kaempferol and its 7′-glucoside and 3-sulphate, luteolin and its 7-glucoside [1, 2]. Sitosterol and its glucoside, a triterpene acetate [1], polyacetylenes [3], fumaric acid.

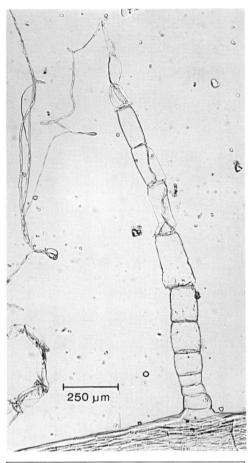

Fig. 4: Characteristic trichome with bulging cells and a very long, slender and tortuous terminal cell

Indications: As a cholagogue in supportive treatment of hepatic and biliary functional disorders. Pharmacological and clinical data to substantiate these applications are lacking. Formerly, in *folk medicine,* the drug was also used as an antimalarial, emmenagogue, and in disorders of the uterus and spleen.

Side effects: Poisoning, sometimes with a fatal outcome, has been observed in sheep and cattle [4]. There are no reports of its being toxic in man.

Making the tea: Not usual, or only in *folk medicine* for bile and liver complaints. Boiling water is poured over ca. half-a-teaspoonful of the finely chopped drug and after 5–10 min. passed through a tea strainer. Two or three cups a day are drunk.
1 Teaspoon = ca. 1.5 g.

Phytomedicines: The drug is an infrequent component of mixed herbal teas. Extracts are present in several prepared cholagogues, e.g. Hepafungin®-Tropfen (drops), Cholhepan®, etc.

Authentication: Macro- (see: Description) and microscopically. The spinous leaf margin is a distinct feature, especially on examination with a hand lens (Fig. 3). The epidermal cells are wavy-walled and the stomata on both surfaces have 3–5, but mostly 4, subsidiary cells. On the upper and the lower leaf surfaces, there are occasional uniseriate, multicellular trichomes which have very broad and short, somewhat bulging, cells towards the base and very thin-walled cells, which are therefore often collapsed, towards the tip; the very long terminal cells are slender and tortuous (Fig. 4). There are also three rows of rather wide palisade cells and the spongy mesophyll is very porous – almost like aerenchyma. The pollen grains have spines and are ca. 50 µm in diameter.

Adulteration: Rare. The suspicion of admixture or confusion with Cnicus benedicti herba (Holy thistle), which has sometimes been expressed, has not been confirmed.

Literature:
[1] S.M. Khafagy, N.A. Abdel Salam, and R. Abdel Hamir, Sci. Pharm. **49**, 157 (1981).
[2] A.H. Mericli, Planta Med. **54**, 44 (1988).
[3] K.E. Schulte, G. Rücker, and H. Stigler, Arch. Pharm. (Weinheim) **303**, 7 (1970).
[4] Hager, vol. **6**, 403 (1979).
[5] Report from Deutsches Arzneiprüfungs-Institut, Pharm. Ztg. **130**, 699, 2997 (1985).

Carlinae radix   Stemless carlina root

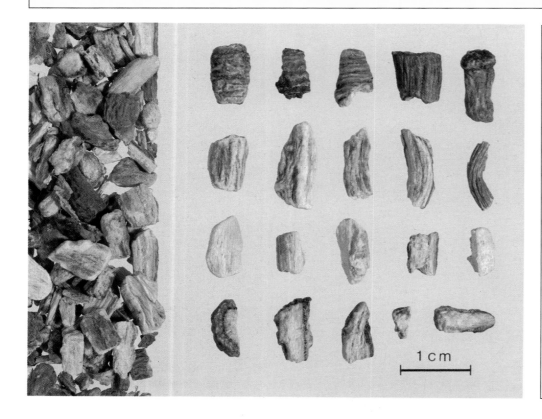

1 cm

Fig. 1: Stemless carlina root

Description: The drug consists of large, often twisted, short pieces of greyish brown to pale brown root, with coarse longitudinal wrinkles on the outer surface. The fracture is horny and not fibrous. The tranverse section shows a narrow brown cortex becoming lighter towards the inside, sometimes resinous and shiny, and a broad, light yellow xylem, radially striated by brownish medullary rays, and fissured in a characteristic fashion, owing to disruption of the vascular bundles during the drying process. Brownish red secretory glands can be seen in the narrow cortex and in the medullary-ray tissue (hand lens; Fig. 3).

Odour: Faintly aromatic, unpleasant.

Taste: Initially bitter-sweet, then pungent and acrid.

Fig. 2: *Carlina acaulis* L.

Thistle-like, short-stemmed, perennial herb with spiny, toothed, partly pinnate, leaves. Flower-heads up to 12 cm in diameter, with silvery involucral bracts.

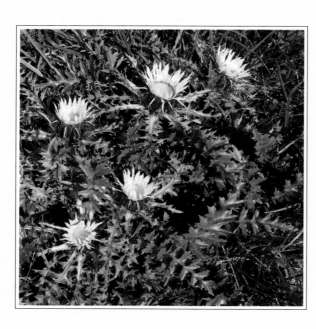

Erg. B. 6: Radix Carlinae

Plant source: *Carlina acaulis* L., stemless carline thistle (Asteraceae).

Synonyms: Radix Cardopatiae, Radix Chamaeleontis albae (Lat.), Eberwurz, Silberdistelwurz(el) (Ger.), Racine de carline acaule (Fr.).

Origin: Native in the mountains of central and southern Europe, in the Balkans, and in southern Russia. The drug comes entirely from the wild. In Germany, its collection is prohibited, as the plant is a protected species, and the drug is imported from former Yugoslavia and Bulgaria.

Constituents: The roots have not been adequately studied chemically. A number of early observations indicate that the drug has 1.5–2% essential oil, comprising up to 80% carlina oxide (benzyl-2-furylacetylene) and ca. 15% carilene ($C_{15}H_{24}$), as well as a phenol and palmitic acid. In addition, the drug contains tannins, resins, and 18–22% inulin.

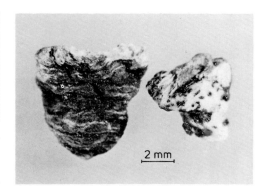

Carlina oxide

Fig. 3: **Numerous brownish red excretory glands in the paler cortex of *Carlina acaulis* root**

2 mm

Indications: The drug is now rarely employed. In *folk medicine,* it still finds very occasional use as a diuretic, diaphoretic, and stomachic, and sometimes also as a gargle against catarrh.

Externally, acetic extracts of the root are used to wash herpetic eruptions, suppurating rashes (pyodermias), and other skin conditions, as well as against toothache. In *folk medicine,* extracts prepared with wine and water are said to be good for washing out wounds and sores. The acetone extract, the essential oil, and carlina oxide have strong antibacterial activity, but not so the aqueous extract [1, 2]; among the bacteria tested were *Staphylococcus, Enterococcus, Salmonella,* and *Shigella.*

Making the tea: Cold water is added to 1.5 g of the finely cut or coarsely powdered drug, boiled for a short while, and then passed through a tea strainer. A cupful is drunk one to three times a day.

1 Teaspoon = ca. 2.8 g.

Phytomedicines: Extracts of stemless carlina root are a component of the multi-ingredient preparation Infi®-tract-Tropfen (drops) which finds use in gall-bladder disorders, digestive insufficiency, and gastrointestinal spasms. The drug is a component of the (gastrointestinal) remedy "Swedish bitters"; see the note under: Aloe capensis.

Authentication: Macro- (see: Description) and microscopically. Schizogenous secretory glands occur in the cortex and in the medullary rays; the xylem consists of broad medullary rays and narrow, light yellow rows of cells with large, thick-walled vessels; the parenchyma contains inulin masses (red coloration with α-naphthol/sulphuric acid reagent) and calcium oxalate in the form of small, single and twinned prisms.

Quantitative standards: <u>Erg. B. 6</u>: *Volatile oil,* not less than 1%. *Ash,* not more than 12%.

Adulteration: Very rare. Roots of other *Carlina* species can be recognized by their deviating diagnostic features: Carlinae sylvestris radix has no secretory glands and Carlinae gummiferae radix, which closely resembles the genuine drug, has laticifers in the phloem and also numerous fibres in the xylem. See also [3].

Recent examination of commercial samples of Carlinae radix has shown that most of them did not come from *C. acaulis,* as required by the Erg. B. 6, but that they consisted largely of the roots of *C. acanthifolia* ALL., a species which in France has much the same applications. The plant is to be looked upon as a substitute rather than an adulterant. Fingerprint chromatograms of various extracts from *C. acaulis* and *C. acanthifolia* are almost identical. However, the phytochemistry of carlina oxide, the active principle, in this latter species would need detailed study before official acceptance of it as an additional source of Carlina radix. The current situation is perhaps best described as a "commercial compromise" [3].

Storage: Protected from light and moisture in well-sealed containers (not made of plastic).

Literature:
[1] J. Schmidt-Thomé, Z. Naturforsch. **5b**, 409 (1950).
[2] H.D. Stachel, Dtsch. Apoth. Ztg. **101**, 1233 (1960).
[3] H. Schilcher and H. Hagels, Dtsch. Apth. Ztg. **130**, 2186 (1990).

Carvi fructus   (DAB 10), Caraway (*BAN*, BP 1988; *USAN*), Carum (BHP 1983)

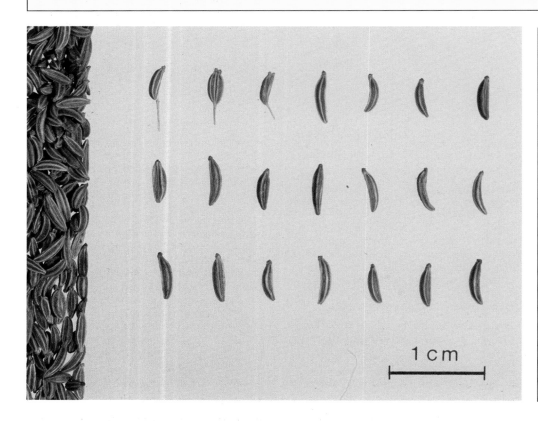

1 cm

Fig. 1: Caraway

<u>Description:</u> **The drug consists of the mericarps of the original cremocarps (double achenes). They are glabrous, 3–6 mm long, ca. 1 mm thick, greyish brown, and mostly slightly crescent-shaped with both ends pointed. On the somewhat convex outer surface there are three, and on the edge of the slightly concave commisural surface two, straight and narrow, prominent light-coloured ridges. At the upper end, the pistil with its roundish cushion (pulvinus) is often still present.**

<u>Odour:</u> **Aromatic.**

<u>Taste:</u> **Spicy and aromatic.**

Fig. 2: *Carum carvi* L.

A perennial, up to 1 m in height with finely lacerate (2–3 times pinnately divided) leaves, occurring in meadows and along roadsides. Small white to faint pink flowers arranged in compound umbels, often without bracts and bracteoles.

Fig. 3: *Carum carvi* L.

Fruiting and showing the oblong cremocarps (double achenes)

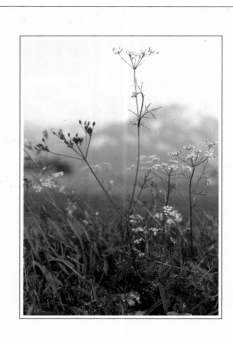

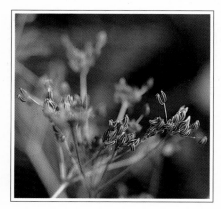

DAB 10: Kümmel
ÖAB: Fructus Carvi
Ph. Helv. VII: Carvi fructus
St.Zul.: 1109.99.99

Plant source: *Carum carvi* L., caraway (Apiaceae = Umbelliferae).

Origin: Native in Europe; the drug comes from cultivated plants, especially from Poland, the eastern part of Germany, and Egypt. The fruits are usually harvested before they are fully ripe – when the essential-oil content is at its greatest.

Synonyms: Semen Cumini pratensis (Lat.), Caraway fruit or seeds (Engl.), Kümmel, Wiesen- or Feldkümmel, Kümmich (Ger.), Semences (Fruits) de carvi, Cumin des prés, Anis des Vosges (Fr.).

Constituents: 3–7% essential oil, with as main odoriferous component (S)-(+)-carvone (up to 65%); also (*R*)-(+)-limonene (up to ca. 50%) and other terpenes (including α- and β-pinene, sabinene, car-3-ene, isomers of dihydrocarvone, dihydrocarveol, and

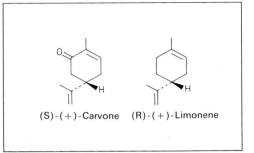

(S)-(+)-Carvone   (R)-(+)-Limonene

carveol). Further, 10–18% fixed oil, ca. 20% protein, ca. 20% carbohydrate; flavonoids [1, 2, 5].

Indications: As a stomachic, since the essential oil promotes gastric secretion and stimulates the appetite. Because of its good spasmolytic activity (like fennel, aniseed, and coriander), as a carminative, e.g. in tympanites (meteorism) and flatulence; also as a cholagogue. Caraway oil has been shown to have marked fungicidal activity (stronger than that of nystatin) [3].
In *folk medicine*, caraway is also employed as a galactagogue. The essential oil is included in mouth washes for gargling and in skin frictions (to bring about hyperaemia). The bulk of caraway is used as a spice and taste enhancer, as well as to improve the tolerance to foods causing flatulence, e.g. cabbage, fresh bread, and in the preparation of liqueurs and spirits, e.g. Kümmel, etc. [2, 4].

Making the tea: Boiling water is poured over 1–5 g of freshly crushed caraway, covered and allowed to stand for 10–15 min., and then passed through a tea strainer.
1 Teaspoon = ca. 3.5 g.

Phytomedicines: As a component of gastrointestinal remedies (carminatives, laxatives) in the form of alcoholic distillates and drops, often together with other drugs containing essential oils, such as aniseed, coriander, fennel, etc.

Regulatory status (UK): General Sales List – Schedule 1, Table A.

Authentication: Macro- (see: Description) and microscopically, following the DAB 10; see also the BP 1988. The detailed mi-

croscopy of the powder is described and illustrated in [6].
The DAB 10 TLC test of identity is as follows:

Test solution: 0.5 g freshly powdered drug shaken for 2–3 min. with 5.0 ml dichloromethane and filtered over ca. 2 g anhydrous sodium sulphate; filtrate = test solution.

Reference solution: 2 µl carvone + 5 µl olive oil dissolved in 1.0 ml dichloromethane.

Loadings: 20 µl test solution and 10 µl reference solution, as 2-cm bands on silica gel GF_{254}.

Solvent system: dichloromethane, 2 × 10 cm run.

Detection and Evaluation: examination in UV 254 nm light and quenching zones noted; then sprayed with anisaldehyde reagent, heated for 5–10 min. at 100–105 °C while under observation and examined in daylight. Reference solution: at about the middle, the quenching, but after spraying, strong orange-brown carvone zone and slightly above it the violet triglycerides zone.

Test solution: zones of similar intensity, size, colour, and position; near the solvent front, an inconspicuous violet zone, due to terpene hydrocarbons; in the lower part, a few faint, mostly greyish violet and brownish zones.

Quantitative standards: BP 1988: *Volatile oil*, not less than 3.5%. *Foreign matter*, not more than 2.0%. *Acid-insoluble ash*, not more than 1.5%.
DAB 10: *Volatile oil*, not less than 3.0%. *Foreign (vegetable and/or mineral) matter*, not more than 2%. *Loss on drying*, not more than 12.0%. *Ash*, not more than 7.0%.

Adulteration: Rare.

Storage: Protected from moisture and light in well-closed metal or glass, but not plastic, containers (BP 1988, not above 25 °C).

Literature:
[1] V. Formácek and K.-H. Kubeczka, Essential oils analysis by capillary gas chromatography and carbon-13 NMR spectroscopy, Wiley, Chichester, 1982.
[2] Kommentar DAB 10.
[3] G.G. Ibragimov and O.D. Vasilev, Azerb. Med. **62**, 44 (1985); C.A. **103**, 138380 (1985).
[4] Hager, vol. **3**, 727 (1972); vol. **4**, 693 (1992).
[5] M. Gorunovic, Acta Pharm. Jugoslav. **41**, 267 (1991).
[6] B.P. Jackson and D.W. Snowdon, Atlas of microscopy of medicinal plants, culinary herbs and spices, Belhaven Press, London, 1990, p. 42.

Caryophylli flos   (DAB 10, Ph. Eur. 2), Clove (BAN; BP 1988)

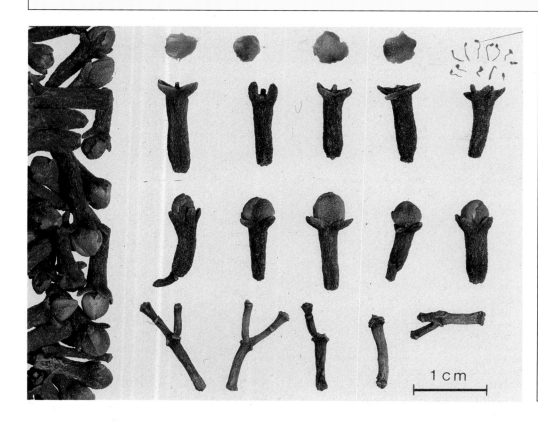

Fig. 1: Clove

Description: The drug consists of the dried buds. These are dark brown, 12–17 mm long, and comprise the elongated and up to 4 mm wide hypanthium, with its four stout, projecting, calyx lobes. The four paler, yellowish brown petals form a hood (middle row) underneath which are numerous stamens (above right). In the upper part of the hypanthium there is the inferior bilocular ovary with numerous ovules.
On bruising the clove with the fingernail, essential oil exudes from the spot where the pressure was applied.

Odour: Strongly aromatic.

Taste: Pungently spicy.

Fig. 2: *Syzygium aromaticum* (L.) MERR. et L.M. PERRY

An up to 20 m tall, slender, evergreen tree, with entire, leathery leaves. Flowers in compact repeatedly branching cymes. The illustration shows the buds immediately before harvesting.

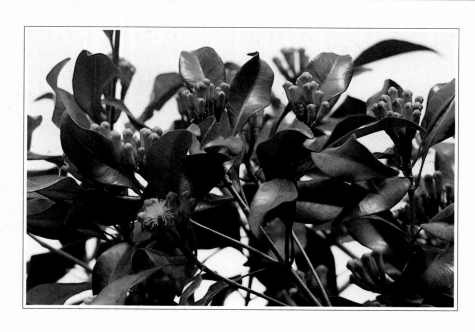

DAB 10: Gewürznelken
Ph. Helv. VII: Caryophylli flos
ÖAB: Flos Caryophylli

Plant source: *Syzygium aromaticum* (L.) MERR. et L.M. PERRY (syn. *Caryophyllus aromaticus* L., *Jambosa caryophyllus* (SPRENG.) NIED., *Eugenia caryophyllus* (SPRENG.) BULLOCK et S.K. HARRIS), clove (Myrtaceae).

Synonyms: Flores caryophylli (Lat.), Caryophyllum (Engl.), Gewürznelken, Nägelein (Ger.), Clous de girofle (Fr.).

Origin: Native in the Moluccas and the southern Philippines, but nowadays cultivated in many tropical countries. Imports come from Madagascar, Indonesia, Malaysia, East African islands (Zanzibar and Pemba), Sri Lanka, and South America.

Constituents: 15% to more than 20% essential oil with eugenol as the main component (85–95% of the oil), a little eugenol acetate, β-caryophyllene and its oxide, α-humulene and its epoxide, etc.; flavonoids (quercetin

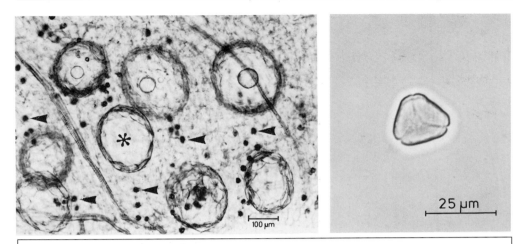

Fig. 3: Large schizogenous oil glands (*) and numerous calcium oxalate cluster crystals (◄) in the petal of *Syzygium aromaticum*

Fig. 4: Characteristic, tetrahedral pollen grain of *Syzygium aromaticum*

Extract from the German Commission E monograph (BAnz no. 223, dated 30.11.1985)

Uses

Inflammation of the mucous membranes of the mouth and throat.
In dentistry, as a topical analgesic.

Contraindications

None known.

Side effects

In concentrated form, clove oil irritates the tissues.

Interactions with other remedies

None known.

Dosage

Unless otherwise prescribed: in mouth washes, equivalent to 1–5% essential oil; in dentistry, the undiluted oil.

Mode of administration

Powdered, comminuted, or whole drug to obtain the essential oil, and other galenical preparations for topical use.

Effects

Antiseptic, antibacterial, antifungal, antiviral, local-anaesthetic, spasmolytic.

and kaempferol derivatives); tannins; phenolic carboxylic acids (gallic acid, protocatechuic acid, etc.); small amounts of sterols and sterol glycosides; ca. 10% fixed oil [1, 3].

Indications: The drug is used primarily as a spice. The essential oil has marked antibacterial activity and as such (clove oil: Ph. Eur. 2, BP 1988, etc.) is much used as an antiseptic in dentistry.

Besides its use as an aromatic, it has a modest role, almost always in combination with other drugs, as a carminative, stomachic, and tonic.

Cloves are said to have a positive effect on the healing of stomach ulcers [2]. The sesquiterpenes cited above (section on constituents) have been shown to have significant activity in inducing the detoxifying enzyme glutathione *S*-transferase in mouse liver and small intestine; the ability of natural anticarcinogens to induce such detoxifying enzymes correlates well with their ability to inhibit chemical carcinogenesis [3].

Making the tea: Not applicable.

Herbal preparations: Cloves are a more or less regular component of spice mixtures intended for making mulled wine.

Phytomedicines: Occasionally, in antitussives and expectorants, as well as gastrointestinal remedies.

OH
OCH₃

Eugenol

Regulatory status (UK): General Sales List – oil: Schedule 1, Table A.

Authentication: Macro- (see: Description) and microscopically. Prominent features are the numerous, fairly large (up to 200 µm in diameter) schizogenous oil glands in the parenchyma of the hyphanthium, petals, and ovary, and the numerous small calcium oxalate cluster crystals (Fig. 3). The mostly still closed anthers have a stellate endothecium. The pollen grains, which often adhere to the material, are tetrahedral and the pores can be seen at the truncated corners (Fig. 4). The detailed microscopy of powdered cloves is described and illustrated in [4].
The Ph. Eur. 2, etc. require a TLC identity test.

Quantitative standards: <u>Ph. Eur. 2, etc.</u>: *Volatile oil*, not less than 15.0% (BP 1988: powdered cloves, not less than 12%). *For-*

eign matter, not more than 4% blown (opened) cloves, peduncles (Fig. 1, bottom row), and fruits; not more than 2% fermented cloves; not more than 0.5% other foreign matter. *Sulphated ash*, not more than 8.0%.

Adulteration: Nowadays, rare. "Exhausted" cloves can be recognized by the "fingernail test" (see: Description); in distilled water, to some extent they float or lie horizontally, while the genuine drug sinks or floats vertically.
The fruits of *Syzygium aromaticum* are ca. 25 mm long and this alone, as well as their ventricose shape, allows them to be easily recognized. Since they are more expensive than cloves, they play no part as an adulterant.

Literature:
[1] Kommentar DAB 10.
[2] S.H. Zaidi, Ind. J. Med. Res. **46**, 732 (1958).
[3] G.-Q. Zheng, P.M. Kenney, and L.K.T. Lam, J. Nat. Prod. **55**, 999 (1992).
[4] B.P. Jackson and D.W. Snowdon, Atlas of microscopy of medicinal plants, culinary herbs and spices, Belhaven Press, London, 1990, p. 64.

Castaneae folium   Castanea (BHP 1983), Chestnut leaf

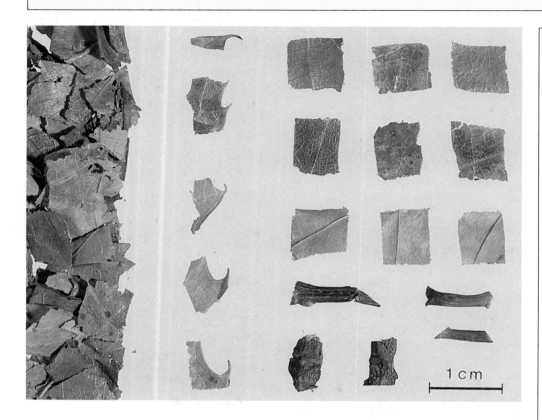

Fig. 1: Chestnut leaf

<u>Description:</u> The leaves gathered in September/October are up to 20 cm long and up to 7 cm wide, with a distinctly serrate and mucronate and, on the lower surface, swollen margin. One of the parallel lateral nerves runs into each mucro, which is often curved inwards. In contrast to the young leaves, the mature ones are only slightly pubescent (Fig. 3). The cut drug consists mainly of tough, leathery pieces of leaf with a green upper surface; the midrib and lateral nerves stand out conspicuously from the lower surface. Occasionally, petiole fragments are present.

<u>Taste:</u> Astringent.

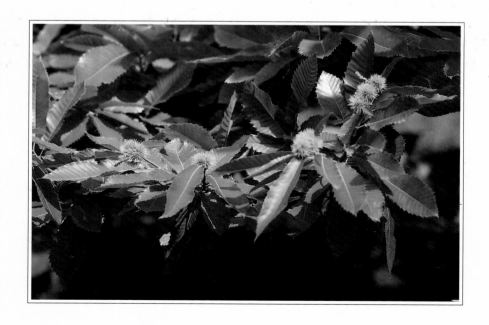

Fig. 2: *Castanea sativa* MILL.

A tree up to 30 m in height with oblong lanceolate, mucronate and serrate leaves. Male flowers in erect catkins; 1–3 female flowers grouped in a scaly receptacle. Fruit densely spiny with brown seeds.

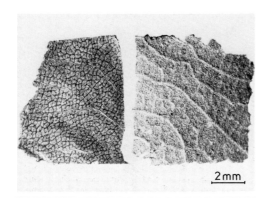

Fig. 3: *Castanea sativa* **leaf: mature, sparsely hairy (left), and young, very hairy lower surface (right)**

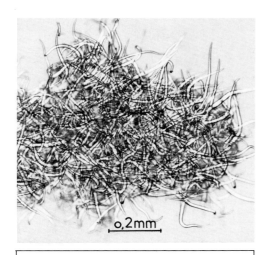

Fig. 4: The matted trichomes on the lower surface of a young leaf

Plant source: *Castanea sativa* MILL. (syn. *C. vesca* GAERTN., *C. vulgaris* LAM.), sweet or Spanish chestnut (Fagaceae).

Synonyms: Edelkastanienblätter (Ger.), Feuilles de châtaigner (Fr.).

Origin: A decorative and useful plant of the Mediterranean region and south-eastern Europe. The drug comes mostly from plantations and is imported from the former USSR, former Yugoslavia, and Hungary.

Constituents: Ca. 9% tannins whose nature is not precisely known (both gallic and ellagic acids have been detected); flavonoids, especially quercetin derivatives [1]; triterpenes, e.g. ursolic acid [2]; ca. 0.2% vitamin C [3]; other ubiquitous substances.

Indications: Like other tannin-containing drugs, chestnut leaf can be used as an astringent. So far, no substances have been detected that support the use in *folk medicine* as an expectorant and whooping-cough reme-dy. As the availability of many commercial phytomedicines shows, this fact does not appear to be an obstacle to making use of the drug (as extract).

Making the tea: Boiling water is poured over 2–4 g of the finely cut leaves and after standing for a short time passed through a tea strainer, or cold water is added to the same amount of drug, boiled for a short time, and then strained.
1 Teaspoon = ca. 1.0 g.

Phytomedicines: More than 20 multi-ingredient preparations, chiefly antitussives and expectorants, contain the extract or fluid extract of the drug; they include Guakalin® (cough cordial, drops), Respirogutt®-Tropfen (drops), Equisil® (juice), etc.

Authentication: Apart from the macroscopic characters, among the microscopically observable diagnostic features are: thick-walled trichomes on the lower surface of the leaf (Fig. 4); epidermal cells which are wavy-walled on the lower surface, but polygonal and pitted on the upper surface; in the mesophyll, cluster crystals of calcium oxalate up to 60 mm in diameter.
Descriptions of the macro- and microscopical features are also to be found in the BHP 1983.

Quantitative standards: BHP 1983: *Foreign organic matter*, not more than 5%. *Acid-insoluble ash*, not more than 2%.

Adulteration: Almost never.

Literature:
[1] G. Romussi, L. Mosti, and G. Ciarallo, Pharmazie **36**, 718 (1981).
[2] A. Marsili and I. Morelli, Phytochemistry **11**, 2633 (1972).
[3] E. Jones and R.E. Hughes, Phytochemistry **23**, 2366 (1984).

Centaurii herba   (DAB 10), Lesser centaury, Centaurium (BHP 1983)

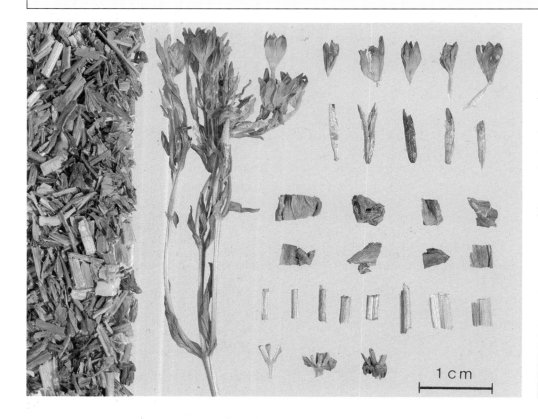

Fig. 1: Lesser centaury

<u>Description</u>: **Prominent features of the drug, which consists of the aerial parts of the flowering plant, are the mostly yellowish, 4-angled, hollow pieces of stem and the up to 8 mm long reddish flowers. Fragments of the small, entire, and glabrous opposite leaves, on the other hand, are less conspicuous. Occasionally, two-valved dehiscent fruits are present (Fig. 3), together with the loose, very small seeds discharged from them. Another characteristic feature is the anthers which become spirally twisted after releasing their pollen (Fig. 4).**

<u>Odour</u>: **Faint and characteristic.**

<u>Taste</u>: **Very bitter.**

Fig. 2: *Centaurium erythraea* RAFN

A biennial, only 30 cm in height, producing a basal rosette of elliptical to spathulate leaves in the first year and a branched flowering stem bearing small sessile, 5-part, pinkish red, tubular flowers in flat umbels in the second year.

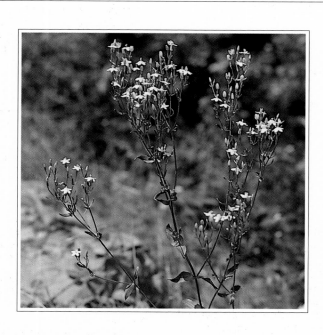

DAB 10: Tausendgüldenkraut
Ph. Helv. VII: Centaurii herba
ÖAB: Herba Centaurii
St. Zul. 1319.99.99

Plant source: *Centaurium erythraea* RAFN subsp. *erythraea* (syn. *C. minus* MOENCH [thus in the DAB 10], *C. umbellatum* GILIB., *Erythraea centaurium* (L.) PERS.), common centaury (Gentianaceae).

Synonyms: Herba Chironiae or Felis terrae (Lat.), Centaury herb (Engl.), Tausendgüldenkraut, Fieberkraut, Bitterkraut (Ger.), Herbe de petite centaurée, Gentianelle (Fr.).

Origin: Scattered to widespread in Europe, North America, North Africa, and western Asia. The drug is imported from Morocco, former Yugoslavia, Bulgaria, and Hungary.

Constituents: Small amounts of intensely bitter-tasting secoiridoid glycosides, especially centapicrin (bitterness value ca. 4,000,000), swertiamarin, sweroside, and gentiopicroside [1, 2], and in smaller amounts the dimeric secoiridoid centau-

Sweroside: $R^1 = H$, $R^2 = H$
Centapicrin: R^1 = m-Hydroxybenzoyl
R^2 = Acetyl

Swertiamarin   Gentiopicroside

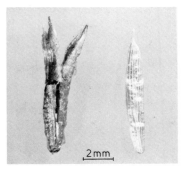
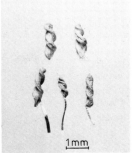
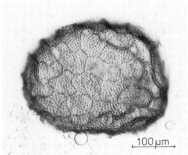

Fig. 3: Fruit of *Centaurium erythraea*, a capsule (left, ripe; right, unripe)

Fig. 4: Spirally-twisted anthers from the flower

Fig. 5: Typical seeds with a verrucose testa

roside [3]. The drug contains up to 0.4% flavonoids, methoxylated xanthone derivatives, e.g. methylbellidifolin, phenol-carboxylic acids, triterpenes, sterols, and traces of pyridine and actinidine alkaloids [4]. 2-Hydroxy- and 2,5-dihydroxyterephthalic acids are present in the aerial parts and the roots [6].

Indications: As a bitter, for stimulating the appetite and increasing the secretion of the gastric juice, especially in chronic dyspeptic states and achylia; it is less active than comparable drugs, e.g. gentian root.
In *folk medicine*, it is also employed as a roborant and tonic.

Making the tea: Boiling water (ca. 150 ml) is poured over 2–3 g of the finely chopped drug and after 10 min. strained. Some authors recommend extracting the drug with cold water for several hours.
1 Teaspoon = ca. 1.8 g.

Herbal preparations: The drug is also offered in tea bags (1.0 or 1.8 g). Dry extracts of the drug are present in instant teas for use as gastrointestinal remedies and liver and bile remedies.

Phytomedicines: About 40 prepared remedies with extracts of the drug, as gastrointestinal remedies and cholagogues, as well as urological remedies, e.g. Canephron®, Nephro-Tonikum®.

Authentication: Macro- (see: Description) and microscopically, following the DAB 10; see also the BHP 1983. The numerous single oxalate crystals in the mesophyll, the crisscross layers of fibres of the testa, and the small brown seeds with a finely punctate epidermis (Fig. 5) are diagnostic features. The DAB 10 method for the TLC test of

identity (detection of the bitter substances) is as follows:

Test solution: 1.0 g powdered drug refluxed for 10 min. with 20 ml methanol and filtered when cold.

Reference solution: 10 mg rutin dissolved in 10 ml methanol.

Loadings: 30 µl test solution and 10 µl reference solution, as 2-cm bands on silica gel GF_{254}.

Solvent system: ethyl acetate + glacial acetic acid + water (69 + 16 + 16), 2×12 cm run with in between 5 min. drying in a current of cold air.

Detection and Evaluation: In UV 254 nm light. <u>Test solution:</u> the main quenching zone (swertiamarin) at about the same Rf as the rutin reference zone; other quenching zones all very faint.

Then sprayed with anisaldehyde reagent and kept under observation while being heated at 100–105 °C for 5–10 min. Reference solution: rutin as a yellowish brown, green fluorescent zone. Test solution: swertiamarin as a brown zone; a little above it, a faint yellowish zone and above that, as far as the reddish violet zone at the solvent front, only a few very faint, mostly grey zones; a strong, somewhat diffuse yellow zone slightly below the swertiamarin zone.

After spraying and heating, in UV 365 nm light. Test solution: swertiamarin as a strong brown to brownish yellow fluorescent zone; just above it, a bright green to yellowish green fluorescent zone; as far as the faint reddish violet fluorescent zone, only a few weak bluish or yellowish fluorescent zones; below the swertiamarin zone, bright green to yellowish green (some intense) fluorescent zones, along with a couple of faint brownish fluorescent zones.

Other TLC systems are to be found in [7].

Quantitative standards: DAB 10: *Bitterness value*, not less than 2000. *Foreign matter*, not more than 3%. *Loss on drying*, not more than 10.0%. *Ash*, not more than 6.0%.
ÖAB: *Bitterness value*, not less than 2000. *Foreign matter*, not more than 1%. *Ash*, not more than 4.0%.
Ph. Helv. VII: *Bitterness value*, not less than 100 Ph. Helv. units/g. *Foreign matter*,

not more than 3%. *Sulphated ash*, not more than 8%.
BHP 1983: *Foreign organic matter*, not more than 2%. *Total ash*, not more than 8%. *Acid-insoluble ash*, not more than 2%.
The bitterness values are only attained with an appropriate proportion of flowers, which have the highest content of bitter substances.

Adulteration: Very rare, with other *Centaurium* species, e.g. *C. pulchellum* (SCHWARTZ) DRUCE, lesser centaury, recognizable by the distinctly pedicelled flowers. Since this species contains very similar iridoids [5], it can be regarded rather as a substitute. It can be differentiated by TLC [5]: a methanolic extract of *C. pulchellum*, when separated on silanized silica gel 60F$_{254}$ with ethyl formate saturated with water as solvent system, shows a distinct xanthone spot in the middle Rf range which is absent from extracts of *C. erythraea*.

The question of adulteration is not as simple as portrayed in the previous paragraph. According to Länger [8], it is not possible to identify the cut drug unequivocally by morphological- anatomical studies on their own. Not only that, but the hierarchical (taxonomic) rank of the various plants raises problems: thus, the DAB 10 only permits *C. minus* – the correct name for which is *C. erythraea* – and all other species are adul-

terants. But, depending on its rank, the particularly good drug from Morocco (so-called "Atlas quality") is either an adulterant, if it is called *C. majus* (HOFFMANNS. et LINK) ZELTNER, or admissible, if it is named *C. erythraea* subsp. *majus* (HOFFMANNS. et LINK) MELDERIS. Länger therefore proposes that all species of the genus *Centaurium* are worth considering as source plants for the pharmacopoeial drug Centaurii herba, provided they have the required bitterness value (not less than 2000). It is worth pointing out that so far no injurious constituents have been reported from *Centaurium* species. As regards active principles, Länger [see 8], distinguishes between less satisfactory and satisfactory taxa.

Literature:
[1] W.G. van der Sluis and R.P. Labadie, Pharm. Weekbl. **113**, 21 (1978).
[2] W.G. van der Sluis and R.P. Labadie, Planta Med. **41**, 150 (1981).
[3] S. Takagi et al., Yakugaku Zasshi **102**, 313 (1982); C.A. **97**, 52511 (1982).
[4] Kommentar DAB 10.
[5] W.G. van der Sluis and R.P. Labadie, Planta Med. **41**, 221 (1981).
[6] M. Hatjimanoli et al., J. Nat. Prod. **51**, 977 (1988).
[7] H. Wagner, S. Bladt, and E.M. Zgainski, Plant drug analysis, Springer-Verlag, Berlin, Heidelberg, New York, Tokyo, 1984, p. 132.
[8] R. Länger, Dtsch. Apoth. Ztg. **130**, 2366 (1990).

Cetrariae lichen   (DAB 10), Iceland moss

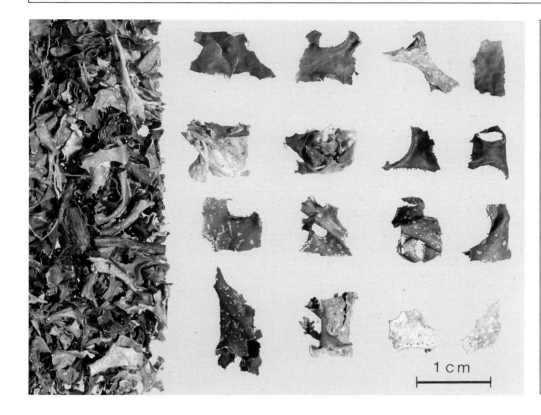

Fig. 1: Iceland moss

The usual name in English ("moss") and German ("Moos") is incorrect, since the plant concerned is not a moss (member of the Bryophyta) but a lichen (member of the Lichenes).

<u>Description:</u> The drug consists of the dried thallus, which is foliaceous, with irregular dichotomous branching and broader or narrower, channelled or almost flat, sometimes curled, segments. The side turned towards the light is greenish brown, while the side away from the light is whitish to pale brownish. The thallus is glabrous on both sides and has a fringed margin (Fig. 3). When dry, it is brittle, but on moistening with water it becomes soft and cartilaginous. The chopped drug consists of irregular, sometimes curled, fragments.

<u>Odour:</u> Faint and characteristic.

<u>Taste:</u> Bland, mucilaginous and bitter.

Fig. 2: *Cetraria islandica* (L.) ACH. s.l.

A ca. 10 cm high lichen, growing on the ground, the brown shrubby thallus lobed and forked and with a fringed margin. Upper surface olive-green to brown and lower surface whitish grey and flecked with white.

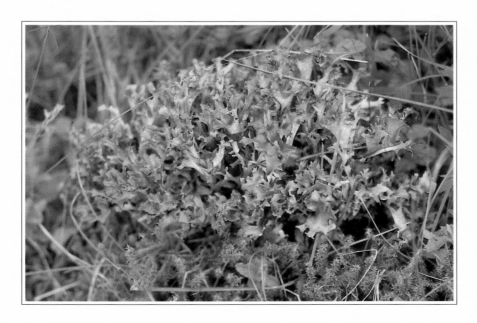

DAB 10: Isländisches Moos
ÖAB, Ph. Helv. VII: Lichen islandicus
St.Zul. 1049.99.99

Plant source: *Cetraria islandica* (L.) ACH. s.l. (Parmeliaceae – Lichenes). *C. ericetorum* OPIZ (syn. *C. tenuifolia* (RETZ.) HOWE), at one time considered to be no more than a smaller form of *C. islandica*, is also permitted as a source of the drug.

Synonyms: Fucus or Muscus or Lichen islandicus or catharticus, Thallus Cetrariae islandicae (Lat.), Cetraria (Engl.), Isländisches Moos, Isländische Flechte, Heide-, Blätter-, or Fieberflechte, Fieber-, Lungen- or Purgiermoos (Ger.), Lichen d'Islande (Fr.).

Origin: In the higher mountains of northern, central, and eastern Europe. The drug is collected in the wild and imported principally from Bulgaria, former Yugoslavia, the former USSR, and Romania.

Constituents: Ca. 50% water-soluble polysaccharides, with as main component lichenin, a linear cellulose-like polymer of β-D-glucose with alternating 1 → 3 and 1 → 4 linkages (which is only soluble in hot water and which on cooling forms a gel that is not stained with iodine reagent) and isolichenin, a linear starch-like polymer of α-D-glucose with 1 → 3 and 1 → 4 linkages (which is soluble in cold water and which is stained blue with iodine reagent [1–3]). In addition, alkali-soluble polysaccharides, which are polymers of D-glucose and D-glucuronic acid [4], and galactomannans, have been identified [5]. There are also bitter-tasting lichen acids, e.g. depsidones such as cetraric acid and fumaroprotocetraric acid (2–3%), which are probably converted to protocetraric and fumaric acids during storage and processing of the drug; also protolichesteric acid, which on drying forms lichestearic acid; further, usnic acid (?) [6]; for additional information about the constituents, see [3, 7].

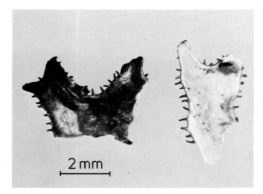
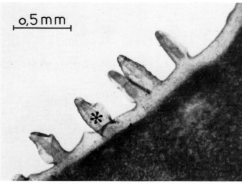

Fig. 3: Fragment of the thallus of the lichen *Cetraria islandica*, showing the fringed margin

Fig. 4: Margin of the thallus, showing cylindrical spermogonia (*) and the colourless cortical layer (loose hyphal tissue without algae)

Indications: In the form of decoctions, as a demulcent and expectorant for alleviating irritation of the throat in coughs (here, the antibiotic and bacteriostatic lichen acids may be of significance [8]; the immunostimulant effects of extracts of the drug, observed by Japanese workers, may also contribute to a more rapid recovery from disorders of the respiratory tract [cf. 7]; for lack of appetite and gastroenteritis (in this case, the lichen acids function as a bitter tonic). A review of the therapeutic applications of the drug is given in [7].

In *folk medicine*, the drug is also used for pulmonary complaints, as a galactagogue, as a roborant, and for kidney and bladder disorders; externally, it is applied to poorly healing wounds (antibiotic effect of the lichen acids). Boiling removes the bitterness from the drug, and its effects are then due only to the mucilage present [9, 10].

Making the tea: Boiling water is poured over 1.5–2.5 g of the finely chopped drug and after 10 min. passed through a tea strainer.

To obtain an expectorant which has plenty of mucilage, but which is less bitter, it has been suggested that, after pouring the hot water over the drug, the water should be immediately discarded (it contains most of the lichen acids) and then more hot water added [6]; However, doing this also removes the antibiotically active constituents!
1 Teaspoon = ca. 1.3 g.

Herbal preparations: A spray-dried extract is a component of instant bronchial and cough teas, e.g. Isla-Mint®, Isla-Moos®, etc.

Phytomedicines: Together with other "cough remedies", in various preparations for coughs (expectorants, antitussives) and colds, chills, etc., e.g. in teas; as an extract in cough sweets and lozenges for throat infections, e.g. Isla-Moos® (pastilles), etc.
Among the UK products is the multi-ingredient Gerard House Iceland Moss Compound Tablets.

Authentication: Macro- (see: Description) and microscopically: the transverse section shows a cortical layer on both sides, comprising interwoven and compressed hyphae (Fig. 4), below each of which is a layer of looser hyphal tissue with the roundish conidia. The centre consists of a loose tissue of thread-like hyphae. Spherical greenish to brownish cells, 10–15 μm in diameter, are embedded in the hyphal tissue. The distal ends of the projections at the margin of the thallus are often more or less narrowed (Fig. 3).

Other simple tests: Powdered Icelandic moss boiled with 10 parts water for 2–3 min. gives a bitter-tasting mucilage that solidifies on cooling. – Microsublimation yields a white, very finely granular, microcrystalline

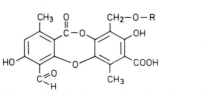

Fumaroprotocetraric acid: R = −CO−CH=CH−COOH
Cetraric acid: R = −C₂H₅
Protocetraric acid: R = −H

Protolichestearic acid

sublimate of fumaric acid and lichestearic acid, dissolving readily in ammonia to give a colourless solution; soon after, acicular, often branched, clusters of ammonium fumarate and ammonium lichestearate crystals appear. – 0.5 g tannin added to 10 ml of a 1% decoct of Icelandic moss furnishes a white turbidity that disappears on warming and reappears on cooling (lichenin). – Boiled-up fragments of thallus exhibit white spots on the surface and when saturated with iodine reagent and washed with water the fragments are stained blue (isolichenin). The DAB 10 includes a specially developed TLC test of identity which produces a characteristic lichen-acid profile [3]:

Test solution: 0.10 g powdered drug warmed for 2–3 min. at ca. 50 °C with 2.0 ml acetone, then cooled and filtered.

Reference solution: 5 mg caffeic acid in 2.0 ml methanol.

Loadings: 20 µl test solution and 10 µl reference solution, as 2-cm bands on silica gel GF$_{254}$.

Solvent system: glacial acetic acid + methanol + chloroform (10 + 10 + 80), 10 cm run.

Detection and Evaluation: in UV 254 nm light. Reference solution: in the lower third, the caffeic-acid quenching zone (fluorescing blue in UV 365 nm light). Test solution: a relatively large quenching zone (fumaroprotocetraric acid) at about the same Rf as the reference caffeic acid.
Sprayed with 0.1% ethanolic *p*-phenylenediamine. Test solution: the fumaroprotocetraric acid zone ochre-yellow (showing intense fluorescence of the same colour in UV 365 nm light); other, weak fluorescent zones present.

Quantitative standards: DAB 10: *Swelling index* (determined on the powdered drug), not less than 4.5. *Foreign matter*, not more than 5%. *Loss on drying*, not more than 12.0%. *Ash*, not more than 3.0%.
ÖAB: *Foreign matter*, not more than 3%. *Ash*, not more than 3.0%.

Ph. Helv. VII: *Swelling index*, not less than 5. *Foreign matter*, not more than 3%. *Sulphated ash*, not more than 3.0%.
BHP 1983: *Foreign organic matter*, not more than 3%. *Total ash*, not more than 2%.

Adulteration: Very rare, e.g. with *Cladonia* species. These, however, can be detected by the tests set out above. Contamination with mosses, grass, or other foreign matter should be checked.

Literature:
[1] M. Luckner, O. Bessler, and P. Schröder, Pharmazie **20**, 80 (1965).
[2] Hager, vol. **3**, p. 824 (1972); vol **4**, 790 (1992).
[3] Kommentar DAB 10.
[4] M. Hranisavljević-Jakovljević et al., Carbohydrate Res. **80**, 291 (1980).
[5] P.A.J. Philip and M. Iacomini, Carbohydrate Res. **128**, 119 (1984).
[6] F.-C. Czygan, unpublished (1987): 15 commercial (wholesale) samples, along with 36 samples and herbarium specimens collected by the writer, and all unequivocally identified as *Cetraria islandica*, were compared by TLC with authentic usnic acid. 6 of the commercial samples and 16 of the other samples contained usnic acid. Either there are chemical races or the content varies as a result of still undetermined factors.
[7] Th. Kartnig, Z. Phytotherap. **8**, 127 (1987).
[8] O. Sticher, Pharm. Acta Helv. **40**, 385 (1965).
[9] H. Braun and D. Frohne, Heilpflanzenlexikon für Ärzte und Apotheker, G. Fischer, Stuttgart – New York, 1987.
[10] R.F. Weiß, Herbal Medicine, Arcanum, Gothenburg, and Beaconsfield Publishers, Beaconsfield, 1988.

Chamomillae romanae flos

(DAB 10, Ph. Eur. 2, etc.), Chamomile flowers (*BAN*; BP 1988), Roman chamomile flower (BHP 1/1990)

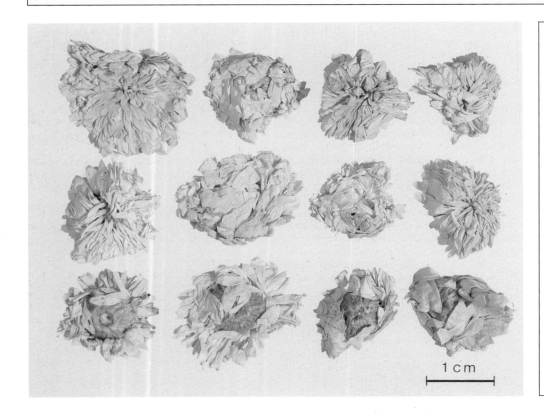

1 cm

Fig. 1: Roman chamomile flowers

<u>Description:</u> The white to yellowish white flower-heads of the double variety are 2–3 cm in diameter and have 2–3 rows of erect, imbricate, pale green, narrowly lanceolate, membranaceous, involucral bracts. The up to 7 mm long, female ray-florets have four more or less parallel nerves, an irregular three-toothed tip, and a short, yellowish brown ovary (achene). In the centre of the flower-head, there are a few disk-florets, but these may also be entirely absent. The base of the conical receptacle is covered with numerous oblong scales (paleae).

<u>Odour:</u> Characteristic and pleasant.

<u>Taste:</u> Bitter and aromatic.

Fig. 2: *Chamaemelum nobile* (L.) ALL.

Cultivated form of this low plant, only about 30 cm in height, with 2–3 times pinnately divided leaves; flower-heads, up to 3 cm in diameter, comprising almost exclusively white ray-florets.

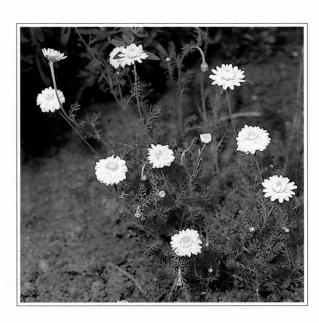

DAB 10: Römische Kamille
ÖAB: Flos Chamomillae romanae
Ph. Helv. VII: Chamomillae romanae flos
St.Zul. 1069.99.99

Plant source: *Chamaemelum nobile* (L.) ALL. (syn. *Anthemis nobilis* L., *Chamomilla nobilis* (L.) GODR., *Anthemis odorata* LAM.), chamomile (Asteraceae).

Synonyms: Flores anthemidis (Lat.), Roman or English or Sweet chamomile (Engl.), Römische Kamille, Große Kamille (Ger.), Fleur de camomille romaine (Fr.).

Origin: Native in southern and western Europe (England, Belgium, France, Germany, Italy, Spain) and North Africa. For the drug, a variety that forms almost exclusively ray-florets is cultivated, especially in Belgium, France, and England, and also in the USA and Argentina.
Imports come primarily from France, Poland, and former Czechoslovakia.

Constituents: 0.6–2.4% essential oil, consisting principally of the angeloyl, methacryl,

sylglucoside), etc.; polyacetylenes, among them dehydromatricaria ester; phenolic compounds such as *trans*-caffeic and ferulic acids and their glucose esters; scopoletin 7β-glucoside; triterpenes.

Indications: The applications of Roman chamomile flowers are the same as those of genuine chamomile (see: Matricariae flos = matricaria flowers) which they replace particularly in Great Britain, France, and Belgium, especially for menstrual problems and as a carminative. It also finds use as an aromatic bitter to stimulate the appetite and the digestion, and externally, for washing out the mouth and wounds. Compared with matricaria flowers, chamomile flowers have been less thoroughly examined pharmacologically. In addition to the essential oil and the flavonoids, the germacranolides probably also make an essential contribution to the overall picture of activity, for other representatives of this group of compounds with an exocyclic methylene group on the

γ-lactone ring have proved to be potent antiphlogistic and antibacterial substances [3–6]. Some of the hydroperoxides have been shown to have moderate antibacterial activity [11].

Making the tea: Boiling water is poured over 1.5–2 g of the finely chopped drug and after 10 min. strained. A 3% infusion is made for external use.
1 Teaspoon = ca. 0.8 g; 1 tablespoon = ca. 1.8 g.

Phytomedicines: In just a few gastrointestinal remedies, e.g. Stovalid® (drops), etc. In prepared remedies, usually matricaria flowers are used.
An extract of chamomile flowers is a component of Potter's Appetiser Mixture (oral liquid).

Regulatory status (UK): General Sales List – flowers: Schedule 1, Table A; oil: Schedule 1, Table B (for external use only).

tigloyl, and isobutyryl esters of aliphatic C_4- to C_6-alcohols; ca. 0.6% germacranolide-type sesquiterpene lactones (bitter substances) [1]: nobilin, 3-epinobilin (3α-OH), sesquiterpene peroxides such as 1β-hydroperoxyisonobilin [2], etc.; flavonoids, including apigenin and luteolin 7-*O*-glucosides, quercitrin, apiin (apigenin 7-apio-

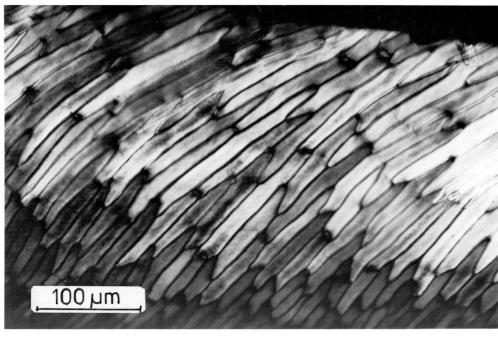

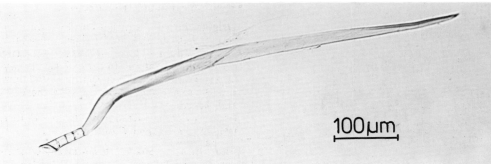

Fig. 3: Thin-walled cells of the scales (paleae) on the receptacle, in polarized light

Fig. 4: Covering trichome from the involucral bract, showing the pennant-like terminal cell

Authentication: Macro- and microscopically [7]. The paleae, especially when viewed in polarized light, afford a diagnostic feature (Fig. 3); the covering trichomes of the involucral bracts are also characteristic (Fig. 4). The detailed microscopy of the powdered drug is described and figured in [9].
The BHP 1990 requires the drug to comply with the appropriate monographs of the Ph. Eur. 2 and BP 1/1988.
The Ph. Eur. 2 TLC method of examination is as follows:

Test solution: 0.5 powdered drug shaken with 10 ml methanol on the water-bath at 60 °C for 5 min., cooled, and filtered.

Reference solution: 1 mg caffeic acid and 2.5 mg rutin in 10 ml methanol, prepared immediately before use.

Loadings: 10 µl each of the test and reference solutions, as 2-cm bands on silica gel G.

Solvent system: butan-1-ol + glacial acetic acid + water (66 + 17 + 17).

Detection: after drying at 80–100 °C for 5 min., sprayed with 1% methanolic diphenylboric acid aminoethyl ester, followed by 5% methanolic polyethylene glycol 400.

Evaluation: after 30 min. examined in UV 365 nm light. Reference solution: in the upper part, a bright blue fluorescent zone (caffeic acid); about the middle, a brownish yellow fluorescent zone (rutin). Test solution: a yellowish green fluorescent zone with the highest Rf (apigenin) and below it a faint, bright blue fluorescent zone corresponding in position and fluorescence with caffeic acid; directly below this zone, a brownish fluorescent zone (luteolin); at an Rf slightly greater than that of the reference rutin, a light brown fluorescent zone (apiin) with immediately above it a yellowish fluorescent zone (apigenin 7-glucoside) and immediately below it a strong bright blue fluorescent zone; at an Rf below that of reference rutin, a bright blue fluorescent zone; other faint bluish fluorescent zones possibly also present.

An aid to the assignment of the TLC spots is given in [8].

Quantitative standards: Ph. Eur. 2, etc.: *Volatile oil*, not less than 0.7%. *Flowerheads*, not more than 3% with a diameter less than 8 mm. *Condition*, brown or darkened flower-heads must be absent. *Water*, not more than 10.0%. *Sulphate ash*, not more than 12.0%.

Adulteration: Rare, and mostly detectable by the absence of paleae.

Storage: Protected from light and moisture, but not in plastic containers.

Literature:

[1] M. Holub and Z. Samek, Collect. Chem. Comm. **42**, 1053 (1977).
[2] R. Mayer and G. Rücker, Arch. Pharm. (Weinheim) **320**, 318 (1987).
[3] I.H. Hall et al., J. Pharm. Sci. **68**, 537 (1979).
[4] I.H. Hall et al., J. Pharm. Sci. **69**, 537 (1980).
[5] K.H. Lee et al., Phytochemistry **16**, 1177 (1977).
[6] G. Willuhn, Dtsch. Apoth. Ztg. **127**, 2511 (1987).
[7] P. Rohdewald, G. Rücker and K.-W. Glombitza, Apothekengerechte Prüfvorschriften, S. 937. Deutscher Apothekerverlag Stuttgart 1986.
[8] P. Pachaly, Dünnschichtchromatographie in der Apotheke, Wiss. Verlagsges., 2nd ed., Stuttgart 1983.
[9] B.P. Jackson and D. W. Snowdon, Atlas of microscopy of medicinal plants, culinary herbs and spices, Belhaven Press, London, 1990, p. 54.
[10] G. Rücker, K.-R. Lee, and R. Mayer, Arch. Pharm. (Weinheim) **320**, 867 (1987).
[11] G. Rücker, R. Mayer, and K.-R. Lee, Arch. Pharm. (Weinheim) **322**, 821 (1989).

Chelidonii herba   (DAB 10), Greater celandine, Chelidonium (BHP 1983)

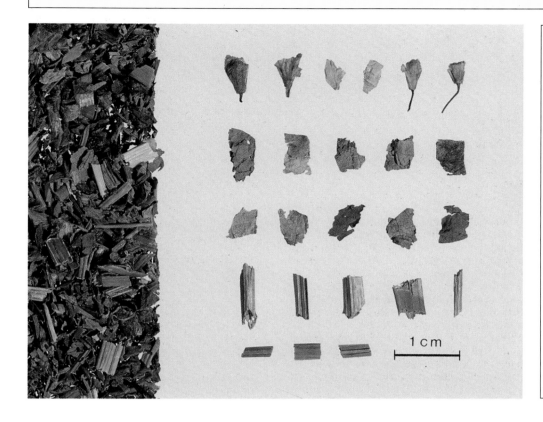

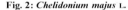

1 cm

Fig. 1: Celandine

<u>Description</u>: The drug consists of the aerial parts of the plant collected at the time of flowering. The yellow to greenish brown, sparsely pubescent pieces of stem are hollow and mostly flattened (bottom row), while the much crumpled, very thin pieces of leaf have a matt, bluish green upper surface and a distinctly lighter bluish green lower surface with a darker reticulate venation. The very fragile flowers have two sepals, which fall off when the flower opens and are therefore only visible in the bud, four yellow petals (top row), numerous stamens, and an elongated ovary. The drug also has a few fruits (pod-like capsules) containing small dark-coloured seeds.

<u>Odour</u>: Peculiar and unpleasant.

<u>Taste</u>: Bitter and somewhat pungent.

Fig. 2: *Chelidonium majus* L.

A ca. 60 cm tall, branched plant, with spreading pubescent stems and blue-green pinnately divided leaves with the leaflets having a lobed margin. Flowers with four yellow petals and numerous stamens, losing the two sepals on opening. Fruit a narrow, pod-shaped capsule. Entire plant with yellow to orange alkaloid-containing latex.

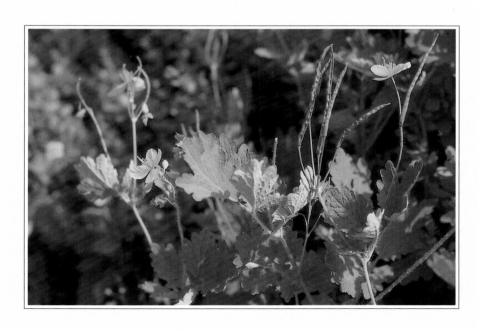

DAB 10: Schöllkraut

Plant source: *Chelidonium majus* L., greater celandine (Papaveraceae).

Synonyms: Celandine (Engl.), Schöllkraut, Goldwurz (Ger.), Chélidoine (Fr.).

Origin: A plant of waste places, widely distributed in Europe and Central and northern Asia; introduced into North America. The commercial product comes mainly from eastern Europe. About the cultivation, see [1].

Constituents: 0.1–1% alkaloid; more than 20 benzylisoquinoline alkaloids are known, of which chelidonine, sanguinarine, coptisine [15] and chelerythrine are quantitatively the most important; berberine, protopine, and stylopine are also worth mentioning [10–12]. The alkaloid content varies considerably; in the roots and rhizomes, the raw material for the industrial preparation of extracts, the alkaloid content is distinctly higher – according to our investigations, up to more than

3%. Other constituents: chelidonic acid and other plant acids, such as malic and citric acids, flavonoids, a saponin [4–6], carotenoids, and other ubiquitous substances. Proteolytic enzymes have been detected in the yellowish orange latex of the plant.

Indications: In dysfunction of the gall bladder and bile duct as cholagogue, spasmolytic, and (weak) analgesic. The pharmacodynamics of some of the alkaloids have been studied: the main alkaloid chelidonine has a direct spasmolytic action on smooth muscle, but weaker than that of papaverine; a weak analgesic and central sedative effect has also been reported. Berberine is said to have a cholekinetic action, while sanguinarine (an acetylcholinesterase inhibitor) and chelerythrine have local irritant properties. Several of the alkaloids have antibacterial activity. However, all in all, no doubt because of the small amount of alkaloid present, the effects of the total alkaloid complex do not appear to be very pronounced [3]. This is also true of the many prepared remedies (q.v.), in which the proportion of *Chelidonium* extracts is usually very small.
Chelidonium (*baiqucai = pai-ch'ü-tsai*) is an important drug in Chinese medicine and is considered to have analgesic, antitussive, anti-inflammatory, and detoxicant properties; an extract is reported to be effective in treating bronchitis and whooping cough [13]; this reference reviews the pharmacology of the drug and its constituent alkaloids. Alcoholic extracts of the drug are indicated to have antihepatotoxic activity in pharmacological models in rats [14].
In *folk medicine,* the fresh latex is dabbed on warts. The demonstrated antimitotic and skin-irritant properties of sanguinarine and chelerythrine may perhaps provide an ex-

planation for this old use, and it is possible that the proteolytic enzymes also play a part.

Side effects: Unlikely if used according to the directions. This is also true of the occasionally recommended external use of the drug (against psoriasis? [7]): old reports regarding irritation of the skin have not been confirmed by Schmaltz [8].

Making the tea: Not very usual. For cramp-like gastrointestinal and biliary disorders, boiling water is poured over $1/2$–1 teaspoon of the finely chopped drug and after 10 min. strained. Two to three cups a day.
1 Teaspoon = ca. 1.2 g.

Herbal preparations: Greater celandine is included in various bile and liver teas, and in herbal mixtures for other indications, as well as in prepared teas.

Phytomedicines: Panchelidon® capsules and drops are monovalent preparations. The powdered drug, extracts, or tinctures are present in many polyvalent preparations, e.g. Cefachol®, Cholhepan® S, Chelidophyt® N, Esberigal® N, Hepaticum Medice®, Cholagogum-Nattermann®, Aristochol®, Gallemollan forte, etc. Liver and bile preparations predominate, but there are also prepared remedies for other indications. There is also a series of preparations containing homoeopathic dilutions of the drug; the mother tincture is made from the fresh roots (and rhizomes). It must again be pointed out, however, that in many allopathic products the amounts of *Chelidonium* present are so small that the drug is unlikely to exert any useful effect [2].

Authentication: Macro- (see: Description) and microscopically, following the DAB 10. The covering trichomes on the stem frag-

ments are 0.4–2 mm long and comprise 5–20 thin-walled, often collapsed, cells. The 10–25 μm wide laticifers that are always associated with the vascular bundles (Fig. 3) are characteristic; they have a yellowish brown, granular content.
The DAB 10 TLC test of identity is as follows:

Test solution: 0.75 g powdered drug extracted with 200 ml 12% aq. acetic acid on the water-bath with frequent swirling for 30 min., then diluted to 250 ml with 12% aq. acetic acid and filtered; 50 ml filtrate basified with 26% ammonia solution and shaken out with 2 × 30 ml chloroform; combined extracts dried over anhydrous sodium sulphate, taken to dryness, and the residue dissolved in 1 ml methanol.

Reference solution: 2.0 mg papaverine hydrochloride and 10 mg methyl red in 10 ml 96% ethanol.

Loadings: 20 μl test solution and 10 μl reference solution, as 2-cm bands on silica-gel GF$_{254}$.

Solvent system: anhydrous formic acid + water + propan-1-ol (1 + 9 + 90), 10 cm run.

Detection and Evaluation: In UV 254 and 365 nm light. <u>Reference solution:</u> quenching zone of papaverine in the lower Rf region and methyl-red zone in the middle Rf region. <u>Test solution:</u> a quenching zone at the

Chelidonine

R¹	R²	
CH$_3$	CH$_3$	Chelerythrine
	– CH$_2$ –	Sanguinarine

Berberine

Protopine

Chelidonic acid

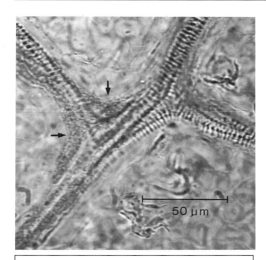

Fig. 3: Laticifer with granular content (arrow), associated with the vascular bundles

same Rf value as papaverine and, immediately below it, a broad reddish yellow fluorescent zone (showing strong orange fluorescence in UV 365 nm light), assigned to sanguinarine (upper zone) and chelerythrine (lower zone), and below that a narrow zone fluorescing reddish yellow (and yellow in UV 365 nm light); in the Rf region between papaverine and methyl red, a distinct quenching zone belonging to chelidonine (not fluorescing in UV 365 nm light); directly above it, a faint zone fluorescing in UV 365 light may be present and above that a broad quenching zone (seen under UV 365 nm light to comprise in order of increasing Rf value a yellow, a blue-violet, and an orange to reddish fluorescing zone).

After spraying with Dragendorff reagent: the papaverine and chelidonine zones yellowish orange, the sanguinarine and chelerythrine zones orange to greyish brown; further yellowish orange to orange may be present. After complete drying (zones fading), on overspraying with sodium nitrite solution the zones already described become brown to greyish brown. Additional zones may occur.

The alkaloid content can be determined spectrophotometrically: the formaldehyde liberated from the methylenedioxy function of chelidonine under strongly acid conditions forms a coloured dibenzoxanthylium cation with chromotropic acid which is stabilized by mesomerism. For the quantitative determination of the main alkaloids after TLC separation, see [9].

Quantitative standards: <u>DAB 10</u>: *Total alkaloid*, not less than 0.6% calculated as chelidonine (M_r 353.4). *Foreign matter*, not more than 10%. *Loss on drying*, not more than 10.0%. *Ash*, not more than 13.0%.

<u>BHP 1983</u>: *Water-soluble extractive*, not less than 20%. *Total ash*, not more than 15%. *Acid-insoluble ash*, not more than 2%.

Adulteration: In practice, rare.

Literature:
[1] C. Franz and D. Fritz, Planta Med. **36**, 246 (1979).
[2] R. Hänsel, Dtsch. Apoth. Ztg. **127**, 2 (1987).
[3] H. Kreitmair, Pharmazie **13**, 85 (1950).
[4] V. Kwasniewski, Pharmazie **13**, 363 (1958).
[5] V. Kwasniewski, Arch. Pharm. (Weinheim) **291**, 209 (1958).
[6] V. Kwasniewski, Arzneim.-Forsch. **8**, 245 (1958).
[7] L.J. Potopalskaja and A.I. Ptopalskii, Vrac. delo Kiew **8**, 129 (1964); according to Harnischfeger/Stolze: Bewährte Pflanzendrogen in Wissenschaft und Medizin, notamed Verlag, Melsungen (1983).
[8] D. Schmaltz et al., Hippokrates, Heft 5, 105 (1940).
[9] C. Scholz, R. Hänsel and C. Hille, Pharm. Ztg. **121**, 1571 (1976).
[10] M. Tin-Wa et al., Lloydia **35**, 87 (1972).
[11] G. Kadan, T. Gözler, and M. Shamma, J. Nat. Prod. **53**, 531 (1990).
[12] S. De Rosa and G. Di Vincenzo, Phytochemistry **31**, 1085 (1992).
[13] H.-M Chang and P.P.-H. But (eds.) Pharmacology and the applications of Chinese materia medica, World Scientific, Singapore – Philadelphia, 1986, vol. 1, p. 390.
[14] S. Mitra et al., Internat. J. Pharmacog. **30**, 125 (1992).
[15] G. Fulde, thesis, Marburg 1993.

Cinchonae cortex   (Ph. Eur. 2), Cinchona bark (*BAN*; BP 1988, BHP 1/1990)

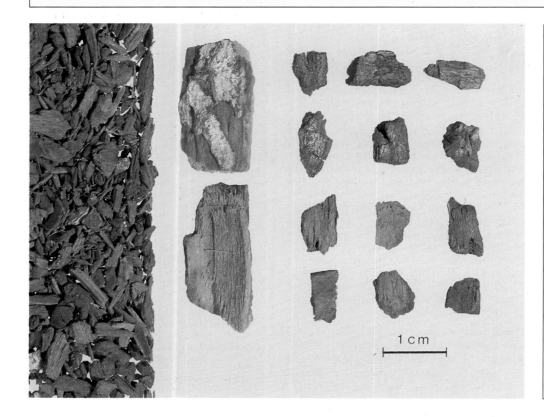

Fig. 1: Cinchona bark

<u>Description:</u> The drug is derived exclusively from cultivated trees and consists of ca. 2–3 mm thick, somewhat curved or channelled pieces of bark with a greyish brown to grey outer surface that is often covered with pale-coloured lichens and a reddish brown inner surface with fine longitudinal striations; the fracture is short and fibrous.

<u>Odour:</u> Faint, characteristic.

<u>Taste:</u> Intensely bitter and somewhat astringent.

Fig. 2: *Cinchona pubescens* VAHL, with bark removed from part of the trunk
Trees up to more than 20 m in height, with leaves up to 30 cm in length and elliptical in shape. Flowers up to 2 cm long and light pink in colour.

Fig. 3: Leaves and flowers of *Cinchona pubescens* VAHL

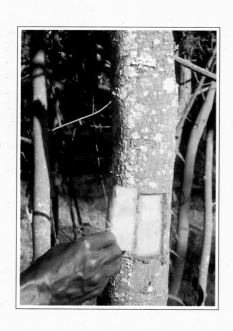

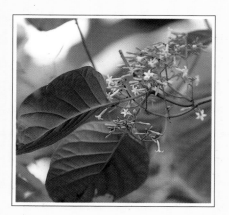

ÖAB: Cortex Chinae
Ph. Helv. VII: Cinchonae cortex
St.Zul. 1459.99.99

Plant source: *Cinchona pubescens* VAHL (syn. *Cinchona succirubra* PAVÓN) or its varieties and hybrids with related *Cinchona* species (Rubiaceae).

Synonyms: Cinchona, Jesuit's bark, Peruvian bark, Red cinchona bark (Engl.), Chinarinde, Fieberrinde (Ger.), Écorce de Quina (Fr.).

Origin: From plantations in South-East Asia, South America, and Central and East Africa. The drug is imported from Indonesia, India, and Sri Lanka and to a limited extent also from South America.

Constituents: 5–15% Alkaloids, with quinine, quinidine, cinchonine, and cinchonidine the most important quantitatively; a further 30 or so alkaloids are also present. Ca. 8% catechol tannins. Bitter substances (glycosides of triterpene acids, e.g. quinovic acid). Traces (ca. 0.005%) of essential oil [1].

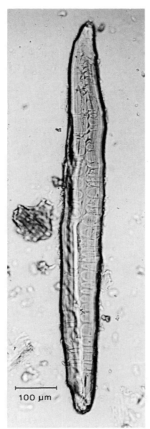

100 µm

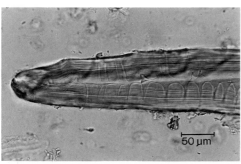

50 µm

Fig. 4: A bark fibre, showing the thick walls and blunt ends

Fig. 5: Detail of bark fibre: striated wall with characteristic funnel-shaped pits

Indications: As a bitter for stimulating the appetite and promoting gastric secretion. In *folk medicine,* also for mild attacks of influenza and very occasionally also as a component of cholagogues.

Side effects: With hypersensitivity to quinine, skin allergies and fever may occur, but with prescribed doses such symptoms are rare. This is also true of the increased tendency to bleeding mentioned in the Standard Licence. It goes without saying that in

such cases medical help is required at once. Cinchona bark is contraindicated during pregnancy and when gastric or intestinal ulcers are present.

Making the tea: Boiling water is poured over ca. 1 g of the finely cut drug, allowed to stand for 10 min. and strained. A cupful, if desired slightly sweetened, is drunk about half-an-hour before meals to stimulate the appetite, but after meals in digestive disorders.

1 Teaspoon = ca. 1.7 g.

Phytomedicines: The drug itself is not used, but extracts are included in (about 100) prepared remedies, especially in those used as stomachics and roborants.

Authentication: Following the Ph. Eur. 2, BP 1988, etc., macro- and microscopically, and by means of TLC. The yellow, thick-walled, 600–1300 µm long bark fibres, with distinctly striated and pitted walls, are characteristic; a detailed description of the microscopy of the powdered drug is given in [2].

The four major cinchona alkaloids and their dihydro derivatives can be separated and quantified by HPLC [3].

Quantitative standards: Ph. Eur. 2: *Total alkaloids*, not less than 6.5%, of which not less than 30% and not more than 60% consists of quinine-type alkaloids. *Foreign vegetable*

and mineral matter, not more than 2%. *Sulphated ash*, not more than 4.0%.

BHP 1/1990: Cinchona Bark complies with the Eur. Ph. 2 monograph on Cinchonae cortex or the BP 1988 monographs on Cinchona bark or Powdered Cinchona bark.

Adulteration: In practice, adulteration with bark from other *Cinchona* species which are used for the production of quinine is observed. These barks are easily recognized by the usually distinct yellow-brown, rather than reddish brown, colour of the inner surface; the fibres are mostly shorter than those present in the official bark and they are blunt-ended.

Storage: Protected from light and kept dry.

Literature:
[1] W.C. Evans, Trease and Evans' Pharmacognosy, 13th ed., Baillière Tindall, London – Philadelphia – Toronto – Sydney – Tokyo, 1989, pp. 620–625 and references cited therein.
[2] B.P. Jackson and D.W. Snowdon, Atlas of microscopy of medicinal plants, culinary herbs and spices, Belhaven Press, London, 1990, p. 60.
[3] D.V. McCalley, Analyst **115**, 1355 (1990).

Cinnamomi cortex (DAB 10, Ph. Eur. 2), Cinnamon (*BAN, USAN*; BP 1988), Cinnamomon, Ceylon

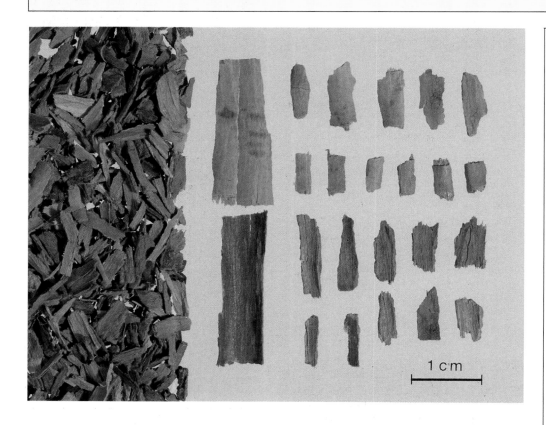

Fig. 1: Cinnamon

The drug consists of the dried bark of the shoots of coppiced trees, freed from the outer cork and underlying parenchyma by scraping.

Description: The matt pieces of bark, 0.2–0.7 mm thick and in the form of single or double compound quills, are light brown on the outside and somewhat darker on the inside; the surface is longitudinally striated and the fracture is short and splintery. See further [1].

Odour: Characteristic and pleasantly aromatic.

Taste: Pungently spicy, somewhat sweet and mucilaginous, and only slightly sharp.

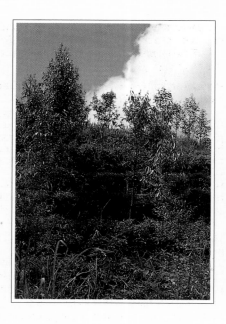

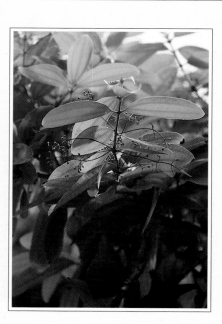

Fig. 2: *Cinnamomum* sp. NEES
Densely leafy, evergreen trees, up to 10 m tall, in plantations mostly kept as bushes by coppicing. Bark taken from the 2–3 cm thick branches of ca. 6-year old trees or from ca. 2-year old root suckers of older plants.

Fig. 3: *Cinnamomum* sp. NEES
Stout, leathery, ovate-lanceolate, and acuminate leaves, up to 20 cm long, with arcuate main veins; on rubbing, smelling of cloves. Flowers, ca. 0.5 cm in diameter and silky-haired, arranged in loose panicles.

DAB 10: Zimtrinde
ÖAB: Cortex Cinnamomi ceylanici
Ph. Helv. VII: Cinnamomi cortex
St.Zul. 1709.99.99 (Zimt)

Plant source: *Cinnamomum verum* J. PRESL (syn. *C. zeylanicum* GARCIN ex BLUME, according to the Ph. Eur. 2, etc.: *C. zeylanicum* NEES), Ceylon cinnamon (Lauraceae).

Synonyms: Cinnamomum, Cinnamon bark (Engl.), Zimtrinde, Echter Kanel (Ger.), Cannellier de Ceylan, Écorce de cannellier de Ceylan (Fr.).

Origin: Native to Sri Lanka (?); cultivated in Sri Lanka, the Seychelles, south-eastern India, Indonesia, the West Indies, and South America. The drug is imported mainly from Sri Lanka, but also Malaysia, Madagascar, and the Seychelles.

Constituents: 0.5–2.5% Essential oil, the main components of which are cinnamaldehyde (65–80%), eugenol, and *trans*-cinnamic acid (5–10%); in addition, other phenylpropanes, including hydroxycinnamaldehyde, *o*-methoxycinnamaldehyde, cinnamyl alcohol and its acetate, and terpenes, among them limonene, α-terpineol; also, tannins, mucilage, oligomeric procyanidins, and traces of coumarin [2–5].

Indications: Occasionally, in combination with other drugs, as a stomachic and carminative.
However, the drug is used primarily as a taste enhancer and as a spice, and to some extent also in the preparation of liqueurs.
In *folk medicine,* the essential oil is used drop-wise ("cinnamon drops") as a remedy in dysmenorrhoea and as a haemostyptic.
The essential oil has antimicrobial and fungicidal properties [4], which are probably due to the *o*-methoxycinnamaldehyde content.

Extract from the German Commission E monograph
(BAnz no. 22a, dated 01.02.1990)

Uses
Lack of appetite; dyspeptic complaints such as mild, colicky upsets of the gastrointestinal tract, a feeling of distension, and flatulence.

Contraindications
Allergy to cinnamon or Peru balsam. Pregnancy.

Side effects
Often, allergic reactions by the skin and mucous membranes.

Interactions with other remedies
None known.

Dosage
Unless otherwise prescribed: daily dose, 2–4 g drug or 0.05–0.2 g essential oil; preparations correspondingly.

Mode of administration
Pulverized drug for infusions; essential oil and other galenical preparations for internal use.

Effects
Antibacterial, fungistatic, motility-stimulating.

Side effects: None, when properly used. In large amounts, cinnamon bark (and in moderate doses, cinnamon oil) bring about tachycardia and increased intestinal peristalsis, respiration, and perspiration, through stimulation of the vasomotor centre; this excitation state follows a central sedative phase characterized by sleepiness and depression [5].

Making the tea: Not very usual; see the Standard Licence.

Herbal preparations: The drug is a component of herbal mixtures for different indications, as well as of mixtures for making mulled wine (Glühwein), and is also available in tea bags.

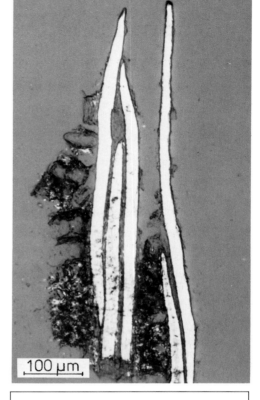

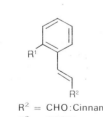

Fig. 4: Thick-walled phloem fibres and very fine calcium oxalate needles in the adjacent parenchyma (in polarized light)

Phytomedicines: Cinnamon bark is included in some prepared remedies, especially stomachics and carminatives, mainly to improve the taste and as an aromatic.

Regulatory status (UK): General Sales List – bark and oil: Schedule 1, Table A.

Authentication: Macro- (see: Description) and microscopically. The drug contains long, slender phloem fibres (Fig. 4) which shine in polarized light, very fine needles of calcium oxalate in the parenchyma, and stone cells that are mostly thickened all round. Cork or lignified cork should be absent, but if present it points to adulteration with Chinese cinnamon. For the detailed microscopy of powdered Ceylon cinnamon, see [6].
The TLC examination for purity given in the Ph. Eur. 2, BP 1988, etc. (q.v.), is also a proof of identity, based on the detection of the characteristic substances: cinnamaldehyde, eugenol, and *o*-methoxycinnamaldehyde:

R¹ = H,   R² = CHO:Cinnamaldehyde
R¹ = H,   R² = COOH:trans-Cinnamic acid
R¹ = OCH₃, R² = CHO:o-Methoxycinnamaldehyde
R¹ = H,   R² = CH₂OH:Cinnamyl alcohol

Eugenol

Coumarin

Test solution: 0.1 g pulverized drug shaken for 15 min. with 2 ml dichloromethane, filtered, the filtrate taken almost to dryness on the water-bath, and the residue dissolved in 0.4 ml toluene.

Reference solution: 50 μl cinnamaldehyde and 10 μl eugenol made up to 10 ml in toluene.

Loadings: 10 μl of each solution, as 2–cm bands on silicia gel GF$_{254}$.

Solvent system: dichloromethane, 10 cm run.

Detection: in UV 254 and 365 nm light, both quenching and fluorescent zones marked.

Evaluation: in UV 254 nm light. Reference and Test solutions: in the middle, a quenching zone (cinnamaldehyde) and directly above it a weak quenching zone (eugenol). In UV 365 nm light. Test solution: just below the cinnamaldehyde zone, a bright blue fluorescent zone (*o*-methoxycinnamaldehyde); sprayed with dianisidine (2.5 g in 10 ml 98% acetic acid), the cinnamaldehyde zone becomes yellowish brown.

On the TLC, adulterants containing more than 0.03% coumarin (pharmaceutical cinnamon bark has less than 0.0008%) exhibit an intense green fluorescent zone at Rf ca. 0.28, just below the one belonging to *o*-methoxycinnamaldehyde at Rf ca. 0.35.

Quantitative standards: Ph. Eur. 2: *Volatile oil*, not less than 1.2%. *Sulphated ash*, not more than 6.0%.

Adulteration: Occurs, especially with the powdered drug. It involves the bark of other *Cinnamomum* species: *C. aromaticum* NEES (syn. *C. cassia* BLUME), Cassia, cassia bark, cassia lignea, Chinese or bastard cinnamon, is distinguished by being much thicker (1–2 mm) and having a cork, the inner part of which comprises thick-walled cells. Large numbers of cork cells and groups of such cells are also typical of adulteration with insufficiently scraped cinnamon or by scrapings. For the detailed microscopy of powdered cassia bark, see [6].

Another adulterant, Padang cinnamon (also known as Java or Indonesian cinnamon), which comes from *C. burmanii* has plates of calcium oxalate in the cells of the medullary rays, unlike Ceylon cinnamon.

To distinguish Chinese and Ceylon cinnamon, the reaction of the powder with baryta water can be used. A specimen of each drug is placed on a microscope slide and moistened with 2–3 drops of 10% aqueous barium hydroxide solution; after 1–2 min., different fluorescence colours are observed when examined under UV 365 nm light: Chinese cinnamon exhibits an intense yellowish green fluorescence, some fibres are bright yellowish, while others are light blue to bluish violet, and the parenchyma appears dark reddish brown. Ceylon cinnamon shows a pale, bluish green colour; the fibres and parenchyma have the same fluorescence colours as the Chinese cinnamon. For the TLC detection of adulterants on the basis of a too high content of coumarin, see: Authentication.

Storage: Protected from light and moisture, in well-closed metal or glass (but not plastic) containers.

Literature:

[1] W.C. Evans, Trease and Evans' Pharmacognosy, 13th ed., Baillière Tindall, London – Philadelphia – Toronto – Sydney – Tokyo, 1989, p. 453.
[2] Kommentar DAB 10.
[3] V. Formácek and K.-H. Kubeczka, Essential oil analysis by capillary gas chormatography and carbon-13 NMR spectroscopy, Wiley, Chichester, 1982.
[4] S. Morozumi, Appl. Environm. Microbiol. **4**, 54 (1973).
[5] Hager, vol. **4**, p. 54 (1973); vol **4**, 884 (1992).
[6] B.P. Jackson and D.W. Snowdon, Atlas of microscopy of medicinal plants, culinary herbs and spices, Belhaven Press, London, 1990, pp. 50 (*C. aromaticum* = *C. cassia*), 62 (*C. verum* = *C. zeylanicum*).

Citri pericarpium   Dried lemon peel (BP 1988)

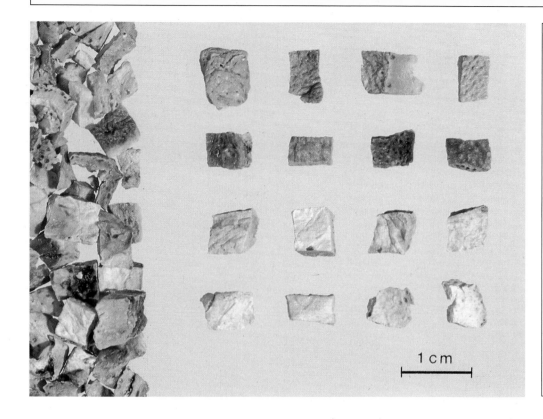

1 cm

Fig. 1: Dried lemon peel

Description: The drug is derived from fully developed, but not yet fully ripe, lemons. The outer layer of the fruit wall is usually removed in the form of a spiral and dried. The 2–3 mm thick pieces are brownish yellow and dimpled on the outside and whitish on the inside.

Odour: Characteristic.

Taste: Spicy, somewhat acid and slightly bitter.

Fig. 2: *Citrus limon* (L.) BURM. f.

Shrubs or small trees, 5–10 m in height, generally with reddish branches and 15 cm long, acuminate and, in contrast to *C. aurantium*, scarcely winged leaves. Axillary flowers, single or in small clusters, with petals white on the inside and reddish on the outside, and readily dropped. Yellow, 8–10-locular fruit narrowing to a point at the upper end.

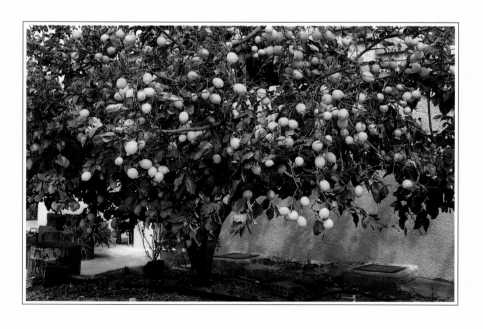

DAB 6: Pericarpium citri
Ph. Helv. VII: Limonis flavedo recens

Plant source: *Citrus limon* (L.) BURM.f. (syn. *C. medica* L. subsp. *limonum* (RISSO) HOOK.F. or var. *limonum* (RISSO) WIGHT et ARN.), lemon (Rutaceae).

Synonyms: Zitronenschale, Limonenschale (Ger.), Écorce de citron (Fr.).

Origin: From plantations in the Mediterranean region, especially southern Italy and Spain. The drug is mainly imported from Spain.

Constituents: 0.2–0.6% essential oil, which contains (+)-limonene as the principal component, also citral (a mixture of neral and geranial), which largely determines the odour, and other monoterpenes [1]; flavonoids, especially neohesperidosides and rutinosides of hesperetin and naringenin, along with many other flavonoids; so far, 44 flavone glycosides have been detected [2]; carotenoids [3]; citric acid and many other plant acids [4]; coumarin derivatives; abundant pectins [5].

Indications: The drug is used chiefly as an aromatic and stomachic. The (bio-)flavonoids of the drug reduce the permeability of the blood vessels, especially of the capillaries, so that it or extracts from it are also included in remedies for phlebitis. The flavonoids, in particular 5,6-di-*C*-glucosylapigenin, are strongly hypotensive on i.v. administration in the rat [2].

Making the tea: Not at all usual. However, the drug is often a component of so-called fruit tea mixtures.
1 Teaspoon = ca. 2.5 g.

Phytomedicines: Lemon peel, extracts prepared from it, or the isolated essential oil (lemon oil DAB 10 (Ph. Eur. 2, BP 1988, etc.)) are present in some polyvalent stomachic and roborant preparations, e.g. Marvina® Lösung (solution), etc.

Regulatory status (UK): General Sales List – oil: Schedule 1, Table A.

Authentication: Macroscopically (see: Description); as with Aurantii pericarpium (Bitter orange peel) (q.v.), microscopy is of little use. The two peels can be differentiated by means of their flavonoid profiles [6]:

Test solution: 1 g powdered drug extracted for 5 min. with 10 ml methanol on the water-bath at ca. 60 °C, then filtered.

Reference solution: 0.05% rutin in methanol.

Loadings: 25–30 µl test solution and 10 µl reference solution, as bands on silica gel 60F$_{254}$.

Solvent system: ethyl acetate + formic acid + glacial acetic acid + water (100 + 11 + 11 + 27), 15 cm run.

Detection: sprayed with 1% methanolic diphenylboryloxyethylamine, then 5% ethanolic polyethylene glycol 400.

Evaluation: in daylight. Test solution: at Rf ca. 0.4, a violet zone (eriocitrin) and above it a very faint ochre-coloured zone (traces of neohesperidin and hesperidin). In UV 365 nm light. Reference solution: at Rf ca. 0.3, an intense yellow fluorescent zone (rutin). Test solution: at Rf 0.4, an intense reddish orange fluorescent zone (eriocitrin); just below it an intense yellow fluorescent zone (rutin) and directly above it a broad dark green fluorescent zone (neohesperidin and hesperidin).

Note: after ca. 15 min. exposure to UV 365 nm light, the eriocitrin zone becomes intense red.

TLC examination of the carotenoids can also be carried out [7].

Quantitative standards: BP 1988: *Volatile oil*, not less than 2.5%. Ph. Helv. VII: *Volatile oil*, not less than 1.2%.

Adulteration: In practice, rare. Adulteration with Aurantii pericarpium (Bitter orange peel) can also be recognized by spotting with conc. hydrochloric acid: Bitter orange peel turns green, while Lemon peel remains unchanged in colour. As indicated above, TLC of the flavonoids enables the two materials to be distinguished (see also, Aurantii pericarpium: Authentication).

Storage: Protected from light, in well-closed containers (not made of plastic).

Literature:
[1] I. Calvarano, Essenze Deriv. Agrum. **36**, 5 (1966).
[2] Y. Matsubara et al., Termen Yuki Kagobutsu Toronkai Koen Yoshishu **27**, 702 (1985); C.A. **104**, 183261 (1986).
[3] G. Noga and F. Lenz, Chromatographia **17**, 139 (1983).
[4] C.E. Vandercook, Citrus Sci. Technol. **1**, 208 (1977).
[5] E. Postorino, F. Gionfriddo, and A. Di Giacomo, Essenze Deriv. Agrum. **52**, 367 (1982).
[6] H. Wagner, S. Bladt, and E.M. Zgainski, Plant drug analysis, Springer-Verlag, Berlin, Heidelberg, New York, Tokyo, 1984, p. 188.
[7] J. Gross, Chromatographia **13**, 572 (1980).

Cnici benedicti herba   Holy thistle (BHP 1/1990)

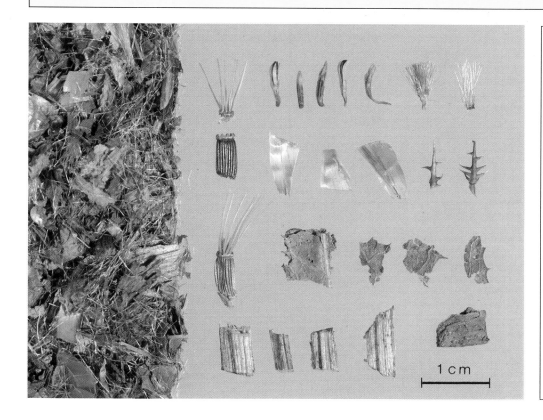

Fig. 1: Holy thistle

Description: Because of the abundant pubescence, particularly of the bracts, the cut drug consists of pieces matted together. There are numerous long filiform paleae from the receptacle of the inflorescence and occasional yellowish disk florets; yellowish straw-coloured fragments of the involucral bracts, which are shiny and whitish on the inner surface, are a prominent feature. The outer involucral bracts are short, with a simple spine, while the inner ones are longer and each one has a geniculate, pinnately divided spine. The leaves have a spinous margin. There are broad stem fragments which have longitudinal grooves and a few achenes with a conspicuous double, woody pappus.

Taste: Bitter.

Fig. 2: *Cnicus benedictus* L.
A low annual, up to 40 cm, with a thistle-like appearance. Leaves with a runcinate, spinous margin and flower-heads consisting almost entirely of ray florets surrounded by numerous, very spiny, imbricated, coriaceous bracts.

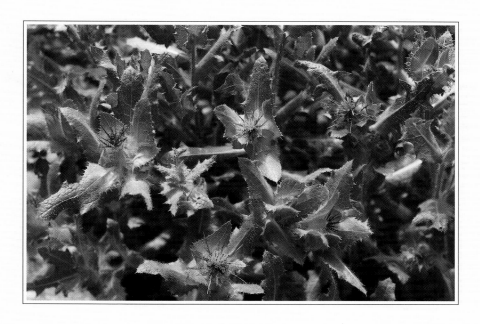

DAC 1986: Benediktenkraut
ÖAB: Herba Cardui benedicti

Plant source: *Cnicus benedictus* L., holy thistle (Asteraceae).

Synonyms: Cnicus, Blessed thistle (Engl.), Kardobenediktenkraut, Benediktenkraut (Ger.), Herbe de chardon bénit (Fr.).

Origin: Native in the Mediterranean region. The drug is collected and imported from eastern and southern Europe, as well as Italy and Spain.

Constituents: Bitter substances of the sesquiterpene lactone type, probably occurring in glycosidic form [1]; the principal constituent is the germacranolide cnicin, which was already isolated from the plant in 1837 [2] and 0.2–0.7% of which may be present in not-too-old commercial material [3]. Lignan lactones, such as trachelogenin, also contribute to the bitterness of the drug.
The essential oil, up to 0.3%, comprises, among other things, terpenes, e.g. *p*-cymene, fenchone, and citral, and phenylpropanes,

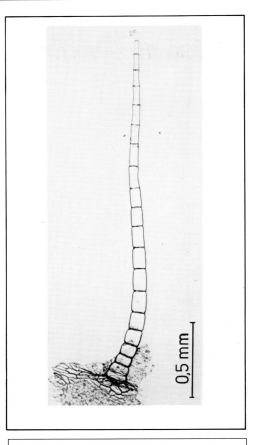

Cnicin

e.g. cinnamaldehyde, and benzoic acid [4]. Other constituents, like triterpenes and flavonoids, are probably not of any importance, as far as the activity of the drug is concerned.

Indications: As an aromatic bitter to stimulate the appetite and to increase the secretion of gastric juice, but somewhat weaker in action than other bitter drugs.

In *folk medicine*, it is also used as a cholagogue.

Pure cnicin is a strong anti-inflammatory, but is also rather toxic and i.p. injection results in considerable irritation of the tissue [3].

Making the tea: Boiling water is poured over 1.5–2 g of the finely chopped drug, or cold water is added and brought to the boil, and after 5–10 min. strained. As an aromatic bitter, a cup of the unsweetened tea is drunk half-an-hour before meals.

1 Teaspoon = ca. 1 g.

Phytomedicines: The drug is a component of several tea mixtures. Extracts are present in

---

Extract from the German Commission E monograph [Benediktenkraut] (BAnz no. 193, dated 15.10.1987)

Uses

Lack of appetite, dyspeptic complaints.

Contraindications

Allergy towards the holy thistle and other members of the daisy family.

Side effects

Allergic reactions are possible.

Interactions with other remedies

None known.

Dosage

Unless otherwise prescribed: average daily dose, 4–6 g drug; preparations correspondingly.

Mode of administration

Chopped drug and dry extracts for infusions; bitter-tasting galenical preparations for internal use.

Effects

Promoting the secretion of saliva and gastric juice.

---

prepared gastrointestinal remedies, e.g. Digestivum Hetterich®, and cholagogues, e.g. Esberigal®, Gallexier®, etc.

The powdered drug is a component of the UK product Gerard House Gladlax tablets.

Regulatory status (UK): General Sales list – Schedule 1, Table A; maximum dose 1.5 g.

Authentication: Macro- and microscopically, following the DAC 1986; detailed descriptions are also given in the BHP 1/1990. Besides glandular trichomes, woolly trichomes, and involucral spines, the multicellular covering trichomes (Fig. 3), especially, are prominent.

The following TLC procedure separates the bitter principles [5]:

Test solution: 1 g powdered drug extracted for 10 min. on the water-bath with 10 ml methanol at 60 °C, filtered, and the filtrate reduced to ca. 2 ml.

Reference solution: 1% cnicin in methanol.

Loadings: 40 µl test solution and 20 µl reference solution, as bands on silica gel 60F$_{254}$.

Solvent system: chloroform + methanol (95 + 5), 15 cm run.

Detection: sprayed with freshly prepared Liebermann-Burchard reagent (5 ml acetic anhydride + 5 ml sulphuric acid carefully added to 50 ml absolute ethanol cooled in ice), heated to 100 °C for 5–10 min.

Evaluation: in UV 365 nm light. Test solution: at least 14 fluorescent zones (mostly light blue, red-brown, or yellow green); cnicin, a yellow green fluorescent zone at Rf ca. 0.05 (in the solvent system: chloroform + acetone (40 + 30), at Rf ca. 0.4).

For its identification test, the BHP 1990 indicates: chloroform + methanol (90 + 10) as the solvent system and freshly prepared anisaldehyde reagent as the spray; after heating for 5–10 min. at 105 °C, examination in daylight. Test solution: relative to the methyl red reference, major bands at Rx 2.2 (purple), 1.75 (pink), 0.8 (purple), and 0.75 (light green, cnicin?).

Quantitative standards: DAC 1986: *Bitterness value*, not less than 800. *Foreign matter*, not more than 2%; absence of the glabrous white-flecked leaves of *Silybum marianum* (L.) GAERTN. (milk thistle), the sparsely pubescent, somewhat spiny leaves of *Cirsium oleraceum* (L.) SCOP. (cabbage thistle), and the white woolly leaves of *Onopordum acanthium* L. (cotton or Scotch thistle). *Loss on drying*, not more than 12.0%. *Ash*, not more than 15.0%.

ÖAB: *Bitterness value*, not less than 800. *Foreign matter*, not more than 5% (stem fragments thicker than 3 mm). *Ash*, not

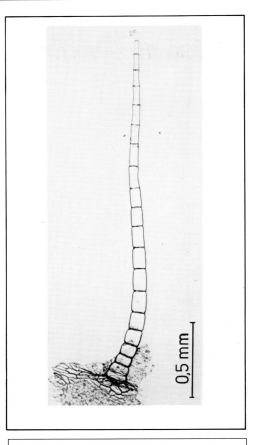

Fig. 3: Multicellular covering trichome from the leaves

more than 15.0%. *Acid-insoluble ash*, not more than 2.0%.

BHP 1990: *Water-soluble extractive*, not less than 20%. *Foreign matter*, not more than 3%. *Total ash*, not more than 15%. *HCl-insoluble ash*, not more than 3%.

For the photometric estimation of cnicin with the Baljet reagent (alkaline picrate), see [3].

Adulteration: Very rare. Leaves from other plants with a thistle-like appearance can generally be recognized macroscopically and with more certainty by microscopical examination.

Literature:
[1] G. Harnischfeger and H. Stolze, notabene medici **11**, 652 (1981).
[2] M. Šucha et al., Chem. Ber. **93**, 2449 (1960).
[3] G. Schneider and I. Lachner, Planta Med. **53**, 247 (1987).
[4] R. Vanhaelen-Fastre, Planta Med. **24**, 165 (1973).
[5] H. Wagner, S. Bladt, and E.M. Zgainski, Plant drug analysis, Springer-Verlag, Berlin, Heidelberg, New York, Tokyo, 1984, p. 134.

Condurango cortex

Condurango, Marsdenia (BHP 1983)

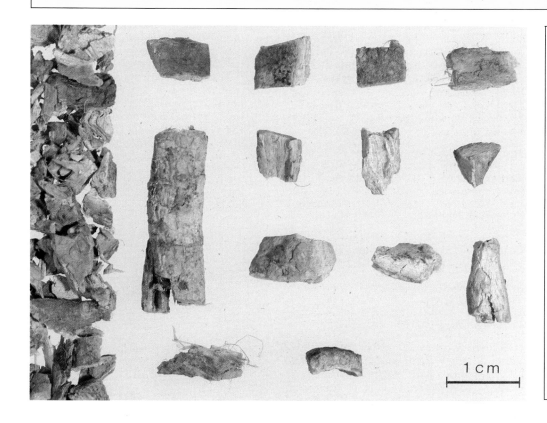

1 cm

Fig. 1: Condurango bark

Description: **The drug consists of quilled pieces of bark up to 5 mm thick, with a grey periderm on the outside; there are large horizontal lenticels and occasionally also some cortex. The inner surface is greyish brown and the fracture is fibrous (primary, unlignified fibres below the periderm). Groups of stone cells in the secondary phloem can be seen with a hand lens.**

Taste: **Slightly bitter and acrid.**

DAC 1986: Condurangorinde
ÖAB: Cortex Condurango
Ph. Helv. VII: Condurango cortex

Plant source: *Marsdenia cundurango* (also *condurango*) RCHB. fil. (Asclepiadaceae).

Synonyms: Condurango or Eagle-vine bark (Engl.), Condurangorinde (Ger.), Écorce de condurango (Fr.).

Origin: A liane occurring in the Andes of Ecuador, Peru, and Colombia. The drug is imported from these countries.

Constituents: 1–3% of a mixture of various condurango glycosides (pregnane derivatives) known as condurangin. In the sugar part, besides glucose, there are rarer sugars such as oleandrose, cymarose, and 6-desoxy-3-O-methylallose [1–3]. These constituents of Condurango can be called bitter substances with a saponin-like character; unusually, their solubility in water decreases on warming (the decoction should therefore be filtered cold). Further constituents: condurangamines A and B (hydroxylated preg-

OR^2

R^{1}O

O

H

H

OH

H

Cymarose

O

Condurango glycoside A
R^1 = Acetyl
R^2 = Cinnamoyl

Oleandrose

3-O-Methyl-6-desoxyallose

nane derivatives esterified with nicotinic acid), chlorogenic and caffeic acids, various cyclitols (including conduritol), various flavonoids, and coumarin derivatives, as well as vanillin [2].

Indications: Like other bitters, to increase gastric secretion and to stimulate the appetite. Formerly, it was (and in many present-day books on *folk medicine* still is)

recommended against stomach cancer. True, a Japanese group when testing the pure condurango-bark glycosides has demonstrated anti-tumour activity in the Ehrlich carcinoma- and sarcoma-180 system [4]. But to assume from these experiments that the drug has a cancerostatic action is certainly premature, especially as experiments with extracts of the drug have not led to any positive results (cited from [5]).

Making the tea: 1.5 g of the finely cut or coarsely powdered drug is added to cold water, brought to the boil for a short time, and, after cooling to room temperature, strained (according to the ÖAB, it can also be prepared as a macerate). Another common procedure is to leave the drug in wine for several days (50–100 g drug per litre).
As a bitter, a cupful of the tea or a liqueur-glass of the wine tincture is drunk half-an-hour before meals.
1 Teaspoon = ca. 3 g.

Phytomedicines: A number of gastrointestinal remedies contain condurango bark, or extracts, fluid extracts, or tinctures made

from it, e.g. Gastrocaps®, Nervogastrol®,
Pankreaplex N® (drops, dragees), etc.

Authentication: Macro- (see: Description)
and microscopically. Material can be
scraped off pieces of the drug and the powder examined. The stone cells (singly or in
groups) with their strongly thickened, somewhat yellowish walls, fragments of unlignified fibres, and the numerous clusters of calcium oxalate, up to 45 μm in diameter, are
particularly conspicuous. Besides small
starch grains, there are occasional fragments
of parenchyma with laticifers (and often
their exuded granular content), and fragments of periderm (with single crystals). See
also the BHP 1983.

Condurango glycosides dissolve better in
cold water than in hot: if 2 g of the powdered drug in 10 ml water is frequently
shaken over a period of 2 hours and then
filtered, the filtrate becomes cloudy at 80 °C
and on cooling becomes clear again (DAC
1986).

The DAC 1986 TLC test of identity has little specificity. The method given in [8] is as
follows:

Test solution: 1 g powdered drug extracted
for 10 min. on the water-bath with 10 ml
methanol at 60 °C, filtered, and the filtrate
evaporated to ca. 2 ml.

Reference solution: 1% neohesperidin in
methanol.

Loadings: 40 μl test solution and 20 μl reference solution, as bands on silica gel $F60_{254}$.

Solvent system: (a) ethyl acetate + methanol + water (77 + 18 + 5).
(b) ethyl acetate + formic acid + glacial
acetic acid + water (100 + 11 + 11 + 26).

Detection: for solvent system (a): vanillin/
sulphuric acid reagent, and for (b): anisalde-
hyde/sulphuric acid reagent, followed by
heating at 100 °C for 10 min.

Evaluation: in daylight. Test solution: several intense greenish black zones in the Rf
range 0.45–0.5, due to conduragins; dark
blue zones below the solvent front derive
from essential oils and aromatic acids;
brown and/or black zones at or just above
the start originate in part from sugars.
Spectrophotometric assay of the condurango glycosides is also possible [6, 7].

Quantitative standards: DAC 1986: *Condurangin*, not less than 1.8% calculated as
condurango glycoside A (M_r 987). *Foreign
matter*, not more than 2%; starch grains
greater than 20 μm in diameter, clusters
crystals of calcium oxalate greater than
60 μm in diameter and single crystals must
be absent. *Loss on drying*, not more than
8.0%. *Ash*, not more than 12.0%. *Acid-insoluble ash*, not more than 1.0%.
ÖAB: *Foreign matter*, not more than 2%.
Ash, not more than 12.0%. *Acid-insoluble
ash*, not more than 1.0%.
Ph. Helv. VII: *Condurango glycosides*, not
less than 1.8% calculated as condurango
glycoside A (M_r 987.3). *Foreign matter*, not
more than 2%; starch grains with a diameter greater than 16 μm or twinned or single
calcium oxalate crystals greater than 45 μm
are not present (false condurango barks).
Sulphated ash, not more than 12.0%.
BHP 1983: *Content of stalks*, not more than
2%. *Foreign organic matter*, not more than
1%. *Total ash*, not more than 12%. *Acid-insoluble ash*, not more than 2%.

Adulteration: Rare, but possibly with the
bark of *Asclepias umbellata* L. or *Elco-
marrhiza amylacea* BARB. RODR.

Literature:
[1] R. Tschesche and H. Kohl, Tetrahedron **24**, 4359
(1968).
[2] H. Koch and E. Steinegger, Pharm. Act. Helv. **56**, 244
(1981) und **57**, 211 (1982).
[3] S. Berger, P. Junior and L. Kopanski, Arch. Pharm.
(Weinheim) **320**, 924 (1987).
[4] K. Hayashi et al., Chem. Pharm. Bull. **28**, 1954 (1980)
und **29**, 2725 (1981).
[5] I. Koch-Heitzmann, Z. Phytother. **8**, 38 (1987).
[6] H. Koch and E. Steinegger, Pharm. Act. Helv. **53**, 56
(1978).
[7] E. Steinegger and P. Brunner, Pharm. Act. Helv. **52**,
139 (1977).
[8] H. Wagner, S. Bladt, and E.M. Zgainski, Plant drug
analysis, Springer-Verlag, Berlin, Heidelberg, New
York, Tokyo, 1984, pp. 129, 132.

Consolidae regalis flos Forking larkspur flowers

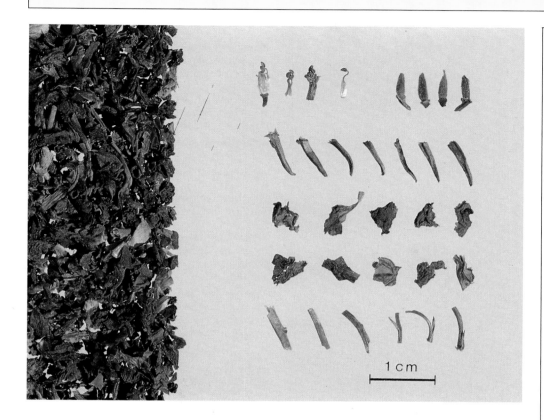

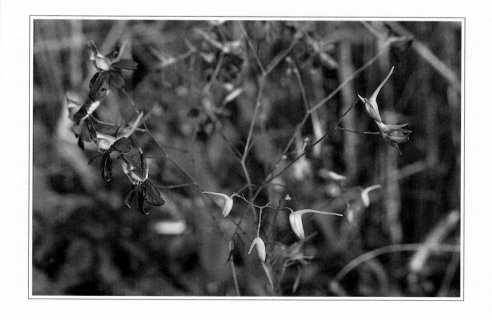

Fig. 1: Forking larkspur flowers

<u>Description</u>: The whole drug consists of the blue, shrivelled flowers. The 5-part calyx is petaloid and zygomorphic. The sepals are violet-blue on the outside, azure-blue on the inside, more or less finely pubescent, and marked with a greenish spot below the tip; the top one is sessile and ends in a spur, while the others are ovate and narrow towards the base. In contrast, the petals are a lighter violet, gamophyllous and prolonged into a spur (2nd row from the top) which lies in the spur of the calyx, and three-lobed with an emarginate middle lobe. The numerous brownish violet stamens have broad filaments and greenish yellow anthers (upper left), and there is only one style. Occasionally, green pubescent pedicels and follicles are present.

The cut drug consists of the somewhat wrinkled, azure-blue, sometimes bluish violet, fragments of the sepals and petals, as well as occasional broad stamens with green anthers. Pedicels (bottom row) are present here and there.

<u>Odour</u>: Faintly honey-like.

Fig. 2: *Consolida regalis* S.F.Gray

A chalk-loving decorative annual, ca. 30 cm in height, with a loose inflorescence of dark blue, 5-part flowers bearing a long spur. Leaves petiolate and pinnate, with fine, narrow segments.

Plant source: *Consolida regalis* S.F. GRAY (syn. *Delphinium consolida* L.), forking larkspur (Ranunculaceae).

Synonyms: Calcatrippae flos, Flores Calcatrippae or Delphinii consolidae (Lat.), Lark's claw or Knight's spur flowers (Engl.), Ritterspornblüten (Ger.), Fleurs de pied d'alouette (Fr.).

Origin: In temperate Europe, in fields and along roadsides; introduced into North America; imports come from plants collected in the wild in eastern Europe.

Constituents: Anthocyan glycosides, particularly those with delphinidin as aglycone, e.g. delphinidin glucoside (delphin) [1]; flavonoids, e.g. kaempferol and quercetin glycosides. Occasionally, in the literature, alkaloids are mentioned as a constituent of the flowers [2], but in a study carried out in 1986 no Dragendorff-positive substances could be detected in 35 samples (own collections and imports) [3].

Indications: The inclusion in herbal mixtures is primarily to enhance the appearance. In *folk medicine*, the drug is occasionally employed as a diuretic, and formerly it was also used as an anthelmintic and to dye wool [4].

Side effects: When used simply to improve appearances, no side effects are to be expected. It should be noted, however, that some parts of the forking larkspur – roots, seeds, herb – contain toxic diterpene alkaloids, which may elicit symptoms similar to those caused by *Aconitum* alkaloids [5].

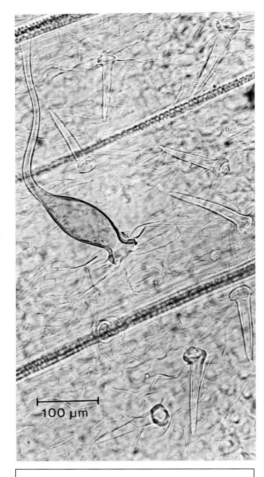

Fig. 3: Unicellular trichomes, somewhat broadened at the base, and a lageniform glandular trichome (with yellow content)

Making the tea: Not usual with the drug on its own. In the Erg. B. 6, the average dose for internal use was indicated to be 1.5 g.

Phytomedicines: Forking larkspur flowers are used almost exclusively to enhance the appearance of herbal mixtures destined for a variety of different indications.

Authentication: Macro- (see: Description) and microscopically, following the Erg. B. 6. Noteworthy are the numerous small unicellular trichomes, the lageniform glandular trichomes with yellow content (Fig. 3), the strongly sinuate cuticular striations, and the papillose epidermal cells of the petals.

Quantitative standard: Erg. B. 6: Ash, not more than 10%.

Adulteration: Rare. In imports from Hungary, occasionally flowers of the eastern larkspur, *Consolida orientalis* (S.F. GAY) SCHROEDINGER (syn. *Delphinium orientale* S.F. GAY) have been found. They are dark violet and the spur is not more than 1 cm long; the seeds are dark red, in contrast to the brownish or yellowish grey seeds of *Consolida regalis* [4].

Storage: Protected from light and moisture; not to be stored for more than one year, since the drug becomes discoloured and unsightly.

Literature:
[1] R. Willstätter and W. Mies, Liebigs Ann. Chem. **408**, 61 (1915).
[2] W. Schneider and A. Enders, Arzneim.Forsch. **5**, 324 (1955).
[3] F.-C. Czygan, unpublished work (1986).
[4] Hager, vol. **6**, p. 483 (1977).
[5] D. Frohne and H.J. Pfänder, A colour atlas of poisonous plants, Wolfe Publishing, London, 1984, p. 180.

Coriandri fructus

(DAB 10), Coriander (*BAN*; BP 1988)

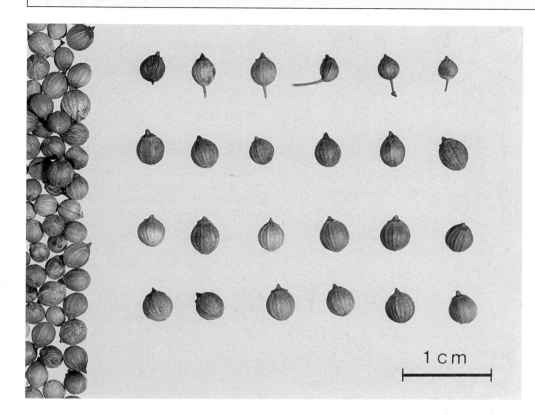

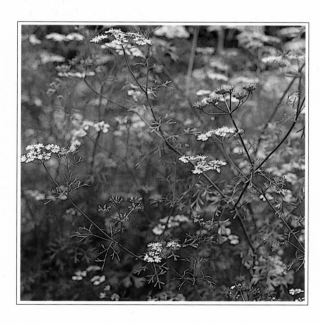

Fig. 1: Coriander

Description: The drug consists of the ripe, more or less spherical (diameter: var. *vulgare* 3–5 mm, var. *microcarpum* 11.5–3 mm) fruits (cremocarps or double achenes), which have mostly not split into the mericarps. The ridges first become visible on drying: 10 wavy, inconspicuous primary ridges and 8 straight, more conspicuous secondary ridges.

Odour: Spicy and aromatic.

Taste: Spicy and aromatic.

Fig. 2: *Coriandrum sativum* L.

An annual, unpleasant smelling plant, up to 60 cm tall, with 1–3 times pinnately divided leaves. Small white 5-merous flowers, with the petals pointing towards the outside mostly somewhat larger; flowers arranged in double umbels.

DAB 10: Koriander
ÖAB: Fructus Coriandri
St.Zul.: 1079.99.99

Plant source: *Coriandrum sativum* L., coriander: var. *vulgare* ALEF. (= var. *macrocarpum* DC.) and/or var. *microcarpum* DC. (Apiaceae = Umbelliferae).

Synonyms: Coriander seed or fruit (Engl.), Koriander(früchte) (Ger.), Fruit de coriandre (Fr.).

Origin: Originally in the eastern Mediterranean region and the Near East (?). Widely cultivated as a spice. Imports of the drug come from Morocco, the former USSR, Romania, Bulgaria, and Turkey.

Constituents: Up to ca. 1% essential oil; 60–70% D-(+)-linalool, 20% monoterpene hydrocarbons (α-pinene, limonene, γ-terpinene, *p*-cymene etc.); camphor; geraniol and geranyl acetate [1, 2]. *trans*-Tridec-2-en-1-al is responsible for the "bedbug" smell of the unripe fruit and of the herb [2].

Indications: Because of the essential oil, as a stomachic, spasmolytic, and carminative, which also has bactericidal and fungicidal properties; also for sub-acid gastritis, diarrhoea, and dyspepsia of various origins. The addition of coriander to preparations of Rhei radix, Frangulae cortex, Rhamni purshiani cortex, and Sennae folia is supposed to prevent the colicky pains that may sometimes occur when anthraquinone drugs are used.

In *folk medicine,* the drug finds use against worms and as a component of embrocations for rheumatism and pains in the joints.

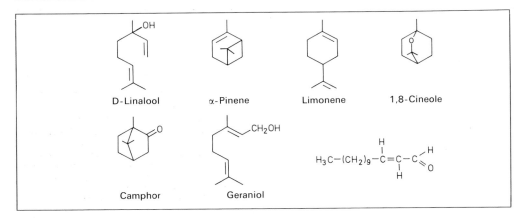

D-Linalool   α-Pinene   Limonene   1,8-Cineole

Camphor   Geraniol

However, coriander is employed more especially as a spice, e.g. in bread in order to make it more wholesome when fresh, in certain kinds of curry powders, and in gingerbread, and as an ingredient in liqueurs, e.g. Danziger Goldwasser, Boonekamp (a digestive), etc., and in certain "spirits", e.g. Spiritus Melissae compositus (Karmelitergeist) and Spiritus aromaticus [3]. – The essential oil is also used as an aroma substance in the tobacco and perfumery industries.

Side effects: Powdered coriander, and more particularly the oil, is known to give rise to allergic reactions. 5- and 8-methoxypsoralen and imperatorin and other photo-active compounds are present in various parts of the plant, including the fruit [6].

Making the tea: Boiling water is poured over 1–3 g of coriander which has been pounded or crushed immediately before use, covered and allowed to stand for 10–15 min., and finally strained.
1 Teaspoon = ca. 2.3 g.

Phytomedicines: As a component of carminative and laxative remedies, in the form of alcoholic distillates and drops, often in combination with other essential-oil drugs, such as anise, caraway, and fennel.

Regulatory status (UK): General Sales List – oil: Schedule 1, Table A.

Authentication: Macro- (see: Description) and microscopically. The yellowish brown powdered drug is characterized particularly by fragments of the 50–75 µm thick layers of sclerenchyma from the mesocarp, which comprise groups of fusiform, sinuous, strongly thickened and pitted, lignified cells oriented in various directions; see further [5].
The TLC test of identity given in the DAB 10 is as follows:

Test solution: 0.5 g freshly powdered drug shaken for 2–3 min. with 5.0 ml dichloro-

methane and filtered over ca. 2 g anhydrous sodium sulphate; the filtrate (= test solution) to be used immediately.

Reference solution: 15 µl linalool and 25 µl olive oil freshly dissolved in 5.0 ml dichloromethane.

Loadings: 20 µl test solution and 10 µl reference solution, as 2 cm bands on silica gel G.

Solvent system: ethyl acetate + dichloromethane (3 + 97), 10 cm run.

Detection: sprayed with anisaldehyde reagent (0.5 ml anisaldehyde mixed successively with 10 ml 98% acetic acid, 85 ml methanol, and 5 ml 96% sulphuric acid), followed by heating at 100–105 °C for 5–10 min. while under observation.

Evaluation: immediately in daylight. Reference solution: the violet linalool zone in the lower third and the violet triglyceride zone just above the middle. Test solution: the main violet to greyish violet zone at the

same Rf as the reference linalool zone; the reddish to reddish violet triglyceride zone at the same Rf as the corresponding reference zone; slightly below the triglyceride zone, the mostly faint violet-grey geranyl acetate zone; in between the linalool zone and the starting line, several faint zones, the uppermost one (not always visible) the brownish yellow borneol zone and below it the violet-grey geraniol zone and several more violet-grey or brownish zones; between the triglyceride zone and the solvent front, a faint violet monoterpene hydrocarbon zone.

Quantitative standards: DAB 10: *Volatile oil*, not less than 0.6%. *Foreign (vegetable and mineral) matter*, not more than 2%. *Loss on drying*, not more than 13%. *Ash*, not more than 12%.
BP 1988: *Volatile oil*, not less than 0.3% (powdered coriander, 0.2%). *Foreign matter*, not more than 2.0%. *Acid-insoluble ash*, not more than 1.5%. *Storage*, not above 25 °C.
ÖAB: *Volatile oil*, not less than 0.5%. *Foreign matter*, not more than 1%. *Ash*, not more than 7.0%.
For the TLC of coriander oil, see [4].

Adulteration: In practice does not occur.

Storage: Protected from moisture and light in well-closed metal or glass (not plastic) containers.

Literature:
[1] V. Formáček and K.-H. Kubeczka, Essential Oils Analysis by Capillar Gas Chromatography und Carbon-13 NMR Spectroscopy. John Wiley & Sons, Chichester etc. 1982.
[2] E. Schratz and S.M.J.S. Quadry, Planta Med. **14**, 310 (1966).
[3] Hager, vol. **4**, 300 (1973); vol. **4**, 996 (1992).
[4] H. Wagner, S. Bladt, and E.M. Zgainski, Plant drug analysis, Springer-Verlag, Berlin, Heidelberg, New York, Tokyo, 1984, p. 30.
[5] B.P. Jackson and D.W. Snowdon, Atlas of microscopy of medicinal plants, culinary herbs and spices, Belhaven Press, London, 1990, p.76
[6] O. Ceska et al., Phytochemistry **27**, 2083 (1988).

Crataegi folium cum flore (DAB 10), Hawthorn leaf/flower

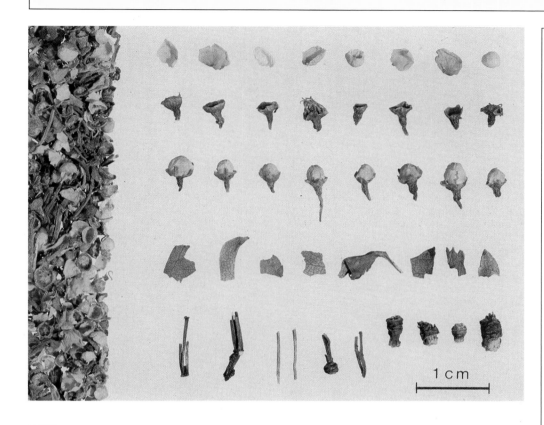

Fig. 1: Hawthorn leaf/flower

Description: The drug consists of dark brown, woody pieces of stem with petiolate, more or less deeply lobed leaves, the margin of which is only slightly serrate or almost entire; the close reticulate venation is prominent, especially on the paler, lower surface of the leaves, which, depending on the *Crataegus* species, are pubescent to a greater or lesser degree (see: Authentication). The flowers have a brownish or greyish green hypanthium, on the upper margin of which can be seen the five triangular calyx lobes. The five yellowish white to brownish petals are free (top row) and roundish or broadly ovate, with a short acumen. Depending on the species, the ovary, which is fused with the hypanthium, bears 1–5 long styles.

Odour: Faintly scented, characteristic.

Taste: Sweetish, and slightly bitter and astringent.

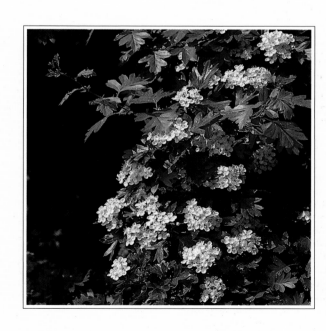

Fig. 2: *Crataegus monogyna* JACQ.

Usually a much branched 2–5 m tall shrub, or up to 10 m tall tree, with thorny branches bearing oval to rhombic, deeply 3–5-lobed (*C. monogyna*) or only slightly 3-lobed but finely serrate (*C. laevigata*) leaves. Broad cymes of white flowers, with one or more styles, depending on the species, and numerous stamens with red anthers. (*Crataegus* species readily hybridize, so that precise identification of the species is often not possible.)

DAB 10: Weißdornblätter mit Blüten
Ph. Helv. VII: Crataegi folium cum flore
St.Zul. 1349.99.99

Plant sources: *Crataegus laevigata* (POIRET) DC. (syn. *C. oxyacantha* auct., *C. oxyacanthoides* THUILL.), Midland hawthorn, or *C. monogyna* JACQ., hawthorn; and less often *C. pentagyna* WALDST. et KIT. ex WILLD., *C. nigra* WALDST. et KIT., and *C. azarolus* L. (Rosaceae).

Synonyms: Hawthorn tops, Haw, May, or Whitethorn herb (Engl.), Weißdornblätter mit Blüten, Hagedorn (Ger.), Herbe d'aubépine avec fleurs (Fr.).

Origin: *Crataegus laevigata* and *C. monogyna* occur throughout Europe; *C. pentagyna* is native in the Balkan Peninsula, *C. azarolus* in the eastern Mediterranean region, and *C. nigra* in Hungary and former Yugoslavia; there is some cultivation. The drug is imported from Bulgaria, Albania, former Yugoslavia, the former USSR, Romania, and Poland.

Dimeric procyanidin (B-2)

Hyperoside

Vitexin

Constituents [1, 9]: 1–3% oligomeric procyanidins (also called leucoanthocyanidins or pycnogenols), of only partially known structure; their profile is qualitatively and quantitatively much the same for all five official species [10].

On the other hand, the composition of the 1–2% flavonoids present differs with each species [2]; moreover, the flavonoid profile of the leaves and flowers also varies within each species. In *C. monogyna* and *C. laevigata*, the flower buds are richer in total flavonoids and in hyperoside, and the leaves collected just before flowering have the highest total flavonoid content [10]; the young leaves contain more acetylated and unacetylated vitexin 2''-rhamnoside than old leaves [11].

The principal flavonoid in the flowers of *C. monogyna* and *C. laevigata* is hyperoside (ca. 1%); while the leaves of *C. monogyna* contain vitexin 2-rhamnoside and 4'''-acetyl-2''-rhamnoside (together ca. 1%), those of *C. laevigata* have only the unacetylated derivative; in both species, rutin and spiraeoside are present in small amounts in the leaves; however, rutin occurs in traces in and spiraeoside is absent from the flowers [12]. Many other flavonoids and glycosyl-flavones are present. For the TLC analysis of all five official species, see under: Authentication.

Other constituents: amines (some with a cardiotonic action [3]), catechols, phenol-carboxylic acids (especially chlorogenic acid), triterpene acids, sterols, amines (among them N^1,N^5,N^{10}-tri-4(*E*)-coumaroylspermidine [13]), and purines. See further the detailed review in [9].

Indications: Against incipient cardiac insufficiency, especially coronary insufficiency, and for mild cardiac muscular insufficiency (stages I-II of the New York Heart Association), as well as for the ageing heart not yet requiring cardiotonic glycosides, against a feeling of pressure and tightness in the cardiac region, and in mild bradyarrhythmia. Before use, it must be ascertained that the aforementioned symptoms do not have an organic cause (in which case other medication is required); accordingly, hawthorn must not be recommended uncritically for self-medication.

Extensive pharmacological and clinical tests [4–6] have demonstrated that the oligomeric procyanidins and flavonoids are the active substances largely (but not entirely) responsible for the action of the drug. Standardized hawthorn extracts bring about characteristic effects, particularly improved myocardial and coronary circulation, which can be measured against the raised tolerance of the myocardium to oxygen deficiency. More

precise pharmacological analysis suggests rather that the positive inotropic action is antagonism to a negative inotropism (that can be induced by beta-blockers). These effects have their molecular basis in the inhibition of c-AMP-phosphodiesterase which takes place even with low doses; in addition, the *Crataegus* flavones have a measurable effect on the control of the intracellular Ca^{++} concentration.

Central effects have also been demonstrated with extracts of *C.laevigata*: in the mouse, after oral administration of an ethanolic extract, there is a modest, but definite depressant effect (determined using four different tests) [7]. Although it has been shown that the oligomeric procyanidins are absorbed on oral administration, the recommended daily dose of not less than 5 mg is so small that, in spite of their pharmacologically proved potency, there must be scepticism regarding their therapeutic significance (at least as the only supposedly active substances); evidently, the therapeutic application of *Crataegus* depends on the combined effects of several different constituents or groups of constituents [4, 8]. It has been observed empirically that with the combination of *Crataegus* extract and cardiotonic glycosides, the dose of the latter can be reduced; such preparations are being used therapeutically, e.g. Crataelanat®, etc.

Side effects: Not known in therapeutic doses.

Making the tea: Boiling water (ca. 150 ml) is poured over 1–1.5 g finely chopped drug and after 15 min. strained. During the treatment, the infusion is taken three or four times a day, over a period of several weeks. 1 Teaspoon = ca. 1.8 g.

Phytomedicines: The drug, but more especially extracts prepared from it, are present in more than 100 prepared remedies, particularly in the groups cardiotonics, coronary remedies, and antihypertonics, as well as geriatric preparations, tonics, arteriosclerosis remedies, etc.; products containing only *Crataegus* extracts are usually standardized on the basis of their oligomeric procyanidins, e.g. Crataegutt® (dragees, drops, ampoules), Eurython® (drops), etc., or adjusted to a given flavonoid content, e.g. Esbericard® (dragees, drops, injection), Cratamed®, Oxacant® (drops), Melicedin® (capsules), etc. The number of preparations which have hawthorn extracts as a component in combination with other drug extracts is very much larger; here also, preference should be given to standardized preparations.

Note: Crataegus is the subject of an ESCOP proposal for a European harmonized monograph which combines elements of hawthorn leaves/flowers and fruits (haws).

Authentication: Macro- (see: Description) and microscopically, following the DAB 10. The leaves of the various *Crataegus* species have very different degrees of pubescence (Fig. 3). *C. nigra* and *C. azarolus* are densely pubescent, especially on the lower surface, the other species less so; the trichomes are unicellular, thick-walled, and long (Fig. 4). There are clusters of calcium oxalate crystals in the mesophyll; single crystals are less frequent.
The TLC examination of the flavonoids is carried out according to DAB 10:

Test solution: 1.0 g powdered drug shaken with 10 ml methanol for 5 min. on the water-bath at 60 °C and filtered.

Reference solution: 1.0 mg chlorogenic acid and 2.5 mg each of hyperoside and rutin dissolved in 10 ml methanol.

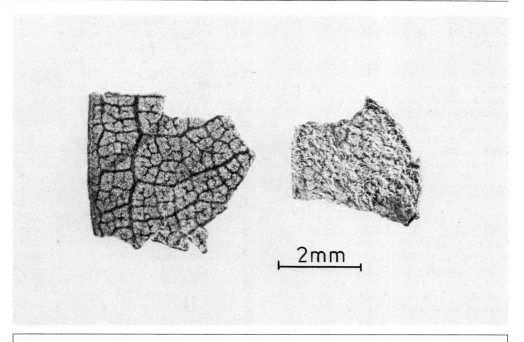

Fig. 3: Lower leaf surface of *Crataegus laevigata* (left) and *Crataegus nigra* (right; densely pubescent)

Loadings: 30 µl test solution and 10 µl reference solution, as 2 cm bands on silica gel G.

Solvent system: water + anhydrous formic acid + ethyl methyl ketone + ethyl acetate (10 + 10 + 30 + 50), 15 cm run.

Detection: after drying at 100–105 °C, while still warm sprayed with 1% methanolic diphenylboryloxyethylamine and then with 5% methanolic polyethylene glycol 400.

Evaluation: after 30 min., in UV 365 nm light. Reference and Test solutions: lowest zone, the moderately intense yellowish brown fluorescent zone of rutin; towards the

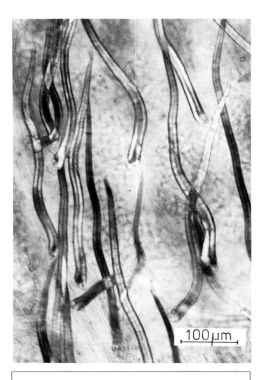

Fig. 4: Thick-walled trichomes from *Crataegus nigra*

Wording of the package insert, from the German Standard Licence:

5.1 **Uses**
Cardiac insufficiency; a feeling of pressure and tightness in the cardiac region.

5.2 **Dosage and Mode of administration**
Hot water (ca. 150 ml) is poured over a teaspoonful of **Hawthorn leaves/flowers** and after 20 min. passed through a tea strainer.
Unless otherwise prescribed, a cup of the freshly prepared tea is drunk two or three times a day.

Note
Store protected from light and moisture.

solvent front, the pale blue fluorescent chlorogenic-acid zone and the intense yellowish brown-orange fluorescent hyperoside zone. Test solution: directly above the hyperoside zone, a similarly coloured fluorescent zone and, near the solvent front, a light blue fluorescent zone; other, fainter zones present.

TLC on silica gel 60F$_{254}$ of the procyanidins and flavonoids in methanol leaf extracts enables all five official *Crataegus* species to be differentiated. The solvent systems are: (a) procyanidins, ethyl acetate + glacial acetic acid + water (10 + 2 + 3; upper phase) and detection with 1% methanolic vanillin, followed by conc. hydrochloric acid, and examination in daylight; (b) flavonoids, ethyl acetate + formic acid + water (30 + 2 + 3) and detection as set out above. For details and illustrations of the chromatograms, see [10].

A reverse-phase HPLC method is also available for the identification and semi-quantitative standardization of the procyanidins in *Crataegus* extracts [13].

Quantitative standards: DAB 10: *Flavonoids*, not less than 0.7% calculated as hyperoside (M_r 464.4). *Foreign matter*, not more than 2%; flowers of other genera (*Sorbus, Prunus*) must not be present. *Loss on drying*, not more than 10.0% *Ash*, not more than 9.0%.

Ph. Helv. VII: *Flavonoids*, not less than 0.7% calculated as hyperoside (M_r 464.4). *Foreign matter*, not more than 8% lignified elements; flowers of other genera (*Sorbus, Robinia*) must not be present. *Sulphated ash*, not more than 12%.

Adulteration: Extremely rare. Flowers of other *Crataegus* species, of *Sorbus aucuparia* L., rowan tree, of *Prunus spinosa* L., blackthorn, can be recognized by their deviating morphological and anatomical characters [1].

Drugs consisting only of the flowers of *Crataegus*, (Crataegi flos, Flores Crataegi) are sometimes adulterated with the very similar looking flowers of blackthorn (Prunus spinosae flos, q.v.). An easily ascer-tained difference: the endothecium of *Crataegus* appears red in cold chloral hydrate solution, that of *Prunus spinosa* does not.

Literature:
[1] Kommentar DAB 10.
[2] A. Hecker-Niediek, Thesis, Univ. Marburg, 1983.
[3] H. Wagner and J. Grevel, Planta Med. **45**, 98 (1982).
[4] F. Occhiuto et al., Plantes Méd. Phytothérap. **20**, 37, 52, 115 (1986).
[5] H.P.T. Ammon and M. Händel, Planta Med. **43**, 105, 209, 313 (1981).
[6] A. Beretz, M. Haag-Berrurier, and R. Anton, Plantes Méd. Phytothérap. **12**, 305 (1978).
[7] R. Della Loggia et al., Sci. Pharm. **51**, 319 (1983).
[8] M. Iwamoto, T. Sato, and T. Ishizaki, Planta Med. **42**, 1 (1981).
[9] C. Hobbs and S. Foster, Herbal Gram no. **22**, 21 (1990).
[10] M. Schüssler and J. Hölzl, Dtsch. Apoth. Ztg. **132**, 1327 (1992).
[11] J.L. Lamaison and A. Carnart, Plantes Méd. Phytothérap. **25**, 12 (1991)
[12] J.L. Lamaison and A. Carnart, Pharm. Acta Helv. **65**, 315 (1990).
[13] D. Strack et al., Phytochemistry **29**, 2893 (1990).
[14] U. Krawczyk, G. Petri, and A. Kéry, Arch. Pharm. (Weinheim) **324**, 97 (1991).

Crataegi fructus   Hawthorn berry

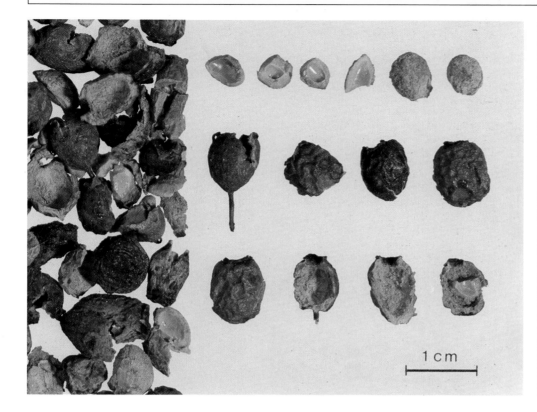

Fig. 1: Hawthorn berry

<u>Description:</u> **The drug consists of the wine-red to yellowish brown, ovoid, coarsely to finely wrinkled, berry-like false fruit (pome) which at the upper end bears five reflexed calyx lobes. Inside, there is a brownish yellow tissue (fruit flesh) in which are embedded 1–3 hard, yellow stones (seeds), partly broken (top row).**

<u>Taste:</u> **Sweetish and mucilaginous.**

Fig. 2: *Crataegus laevigata* (POIRET) **DC.**

Flowers with 2–3 styles (*C. laevigata*). *Crataegus* – a genus with an inferior ovary (characteristic of the subfamily Maloideae) fused with the tissues of the floral axis and ripening into a red, fleshy false fruit with 1 (*C. monogyna*) or 2–3 (*C. laevigata*) stones.

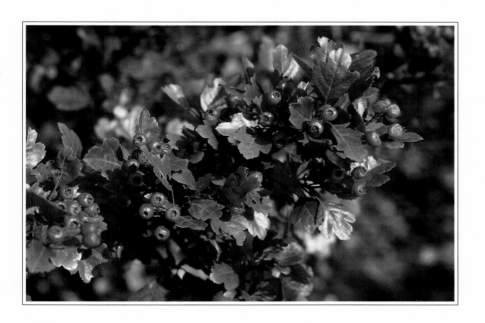

DAC 1986: Weißdornbeeren

Plant sources: *Crataegus laevigata* (POIRET) DC., Midland hawthorn, and *C. monogyna* JACQ., hawthorn (Rosaceae). The three other species permitted by the DAB 10 for the leaf and flower drug are excluded by the DAC 1986, no doubt because there was insufficient experience with them.

Synonyms: Fructus oxyacanthae, Fructus spinae albae (Lat.), Crataegus fruit (BHP 1983), Weißdornfrüchte, Hagedornbeeren (Ger.), Fruits d'aubépine (Fr.).

Origin: See, Crataegi folium cum flore. The drug is imported from Bulgaria, Romania, the former USSR, Poland, Hungary, and former Yugoslavia.

Constituents: Very similar to those of Crataegi folium cum flore (q.v.); the relative amounts of the individual flavonoids and oligomeric procyanidins is, however, different from the leaves – the fruits contain relatively more hyperoside, the leaves relatively more vitexin rhamnoside.

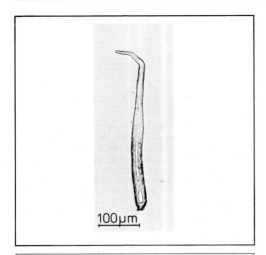

Fig. 3: Thick-walled trichome from the styles

Indications: As for Crataegi folium cum flore (q.v.). Unlike the leaves and flowers, the fruits are not used to prepare infusions, but they play a greater role in the manufacture of prepared remedies.

Making the tea: Not usually done with the fruit.

Phytomedicines: There are many prepared remedies in which extracts of this drug, often combined with extracts from hawthorn leaf and flower, form an essential part. The more than 100 preparations are mainly in the groups cardiotonics, coronary remedies, antihypertonics, and arteriosclerosis remedies, geriatric remedies, and tonics.

Authentication: Macro- (see: Description) and microscopically, following the DAC 1986. The unicellular, thick-walled trichomes of the styles (Fig. 3), which are partly geniculate and end in a point, are characteristic. Sclereids, partly in groups, and clusters, as well as single crystals, of calcium oxalate are also present.
The TLC examination of the flavonoids, catechins, and triterpenes is carried out according to the DAC 1986.

Note: The DAC 1986 monograph has been temporarily withdrawn, pending redrafting. About the ESCOP proposal for a harmonized European monograph on hawthorn, see: Crataegi folium cum flore.

Adulteration: In practice, very rare. According to the DAC 1986, fruits of *Crataegus* species other than those mentioned should be absent. *C. nigra* fruits are black, while those of *C. azarolus* are bigger and yellowish red; they very rapidly become mouldy. The fruits of *C. pentagyna* are very much smaller and more slender than the fruits of the permitted species; all these fruits contain more than three stones.

Croci stigma (Ph. Eur. 1/III), Saffron

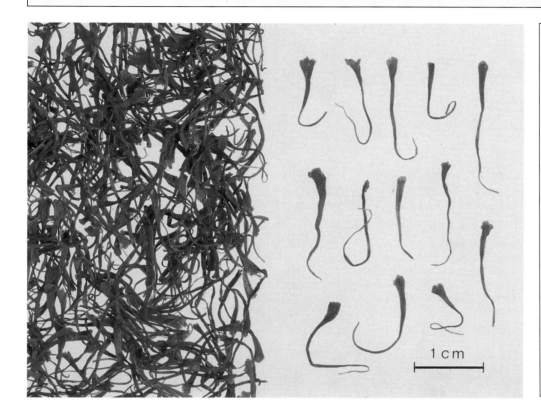

Fig. 1: Saffron

<u>Description:</u> Saffron consists of a loose mass of stigmas mostly still attached to the top part of the style of the autumn-flowering *Crocus sativus*. The sealing-wax red stigmas in the dry condition are 20–40 mm long and when wet 35–50 mm long. The tubes of the styles are split open on one side and widen into a narrow funnel towards the apex, which is open and finely notched along the upper edge. The top part of the style to which the stigmas are attached is pale yellow and not more than 5 mm in length.

Odour: Strongly aromatic.

<u>Taste:</u> Spicy, aromatic, somewhat pungent, slightly bitter and not sweet, reminiscent of iodoform. The saliva takes on a strong yellow colour.

Fig. 2: *Crocus sativus* L.

A bulbous plant, flowering in the autumn, with very narrow, long leaves. Flowers comprising a long tube topped by a lilac perigone with violet veins, three yellow stamens, a thin yellow stigma and three long, protruding, funnel-shaped, red styles.

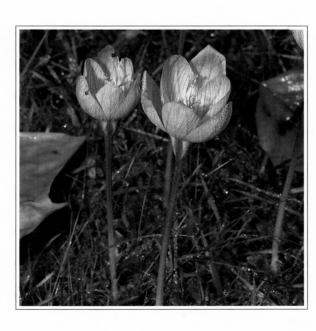

ÖAB: Flos Croci
Ph. Helv. VI: Crocus

Plant source: *Crocus sativus* L., saffron crocus (Iridaceae).

Synonyms: Crocus orientalis or hispanicus (Lat.), Hay saffron (Engl.), Safran, Gewürzsafran (Ger.), Safran (Fr.).

Origin: An ancient cultivated plant, and probably native to southern Europe and south-western Asia; nowadays, the drug comes almost exclusively from sterile *Crocus* plants cultivated in southern Spain. There are various commercial forms: in particular, crocus naturalis, which is mixed with style remains, and crocus electus, a selected product, which has been freed from style remains; for other commercial varieties, see [1]. About the cultural history of saffron, see [2].

Constituents: Yellow, water-soluble pigments derived from crocetin, which formally is a diterpene but which biosynthetically be-

Crocetin: R = H
Crocin: R = Gentiobiose

Glucose—O Picrocrocin → HO 4-Hydroxycyclocitral → Safranal

longs to the carotenoids, e.g. crocin (crocetin di-β-D-gentiobiosyl ester); further, bitter substances, e.g. picrocrocin, and the characteristic aroma substance safranal, which arises from the aglycone picrocrocin, β-hydroxycyclocitral, by the splitting off of water during the drying process. It is the main component of the essential oil which may form up to 1% of the drug. In addition, fixed oil (up to 10%) and oleanolic-acid derivatives [3].

Indications: The drug *no longer has any medicinal importance.* Its inclusion in the Eur. Ph. 1/III at the time was due to the fact that it was intended to prepare a monograph on "Tinctura Opii crocata" which has since been abandoned.
According to animal experiments, crocetin has lipid-lowering properties; it inhibits artificially induced hypercholesterolaemia in rabbits, considerably raises oxygen diffusion in the plasma (by up to 80%), and leads to a decrease in serum cholesterol levels by ca. 30% [5].
In *folk medicine,* saffron is still occasionally used as a sedative, spasmolytic, and stomachic.
The main importance of the drug nowadays is as an aroma and taste enhancer: in the kitchen, as a spice, e.g. added to curried rice, bouillabaise, paella, etc., and especially in industry as a colouring agent for bakery products, liqueurs, cosmetics, and medicines.

Side effects: Saffron taken in large amounts is highly toxic. The lethal dose is ca. 20 g; but smaller amounts give rise to intoxication, with the following symptoms: vomiting, uterine bleeding (formerly, because of its stimulating action on smooth muscle, saffron was misused as an abortifacient), bloody diarrhoea, haematuria, bleeding from the nose, lips, and eyelids, vertigo,

numbness, yellowing of the skin and mucous membranes (simulating icterus).

Making the tea: Not applicable.

Phytomedicines: Extracts of saffron are present in so-called "Swedish bitters" made by various manufacturers (see the note under: Aloe capensis) and also in a very few prepared remedies belonging to different indications.

Authentication: As the drug is very expensive, authentication is particularly important, because, especially when in the powdered form, it is very often adulterated. Macro- (see: Description) and microscopical examination is therefore essential.
The epidermal cells are elongated and in the middle often have a short papilla; when mounted in water, a yellow pigment leaches

---

Extract from the German Commission E monograph
(BAnz no. 76, dated 23.04.1987)

Uses

Saffron is used to calm the nerves and against cramps and asthma.
There is no evidence for the efficacy of the drug in the conditions indicated.

Risks

With a maximum daily dose of 1.5 g, so far no risks have been documented.
The lethal dose for saffron is 20.0 g and the abortifacient dose 10.0 g.
When used as an abortifacient, the effects of the drug are as follows: severe purpura after taking 5 g saffron (in milk), with deep black necrosis of the nose accompanied by thrombocytopaenia (24,000), hypothrombinaemia (41%), and severe collapse with uraemia.
In addition, there may be: vomiting, uterine bleeding, bloody diarrhoea, haematuria, bleeding from the nose, lips, and eyelids, as well as attacks of dizziness and numbness; yellowing of the sclera, skin, and mucous membranes, thus simulating icterus, may also occur.

---

out. The upper edge of the stigma has digitate papillae which are up to 150 μm long. Between the papillae there are single, spherical, thick-walled pollen grains, up to 100 μm in diameter, which have a finely grained exine (Fig. 3, below) without preformed pores. The vascular bundles have narrow vessels with spiral thickening. Fibres and lignified elements should be absent (negative reaction with phloroglucinol and hydrochloric acid). Pollen with three pores (as when adulterated with safflower), fragments of the endothecium of the anthers (adulteration with the stamens and pollen sacks of *Crocus sativus*), and crystals (various yellow flowers) should likewise be absent.
If a drop of conc. sulphuric acid is added to a trace of saffron powder placed on a slide, the powder first becomes dark blue and then changes to reddish brown to reddish violet (detection of carotenoids in saffron, as well as in other carotenoid-containing petals).
The Ph. Helv. VI (not VII) has the following test for crocetin and its precursors: if a few mg of the drug powder on a slide are rubbed with a drop of phosphomolybdic/sulphuric acid reagent and a cover slip at once placed on top, when examined under $100\times$ magnification most of the fragments of powder should turn blue within one min. and become surrounded by a bluish halo.
A rapid test may be useful: sufficient saffron to cover the tip of a spatula are shaken with 50 ml water or 50 ml chloroform for a few minutes; the aqueous solution must be dark yellow (water-soluble crocin) and the chloroform solution must be almost colourless (a yellow colour points to the presence of lipophilic flower and fruit carotenoids of *Capsicum* and of aniline dyes).
The Ph. Eur. 1/III method for the TLC examination is as follows:

Test solution: 10 mg drug crushed with a glass rod and moistened with one drop of water; after 2–3 min. 1 ml methanol added, stood in the dark for 20 min., and filtered through glass wool.

Reference solution: 5 mg Sudan Red G in 5 ml chloroform added to 5 mg Naphthol Yellow in 5 ml methanol.

Loadings: 5 μl each of the test and reference solutions, as 1.5 cm bands on silica gel GF_{254}.

Solvent system: ethyl acetate+propan-2-ol+water (65+25+10), 10 cm run.

Detection: in UV 254 nm light, then daylight, and finally sprayed with anisaldehyde reagent and heated for 5–10 min. at 100–105 °C while under observation.

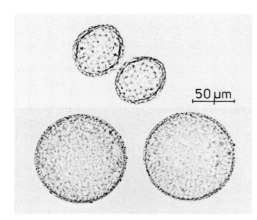

Fig. 3: **Pollen grains of *Carthamus tinctorius* (top) and *Crocus sativus* (bottom)**

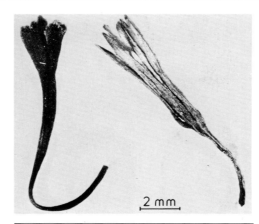

Fig. 4: **Stigmas of *Crocus sativus* (left) and tubular flowers of *Carthamus tinctorius* (right; safflower)**

ers, e.g. of *Calendula officinalis* L. (see: Calendulae flos), *Carthamus tinctorius* L. (safflower), recognizable as tubular flowers even under low magnification (Fig. 4) and by the numerous smaller pollen grains (Fig. 3, top) with a thicker, coarsely verrucose, exine; on microscopical examination, secretory ducts with a brown resinous content can be seen near the vascular bundles.

Falsification with *Tagetes* species (American saffron), with stigmas of *Crocus sativus* L. (meadow saffron), or with paprika powder, *Curcuma* powder (turmeric), batches of faded saffron subsequently coloured with aniline dyes, and red-sandalwood powder, etc. [1, 3, 4, 6], is less frequent. Often, powdered saffron is also loaded with glycerol, barium sulphate, flour, etc.; about this, see: Authentication. – More recently, samples of saffron have been offered on the market which consist entirely of safflower (see above) stained with so far unidentified water-soluble yellow dyes.

Evaluation: Test solution: in *daylight* – in the lower third, three yellow bands with the lowest one the most intense (crocin), corresponding in size and colour with the reference Naphthol Yellow band; no yellow, orange, or red bands, especially at the starting point (absence of crocin decomposition products or foreign colouring matters); in *UV 254 nm light* – at about the same Rf a dark band (picrocrocin); at the Rf of the reference Sudan Red G band, another dark band (β-hydroxycyclocitral); sprayed with *anisaldehyde reagent* – greyish blue crocin and picrocrocin bands, along with other coloured bands.

Coloured illustrations of the TLC are to be found in [7].

Quantitative standards: Ph. Eur. 1/III: *Colouring power*, 0.10 g powdered drug is occasionally shaken with 100 ml water over a period of 2 h, filtered, and 10 ml filtrate diluted to 100 ml with water; the final solution should not be less coloured than a 0.05% aqueous solution of potassium dichromate. *Loss on drying*, not more than 10.0%. *Sulphated ash*, not more than 8.0%.

Adulteration: Very frequent; the powdered drug is usually more or less grossly adulterated or contaminated. It is therefore recommended to buy in only the more easily identified whole drug.

The following adulterants have been encountered: yellow flowers and parts of flow-

Storage: Protected from light and moisture in tightly closed metal or glass (but not plastic) containers, since the drug rapidly fades and the essential oil is rather volatile.

Literature:
[1] Hager, vol. **4**, p. 336 (1973).
[2] F.-C. Czygan, Z. Phytotherap. **7**, 180 (1986).
[3] Commentary Ph. Eur. 1/III, Croci stigma.
[4] Berger, vol. **1**, p. 287 (1949).
     K. Staesche, in: Handbuch der Lebensmittelchemie, Springer, Berlin, 1970, vol. **6** (Gewürze), pp. 426-610, G. Gassner, Mikroskopische Untersuchung pflanzlicher Lebensmittel, 4th ed., G. Fischer, Stuttgart, 1973.
[5] J. Gainer and J. Jones, Experientia **31**, 548 (1978).
[6] F.-C. Czygan, Pharm. Ztg. **125**, 1853 (1980).
[7] H. Wagner, S. Bladt, and E. M. Zgainski, Plant drug analysis, Springer-Verlag, Berlin, Heidelberg, New York, Tokyo, 1984, p. 275.

Cucurbitae semen   (DAB 10), Pumpkin seed

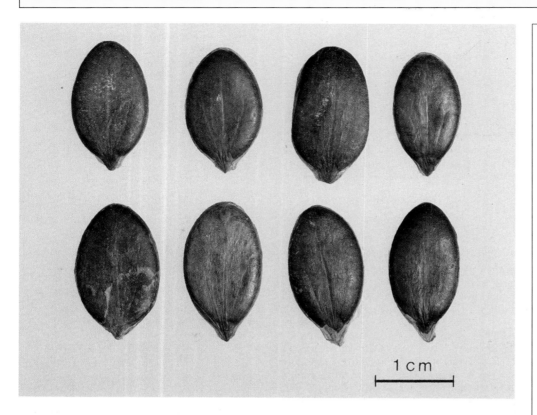

Fig. 1: Pumpkin seed

<u>Description</u>: The greenish to earth-coloured, oval, flattened seeds are ca. 7–15 mm long (in the case of *Cucurbita maxima* up to 24 mm) and usually twice as long as broad, with the micropyle recognizable at the narrow pointed end. Nowadays, the drug comes mainly from cultivated varieties which do not have a testa. Where it is present, the surface has an irregular nap (hand lens). The edge of the seed is more or less distinctly ridged.

<u>Taste</u>: Oily and sweetish.

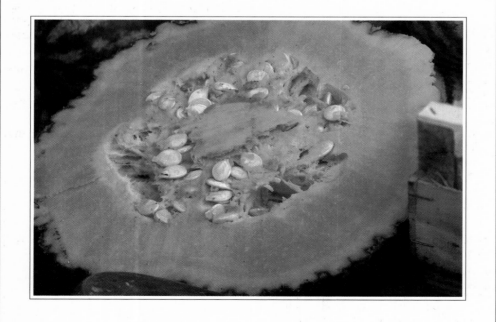

Fig. 2: *Cucurbita pepo* L.

Annuals forming prostrate shoots, up to 10 m long, with very large, more or less clearly 5-lobed leaves and yellow dioecious flowers with a funnel-shaped corolla (monoecious). Huge spherical fruits (berries) containing many flattened seeds.

DAB 10: Kürbissamen
St.Zul. 1559.99.99

Plant sources: Nowadays, especially *Cucurbita pepo* L. convar. *citrullinina* GREB. var. *styriaca* GREB. (Cucurbitaceae) [1]. *C. pepo* is known variously as (a non-keeping) vegetable marrow, summer and autumn squash and pumpkin.
The following taxa are also certainly involved: *C. maxima* DUCHESNE, (a keeping) autumn and winter squash, pumpkin; *C. moschata* DUCHESNE ex POIR., winter squash or pumpkin; *C. argyro- sperma* HUBER (*C. mixta* PANGALO), winter squash, pumpkin; and *C. ficifolia* BOUCHÉ, Malabar gourd.

Synonyms: Semen peponis (Lat.), Kürbissamen (Ger.), Graine de pépon, Graine de courge, Graine de citrouille (Fr.).

Origin: Native to America, but now cultivated worldwide. Imports come from the former USSR, former Yugoslavia, China, Austria, Hungary, and Mexico.

Constituents: Ca. 1% steroids, especially 24β-ethyl-5α-cholesta-7,25(27)-dien-3β-ol and 24β-ethyl-5α-cholesta-7-*trans*-22,25(27)-trien-3β-ol as essential components [1], and to some extent also sterol glucosides [2] and Δ^5- and Δ^8-sterols [3]; tocopherols (vitamin E); trace elements, particularly selenium, manganese, zinc, and copper; 35–40% fixed oil; ca. 30% pectins; ca. 25–30% protein. The nature and amount of the constituents depends to a large extent on the taxon [4, 5].

Indications: Nowadays, mostly for treating problems of micturition, especially those associated with benign prostate adenomas. The use is still largely empirical, but there are reliable medical and clinical reports [6–8]. According to [4], only the seeds of *C. pepo* convar. *citrullinina* var. *styriaca* should be used, since it is only for these seeds that sufficient clinical experience is available. The protective function that α-tocopherol and selenium have towards the oxidative degradation of lipids, vitamins, hormones, and enzymes has been discussed as the possible mechanism of action [4]. The effect of the cucurbitacins on the binding of 5α-dihydrotestosterones to SHBG (sex-hormone binding globulin) has also been considered (prostate complaints are seen as a derangement of this process), but owing to the absence of cucurbitacins, this finding [9, 10] is irrelevant to the use of pumpkin seeds as a drug [11].
Certain protein fractions in pumpkin seeds function as trypsin inhibitors [12]. The use as a vermifuge, especially against tapeworms and roundworms, which was formerly common in *folk medicine*, has now greatly declined.

Making the tea: Not applicable. For internal use, 10–20 g seed (1–2 tablespoons) is well chewed.
1 Teaspoon = ca. 5 g, 1 tablespoon = ca. 10 g.

Phytomedicines: Some prepared urological and prostate remedies, e.g. Prosta Fink N®, Granufink Kürbis-Granulat, Prostatin Kanoldt®, Prostamed®, Uvirgan®, etc. The fixed oil from pumpkin seed is also present in such preparations, e.g. Cysto-Fink®, etc.

Authentication: Macro- (see: Description) and microscopically. The testa of the seed is greatly reduced in most cultivated forms; the tissue of the cotyledons is largely composed of thin-walled parenchyma containing fixed oil and aleurone grains.

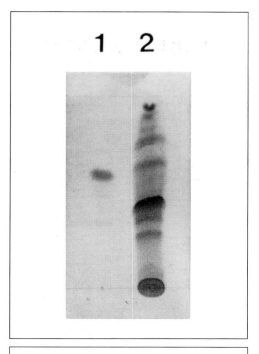

Fig. 3: TLC on 4 × 8 cm silica-gel foil

1: β-Sitosterol (reference compound)
2: Pumpkin seed

For details, see the text

The following is a suitable TLC identification procedure:

Test solution: 2 g powdered drug refluxed for 10 min. with 10 ml methanol at 60 °C, cooled and filtered, washed with methanol, and made up to 10 ml with methanol.

Reference solution: 10 mg β-sitosterol dissolved in 10 ml methanol.

Loadings: 10 µl test solution and 5 µl reference solution, as bands.

Solvent system: chloroform + ethanol (95 + 5), 6 cm run.

Detection: dried in a current of warm air, then sprayed with a mixture comprising 8 ml 2% ethanolic vanillin solution and 2 ml 85% phosphoric acid, followed by heating at 105 °C for 10 min.

Evaluation: in daylight. <u>Reference solution</u>: slightly below the middle , a bluish violet zone (β-sitosterol). <u>Test solution</u>: at roughly the same Rf value, a bluish violet zone (sterols); just below the middle another intense blue zone (linoleic acid); in the upper third and below the linoleic-acid zone, further blue, bluish green, or bluish violet zones (Fig. 3).

Quantitative standards: <u>St.Zul. 1559.99.99</u>: *Diethyl ether-soluble extractive*, not less than 35%. *Phytosterols*, not less than 0.1%. *Foreign matter*, not more than 1%. *Loss on drying*, not more than 12.0%. *Sulphated ash*, not more than 6.0%.

Adulteration: Seed that is unripe or seed that has been attacked by insects can be detected by inspection.

Literature:

[1] W. Sucrow, M. Slopianka and H.W. Kircher, Phytochemistry **15**, 1533 (1976).

[2] H.W. Rauwald, M. Sauter and H. Schilcher, Phytochemistry **24**, 2746 (1985).

[3] T. Akihisa et al., Lipids **21**, 39 (1986).

[4] H. Schilcher, Z. angew. Phytother. **2**, 14 (1981); 7, 19 (1986).

[5] W. Schuster, W. Zipse and R. Marquard, Fette, Seifen, Anstrichm. **85**, 56 (1983).

[6] H. Lützelberger, Ärztl. Praxis **76**, 3278 (1974).

[7] H. Haefele, Ärztl. Praxis **79**, 3321 (1977).

[8] R. Nitsch-Fitz, H. Egger, H. Wutzl and H. Maruna, Erfahrungsheilkunde **28**, 1009 (1979).

[9] K. Schmidt et al., Helv. Chir. Acta **47**, 439 (1980).

[10] K. Schmidt, V. Hagmaier and A. Seebauer, Klin. Exp. Urol. **4**, 152 (1982).

[11] H. Schilcher, personal communication.

[12] A. Szewczuk et al., Hoppe-Seyler's Z. Physiol. Chem. **364**, 941 (1983).

Curcumae longae rhizoma   Turmeric

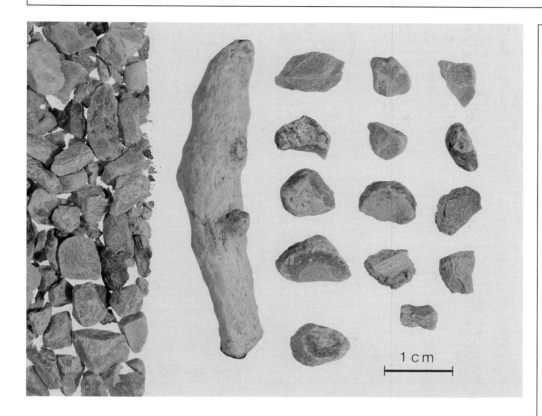

1 cm

Fig. 1: Turmeric

<u>Description:</u> The drug consists of cylindrical or finger-shaped, up to 15 mm thick secondary rhizomes (curcuma longa; finger or long turmeric), bearing scars of lateral branches, or tuberousovoid, up to 4 cm long, primary rhizomes (curcuma rotunda; bulb or round turmeric), bearing transverse annular leaf scars. Owing to the steaming or scalding carried out after harvesting, externally pieces of the drug fragments are yellowish brown, yellow, or greyish brown, and speckled. The fracture is smooth and finely granular; the broken surface is somewhat shiny and orange-yellow throughout, with a narrow, darker cortex on the outside.

<u>Odour:</u> Faintly aromatic and spicy.

<u>Taste:</u> Pungent and bitter.

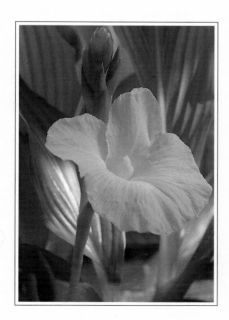

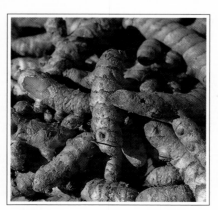

Fig. 2: *Curcuma domestica* VALETON

A rhizomatous tropical shrub with very large, oblong lanceolate, basal, petiolate leaves with more or less parallel nervature starting from the midrib. Zygomorphic flowers appearing at ground level and having three fused sepals and three large yellow petals.

Fig. 3: *Curcuma domestica* VALETON, freshly dug-up secondary rhizomes

With a greyish brown cork layer, Longish fragments of rhizome with a greyish brown cork layer and clearly visible longitudinal leaf scars and round root scars; where broken, intense yellow-orange in colour (curcuminoids).

DAC 1986: Curcumawurzelstock

Plant source: *Curcuma domestica* VALETON (syn. *C. longa* L.), turmeric (Zingiberaceae).

Synonyms: Turmeric rhizome or root, Indian saffron (Engl.), Kurkumawurzelstock, Gelbwurzel (Ger.), Rhizome de curcuma (Fr.).

Origin: Cultivated in tropical Asia and Africa. Drug imports come from China, Indonesia, and India.

Constituents: 3–5% yellow pigments that are not volatile in steam (curcuminoids), consisting of curcumin (diferuloylmethane), monodesmethoxycurcumin, and bisdesmethoxycurcumin [1, 2]. 2–7% essential oil, comprising mainly bisabolane, guaiane, and germacrane sesquiterpenes: turmerone, *ar*-turmerone, zingiberene, curlone, etc.; the high content of bisabolane derivatives distinguishes turmeric from other *Curcuma* species [18]. The earlier described *p*-tolyl methyl carbinol [3] is no doubt an artefact formed during distillation of the essential oil [4]. The abundant starch is largely gelatinized. A complex acidic arabinogalactan, ukonan A, is also present [19].

Indications: Turmeric is used chiefly as a spice and is an essential component of curry powders and other condiments. In addition, it has a role to play as a cholagogue [1, 2, 5–8]. While choleresis-inhibiting properties are ascribed to bisdesmethoxycurcumin, with altogether higher content of curcuminoids the cholagogic effect of the drug is

scarcely inferior to that of Javanese turmeric, *temu lawak*.

Curcuminoids have considerable antiphlogistic activity [9], which is due, at least in part, to inhibition of leukotriene biosynthesis and its consequent effect on prostaglandin production [10, 11, 20]. *ar*-Turmerone has anti-snake venom activity and blocks the haemorrhagic effect of *Bothrops* venom and much of the lethal effect of *Crotalus* venom; it blocks the proliferation and natural killer activity of human lymphocytes – effects possibly related to its anti-inflammatory properties [21]. Antihepatotoxic, as well as antibacterial, effects, both *in vitro* and *in vivo*, have been reported [12]. The polysaccharide ukonan A activates the reticulo-endothelial system and has powerful phagocytic activity in mice [19]. Recent investigations suggest that curcuminoids may be active in the external treatment of certain cancerous conditions [13]; this is presumably connected with the cytotoxicity of these substances, which has been demonstrated on cell cultures, including those of tumour cells [14].

The drug also finds use as a stomachic and carminative.

Side effects Curcuminoids are cytotoxic [14], inhibiting mitosis and leading to chromosome changes [15]. However, nothing is known about the oral toxicity of curcuminoids in man; the cytotoxic effects have been observed in cell cultures. In mice, chronic administration leads to significant changes in heart and lung weights and to falls in the red and white blood corpuscle counts [22]. Curcuminoids may possibily cause the formation of stomach ulcers [16].

Making the tea: Rarely done. It is better to take standardized preparations (low solubility of the essential oil and the curcumins), provided the curcumin content is sufficiently high; concerning this, see the critical remarks in [17]. Dose of the powdered drug: 0.5–1 g, several times a day between meals.

Phytomedicines: Ca. 70 prepared cholagogues and biliary remedies, e.g. Bilgast®, Cholagogum N Nattermann®, Cholhepan N®, etc., etc. The proportion of *Curcuma* in the mixtures is usually small.

Authentication: Macro- and microscopically, following the DAC 1986; for detailed microscopy of the powdered drug, see [23]. The red fluorescence in UV 365 nm light exhibited by an acetic anhydride/conc. sulphuric acid extract of the powder is due to the presence of bisdesmethoxycurcumin. The occurrence of mostly gelatinized starch is characteristic.

The TLC prcedure set out in the DAC 1986 is as follows:

Test solution: 1.0 g powdered drug shaken repeatedly with 4 ml methanol; after 30 min., filtered and made up to 5 ml.

Reference solution: (a) 5 mg thymol dissolved in 10 ml methanol, and 1 ml of this diluted to 10 ml; (b) 2 mg methyl red dissolved in 10 ml methanol.

Loadings: 10 µl of each solution as bands on silica gel 60.

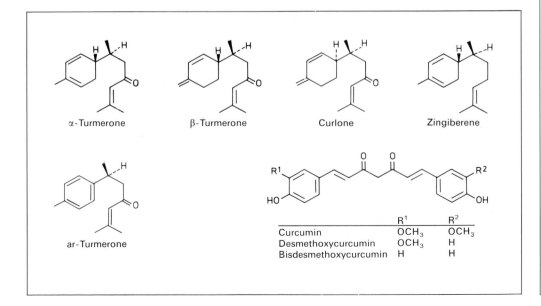

	R¹	R²
Curcumin	OCH₃	OCH₃
Desmethoxycurcumin	OCH₃	H
Bisdesmethoxycurcumin	H	H

α-Turmerone · β-Turmerone · Curlone · Zingiberene · ar-Turmerone

Solvent system: dichloromethane + ethanol + 98% acetic acid (94 + 5 + 1), 10 cm run.

Detection: in daylight, then sprayed with 0.5% Fast Red salt solution and again in daylight.

Evaluation: <u>Test solution:</u> in the middle third, **three** yellow zones (differentiation from Curcumae xanthorrhizae rhizoma = *temu lawak*) (q.v.), with the uppermost one at about the same Rf as the methyl red zone; after spraying, the zones becoming yellowish brown.

See further, Curcumae xanthorrhizae rhizoma.

HPLC is the method of choice for quantification (Nucleosil NH_2 column (200 × 4.6 mm int. diameter; 5 µm particle size; eluant ethanol + water (96 + 4)), but a useful alternative is HPTLC on 10 × 10 cm $NH_2F_{254}S$ plates with double development in ethanol + water (96 + 4) and quantification at 420 µm; Rf curcumin 0.13, monodesmethoxycurcumin 0.21, and bisdesmethoxycurcumin 0.36. To avoid undue decomposition of the curcuminoids on the amino-silica gel, conditions should be standardized and the application of the samples, development of the plate, and quantification should be carried out immediately one after the other; low concentrations of curcuminoids should be avoided, since the decomposition depends on the concentration [24].

Quantitative standards: <u>DAC 1986:</u> *Dicinnamoylmethane derivatives* (curcuminoids), not less than 3.0% calculated as curcumin (M_r 368.4). Essential oil, not less than 3.0%. *Foreign matter*, not more than 2%. *Loss on drying*, not more than 12.0%. *Ash*, not more than 7.0%.

Adulteration: Very rare. Insofar as confusion with *temu lawak* may occur, it can be detected by TLC of the essential oil (xanthorrhizol is characteristic of *temu lawak*).

Storage: Protected from light, in well-closed (but not plastic) containers.

See further: Curcumae xanthorrhizae rhizoma (Javanese turmeric or *temu lawak*).

Literature:

[1] K. Jentzsch, Th. Gonda, and H. Höller, Pharm. Acta Helv. **34**, 181 (1959).
[2] K. Jentzsch, P. Spiegl, and R. Kamitz, Sci. Pharm. **36**, 251 (1968).
[3] H. Dieterle and Ph. Kaiser, Arch. Pharm. (Weinheim) **271**, 337 (1933).
[4] Th.M. Malingré, Pharm. Weekbl. **110**, 601 (1975).
[5] J.C. Baumann, Med. Monatschr. **29**, 173 (1975).
[6] G. Harnischfeger and H. Stolze, notabene medici **12**, 562 (1982).
[7] H. Kalk and K. Nissen, Dtsch. Med. Wochenschr. **57**, 1613 (1931); idem., *ibid.*, **58**, 1718 (1932).
[8] R.C. Srimal and B.N. Dhawan, J. Pharm. Pharmacol. **25**, 447 (1973).
[9] R.R. Satoskar, S.J. Shah, and S.G. Shenoy, Internat. J. Clin. Pharmacol. Toxicol. **24**, 651 (1986).
[10] H. Wagner, M. Wierer, and R. Bauer, Planta Med. **52**, 184 (1986).
[11] R. Srivastava et al., Arzneim.-Forsch. **36**, 715 (1986).
[12] Y. Kiso et al., Planta Med. **49**, 185 (1983).
[13] R. Kuttan, P.C. Sudheeran, and C.D. Josph, Tumori **73**, 29 (1987).
[14] R. Kuttan et al., Cancer Lett. **29**, 197 (1985).
[15] C.E. Goodpasture and F.F. Arrighi, F.Q. Cosmet. Toxicol. **14**, 9 (1982).
[16] B. Gupta et al., Indian J. Med. Res. **71**, 806 (1980).
[17] R. Hänsel, Dtsch. Apoth. Ztg. **125**, 1373 (1985).
[18] M. Ohshiro, M. Kuroyanagi, and A. Ueno, Phytochemistry **29**, 2201 (1990).
[19] M. Tomoda et al., Phytochemistry **29**, 1083 (1990).
[20] H.P.T. Ammon et al., Planta Med. **58**, 226 (1992).
[21] L.A.F. ferreira et al., Toxicon **30**, 1211 (1992).
[22] S. Qureshi, A. H. Shah, and A. M. Ageel, Planta Med. **58**, 124 (1992).
[23] B.P. Jackson and D.W. Snowdon, Atlas of microscopy of medicinal plants, culinary herbs and spices, Belhaven Press, London, 1990, p. 236.
[24] H. Hjorth Tønnesen, A.-L. Grislingaas, and J. Karlsen, Z. Lebensm.-Unters.-Forsch. **193**, 548 (1991).

Curcumae xanthorrhizae rhizoma   (DAB 10), Javanese turmeric

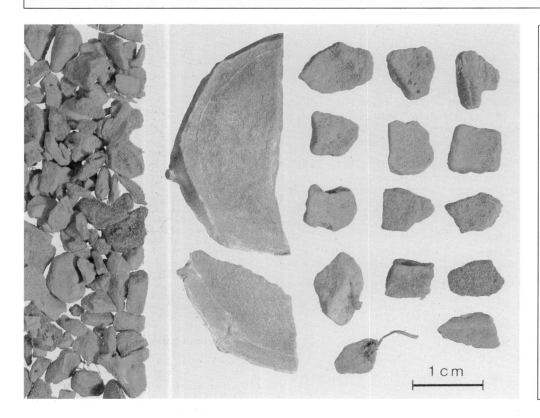

Fig. 1: Javanese turmeric

Description: The drug consists of somewhat crooked orange-yellow to greyish brown slices or fragments of slices, only a few mm thick, which may show the division between the cortex and central stele as a lighter-coloured line. The fracture is smooth and granular.

Odour: Intensely aromatic.

Taste: Spicy, somewhat bitter and pungent.

Fig. 2: *Curcuma xanthorrhiza* ROXB., freshly dug rhizome.

Fig. 3: *Curcuma xanthorrhiza* ROXB.

South-East Asian rhizomatous herb, almost exclusively cultivated. Leaves up to 1.5 m in height, broadly ovate. Flowers in ground-level, conical spikes; individual flowers funnel-shaped with only one fertile stamen.

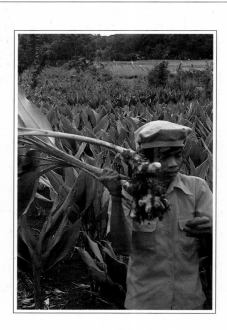

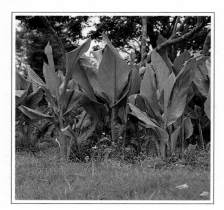

DAB 10: Javanische Gelbwurz

Plant source: *Curcuma xanthorrhiza* ROXB. (Zingiberaceae).

Synonyms: Javanische Gelbwurz (Ger.), Temu (Temoe) lawak (Indon.), Temu lawas (Mal.), Rhizome de Temoé-Lawaq (Fr.).

Origin: From Indonesia, and to a small extent also from India.

Constituents: 1–2% yellow pigments that are not volatile in steam, especially curcumin (= diferuloylmethane), mono- and bisdesmethoxycurcumin (= feruloyl-*p*-hydroxycinnamoylmethane and bis-(*p*-hydroxycinnamoyl)methane), and related compounds, at least one of which has antioxidant properties [1, 9]. 3–12% essential oil, comprising mainly sesquiterpenes, e.g. *ß*- curcumene, *ar*-curcumene, and xanthorrhizol which is characteristic of the drug, etc. The earlier described *p*-tolyl methyl carbinol [2] is an artefact arising during distillation [3]. Abundant non-gelatinized starch (difference from *Curcuma domestica* VALETON = *C. longa* L.).

	R^1	R^2
Curcumin:	OCH_3	OCH_3
Desmethoxycurcumin:	H	OCH_3

β-Curcumene   ar-Curcumene   Xanthorrhizol

Indications: As a choleretic and cholekinetic in treating chronic forms of cholangitis and cholecystitis, as well as gallstones. The choleretic action is ascribed mainly to the essential oil, while the curcumins may be responsible for the cholekinetic effects of the drug [4–6]. The effects described for Curcumae longae rhizoma (q.v.) are also probably valid for *temu lawak*.
Use as a stomachic and carminative is also quite usual.

Side effects: Large doses may cause irritation of the gastric mucous membrane with consequent nausea. Not to be used in acute cholangitis or icterus.

Making the tea: Not usual. Boiling water is poured over 0.5–1 g of the coarsely powdered drug and after 5–10 min. strained. Taking standardized preparations is recommended. As a choleretic, several cupfuls are drunk throughout the day; and as a stomachic and carminative, a cupful is taken before or during meals.
1 Teaspoon = ca. 2.5 g.

Phytomedicines: In the form of extracts, in about 30 prepared cholagogues, e.g. Aristochol®, etc. The proportion of curcuma is mostly small [7]. For some preparations it is not clear which drug has been used (only "Rhiz. Curcumae" is indicated; see: Curcumae longae rhizoma).

Authentication: Macro- and microscopically, following the DAB 10.
The TLC test of identity is as follows:

Test solution: 0.5 g powdered drug shaken for 30 min. with 5 ml methanol and then filtered; filtrate as test solution.

Extract from the German Commission E monograph (BAnz no. 122, dated 06.07.1988)

Uses
Dyspeptic complaints.

Contraindications
Obstruction of the bile duct.
In cases of gallstones, to be used only after consultation with a doctor.

Side effects
On prolonged use, gastric complaints.

Interactions with other remedies
None known.

Dosage
Unless otherwise prescribed: average daily dose, 2 g drug; preparations correspondingly.

Mode of administration
The crushed drug for infusions and other galenical forms for internal use.

Effects
Choleretic.

Reference solution: 5 mg fluorescein and 10 mg each of curcumin and thymol dissolved in 10 ml methanol.

Loadings: 10 µl each of the test and reference solutions, as 2 cm bands.

Solvent system: 98% acetic acid + 96% ethanol + chloroform (1 + 5 + 94), 10 cm run.

Detection and Evaluation: in daylight. Reference solution: in the lower third, the yellow fluorescein zone and about the middle the yellow curcumin zone. Test solution: the curcumin zone the most intense, and below it the likewise yellow, less intense, desmethoxycurcumin zone.
In UV 376 nm light. Test solution: both curcuma pigments with an intense greenish yellow fluorescence; below the desmethoxycurcumin zone, a fainter fluorescent zone possibly present.
Sprayed with 0.04% dichloroquinonechloroimide in propan-2-ol and then carefully exposed to ammonia vapour (from 26% ammonia solution). Test solution: curcuma pigment zones both yellowish brown to brown; at the same level as the violet reference thymol zone, the distinct blue xanthorrhizol zone.
Only two yellow zones corresponding to the curcumins mentioned should be visible; a third yellow zone points to the presence of *C. longa* (see: Curcumae longae rhizoma). Spraying the same plates with dichloroquinonechloroimide detects the xanthorrhizol that is characteristic of the drug [8].

Quantitative standards: DAB 10: *Volatile oil*, not less than 5.%, and dicinnamoylmethane derivatives calculated as curcumin (M_r 368.4) not less than 1.0%. *Foreign matter*, not more than 2%; fragments of *C. domestica* rhizome must not be present. *Loss on drying*, not more than 18.0%. *Ash*, not more than 8.0%.

Adulteration: Especially in the cut or powdered drug, with the rhizome of *Curcuma domestica* Valeton; it contains gelatinized starch grains. TLC (above) provides an unequivocal proof.
C. domestica can also be detected if 2 ml acetic anhydride and 0.2 ml conc. sulfuric acid are added to a small sample (10 mg, or a corresponding amount of extract): under UV 365 nm light, the sample should exhibit only a faint grey or yellowish fluorescence. If, however, *C. domestica* is present, there is an intense red fluorescence due to bisdesmethoxycurcumin.

Literature:
[1] K. Jentzsch, P. Spiegl, and R. Kamitz, Sci. Pharm. **36**, 251 (1968).
[2] H. Dieterle and Ph. Kaiser, Arch. Pharm. (Weinheim) **271**, 337 (1933).
[3] T.M. Malingré, Pharm. Weekbl. **110**, 601 (1975).
[4] J.C. Baumann, Med. Monatsschr. **29**, 173 (1975).
[5] G. Harnischfeger and H. Stolze, notabene medici **12**, 562 (1982).
[6] H. Kalk and K. Nissen, Dtsch. Med. Wochenschr. **57.**, 1613 (1931); idem., *ibid.*, **58**, 1718 (1932).
[7] R. Hänsel, Dtsch. Apoth. Ztg. **125**, 1373 (1985).
[8] H. Rimpler, R. Hänsel, and L. Kochendörfer, Dtsch. Apoth. Ztg. **109**, 1588 (1969).
[9] T. Masuda, J. Isobe, A. Jitoe, and N. Nakatani, Phytochemistry **31**, 3645 (1992).

Droserae longifoliae herba   Long-leaved sundew herb

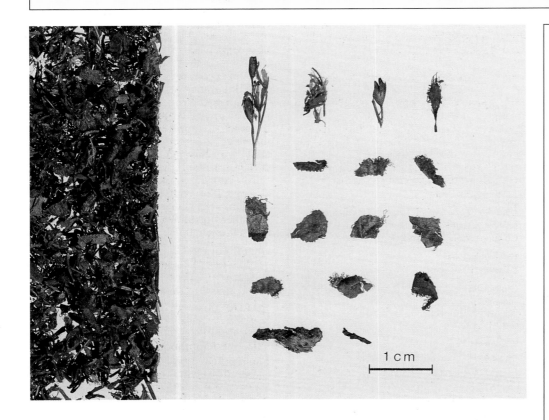

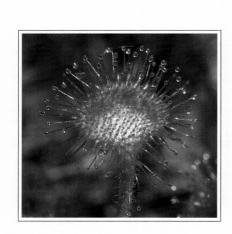

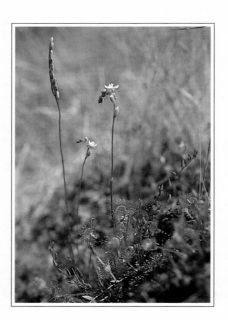

Fig. 1: Long-leaved sundew herb

<u>Description:</u> The alternate leaves of the cut drug are reddish brown to black. The lamina is obovate, up to ca. 15 mm long and up to 4 mm wide, and often compressed. On the upper surface there are red hairs ("tentacles") and on the lower surface small white hairs. The lamina narrows like a spatula towards the ca. 25 mm long petiole. The fragments of stem feel rough owing to the leaf scars (*Drosera ramentacea* does not form a rosette like *D. rotundifolia*). The drug contains additionally fragments of roots, flowers, and fruits.

<u>Taste:</u> Somewhat bitter and astringent.

Figs. 2 and 3: *Drosera rotundifolia* L.

A herb found in bogs, with a basal rosette of long-petiolate, round leaves, 5–8 mm in diameter, covered with numerous red, stalked, sticky glandular hairs ("tentacles"), these containing proteolytic enzymes and ensuring, through the digestion of animal protein, the nitrogen requirement of the plant. 6–10 Small white flowers in spikes on ca. 15 cm long, leafless stalks (habit of other *Drosera* species similar, except for the position and shape of the leaves).

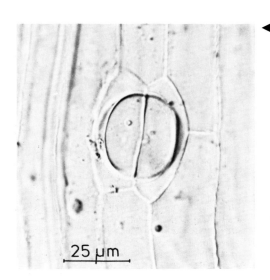

Plumbagin: R = H
Ramentone: R = OH
Ramentaceone

Plant source: *Drosera ramentacea* Burch. ex Harv. et Sond., Madagascar sundew (Droseraceae).

Note: In Germany, all three species of *Drosera*, *D. rotundifolia* L., *D. intermedia* Hayne, *D. anglica* Hudson, as well as hybrids of *D. rotundifolia* and *D. anglica* (= *D. xobovata* Mert. et Koch ex Röhling) are threatened with extinction and are therefore strictly protected. (In the UK, however, *Drosera* species are not protected.) It is for this reason that *D. ramentacea* was long ago admitted to the former East German pharmacopoeia (AB-DDR) [1]; because of its ovate to spathulate, long-petiolate leaves, it has been known in commerce in western Germany under the name Herba droserae longifoliae.
More recently, other *Drosera* species, from Asia and Australia, have come on to the market, e.g. *D. peltata* Sm., which is similar to *D. ramentacea*, and a species which is

probably *D. burmannii* Vahl. For a detailed discussion, see [2].

Synonyms: Sonnentaukraut (Ger.), Herbe de droséra africaine (Fr.).

Note: The oblong-leaved sundew, *D. intermedia*, is sometimes also known as the long-leaved sundew.

Origin: East Africa and Madagascar.

Constituents: The active principles in all *Drosera* species are mainly 1,4-naphthoquinone derivatives [1, 6], in *D. ramentacea*

Extract from the German Commission E monograph
(BAnz no. 228, dated 0.5.12.1984)

Uses
Coughing fits and dry irritating coughs.

Contraindications
None known.

Side effects
None known.

Interactions
None known.

Dosage
Unless otherwise prescribed: average daily dose, 3 g drug.

Mode of administration
Liquid and solid formulations for external and internal use.

Effects
Bronchospasmolytic, antitussive.

---

essentially plumbagin, ramentaceone (occurring in the fresh plant as glucosides, e.g. rossoliside), ramentone, and biramentaceone (= 2,2′-dimer of ramentaceone); the total content in the drug is only ca. 0.25%, which is only half as much as is present in *D. rotundifolia*. There are no reliable data on the constituents of *D. burmannii* and *D. peltata*.

Indications: Alcoholic extracts, as well as plumbagin and its analogues, have broncholytic, secretolytic, and spasmolytic actions [3, 4]; the drug is therefore used against disorders of the respiratory organs, especially bronchitis, whooping cough, and generally against coughing fits and dry irritating coughs (particularly in paediatrics). In addition to the antitussive effect, the antibacterial properties of the nathphoquinones also play a part, e.g. plumbagin inhibits the growth of streptococci, staphylococci, and pneumococci [1, 4].
In *folk medicine*, the drug is used against asthma and (perhaps because of the proteolytic enzymes in the leaf "tentacles"?) against warts [3].

Making the tea: Preparations with *D. ramentacea* have to be given in higher doses than those made from *D. rotundifolia*, since the naphthoquinone content is lower. Boiling water is poured over 1–2 g of the finely chopped drug and after 10 min. strained. As a broncholytic, a cupful of the infusion is drunk three or four times a day. 1 Teaspoon = ca. 0.4 g.

Phytomedicines: Extracts of the drug (the *Drosera* species used is usually not indicated!) are combined with other drug extracts

---

Fig. 4: Small bicellular glandular trichome, in surface view

Fig. 5: Head of a "tentacle", with a large group of tracheids

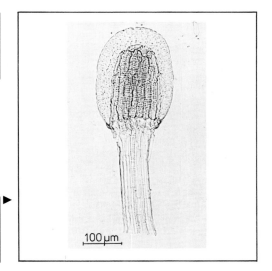

25 µm

100 µm

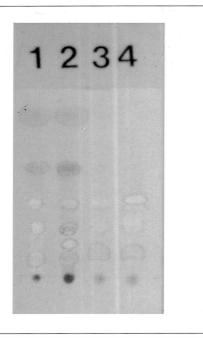

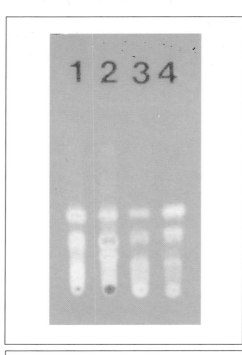

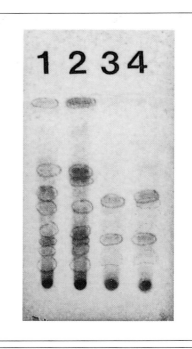

Fig. 6: TLC on 4 × 8 cm silica-gel foil
Evaluation in UV 254 nm light

1: *Drosera intermedia*
2: *Drosera peltata*
3: *Drosera rotundifolia*
4: *Drosera ramentacea*

For details, see the text

Fig. 7: TLC on 4 × 8 cm silica-gel foil
Evaluation in UV 365 nm light
See also Fig. 6

Fig. 8: TLC on 4 × 8 cm silica-gel foil
Evaluation in daylight (after spraying)
See also Fig. 6

(garden thyme, anise, fennel, etc.) in various prepared antitussives, e.g. Pertussin® (drops, juice), Primotussan® (drops), Makatussin-Drosera® (drops, juice), etc.

Authentication: Macro- (see: Description) and microscopy, following [5]: The leaf exhibits the same anatomical structure as that of *D. rotundifolia* (see, e.g. BHP 1983, Erg. B. 6). The epidermis on both surfaces is made up of squat cells. The mesophyll shows no differentiation into palisade and spongy parenchyma, but consists simply of two to three layers of spongy parenchymatous cells. On the upper and lower surfaces, there are very small anomocytic stomata, and small colourless glandular trichomes (Fig. 4), which have a bicellular oval stalk and a head that is almost as wide and comprising one or two sets each of two cells. The lower leaf surface also has colourless, often bent, trichomes with a uni- or biseriate stalk of mostly thickened cells and a pointed terminal cell. Shorter trichomes are biseriate all along their length; in the lower part, the lu-

men is sometimes filled with a yellow granular content. The "tentacles" are ca. 2 mm long and structurally similar to those of *D. rotundifolia*, the epidermis of their stalk being made up of elongated cells, through the middle of which runs a fine vascular strand with spiral thickening. The epidermis of the head consists of radially elongated cells and the layer underneath of polygonal cells. The group of vascular cells terminating the vascular strand of the stalk is surrounded by an additional layer of parenchyma cells (Fig. 5). Sometimes, a narrow hyaline border which is broader at the top can be recognized.
If the drug is extracted with chloroform, a yellow solution is obtained, which, on addition of ammonia, turns purplish red.
The following TLC procedure is a suitable test of identity:

Test solution: 1.0 g powdered drug extracted by frequent shaking with 10 ml chloroform for 30 min. and then filtered; filtrate = test solution.

Reference solution: authentic drug treated similarly.

Loadings: 10 µl each of the test and reference solutions, as spots on silica gel.

Solvent system: tetrachloromethane + ethyl acetate (90 + 10), 5 cm run.

Detection: first observed under UV 254 and 365 nm light, then sprayed with 5% ethanolic sulphuric acid, followed by 1% ethanolic vanillin solution, and heated at ca. 105 °C for 3–5 min.

Evaluation: immediately after spraying. In Figs. 6–8, quenching and fluorescent spots, as well as those visible in daylight, of the four *Drosera* species: *D. intermedia*, *D. peltata*, *D. rotundifolia*, and *D. ramentacea*. Characteristic of the *D. ramentacea* chromatogram: in UV 365 nm light, a blue fluorescent spot at Rf ca. 0.40 and below it weaker fluorescent spots; in daylight, two violet spots at Rf 0.40 and ca. 0.25.

Note: The BHP 1983 monograph on Drosera is based on *D. rotundifolia.*

Adulteration: See under: Plant source (cf. [2]).

Literature:

[1] R. Luckner and M. Luckner, Pharmazie **25**, 261 (1970), and the Kommentar AB-DDR.
[2] W. Schier and W. Schultze, Dtsch. Apth. Ztg. **127**, 2595 (1987).
[3] Hager, vol. **4**, p. 723 (1973).
[4] Symposium report by the firm Zyma GmbH (Munich) on the Pharmacology of Naphthoquinone Derivatives (1978).
[5] Summarizing description by W. Schier, 1988.
[6] T. Schólly and I. Kapetanidis, Pharm. Acta Helv. **64**, 66 (1989).

Echinaceae herba/radix[1]   Echinacea (BHP 1/1990)

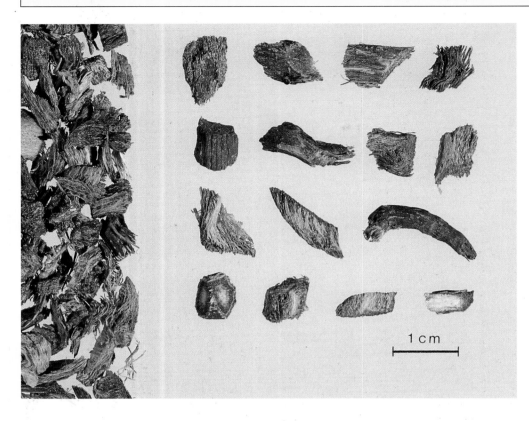

Fig. 1: Echinacea root

Description: The drug comprises more or less cylindrical, ca. 4–20 mm thick, irregular, branched pieces of root, with a greyish brown, longitudinally striated or wrinkled surface. The transverse section shows a thin cortex (up to 1 mm wide) and a whitish yellow xylem which is traversed by radial striations (Fig. 2).

Odour: Faint and characteristic.

Taste: At first slightly sweetish and aromatic, then pungent to bitter, and astringent.

The wide range of alkylamides (mainly isobutyl-amides) occurring in the roots of *Echinacea* species has been investigated in considerable detail; in *E. angustifolia*, the principal components are the isomeric dodeca 2E,4E,8Z,10E/Z-tetraenoic acid isobutylamides; such compounds are also present in the aerial parts.

A series of keto-alkynes and -alkenes is present in *E. pallida*; but not *E. angustifolia*; they are readily oxidized by atmospheric oxygen, so that in stored (commercial) roots hydroxylated derivatives are found and only residual amounts of the native compounds.

Essential oil is present throughout the plants; in the oil from the aerial parts, borneol, bornyl acetate, pentadeca-8(Z)-en-2-one, germacrene D, caryophyllene and caryophyllene epoxide are important components; pentadeca-8(Z)-en-2-one is a also major constituent of the oil from the roots of *E. pallida*. The major anthocyanins of *E. pallida* flowers are cyanidin 3-*O*-β-D- glucopyranoside and 3-*O*-(6-*O*-malonyl-β-D-glucopyranoside) [29]. Traces (0.006%) of the pyrrolizidine alkaloids tussilagine and isotussilagine have been found in *E. angustifolia* and *E. purpurea* [12].

DAB 9: Sonnenhutwurzel (deleted in DAB 10)
St.Zul. 1279.99.99

Plant sources: *Echinacea angustifolia* DC. and *E. pallida* (NUTT.) NUTT. (Asteraceae). Herbaceous plants: *E.angustifolia*, stems, often branching, 10–60 cm in height, with single, more or less hemispherical flower-heads of reddish brown tubular florets surrounded by a few pinkish red spreading ray florets; *E. pallida*, stems rarely branching, 30–100 cm in height, with more or less hemispherical flower-heads of reddish brown tubular florets surrounded by a few pinkish red drooping ray florets [25].

Synonyms: Coneflower, Black sampson (Engl.), Sonnenhutwurzel, Igelkopfwurzel (Ger.), Racine d'Echinacea (Fr.).

Origin: Native in the southern United States; cultivated in Europe to some extent. Most of the drug is imported from North America.

Constituents [25, 26]: Polysaccharides of unknown structure have been isolated from *E. pallida*, but much more is known about two products, PS I (a 4-*O*-methylglucuronoarabinoxylan, M_r 35 kD) and PS II (an acid rhamnoarabinogalactan, M_r 450 kD), from *E. purpurea* herb.

The caffeic acid ester echinacoside is present in *E. angustifolia* (roots, 0.3–1.3%; flowers, 0.1–1.0%) and *E. pallida* (roots, 0.4–1.7%; flowers, traces only); it is present in other *Echinacea* species and in species from other plant families. Cynarin (1,5-di-*O*-caffeoylquinic acid) is characteristic of *E. angustifolia* roots; chicoric acid (2,3-*O*-di-caffeoyltartaric acid) is the major compound in the flowers, leaves, and roots of *E. pallida*. An array of other caffeic acid derivatives is present in *Echinacea* species; see also [27, 28].

Indications: For the prophylaxis and treatment of mild to moderately severe colds, influenza, and septic processes; topically, for treating poorly healing wounds and inflamed skin conditions. The drug comes from the traditional medicine of the original Indian inhabitants of North America, and in the 19th century was the most widely used plant drug in the United States. The action is supposedly due to enhancement of the body's own defences by non-specific stimulation of the immune system, especially activation of phagocytosis and stimulation of fibroblasts. The spread of the causative agents in the body is supposedly lessened through blockade of the tissue and bacterial hyaluronidase [15]. Components of the polysaccharide fraction are thought to be the active substances [1, 2]; up to now, none of these compounds has had its structure determined.

---

[1] Owing to the confused situation on the drug market (see: Adulteration), the German Pharmacopoeial Commission deleted this monograph, which covered only the roots of Echinacea angustifolia, and it has not been included in the DAB 10. However, the Commission E has quite recently published two separate monographs dealing with the aerial parts and roots of both *E. angustifolia* and *E. pallida*. This is taken into account in the treatment presented here.

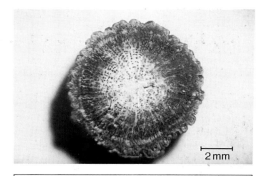

Echinacoside

Cichoric acid

Echinaceine

Echinolone

More detailed investigations have been carried out on *Echinacea purpurea* (L.) MOENCH, purple coneflower, which is used for the same purposes [16–18].

Experimental proof of the immunostimulant action of the polysaccharides has so far only been demonstrated by *in-vitro* studies and *in vivo* only after i.p. administration. The question of whether they are active orally has not yet been clarified. Use of the drug is therefore very often through i.m. or i.v. administration of appropriate preparations. Wound healing is promoted by the polysaccharide fraction echinacin B [19]. The lipophilic amides, as well as the polar caffeic acid derivatives, make a considerable contribution to the immunostimulant activity of alcoholic *Echinacea* extracts. Polysaccharides are implicated in the activity of Echinacin®, the aqueous extracts, and the powdered whole drug when taken orally. Only low concentrations of the polysaccharides are present in the expressed juice and they do not have the same composition as extracts from the aerial parts. The overall immunostimulant activity of alcoholic and aqueous extracts thus depends on the combined effects of several constituents [25, 26].

Topical application of purified aqueous root extracts, as well as of a polysaccharide fraction, leads to inhibition of croton oil-induced oedema of the mouse ear and to a reduction in leucocyte infiltration [20, 21] and, after i.p. administration, to inhibition of rat-paw oedema.

Echinaceine and the other isobutylamides have insecticidal properties [7, 22]. It has also been shown that the root extract has an effect on the juvenile hormone of insects [8] and that *Z*-pen-tadeca-1,8-diene has an effect on tumours *in vivo* [10]. Echinacoside has antibacterial and the polyacetylenes bacterio- and fungistatic activity. Echinacin® and chicoric and caffeic acids have antiviral properties. Pentane-soluble fractions from *E. angustifolia* and *E. pallida* have some oncolytic activity [25, 26]. For other activities and a summary of the results of clinical studies, see [25, 26].

Side effects: The lyophilized expressed juice from *E. purpurea*, Echinacin® Liquidum, has been shown to be non-toxic in rats and mice at doses far in excess of those used in human therapy; *in-vitro* mutagenicity and carcinogenicity tests are also negative [30].

The pyrrolizidine alkaloids found in *E. angustifolia* and *E. purpurea* are unlikely to cause any liver damage, since they lack the 1,2-unsaturated necine ring system required for hepatotoxicity [25, 26].

Making the tea: Not very usual. Boiling water is poured over ca. half a teaspoonful of well reduced or coarsely powdered drug and after 10 min. strained. For colds, etc., and to augment the body's own defences, a cup of the freshly prepared infusion is drunk as warm as possible several times a day, but best between meals.

1 Teaspoon = ca. 2.5 g.

Phytomedicines: Almost 40 specialities as urological remedies, influenza remedies, antiphlogistics, and alteratives, as well as externally as wound remedies, e.g. Pascotox forte-Injektopas®, Esberitox®, Salus®, Echinacea-Tropfen (drops), and further as a component of several mixed herbal teas. Preparations containing the powdered root and/or extracts that are available in the UK include: Potter's Antifect and Skin Clear Tablets, Gerard House Echinacea Tablets (*E.angustifolia* + *E. purpurea* 4 : 1-extract) and Echinacea & Garlic Tablets, Arkopharma Phytokold (*E. purpurea*) and Phytoimmune boost capsules.

Regulatory status (UK): General Sale List – Schedule 1, Table A.

Authentication: Macro- (see: Description) and microscopically. The roots of *E. angustifolia* and *E. pallida* are very similar both macro- and microscopically. The transverse section (cf. Fig. 3) shows in the xylem a few narrow medullary rays which near the large vessels are capped or edged with groups of lignified fibres. In *E. angustifolia* oleo-resin canals are present only outside the central cylinder, but in *E. pallida* they are present both inside and outside. In *E. angustifolia* the narrow, 300–800 μm long, lignified fibres are in scattered groups usually surrounded by phytomelanin deposits, while in *E. pallida* they are present only in the periphery of the cortex and they are mostly single, wider and shorter, being 100–300 μm, and phytomelanin is often absent. See further [25].

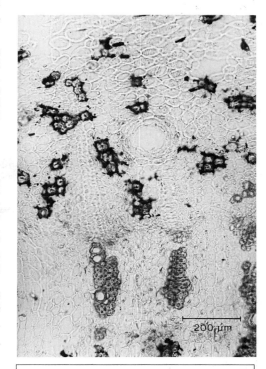

Fig. 2: Radial striations through the black, melanogenic layers (hand lens); see also Fig. 3

Fig. 3: Transverse section through the cambial region. Cortex with oleo-resin canals, and groups of phloem fibres embedded in the melanogenic layers (black intercellular deposit). Vessels together with groups of xylem fibres

A useful TLC identification test is based on the detection of echinacoside and other caffeic acid derivatives in the methanolic root extract [26]:

Test Solution: 1 g powdered drug warmed on the water-bath with 10 ml for 10–15 min., cooled and filtered.

Reference compounds: echinacoside, cynarin, chicoric acid, chlorogenic acid.

Loadings: 20 μl each of the test and reference solutions, as 2-cm bands on silica gel.

Solvent system: ethyl acetate + anhydrous formic acid + glacial acetic acid + water (100 + 11 + 11 + 27), 15 cm run.

Detection: sprayed with 1% methanolic diphenyl-boryloxyethylamine, followed by 5% ethanolic polyethylene glycol 4000.

Evaluation: in UV 365 nm light. Reference compounds: pale blue fluorescent zones – echinacoside, Rf 0.26; chlorogenic acid, Rf 0.50; cynarin Rf 0.74, chicoric acid Rf 0.91. Test solutions: *E. angustifolia* – strong echinacoside zone, other faint pale blue zones above and below, and a faint cynarin zone; *E. pallida*, similar to *E. angustifolia*, but cynarin zone absent; *E. purpurea*, intense chlorogenic and chicoric acid zones and no echinacoside zone.

There is a colour illustration of the chromatogram in [26].

A methanolic extract of the aerial parts can be separated in the system: toluene + ethyl formate + formic acid + water (5 + 100 + 10 + 10), followed by examination in UV 254 nm light and, after spraying as above, in UV 365 nm light. The chicoric acid zone is prominent in the *E. pallida* and *E. purpurea* extracts, but weak in the *E. angustifolia* extract. Isochlorogenic acid zones are present in the *E. angustifolia* and *E. pallida* extracts, but absent in the *E. purpurea* extract.

Rutin is present in all three extracts, but echinacoside, verbascoside, and chlorogenic acid zones are observed only with the *E. angustifolia* and *E. pallida* extracts [26].

Quantitative standards: DAB 9 (*E. angustifolia* root): *Foreign matter*, not more than 3%. *Loss on drying*, not more than 10.0%. *Ash*, not more than 6.0%. *HCl-insoluble ash*, not more than 2.0%.

BHP 1/1990 (*E. angustifolia* root): *Water-soluble extractive*, not less than 15%. *Foreign matter*, not more than 3%. *Total ash*, not more than 9%. *HCl-insoluble ash*, not more than 3%.

Adulteration: Particularly by the roots of *Echinacea purpurea* (L.) MOENCH, which are considered to be equivalent, but which are reported not to contain echinacoside [11] and *Parthenium integrifolium* L., American feverfew [13]. This last plant can be recognized on TLC by the absence of chicoric acid or through the presence of the sesquiterpene esters cinnamoyl-echinadiol, -epoxyechinadiol, -echinaxanthol, and -dihydroxynardol [14]. These new diterpene esters were first described as constituents of *E. purpurea* roots and were also thought perhaps to be responsible for the immunological action of this drug [24]. However, they are only present in *P. integrifolium* root and therefore cannot be utilized for the suggested TLC differentiation of *E. pur-purea* and *E. angustifolia* roots [13].

Microscopically, *E. purpurea* is distinguished by large, wedge-shaped and partly reticulated groups of vessels surrounded by numerous broad, spindle-shaped xylem fibres and parenchyma; sclereids are rare; the 12–20 oil glands are small 50 by 120 µm) and arranged circumferentially in groups of 4 in the inner part of the phloem parenchyma; noteworthy is the absence of black phytomelanin deposits [25]. For the TLC differentiation, see above.

Extracts from the German Commission E monograph (BAnz no. 162, dated 29.08.92)

Echinaceae angustifoliae/pallidae herba
Echinaceae angustifoliae radix

Ingredients of the drug

The fresh or dried roots, or the fresh or dried aerial parts collected at the time of flowering, of *Echinacea angustifolia* DC., as well as their preparations.
The fresh or dried aerial parts, collected at the time of flowering, of *Echinacea pallida* (NUTT.) NUTT., as well as their preparations.
On the market, preparations of *Echinacea pallida* are to some extent incorrectly labelled as "Echinacea angustifolia".

Uses

Preparations from "Echinacea angustifolia" are used to support and promote the natural powers of resistance of the body, especially in infectious conditions (influenza and colds, etc.) in the nose and throat, as an alterative in influenza, inflammatory and purulent wounds, abcesses, furuncles, ulcus cruris (indolent leg ulcers), herpes simplex, inflammation of connective tissue, wounds, headaches, metabolic disturbances, diaphoretic, and antiseptic. Activity in the uses listed has not been substantiated.

Risks

Internal use: not to be used by progressive conditions such as tuberculosis, leukosis, collagenosis, multiple sclerosis, AIDS, HIV infection, and other auto-immune disorders.
Parenteral use: Depending on the dose, chills, short-lived fever, nausea, and vomiting may occur. In a few cases, immediate allergic reactions may take place. With a tendency to allergic reactions, especially against Asteraceae (Compositae; daisy family), and during pregnancy, no parenteral administration.
Warning: With diabetics, on parenteral administration the metabolic situation may worsen.

Evaluation

Since the activity in the conditions listed above has not been substantiated, therapeutic use cannot be recommended. Because of the risks, the use of parenteral preparations is not justified.

Extract from the German Commission E monograph (BAnz no. 162, dated 29.08.92)

Echinaceae pallidae radix
Ingredients of the drug

Echinacea pallida root, consisting of the fresh or dried root of *Echinacea pallida* (NUTT.) NUTT., as well as its preparations at an active dosage level.

Uses

In supportive treatment of influenza-like infections.

Contraindications

In principle, not to be used in progressive conditions such as tuberculosis, leukosis, collagenosis, multiple sclerosis, AIDS, HIV infection, and other auto-immune disorders.

Side effects
None known.

Special precautions for use
None known.

Use during pregnancy and laction
None known.

Interactions with other remedies
None known.

Dosage
Unless otherwise prescribed: daily dose, tincture (1:5) with 50% (v/v) alcohol from original dry extract (50% ethanol, 7–11:1), corresponding to 900 mg drug. Information on dosages for children is not available.

Mode of administration
Liquid preparations for internal use.

Period of use
Not longer than 8 weeks.

Overdosage
Not known.

Special warnings
None.

Effects on drivers and ability to use machines
None known.

Literature

[1] H. Wagner et al., Arzneim.Forsch. **35**, 1069 (2985).
[2] N. Beuscher and K. Kopanski, Acta Agron. Hung. **34** (Suppl.), 89 (1985).
[3] A. Stoll, J. Renz, and A. Brack, Helv. Chim. Acta **33**, 1877 (1950).
[4] H. Becker et al., Z. Naturforsch. **37c**, 351 (1982).
[5] H. Becker and W.Ch. Hsieh, Z. Naturforsch. **40c**, 585 (1985).
[6] M. Jacobson, J. Org. Chem. **32**, 1646 (1967).
[7] F. Bohlmann and M. Genz, Chem. Ber. **99**, 3197 (1966).
[8] M. Jacobson, R.E. Redfern, and G.D. Mills, Lloydia **38**, 473 (1975).
[9] K.E. Schulte, G. Rücker. and J. Perlick, Arzneim.Forsch. **17**, 825 (1967).
[10] D.J. Voaden and M. Jacobson, J. Med. Chem. **15**, 619 (1972).
[11] H. Becker, Dtsch. Apoth. Ztg. **122**, 2320 (1982).
[12] J.H. Röder et al., Dtsch. Apoth. Ztg. **124**, 2316 (1984).
[13] R. Bauer, I.A. Khan, and H. Wagner, Dtsch. Apoth. Ztg. **126**, 1065 (1986).
[14a] R. Bauer, I.A. Khan, and H. Wagner, Dtsch. Apoth. Ztg. **127**, 1325 (1987).
[14b] R. Bauer and H. Wagner, Z. Phytotherap. **9**, 151 (1988).
[15] G. W. Korting and W. Born, Arzneim.Forsch. **4**, 424 (1954).
[16] A. Stimpel et al., Infekt. Immun. **46**, 845 (1984).
[17] A. Proksch and H. Wagner, Phytochemistry **26**, 1988 (1987).
[18] H. Wagner et al., Z. Phytotherap. **8**, 180 (1987).
[19] J. Bonadeo, G. Botazzi, and M. Lavazza, Riv. Ital. Essenze, Perfumi, Pianti Offic., Aromi, Saponi, Cosmet., Aerosol **53**, 281 (1971); C.A. **75**, 108168 (1971).
[20] E. Tragni et al., Food Chem. Toxicol. **23**, 317 (1985).
[21] A. Tubaro et al., J. Pharm. Pharmacol. **39**, 567 (1987).
[22] M. Jacobson, Science **120**, 1028 (1954).
[23] R. Bauer and H. Wagner, Sci. Pharm. **55**, 159 (1987).
[24] R. Bauer et al., Helv. Chim. Acta **68**, 2355 (1985).
[25] R. Bauer and H. Wagner, Echinacea. Handbuch für Apotheker und andere Naturwissenschaftlicher. Wissenschaftliche Verlagsgesellschaft, Stuttgart, 1990.
[26] R. Bauer and H. Wagner, in: H. Wagner and N.R. Farnsworth (eds.) Economic and Medicinal Plants Research, Academic Press, London – San Diego – New York, vol. 5, p. 253 (1991).
[27] H. Soicke, G. Al-Hassan, and K. Görler, Planta Med. **54**, 175 (1988).
[28] A. Cheminat et al., Phytochemistry **27**, 2787 (1988).
[29] A. Cheminat et al., Phytochemistry **28**, 3246 (1989).
[30] U. Mengs, C.B. Clare, and J.A. Poiley, Arzneim.Forsch. **41**, 1076 (1991).

Epilobii herba – Willow-herb　185

Epilobii herba　Willow-herb

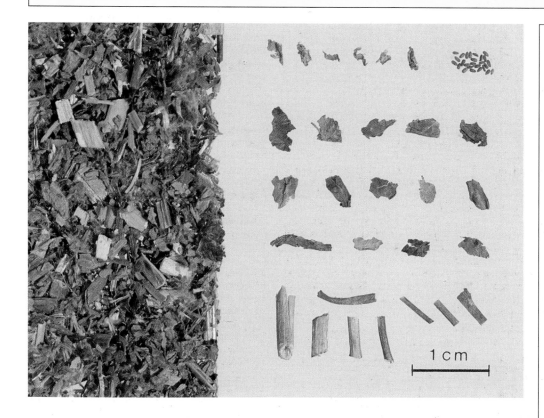

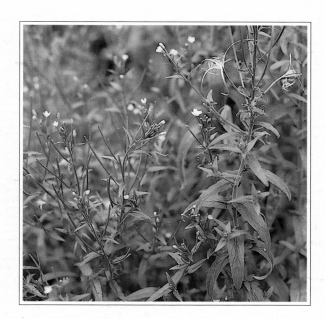

Fig. 1: Willow-herb

Description: The drug consists predominantly of 1–3 mm thick pieces of stem, deep green crumpled fragments of leaves, and only a few flowers and fruits. The stem is longitudinally grooved, and partly covered with a fine, glandular pubescence; the leaves have an indistinct reticulate venation and, depending on the species, are sparsely or distinctly pubescent, and have an entire or finely serrate margin; the flower parts are pale violet. The fruit are long capsules dehiscing on four sides, containing numerous, 0.5–2 mm long, brown to black seeds which often have a tuft of hairs.

Taste: Astringent and somewhat bitter.

Fig. 2: *Epilobium parviflorum* SCHREBER

Small-flowered willow-herb species, all 30–70 cm tall perennials, with opposite leaves (but alternate in *E. angustifolium*, considered an adulterant), mostly sessile (petiolate in *E. roseum*) and more (*E. hirsutum*) or less (*E. parviflorum*, *E. montanum*) pubescent. Perianth comprising four sepals and four pink to purple petals, eight stamens, a style, and a narrow, mostly stalk-like elongated ovary. Long, narrow, pod-like capsules containing many seeds covered with silky hairs.

Plant sources: *Epilobium parviflorum* SCHREB., hoary or lesser hairy willow-herb, *E. montanum* L., broad-leaved willow-herb, *E. roseum* SCHREB., pale or small-flowered willow-herb, *E. collinum* S.G. GMELIN, and other small-flowering *Epilobium* species (Onagraceae).

Synonyms: Weidenröschenkraut (Ger.), Epilobe (Fr.).

Origin: Some of the species mentioned occur widespread or scattered throughout Europe. The drug is mostly collected in the wild in Central Europe, but some is also imported from former Yugoslavia and from Romania.

Constituents: As far as known, all *Epilobium* species contain flavonoids, especially derivatives of kaempferol, quercetin, and myricetin [1–3]. In *E. parviflorum* and *E. angustifolium*, β-sitosterol, various esters of sitosterol, and sitosterol glucoside have been detected [4]. According to our own preliminary studies, large amounts of gallic-acid derivatives are present.

Indications: *Up till now, it has only been used in lay medicine,* for benign prostate adenomas and the associated problems of micturition. There is evidence from various animal experiments that the drug and infusions

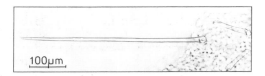

Fig. 3: Long, pointed covering trichome and shorter tubular trichomes

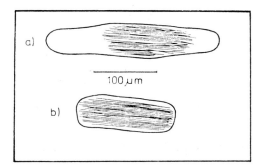

Fig. 4: Raphides incompletely (a) and completely (b) filling the cell

and extracts prepared from it have antiphlogistic activity [5, 6]. Surprisingly, in the rat-paw oedema test *E. angustifolium* has a particularly strong inhibitory action and the liberation of prostaglandins (PGI_2, PGE_2, PGD_2) is greatly reduced. The active principle, myricetin 3-*O*-β-D-glucuronide, is localized in the leaves and reaches its maximum concentration during and just after the flowering period [7, 8]. Whether these findings can be correlated in any way with the treatment of micturition problems is still an open question.

Making the tea: Boiling water (ca. 150 ml) is poured over 1.5–2 g of the finely chopped drug and after 10 min. strained.
1 Teaspoon = ca. 0.8 g.

Phytomedicines: None.

Authentication: This is only possible by microscopy and is very time-consuming, since the distinction between "small-flowered" and "large-flowered" species necessitates close attention to many different characters (measurement of the length and width of the trichomes, raphides, etc.); an added source of difficulty is that *Epilobium* species readily hybridize and nothing is known about the anatomical characters of the hybrids. The trichomes of the leaves are suitable characters for differentiating the various taxa

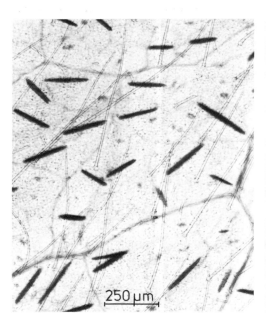
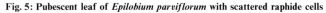

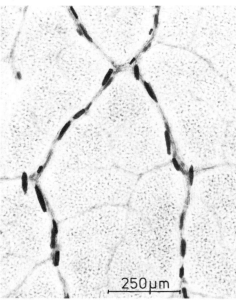

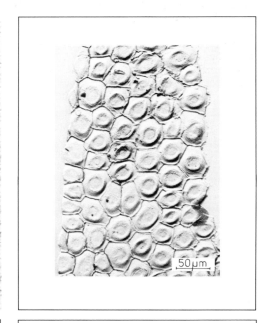

Fig. 5: Pubescent leaf of *Epilobium parviflorum* with scattered raphide cells
Fig. 6: Essentially glabrous leaf of *Epilobium angustifolium* with raphide cells following the course of the veins

Fig. 7: Papillose epidermis of the seed testa

	Covering trichomes	Tubular trichomes	Mucilage cells with raphides	Stigma	Seed epidermis
Epilobium parviflorum	Numerous, straight, 250–500 µm long, cuticle smooth or only slightly warty	Rare, only on young leaves, 80–300 µm long	Numerous, 100–150 µm, raphides fill the cell	Distinctly 4-lobed	Papillose
Epilobium montanum	At leaf margin and along the veins, 150–200 µm long, pointed, bent, warty cuticle	100–200 µm long, partly without protuberances at capitate end	Ca. 150 µm, raphides do not fill the cell	4-Lobed	Papillose
Epilobium collinum	Short, mostly only 80–150 µm long, falcate, cuticle striated or warty	Short, 60–100 µm long, bent at the base	100–150 µm, raphides fill the cell	Indistinctly 4-lobed (hand lens)	Papillose
Epilobium roseum	Bent at the base, 200–300 µm long, cuticle distinctly warty	Very rare, on very young leaves, not at leaf margin	Ca. 150 µm, raphides do not fill the cell	Club-shaped	Slightly papillose

(Fig. 3): covering trichomes and tubular trichomes, often with a small protrusion (these trichomes are absent from the "large-flowered" species, which have been, and sometimes still are, grouped together in their own genus, *Chamerion* or *Chamaenerion*), raphides in mucilage cells, filling the entire cell or much shorter than the cell (Figs. 4, 5, and 6), style (club-shaped or 4-lobed), epidermis of the seed testa (smooth or papillose, Fig. 7), presence or absence of seed plumes.

The above table summarizes some important characters for the most frequently encountered "small-flowered" willow-herbs [4].

A very detailed description of the morphological and anatomical features is to be found in [5].

Adulteration: Drugs originating from "large-flowering" species of *Epilobium* are frequently found on the market [4], mainly *E. angustifolium* L. (= *Chamerion angustifolium* (L.) Holub = *Chamaenerion angustifolium* (L.) Scop.), rose-bay willow-herb, recognizable by the very fine network of veins, the complete absence of tubular trichomes, and the presence of mucilage cells with raphides almost exclusively along the veins (Fig. 6), as well as *E. hirsutum* L., great or great hairy willow-herb, recognizable by the very long (mostly 500–1000 µm) covering trichomes with a smooth cuticle.

Literature:
[1] J.E. Averett, P.H. Raven, and H. Becker, Amer. J. Bot. **66**, 1151 (1979).
[2] A. Hiermann, Sci Pharm. **51**, 158 (1983); idem., *ibid.* **52**, 124 (1984).
[3] M. Wichtl and W. Tadros, Dtsch. Apoth. Ztg. **122**, 2593 (1982).
[4] A. Hiermann and K. Mayr, Sci. Pharm. **53**, 39 (1985).
[5] J. Saukel, Sci. Pharm. **50**, 179 (1982); idem., *Ibid.* **51**, 115 and 132 (1983).
[6] A. Hiermann, H. Juan, and W. Sametz, J. Ethnopharmacol. **17**, 161 (1986).
[7] A. Hiermann, Sci Pharm. **55**, 111 (1987).
[8] A. Hiermann, M. Reidlinger, H. Juan, and W. Sametz, Planta Med. **57**, 357 (1991).

Equiseti herba   (DAB 10), Equisetum (BHP 1/1990)

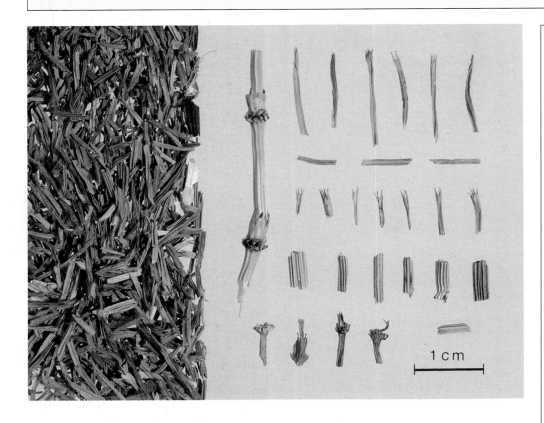

Fig. 1: Equisetum

<u>Description:</u> The drug consists of the dried, sterile, green stems of the field horsetail. The main stem is ca. 1–3.5 mm, rarely up to 5 mm, thick and consists of 2–6 cm long, hollow sections, separated by nodes, with ca. 6–19, but generally 9–13, raised, longitudinal ridges. Each node on the main stems and lateral branches has a membranaceous leaf sheaths with tri-angular-lanceolate, often brown, teeth, the number of which corresponds with the number of ridges of the stem or branch concerned; the first internode of each lateral branch is longer than the leaf sheath of the main stem from which it comes. Both the main stem and lateral branches are green to greyish green, rough, and brittle. The numerous, mostly simple, lateral branches (Fig. 4) are only 1 mm thick, 4-angled with wings (cruciform cross-section), and they have a pith.

<u>Taste:</u> Tasteless; grates on being chewed between the teeth.

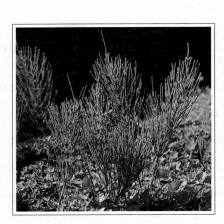

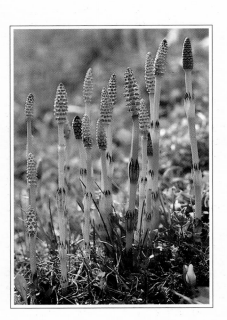

Figs. 2 and 3: *Equisetum arvense* L.

In spring, unbranched fertile stems with characteristic, brownish terminal cones with peltate sporangiophores. In summer, developing up to 50 cm tall, green sterile stems having whorls of usually 4 (rarely 5) winged lateral branches. An important character distinguishing *E. arvense* from *E. palustre* is the difference in size between the internode of the lateral branch and the leaf sheath of the main stem (see: Description, above).

DAB 10: Schachtelhalmkraut
ÖAB: Herba Equiseti
Ph. Helv. VII: Equiseti herba
St.Zul. 1239.99.99

Plant source: *Equisetum arvense* L., field or common horsetail (Equisetaceae).

Synonyms: Horsetail herb, Scouring rush (because of the high silica content, the plant is used for polishing tin and pewter!) (Engl.), Schachtelhalmkraut, Zinnkraut, Pferdeschwanzkraut (Ger.), Herbe de prêle. des champs, Queue de cheval (Fr.).

Origin: Distributed throughout the temperate zone of the northern hemisphere. The drug is imported from the former USSR, former Yugoslavia, Albania, Hungary, and Poland.

Constituents [see also 19]: More than 10% inorganic constituents, two-thirds of which is silicic acid (10% in the form of water-soluble silicates) and potassium salts [1].
The flavonoid composition reveals the existence of two chemotypes: Asian and North American material has flavone (apigenin, luteolin) 5-glucosides and their malonyl esters, while European material is without these constituents; both types have quercetin 3-*O*-β-D-glucopyranoside and its malonyl esters, but only European material has quercetin 3-*O*-sophoroside and genkwanin and protogenkwanin 4'-*O*-β-D-glucopyranoside [2, 14, 15]. Di-*E*-caffeoyl-*meso*-tartaric acid, though present in very small amounts (up to 0.008%), is a marker for both chemotypes, since it is absent from other members of the subgenus Equisetum [16].
Traces of alkaloids, including nicotine and spermidine type bases, also occur [3, 11]. In addition, there are polyenic acids [4] and rare dicarboxylic acids, e.g. equisetolic acid

HOOC—(CH$_2$)$_{28}$—COOH
Equisetolic acid

Palustrine

Extract from the German Commission E monograph (BAnz no. 173, dated 18.09.1986)

Uses

Taken internally: Post-traumatic and static oedema. For irrigating the system in bacterial and inflammatory disorders of the urinary tract and in cases of renal gravel.
Used externally: In supportive treatment of poorly healing wounds.

Contraindications

None known.

Warning: No irrigation therapy where oedema results from impaired heart or kidney function.

Side effects

None known.

Interactions with other remedies

None known.

Dosage

Unless otherwise prescribed:
Internal use: average daily dose, 6 g drug; preparations correspondingly.
External use: for dressings, 10 g drug to 1 litre water.

Mode of administration

For internal use: chopped drug for infusions and other galenical preparations for internal use.
Warning: With irrigation therapy, ensure an abundant fluid intake.
For external use: chopped drug for decoctions and other galenical preparations.

Effects

Weakly diuretic.

[5]. The supposed saponin "equisetonin" is largely a mixture of various sugars (saccharose, and also glucose, fructose, lactose, etc.) and flavonoids; some mannitol and inositol, as well as phenol-carboxylic acids, among them caffeic acid, are also present [6, 17, 18].

Indications: As a diuretic, which, owing to the increased flow through the ureters, is useful in inflammation of the renal pelvis and bacteriuria. The drug brings about water diuresis without altering the electrolyte balance [7, 8].
In *folk medicine*, not only as a diuretic, but also as a haemostyptic and, like many other silicate containing drugs, as an adjuvant in the treatment of tuberculosis. There is, however, no pharmacological or clinical evidence that it has a favourable effect on tuberculosis. Observations indicating that soluble silicates stimulate leucocyte activity are more than 50 years old [9] and since then have been neither confirmed nor disproved. The weak haemolytic activity is due to a combination of surfactant fatty acids (palmitic acid, etc.) and phytosterols [17].

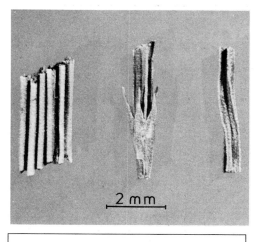

Fig. 4: Hollow, ridged, main stem (left) and fragment of the 4-angled lateral branch (right), with a leaf sheath (centre)

Making the tea: Boiling water is poured over 2–4 g of the drug, boiled for 5 min., and after 10–15 min. strained.
Some authors recommend macerating the drug in cold water for 10–12 hours.
1 Teaspoon = ca. 1.0 g.

Herbal preparations: The drug is available in tea bags (1.5 or 2.0 g). Extracts of the drug are also components of instant diuretic teas. An example of a UK product is Potter's multi-component Kas-bah Herb.

Phytomedicines: The drug is a component of many herbal mixtures with a diuretic action. Extracts of the drug are included in some prepared diuretics.
It is present in such UK preparations as Potter's Antiglan and Antitis Tablets and as a 3:1 extract in Gerard House Waterlax Tablets.

Authentication: Macro- (see: Description) and microscopically, following the DAB 10; see also the BHP 1/1990. The two subsidiary cells which are thickened with cellulose (not silica ridges) and which cover the guard cells of the stomata are a conspicuous feature (Fig. 5).
An even better means of identification (according to [10, cf. 11]) is examination of the epidermal protuberances. A few fragments of the drug, preferably from lateral branches, are cut up and boiled with chloral hydrate solution. In *E. arvense*, the protuberances comprise two cells, while those of *E. palustre* consist of only one cell (Fig. 6). About the microscopical differentiation of other *Equisetum* species, see [10].

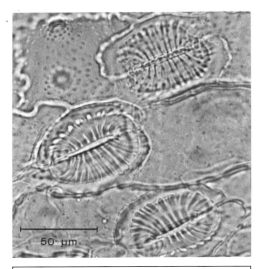

Fig. 5: Paracytic stomata covered over with two subsidiary cells bearing ridges of thickening

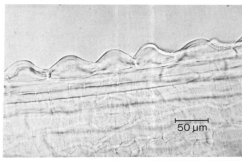

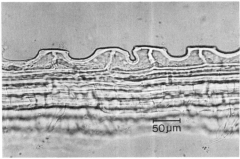

Fig. 6: Epidermal protuberances in *Equisetum palustre* (top) and *Equisetum arvense* (bottom)

The DAB 10 also has a TLC identification
test based on the flavonoid profile; cf. below,
under: Adulteration.

Quantitative standards: DAB 10: *Foreign
matter*, not more than 3% fragments of the

blackish rhizome; not more than 2% other
foreign matter; not more than 10% stems/
branches of hybrids and other *Equisetum*
species. *Loss on drying*, not more than
10.0%. *Ash*, not more than 20.0%.
ÖAB: *Foreign matter*, not more than 3%
black stems; other *Equisetum* species, absent. *Ash*, not more than 15.0–20.0%. *Acid-
insoluble ash*, not more than 6.0–8.0%.
Ph. Helv. VII: *Blackish rhizome fragments
and other foreign matter*, not more than 5%;
TLC for the detection of *E. palustre. Sulphated ash*, 15–24%.
BHP 1/1990: *Water-soluble extractive*, not
less than 15%. *Foreign matter*, not more
than 2%. *Total ash*, not more than 20%.
HCl-insoluble ash, not more than 10%.

Adulteration: Frequent! Usually with other
Equisetum species, especially *E. palustre* L.,
marsh horsetail, which must be excluded because of its content of toxic (?) spermidine
alkaloids (palustrine, etc.). However, the
TLC test for possible admixture with
E. palustre given in the DAB 10 is time-consuming and unsatisfactory (in the second
supplement of DAB 10 the TLC test will be
changed according to [13]): as already mentioned, spermidine-type alkaloids have repeatedly been found in *E. arvense* and contamination with other alkaloidal *Equisetum*
species can only be recognized when at least
15% or more is present [12]. The TLC examination [based on 13] for distinguishing
the species on the basis of their flavonoid
profiles is better suited:

Test solution: 1 g powdered drug refluxed
with 20 ml methanol for 15 min., filtered, the
filtrate concentrated under reduced pressure, and the residue taken up in 2 ml
methanol.

Reference solution: 10 mg rutin and 5 mg
hyperoside dissolved in 10 ml methanol.

Loadings: 3 µl test solution and 2 µl reference solution, on silica gel.

Solvent system: ethyl acetate + anhydrous
formic acid + glacial acetic acid + water
(100 + 11 + 11 + 26).

Detection: solvent completely evaporated in
a current of hot air and the chromatogram
sprayed with 1% methanolic diphenylboryloxyethylamine, followed by 5% ethanolic
polyethylene glycol 400.

Evaluation: ca. 30 min. after spraying, in UV
365 nm light. Reference solution: hyperoside (Rf 0.6) and rutin (Rf 0.45), as orange-
yellow fluorescent spots. Test solution:
E. arvense extract, at Rf 0.65, quercetin 3-

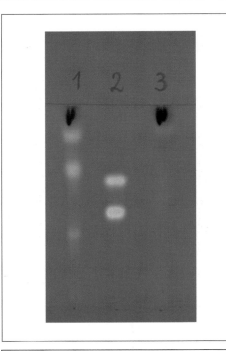

Fig. 7: TLC on 4 × 8 cm silica-gel foil

1: *Equisetum arvense*
2: *Reference compounds*
3: *Equisetum palustre*

For details, see the text

glucoside, the main flavonoid, a bright orange-yellow spot – *E. palustre* extract, absent; *E. arvense* extract, at about Rf 0.45,
faint greenish blue or orange fluorescent
spots; *E. palustre* extract, between Rf 0.1
and 0.4, several weak green fluorescent spots
(kaempferol 3,7-(di)-glycosides) – *E. arvense*
extract, absent (Fig. 7).

*Wording of the package insert, from the
German Standard Licence:*

5.1 Uses

In catarrh of the kidneys and bladder, to increase the
amount of urine.

5.2 Contraindications

Accumulation of water (oedema) as a result of impaired heart or kidney function.

5.3 Dosage and Mode of administration

2–3 Teaspoonfuls (ca. 2–4 g) of **Equisetum** are boiled
in water (ca. 150 ml) for 5–10 min. and after 15 min.
passed through a tea strainer.
Unless otherwise prescribed, a cup of the freshly prepared tea is drunk several times a day between meals.

5.4 Note

Store protected from light and moisture.

Euphrasiae herba

Euphrasia (BHP 1983)

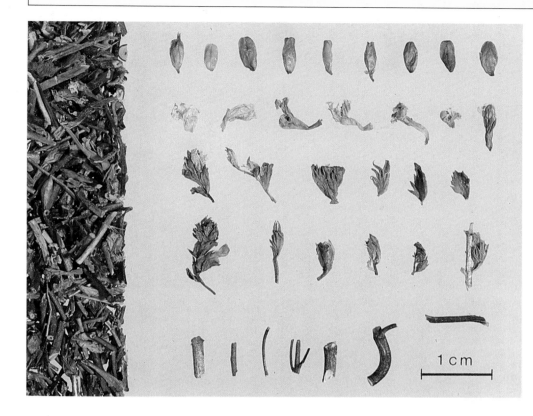

Fig. 1: Eyebright: different parts of the plant – corollas, calyces, leaves, fragments of stem

Description: The cut drug is characterized by the small, shrivelled and brittle, ovate, light to dark green leaves, with 7–10 long pointed teeth along the margin, which often occur in tight clumps; by single brownish white flowers up to 10 mm long, with violet veins and a yellow spot at the throat; by thin and round, bluish violet, slightly hairy fragments of stem; and by a few light brown, bilocular capsules, up to 5 mm long and containing numerous brown ovoid seeds (Fig. 5).

Odour: Not characteristic.

Taste: Somewhat bitter.

Fig. 2: *Euphrasia rostkoviana* HAYNE

A 10–30 cm tall annual with sharply toothed leaves and axillary flowers, white with a yellow spot and violet veins.

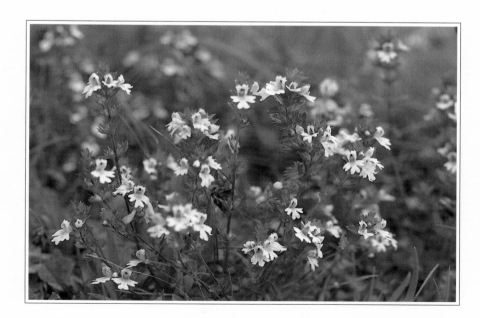

Erg. B. 6: Herba Euphrasiae

Plant sources: Various *Euphrasia* species, but especially taxa grouped round *E. rostkoviana* HAYNE (which includes *E. officinalis* L. – an ambiguous name) and *E. stricta* J.P. WOLFF ex J.F. LEHM., as well as their hybrids (Scrophulariaceae). The classification of the genus *Euphrasia* differs greatly in the literature and is to some extent contradictory. The treatment given in the Flora Europea is followed here; for more detail, see also [10].

Synonyms: Eyebright herb (Engl.), Augentrostkraut (Ger.), Herbe d'euphraise (officinale) (Fr.).

Origin: From European wild plants – particular localities: meadows, pastures, grassy places, heaths, etc.; imported from Bulgaria, Hungary, and former Yugoslavia.

Constituents: Iridoid glycosides such as aucubin, catalpol, euphroside, ixoroside, etc. [1, 2]. Lignans such as dehydrodiconiferylalcohol 4-β-D-glucoside [3], other phenylpropane glycosides, e.g. eukovoside [4], flavonoids, including quercetin and apigenin glycosides [5], tannins (gallotannins?), traces of tertiary alkaloids, steam-volatile substances [6], a range of free and combined phenol-carboxylic acids principally caffeic, *p*-hydroxyphenylpyruvic, and vanillic acids [6, 11].

Indications: Exclusively in *folk medicine*, externally against blepharitis and conjunctivitis, and in poultices for styes; for the general treatment of eye fatigue, functional disturbances of vision of muscular and nervous

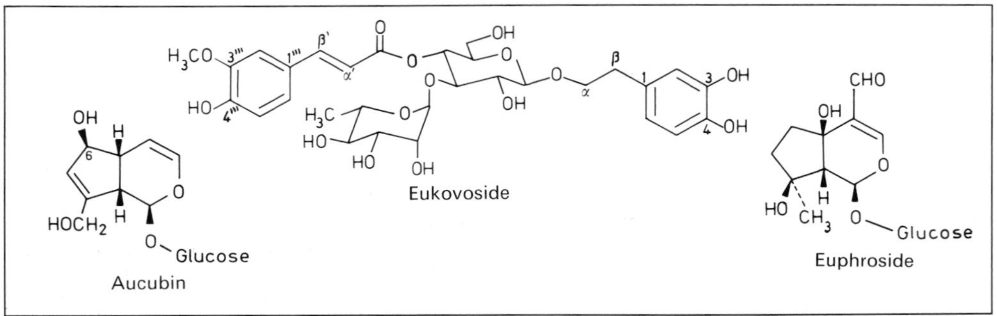

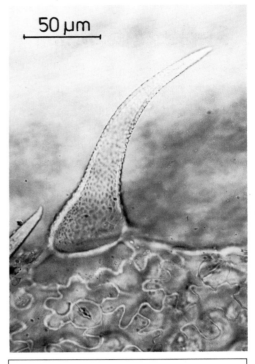

Aucubin
Eukovoside
Euphroside

50 µm

Fig. 3: Thick-walled curved trichomes with rounded base and rough cuticle on the lower leaf surface

Extract from the German Commission E monograph (BAnz no. 162, dated 29.08.92)

Uses

Eyebright (*Euphrasia officinalis*) preparations are used externally as lotions, poultices, and eye-baths, for eye complaints associated with disorders and inflammation of the blood vessels, inflammation of the eyelids and conjunctiva, as a preventive measure against mucus and catarrh of the eyes, "glued" and inflamed eyes, for coughs, colds, catarrh, and as a stomachic and against skin conditions.
Activity in the indications listed has not been substantiated.

Risks

None known.

Evaluation

Since activity against the indications listed has not been substantiated, therapeutic use is unacceptable – on hygienic grounds.

origin. Also, internally for coughs and hoarseness [7–9], as well as in homoeopathy against conjunctivitis. The phenol-carboxylic acids doubtless have a primary role in the antibacterial properties of the drug.

Making the tea: Boiling water is poured over 2–3 g of the finely cut drug or cold water is added and brought to the boil for a short time, and after 5–10 min. passed through a tea strainer. Externally, a 2% decoction is used three or four times daily (for bathing the eyes).
1 Teaspoon = ca. 1.7 g.

Phytomedicines: As the extract, in certain eye drops (ophthalmic remedies); as a tea, together with other components, as a lotion (2% decoction); according to [8], as a hot poultice for styes: $^1/_4$ litre boiling water poured over 5 tablespoonfuls of eyebright, allowed to draw for 10 min., and the mash wrapped in muslin is placed on the stye as hot as possible.

Authentication: Macro- (see: Description) and microscopically; see also the BHP 1983. The diagnostic features of the greyish green powdered drug are: 1–2-celled, thick-walled, curved trichomes with a warty cuticle (Fig. 3); glandular trichomes with a 2–3-celled uniseriate stalk and unicellular head (Fig. 4); very long, unicellular, twisted trichomes; and very short, conical trichomes on the leaf margin. Fragments of the leaf epidermis show cells with very sinuous anticlinal walls (Figs. 3 and 4) and the petal epidermis strongly papillose cells. In chloralhydrate preparations, anther fragments take on a red colour; they have a few, long hooked trichomes with a warty cuticle. The spherical pollen grains are up to 40 µm in diameter and have three pores.

Quantitative standards: Erg. B. 6: *Ash*, not more than 10%.
BHP 1983: *Water-soluble extractive*, not less than 15%. *Foreign organic matter*, not more than 2%. *Total ash*, not more than 10%. *Acid-insoluble ash*, not more than 2%.

Adulteration: Hardly ever occurs.

100 µm

2 mm

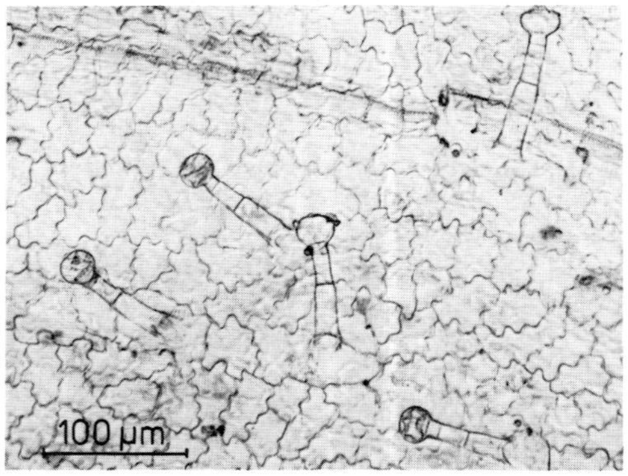

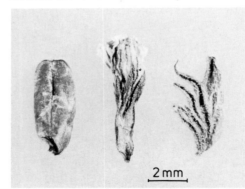

Fig. 4: Numerous glandular trichomes with uniseriate stalk and unicellular rounded heads

Fig. 5: Bilocular fruit capsule (left), flowers (centre), and distinctly serrate leaves (right)

Literature:

[1] M. Królikowska, Acta Polon. Pharm. **17**, 23 (1960); Roczn. Chem. **41**, 529 (1967).
[2] O. Sticher and O. Salama, Planta Med. **39**, 269 (1980); Helv. Chim. Acta **64**, 78 (1981).
[3] O. Salama, R.K. Chaudhuri, and O. Sticher, Phytochemistry **20**, 2603 (1981).
[4] O. Sticher, O.Salama, R.K. Chaudhuri, and T. Winkler, Planta Med. **45**, 159 (1982); Helv. Chim. Acta **65**, 1538 (1982).
[5] I. Matlawska, M. Sikorska, and Z. Kowalewski, Herb. Polon. **31**, 119 (1985).
[6] K.J. Harkiss and P. Timmins, Planta Med. **23**, 342 (1973).
[7] Hager, vol. **4**, p. 886 (1973).
[8] H. Braun and D. Frohne, Heilpflanzenlexikon für Ärzte und Apotheker, G. Fischer Verlag, Stuttgart – New York, 1987.
[9] R. F. Weiß, Herbal Medicine, Arcanum, Gothenburg, and Beaconsfield Publishers, Beaconsfield, 1988.
[10] P.F. Yeo, Bot. J. Linn. Soc. **77**, 223 (1978).
[11] S. Luczak and L. Swiatek, Plantes Méd. Phytothérap. **24**, 66 (1990).

Farfarae folium   (DAB 10), Tussilago (BHP 1983), Coltsfoot

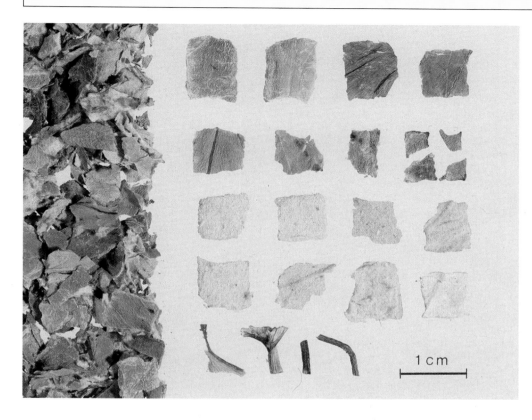

1 cm

Fig. 1: Coltsfoot

Description: The thin leaves are ca. 20 cm across, palmate and lobate, and with a coarsely sinuate-serrate margin and a distinct petiole. They are white-felted on the lower surface (Fig. 4) and yellowish green on the upper surface; only young leaves are pubescent on the upper surface.

Taste: Faintly mucilaginous and sweetish.

Fig. 2: Leaves of *Tussilago farfara* L., with a horseshoe-shaped margin and white-felted lower surface

Fig. 3: *Tussilago farfara* L.

An early flowering perennial herb, up to 30 cm in height. Yellow capitula with narrow ligulate flowers, appearing before the leaves, on densely pubescent and scaly stalks. Fruit with a white pappus.

DAB 10: Huflattichblätter (deleted with the 3. Suppl.)
ÖAB: Folium Tussilaginis
St.Zul. 1039.99.99

Plant source: *Tussilago farfara* L., coltsfoot (Asteraceae).

Synonyms: Huflattichblätter, Brandlattich, Pferdefuß (Ger.), Pas d'âne, Feuilles de tussilage (Fr.).

Origin: Collected exclusively from wild plants in Italy, the Balkans, and eastern Europe (former USSR, former Yugoslavia, Bulgaria, Hungary, Poland, former Czechoslovakia).

Constituents: 6–10% mucilage and inulin [1–3], as well as ca. 5% tannins and small amounts of flavonoids, various plant acids, triterpenes, and sterols. In traces – but only from some sources – pyrrolizidine alkaloids (see: Side effects), e.g. senkirkine and tussilagine [4].

Indications: In catarrhal inflammation, dry cough, and acute and chronic irritation of the mouth and throat.
The mucilage of the drug covers the mucous membranes with a layer that mitigates the effects of chemical and physical irritants and thus lessens the urge to cough.

Side effects: Although several pyrrolizidine alkaloids are known to have hepatotoxic, genotoxic, and/or cancerogenic effects, there is no danger of acute poisoning when the drug is used as prescribed, particularly as the concentration of these alkaloids in a tea is very low [5]. Nevertheless, people should be warned against using the drug for a prolonged period of time [6, 7].

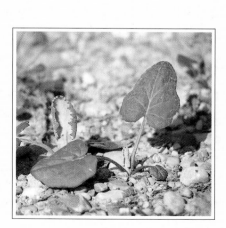

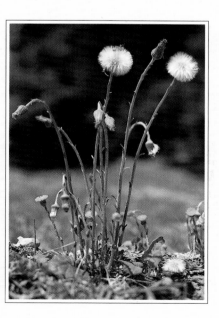

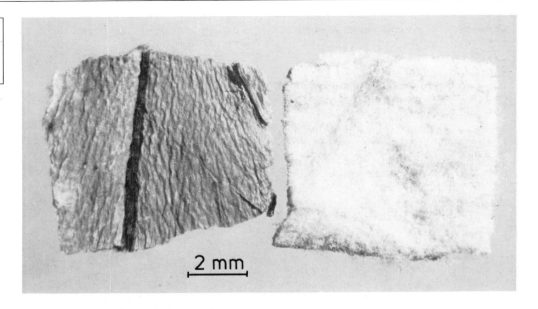

Fig. 4: Glabrous, wrinkled upper surface (left) and white-felted lower surface (right)

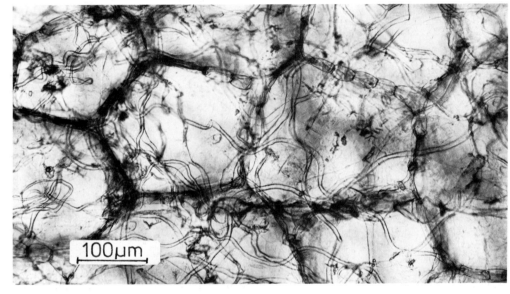

Fig. 5: Long, slender and tortuous trichomes on the lower surface and transparent, large aerenchyma

Meanwhile the German Federal Ministry for Health has limited the medicinal use of coltsfoot by regulation. The oral uptake for pyrrolizidine alkaloids with a 1,2-unsaturated necine-residue must not exceed 100 µg/day [10].

Making the tea: Boiling water is poured over 1.5–2.5 g of the chopped drug and after 5–20 min. strained.
1 Teaspoon = ca. 1 g, 1 tablespoon = ca. 3–4 g.

Herbal preparations: Coltsfoot leaves are present in many bronchial teas and extracts are found in a few instant (bronchial) teas, e.g. Bronchostad®, etc.

Phytomedicines: In the form of the powdered drug, or as extract or percolate, in some prepared cough remedies.

Authentication: Macro- and microscopically, following the DAB 10. Besides the characteristic trichomes on the lower surface of the leaves and the large intercellular spaces in the spongy mesophyll (Fig. 5), the fine wavy striations on the upper epidermis and the absence of trichomes on the upper surface of the leaves are diagnostic. See also the BHP 1983.

The DAB 10 TLC test of identity is as follows:

Test solution: 0.5 g powdered drug shaken on the water-bath at 65 °C with 10 ml methanol for 10 ml and filtered.

Reference solution: 1.0 mg caffeic acid and 2.5 mg each of hyperoside and rutin dissolved in 10 ml.

Loadings: 30 ml test solution and 10 ml reference solution, as 2-cm bands on silica gel G.

Solvent system: Anhydrous formic acid + water + ethyl methyl ketone + ethyl acetate (10 + 10 + 30 + 50), 15 cm run.

Detection: after drying at 100–105 °C, the still warm plate sprayed with 1% methanolic diphenylboryloxyethylamine, followed by 5% methanolic Macrogol 400.

Evaluation: after 30 min. in UV 365 nm light. Reference solution: in order of increasing Rf: yellowish orange to orange-brown rutin and hyperoside fluorescent zones and the greenish blue fluorescent caffeic acid zone. Test solution: in Rf region between caffeic acid and hyperoside, at least 4 yellowish green to orange-brown fluorescent zones, the second from the top being the main one – also seen in daylight as the main zone; in the Rf range between hyeroside and rutin, one or two blue fluorescent zones visible.

Quantitative standards: DAB 10: *Swelling index*, not less than 9. *Foreign matter*, not more than 10% leaf stalks; not more than 2% leaf blades attacked by rusts; not more than 2% other foreign matter. *Loss on drying*, not more than 10.0%. *Ash*, not more than 23.0%.
ÖAB: *Foreign matter*, not more than 3%; leaf fragments of *Arctium* (= *Lappa*) and *Eupatorium* species absent. *Ash*, not more than 20.0%. *Acid-insoluble ash*, not more than 2.0%.

Adulteration: Relatively frequent, especially with the leaves of different *Petasites* species [8, 9]. Particularly in the chopped drug, these are not easy to recognize; microscopic examination reveals the characteristic biseriate glandular (so-called barrel-shaped) trichomes, especially on the upper epidermis; woolly trichomes with a somewhat broader terminal cell, on the lower surface; and the lack of cuticular striations (except in *Petasites albus* (L.) GAERTN. [8, 9]; see further Petasitidis folium.
In the above TLC test of identity, on examination in UV 365 nm light there should be no zone at the same Rf level as rutin; if

present, it points to adulteration with *Petasites*. The DAB 10 also requires conformity with the following TLC examination for purity:

Test solution: 0.5 g powdered drug refluxed with 40 ml light petroleum on the waterbath at ca. 70 °C for 15 min., filtered, the filter washed with a few ml light petroleum, the combined filtrates concentrated and made up to 1.0 ml with light petroleum.

Reference solution: 5 ml each of eugenol and linalool dissolved in 10 ml light petroleum.

Loadings: 20 ml of each solution, as a 2-cm band on silica gel GF$_{254}$.

Solvent system: chloroform, 10 cm run.

Detection and Evaluation: in UV 254 nm light. Reference solution: eugenol quenching zone visible in the middle Rf range. In UV 365 nm light. Test solution: at the level of the eugenol zone and below it no blue or violet fluorescent visible.
After spraying with anisaldehyde reagent and heating at 100–105 °C for 5–10 min. In daylight. Reference solution: in order of increasing Rf value, the greyish red linalool zone and the grey eugenol zone. Test solution: no reddish violet zone visible at the level of the eugenol zone, nor a blue or reddish violet zone in Rf range between the

eugenol and the uppermost reddish violet zones.
In UV 365 nm light. Reference solution: linalool zone red and eugenol zone yellowish green fluorescence. Test solution: no fluorescent zones other than a pale red one should be visible in the region between the Rf values of the two reference substances.
The DAB 10 TLC method for verifying the absence of petasin-containing and petasin-free *Petasites* species is as follows:

Test solution: 0.5 g powdered drug refluxed for 15 min. with light petroleum (b. range 50–70 °C), filtered, and the marc washed with a few ml solvent; the filtrate concentrated and made up to 1.0 ml with light petroleum.

Reference solution: 5 ml each of eugenol and linalool dissolved in 10 ml light petroleum.

Loadings: 20 ml of each solution, as 2-cm bands on silica gel GF$_{254}$.

Solvent system: chloroform, 10 cm run.

Detection and Evaluation: in UV 254 nm light. Reference solution: eugenol quenching zone in the middle Rf range. In UV 365 nm light. Test solution: at the level of the eugenol zone and below it, **no** blue or violet fluorescent zones.
Sprayed with anisaldehyde reagent and heated for 5–10 min. at 100–105 °C while under observation. Reference solution: with increasing Rf value, the greyish red linalool zone and the grey eugenol zone. Test solution: at the level of the linalool zone, **no** reddish violet zone; **no** blue or reddish violet zone in the Rf range between the eugenol zone and the uppermost reddish violet zone.
In UV 365 nm light. Reference solution: red fluorescent zone (linalool) and yellowish green fluorescent zone (eugenol). Test solution: in the Rf range of the two reference substances and in between, **no** fluorescent zones other than pale reddish ones.
Occasionally, there is adulteration with the leaves of the greater burdock, *Arctium lappa* L. These have barrel-shaped trichomes, like *Petasites* species, and cuticular striations like those of *Tussilago farfara*.

Literature:
[1] G. Franz, Planta Med. **17**, 217 (1969).
[2] E. Haaland, Acta Chem. Scand. **26**, 2322 (1972).
[3] E.I. Engalcheva et al., Farmatsiya **33**, 13 (1984); C.A. **101**, 87497 (1984).
[4] E. Röder, H. Wiedenfeld, and E.J. Jost, Planta Med. **43**, 99 (1981).
[5] F.-C. Czygan, Z. Phytotherap. **4**, 630 (1983).
[6] E. Röder, Dtsch. Apoth. Ztg. **122**, 2088 (1982).
[7] H.U. Wolf, Dtsch. Apoth. Ztg. **123**, 2166 (1983); F.-C. Czygan, *ibid.* **122**, 2167 (1983).
[8] J. Saukel, Sci. Pharm. **56**, 47 (1988).
[9] J. Saukel, Sci. Pharm. **59**, 307 (1991).
[10] BGA, Stufenplan, Dtsch. Apoth. Ztg. **130**, VIII/62 (1990).

Foeniculi fructus   (DAB 10), Fennel, Foeniculum (BHP 1983)

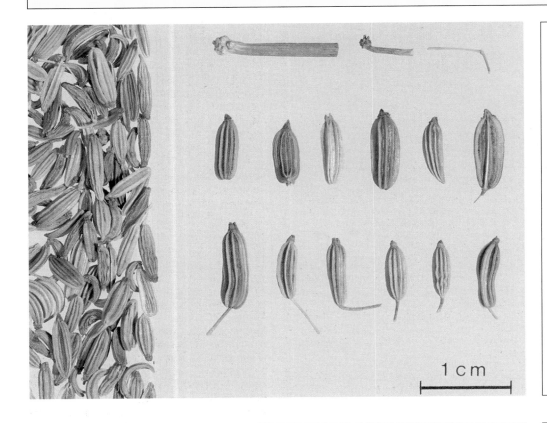

1 cm

Fig. 1: Fennel

Description: The drug consists of the 3–12 mm long and 2–4 mm broad yellowish green to yellowish brown mericarps; occasionally, the mericarps are still attached to each other. Often, the remains of the pistil can be seen at the upper end of the stylopod. Each mericarp has 5 straight, projecting ridges which are particularly prominent on the commissural surface (Fig. 3).

Odour: Intensely spicy.

Taste: Aromatic and spicy, somewhat pungent.

Fig. 2: *Foeniculum vulgare* MILL.

A biennial to perennial plant up to 2 m in height. Feathery leaves with narrow, thread-like segments. Double umbels with mostly unequal rays, lacking involucre and sheath; flowers yellowish.

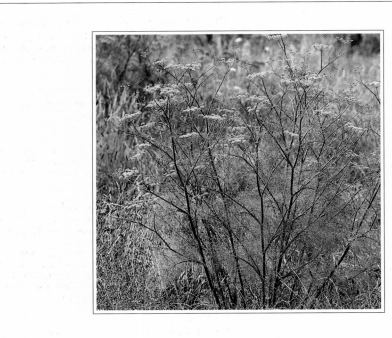

DAB 10: Bitterer Fenchel
ÖAB: Fructus Foeniculi
Ph. Helv. VII: Foeniculi fructus
St.Zul. 5199.99.99

Plant origin: According to the DAB 10, *Foeniculum vulgare* MILL. var. *vulgare* (Apiaceae). The Ph. Helv. VII and ÖAB permit fruits of the two varieties *vulgare* and *dulce* (MILL.) THELL., and the next volume of the Ph. Eur. and the BHP will have two monographs: one for bitter fennel and one for sweet fennel. The two varieties derive from the cultivated subsp. *capillaceum* (GILIB.) HOLMBOE.

Synonyms: Fennel fruit or seed (Engl.), Fenchel, Bitterfenchel (Ger.), Fruit de fenouil, Aneth doux (Fr.).

Origin: Native to the Mediterranean region; nowadays, cultivated in Europe, Asia, parts of Africa and South America. Imports come from China, Egypt, Bulgaria, Hungary, and Romania.
For the cultural history of fennel, see the summary in [6].

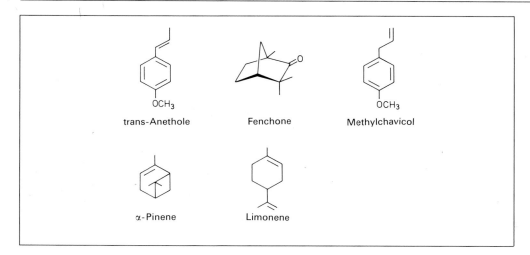

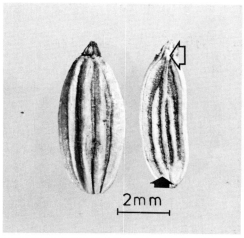

Fig. 3: Mericarp (left, outside surface; right, commissural surface) of *Foeniculum vulgare*, showing the dark secretory canals (vittae) (dark arrow) and carpophore (light arrow)

Constituents: 2–6% essential oil, comprising up to 50–70% of the sweetish *trans*-anethole and up to 20% of the bitter and camphoraceous (+)-fenchone. In addition, there are methylchavicol, anisaldehyde, and some terpenoid hydrocarbons, including α-pinene, α-phellandrene, and limonene. In addition, the fruits contain a fixed oil, protein, organic acids, and flavonoids [1, 2]. – About the occurrence of the oestrogens dianethole and dianisoin, see the data under Anisi fructus.

Indications: As a secretomotor, secretolytic, and antiseptic expectorant, as a spasmolytic and carminative in mild digestive disorders [1, 3, 4]; and therefore often added to laxatives to counteract the mild cramps accompanying their use. It is particularly favoured in paediatrics. The *pure essential oil* reinforces inflammation and has an irritant action on the intestinal musculature. Pure fennel oil must not be used for infants or young children because of the danger of laryngeal spasm, dyspnoea, and excitatory states [1]. In *folk medicine*, it is also used as a galactagogue for lactating women and externally as an eye lotion (decoction) and in functional visual disorders [4]. Fennel is also employed as a taste enhancer.

Making the tea: Boiling water is poured over 2–5 g of the drug crushed or stamped immediately before use, covered, and allowed to stand for 10–15 min. before being passed through a tea strainer.
1 Teaspoon = ca. 2.5 g.

Herbal preparations: The drug is available in tea bags (mostly 2 g); this is pointless, since only very little oil can be extracted from the uncrushed drug. On the other hand, the crushed drug (even in tea bags) rapidly loses its essential oil.
Fennel is also available from various firms in the form of an instant tea.

Phytomedicines: As a component of cough remedies (antitussives, expectorants), stomach and bowel remedies (carminatives, laxatives), especially in paediatrics in the form of

---

Extract from the German Commission E monograph (BAnz no. 74, dated 18/04/91)

Uses

Dyspeptic complaints, such as mild cramp-like gastrointestinal disorders, a feeling of distension, flatulence.
Catarrh of the upper respiratory tract.
Fennel syrup, fennel honey: catarrh of the upper respiratory tract in children.

Contraindications

Drug for infusions and preparations containing an equivalent amount of the essential oil: None known.
Other preparations: Pregnancy.

Side effects

In a few cases, allergic reactions by the skin and the respiratory tract.

Interactions with other remedies

None known.

Dosage

Unless otherwise prescribed: daily dose 5–7 g, fennel syrup or honey (Erg. B. 6) 10–20 g, compound fennel tincture (Erg. B. 6) 5–7.5 g; preparations correspondingly.

Mode of administration

Powdered drug for infusions, tea-like products, and other galenical formulations for internal use.

Duration of use

Preparations of fennel should not be taken for a prolonged period (several weeks) without consulting a doctor or pharmacist.

Warning: Fennel syrup and fennel honey: Diabetics must bear in mind the sugar content of bread exchange-units (according to the manufacturer's information).

Effects

Promotes gastrointestinal motility, in higher concentrations acts as a spasmolytic. Experimentally, anethole and fenchone have been shown to have a secretolytic action in the respiratory tract; in the frog, aqueous fennel extracts raise the muco-ciliary activity of the ciliary epithelium.

Wording of the package insert, from the German Standard Licence:

6.1 **Uses**

Against flatulence and cramp-like pains in the gastrointestinal tract, especially in infants and small children, and to dissolve mucus in the respiratory tract.

6.2 **Dosage and Mode of administration**

Boiling water (150 ml) is poured over 1–3 teaspoonfuls of crushed **Fennel** and after 5–10 min. passed through a tea strainer.
Unless otherwise prescribed, for gastrointestinal complaints a cupful of the freshly prepared infusion is drunk warm between meals two to four times a day. For infants and young children, the infusion may be used to dilute their milk or pap.

6.3 **Note**

Store protected from light and moisture.

teas, tea extracts, dragees, sweets, syrups, and juices; it is often combined with other essential-oil-containing drugs, e.g. aniseed.

Regulatory status (UK): General Sales List – Schedule 1, Table A.

Authentication: Macro- (see: Description) and microscopically, following [1]. Note especially: the reticulately thickened and lignified parenchyma of the mesocarp and the 4–8 μm broad and up to 100 μm long "parquetry" cells of the endocarp. See also the BHP 1983 and [7].

The DAB 10 TLC test of identity is as follows:

Test solution: 0.30 g freshly pulverized drug is shaken for 2–3 min. with 5.0 ml dichloromethane and filtered over ca. 2 g anhydrous sodium sulphate.

Reference solution: 3 μl anethole and 5 μl each of anisaldehyde and olive oil dissolved in 1.0 ml dichloromethane.

Loadings: 20 μl test solution and 10 μl reference solution, as 2-cm bands on silica gel GF$_{254}$.

Solvent system: dichloromethane, 10 cm run.

Detection and Evaluation: in UV 254 nm light. After marking the quenching zones, the plate sprayed with ethanolic phosphomolybdate solution and heated at 100–105 °C while under observation; the still warm layer oversprayed with a freshly and carefully prepared solution of 0.5 g potassium permanganate in 96% sulphuric acid and heated at 100–105 °C, again while under observation for a further 5–10 min.

Reference solution: after the first spray, the anethole and anisaldehyde quenching zones becoming faint bluish grey and brownish yellow, respectively; on heating, the anethole zone (in the upper part of the chromatogram) quickly turning dark blue; between the anethole and anisaldehyde zones, the dark blue triglyceride zone.

Test solution: two dark blue zones corresponding in position, size, and intensity of colour with those of the reference solution; in addition, faint blue zones also visible; after spraying with potassium permanganate/ sulphuric acid, the initially pale fenchone zone, directly above the anisaldehyde zone, rapidly becoming dark blue on heating.

Particular attention should be paid to the distinct blue-coloured fenchone zone on the chromatogram. It allows the official drug, with a fenchone content of 10–20%, to be differentiated from sweet fennel (not permitted by the DAB 10), which has only ca. 1%.

Quantitative standards: DAB 10: *Volatile oil*, not less than 4.0%. *Foreign matter*, not more than 1.5% umbel rays (peduncles) and not more than 1.5% other foreign matter. *Loss on drying*, not more than 13.0%. *Ash*, not more than 8.0%.

ÖAB: *Volatile oil*, not less than 3.5%. *Foreign matter*, not more than 1%; no large amounts of stout fibres or vessels with a wide lumen. *Ash*, not more than 8.0%.

Ph. Helv. VII: *Volatile oil*, not less than 2.0% (and for veterinary purposes, not less than 1.7%). *Foreign matter*, not more than 1.5% (chiefly peduncles and foreign seeds). *Water content*, not more than 7.0%. *Sulphated ash*, not more than 10%.

Adulteration: Rare, but recently fennel imports containing foreign seeds have been encountered (millet [*Sorghum species*], wheat, etc.).

Storage: Protected from moisture and light in glass or lead (but not plastic) containers.

Literature:
[1] Kommentar DAB 10.
[2] V. Formácek and K.-H. Kubeczka, Essential oil analysis by capillary gas chromatography and carbon-13 NMR spectroscopy, J. Wiley, Chichester, 1982.
[3] R. Hänsel and H. Haas, Therapie mit Phytopharmaka, Springer, Berlin – New York, 1983; 2nd ed. 1991.
[4] H. Braun and D. Frohne, Heilpflanzenlexikon für Ärzte und Apotheker, G. Fischer, Stuttgart – New York, 1987.
[5] P. Pachaly, Dünnschichtchromatographie in der Apotheke, 2nd ed., Wissenschaftliche Verlagsgesellschaft, Stuttgart, 1983.
[6] F.-C. Czygan, Z. Phytotherap. **8**, 82 (1987).
[7] B.P. Jackson and D.W. Snowdon, Atlas of microscopy of medicinal plants, culinary herbs and spices, Belhaven Press, London, 1990, p. 98.

Foenugraeci semen   (DAB 10), Fenugreek seed, Trigonella (BHP 1983)

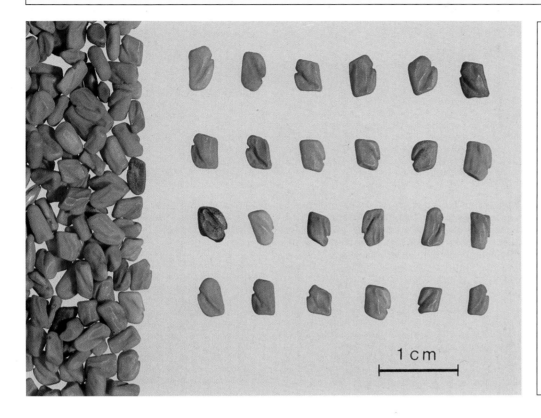

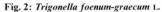

1 cm

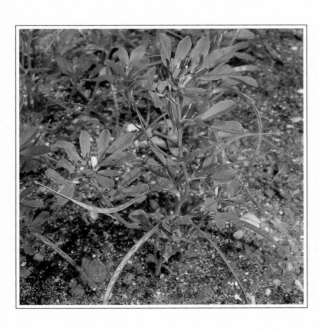

Fig. 1: Fenugreek seed

Description: The very hard, light brown or reddish to yellowish grey seeds are rhombic or flat diamond-shaped, irregularly rounded, 3–5 mm long and 2–3 mm wide and thick. The somewhat sunken light-coloured hilum is situated at about the middle of one of the long narrow sides (hand lens; Fig. 3) and from it there runs a flat diagonal groove which divides the seed into two unequal halves; the radicle is in the smaller half and the cotyledons of the curved embryo are located in the larger half. Placed in water, the seeds swell rapidly and the testa splits open and can be readily separated from the endosperm.

Odour: Characteristic and spicy.

Taste: Somewhat bitter, and on chewing mucilaginous.

Fig. 2: *Trigonella foenum-graecum* L.

An up to 50 cm tall annual herb. Leaves petiolate and in threes. Flowers in the axils of the leaves, pale yellow and towards the base pale violet. Pod up to 20 cm long with numerous seeds.

DAB 10: Bockshornsamen
ÖAB: Semen Foenugraeci
Ph. Helv. VII: Foenugraeci semen ad usum veterinarium

Plant origin: *Trigonella foenum-graecum* L., fenugreek (Fabaceae).

Synonyms: Semen trigonellae (Lat.), Bockshornsamen, Griechische Heusamen (Ger.), Graine de fenugrec (Fr.).

Origin: Native in the Mediterranean region, the Ukraine, India, and China, and in these regions widely cultivated. The drug comes exclusively from cultivated plants and the main supplies originate in India, Morocco, China, and Turkey.

Constituents: Ca. 45–60% carbohydrates, chiefly mucilage located on the cell walls in the endosperm (galactomannans): 1,4-β-gly-cosidically bound mannose chains with α-glycosidically bound galactose chains, together with a small proportion of xylose; fibrous and starchy materials, as well as oligosaccharides are also present. 20–30%

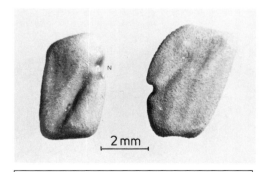

Trigofoenoside A

Foenugraecin

Trigonelline

protein (rich in tryptophan, but poor in S-containing amino acids) and 6–10% fixed oil (rich in unsaturated acids; in the embryo). A range of proteinase inhibitors which act on human trypsin and chymotrypsin is present; ca. 30 components have been detected by electrophoresis. Several steroidal saponins occurring as Δ^5-furostene and 5α-furostane 3,26-bis-glycosides; after removal of the glucose at C-26, they are transformed into spirostanol glycosides and after hydrolysis they afford diosgenin and yamogenin (0.1–2.2%), among others; the 3,26-bis-desmosidic furostanol glycosides trigofoenosides A–G have 22-methoxy-Δ^5-furosten-3β,26-diol, 22-methoxy-5α-furostan-2α,3β,26-triol, and Δ^5-furosten-3β,22,26-triol as aglycones [1–3, 15]. The furostanol glycosides taste bitter and are presumably the bitter principle of the drug. There is also foenugraecin, a 3-peptide ester of diosgenin. Sterols: including cholesterol and sitosterol. Flavonoids: the *C*-glycosylflavones vitexin, saponaretin, homoorientin, etc.; 0.2–0.36% trigonelline (=coffearine, the *N*-methylbetaine of nicotinic acid; traces of nicotinamide); ca. 0.015% essential oil with 51 components, of which 39 have been identified [4]. The typical fenugreek smell is supposed to derive mainly from the presence of 3-hydroxy-4,5-dimethyl-2[5H]-furanone.

Indications: Externally as an emollient in the form of poultices for treating furuncles, boils, inflamed indurations, and eczema. In *folk medicine*, internally as a mucilage in catarrh of the upper respiratory passages and, the powder taken by the tablespoonful several times a day, as a roborant. In rats, orally administered aqueous extracts have been shown to promote the healing of stomach ulcers [5]. Further, in *folk medicine* blood sugar-reducing, lactagogic, and antipella-

gral activities are ascribed to the drug. An antidiabetic action has been observed in diabetic dogs after oral administration of defatted seed extracts [6]. As with the galactomannans of guar gum, the mucilage thickens the diffusion layer of the mucosal cells and the absorption of nutrients is retarded. The same principle may lie at the basis of the demonstrated hypocholesterolaemic effect [7]. In normal and hypercholesterolaemic rats, half of whose food comprised fenugreek seeds, the serum cholesterol level was halved. Adding defatted seed extracts to a hypercholesterolaemic diet prevented a rise in the cholesterol level; the lipid fraction and trigonelline did not show this effect [9]. Foenugraecin may have a hypoglycaemic action, and it is said also to have virostatic, antiphlogistic, and cardiotonic properties [10]. Steroidal saponins have similar antiphlogistic [e.g. 11] and antimicrobial effects [12]. Aqueous extracts of the seeds have been shown to stimulate the uterus and intestine and to have a positive

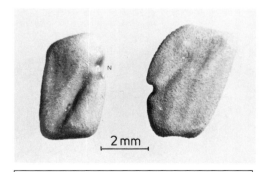

Fig. 3: Seeds showing the diagonal groove, finely punctate surface, and whitish hilum (N)

2 mm

chronotropic effect on the heart [13]. The nicotinamide content is too small to exert an antipellagral effect; the possibility that trigonelline functions as a provitamin has been variously assessed but appears unlikely. Fenugreek seeds have acquired some interest as a possible source of diosgenin for the production of steroid hormones. They are also used in curry and to impart an aroma to tobacco, as well as coffee and vanilla extracts.

Making the tea: The drug is usually only used externally. The powdered seeds are stirred with hot water to give a paste which is used for poultices. For internal use, 0.5 g of the drug is stood in cold water for 3 h and then strained. A cupful, if desired sweetened with honey, is taken several times a day. 1 Teaspoon = ca. 4.5 g.

Phytomedicines: The drug is an infrequent component of prepared gastrointestinal remedies, bronchial remedies, and cholagogues.

Authentication: Macro- (see: Description) and microscopically, following the DAB 10 or [14]; see also the BHP 1983. The transverse section of the seed testa is characteristic and comprises radial palisade-like elongated epidermal cells with thickened external and lateral walls and a more or less bottle-shaped lumen; the cuticle can be seen as a line of light running along the upper ends of the cells. Below the epidermis, the hypodermis is formed by a layer of characteristic

---

Extract from the German Commission E monograph (BAnz no. 22a, dated 01.02.1990)

Uses

Internally: loss of appetite.
Externally: as a poultice for local inflammations.

Contraindications

None known.

Side effects

Repeated external use may bring about undesirable skin reactions.

Interactions with other remedies

None known.

Dosage

Unless otherwise prescribed, daily dose: internally, 6 g drug, and preparations correspondingly; externally, 50 g powdered drug to $^1/_4$ litre water.

Mode of administration

Internally, the crushed drug and other galenical forms; externally, 50 g powdered drug boiled for 5 min. with $^1/_4$ litre water and applied as a moist warm poultice.

pedestal-like cells which narrow at the upper end and have vertical ridges of thickening; in between these cells, there are large intercellular spaces. There follow 2–4 rows of thin-walled cells, slightly elongated tangentially and often compressed. The endosperm comprises large cells with thick, laminated, mucilaginous walls. The embryo consists of thin-walled cells containing oil globules, aleurone, and a little starch (ca. 5 μm). The powdered drug can also be identified by means of these characters; cf. [16]. The DAB 10 TLC test of identity (cf. [14]) is as follows:

Test solution: 1.0 g powdered drug shaken with 5.0 ml methanol for 5 min. on the water-bath at 65 °C, then cooled and filtered.

Reference solution: 3.0 mg trigonelline hydrochloride dissolved in 1.0 ml methanol.

Loadings: 20 μl test solution and 10 μl reference solution, as 2-cm bands on silica gel GF$_{254}$.

Solvent system: water+methanol (30+70), 10 cm run.

Detection and Evaluation: in UV 254 nm light. Reference solution: in the lower half a strongly quenching trigonelline zone. Test solution: a trigonelline quenching zone at the same Rf and of about the same intensity; a few additional weak quenching zones.
Then sprayed with Dragendorff reagent, followed by 0.1N sulphuric acid. Reference and Test solutions: at once, the trigonelline zones intense orange-red on a pale greyish brown background. Test solution: in the upper part, a broad bright yellowish brown zone (triglycerides) and below it one or two yellowish white zones (phospholipids) not always well separated from the triglyceride zone; between the trigonelline zone and the narrow yellowish band at the start line, usually a faint orange-red zone.
With iron(III) chloride, the cotyledons of the embryo become red and with potassium hydroxide yellow (trigonelline reaction).

Quantitative standards: DAB 10: *Swelling index*, not less than 6. *Foreign matter*, not more than 4%. *Loss on drying*, not more than 10.0%. *Ash*, not more than 5.0%.
ÖAB: *Swelling index*, not less than 6. *Foreign matter*, not more than 2%. *Ash*, not more than 5.0%.
Ph. Helv. VII: *swelling index*, not less than 6. *Foreign matter*, not more than 5%; blackened seeds. not more than 2%; at most, only occasional seeds with verrucosities (warts) in rows (*Agrostemma githago* L., corncockle). *Sulphated ash*, not more than 6%.

Adulteration: Not observed in practice.

Literature:
[1] R.K. Gupta, D.C. Thain, and R.S. Thakur, Phytochemistry **23**, 2605 (1984).
[2] R.K. Gupta, D.C. Thain, and R.S. Thakur, Phytochemistry **24**, 2399 (1085).
[3] R.K. Gupta, D.C. Thain, and R.S. Thakur, Phytochemistry **25**, 2205 (1986).
[4] F. Girardou, J.M. Bassiere, J.C. Baccou, and Y. Sauvaire, Planta Med. **51**, 533 (1985).
[5] I. A. Al Meshal, N.S. Parmar, M. Tariq, and A.M. Ageel, Fitoterapia **56**, 236 (1985).
[6] G. Ribes et al., Ann. Nutr. Metabol. **28**, 37 (1984).
[7] G. Valette, Y. Sauvaire, J.C. Baccou, and G. Ribes, Atherosclerosis **50**, 105 (1984).
[8] P.C. Singhal, R.K. Gupta, and L.D. Joshi, Indian Curr. Sci. **51**, 136 (1982).
[9] R.D. Sharma, Nutr. Rep. Int. **33**, 669 (1986); C.A. **104**, 206054 (1986).
[10] S. Ghosal, S. Srivastava, D.C. Chatterjee, and S.K. Dutta, Phytochemistry **13**, 2247 (1974).
[11] S.K. Bhattacharya et al., Rheumatism **6**, 1 (1971).
[12] R. Tschesche and G. Wulff, Z. Naturforsch. **20b**, 543 (1965).
[13] M.S. Abdo and A.A. Al-Kafawi, Planta Med. **17**, 14 (1969).
[14] P. Rohdewald, G. Rücker, and K.W. Glombitza, Apothekengerechte Prüfungsvorschriften, Deutscher Apotheker Verlag, Stuttgart, 1986, p. 663.
[15] J.K.P. Weder and K. Haußner, Z. Lebensmittel-Unters.-Forsch. **192**, 455 (1991).
[16] B.P. Jackson and D.W. Snowdon, Atlas of microscopy of medicinal plants, culinary herbs and spices, Belhaven Press, London, 1990, p. 100

Fragariae folium   Wild strawberry leaf

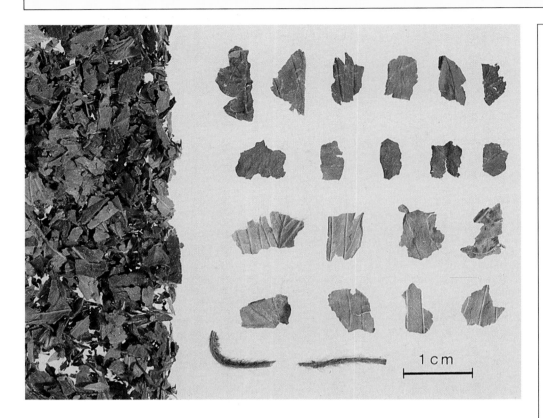

Fig. 1: Wild strawberry leaf

<u>Description</u>: The drug consists mainly of leaf fragments with a silky pubescence on the lower surface; quite often, the sharply serrate margin of the leaf; the lateral nerves are parallel. Occasionally, yellowish white parts of flowers and densely pubescent (green or blue-violet) pieces of stem are present.

<u>Taste</u>: Somewhat mucilaginous and bitter.

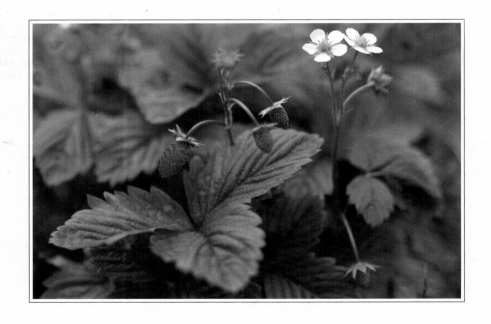

Fig. 2: *Fragaria vesca* L.

A low, perennial, herbaceous plant, forming long rooting runners. Ternate leaves with a sharply serrate margin. Petals white. Ripe red fruit readily falling.

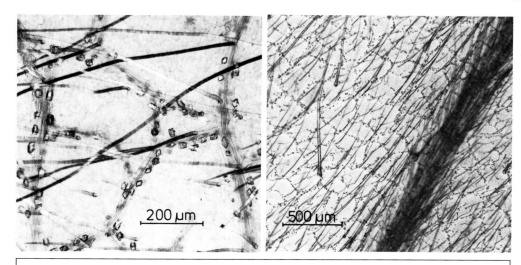

Fig. 3: Oxalate prisms and clusters following the venation of the leaves

Fig. 4: Dense silky pubescence on the lower surface of the leaves

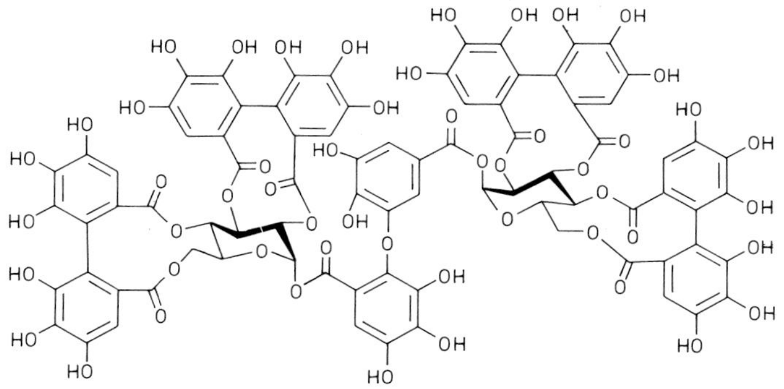

Agrimoniin

Erg. B. 6: Folia Fragariae.

Plant source: *Fragaria vesca* L., wild strawberry (Rosaceae).

Synonyms: Erdbeerblätter (Ger.), Feuilles de fraisier (Fr.).

Origin: Distributed throughout the temperate zones of Europe and Asia. The drug is grown in the eastern part of Germany and is also imported from former Yugoslavia and Bulgaria.

Constituents: Condensed tannins (?), ellagitannins, including pedunculagin and agrimoniin [1, 2]; flavonoids and leucoanthocyans; a little ascorbic acid (?); very small amounts of essential oil [3, 4].

Indications: In *folk medicine*, internally as a mild astringent in diarrhoea. The young leaves are also used as a substitute for ordinary tea [5].

Making the tea: Boiling water is poured over 1 g of the finely chopped drug and after 10 min. strained. As an antidiarrhoeal, a cupful is drunk several times a day.
1 Teaspoon = ca. 1 g.

Extract from the German Commission E monograph (BAnz no. 22a, 01.02.1990)

Uses

Preparations of wild strawberry leaf are used externally for rashes, and internally for treating gastrointestinal catarrh, diarrhoea, intestinal atony, liver disorders, jaundice, catarrh of the respiratory passages, gout, rheumatism, nervousness, renal pain, urinary complaints, gravel, stone, as diuretic, in support of the heart and circulation, in fevers, against night sweats, and for "purifying the blood", to stimulate the digestion, in anaemia, as a tonic, to reduce profuse menstruation, and to "support natural loss of weight".
Activity in the indications listed has not adequately substantiated.

Risks

Strawberry leaf may elicit allergic reactions in people hypersensitive to strawberries.

Evaluation

Since activity against the indications listed has not been adequately substantiated, therapeutic use of the drug is not justified.

There are no objections to use of the drug as a component in tea mixtures. In fact, strawberry leaf in teas and similar products is to be considered rather as a food additive.

Phytomedicines: The drug is a component in a series of mixed herbal teas which are mostly used as ordinary "household" teas. Genuine indications are rare (stomach tea, antiphlebitis tea).

Authentication: Besides the macroscopical characters described above, microscopical study offers further help: calcium-oxalate clusters and occasional single crystals along the nerves (Fig. 3) and unicellular thick-walled trichomes which lie along the leaf surface as if "combed" (Fig. 4). Glandular trichomes with unicellular heads and few-celled stalks are rare.

Quantitative standard: Erg. B. 6: *Ash*, not more than 9%.

Adulteration: Leaves of other *Fragaria* species, including cultivated forms (garden strawberries) are found, but are to be considered as equivalent.

Literature:
[1] E.A. Haddock et al., Phytochemistry **21**, 1049 (1982).
[2] K. Lund, Thesis, Freiburg i. Br. (1986).
[3] Hager, vol. **4**, p. 1046 (1973); vol. **5**, p. 181 (1993).
[4] K. Herrmann, Pharm. Zentralh. **88**, 374 (1949).
[5] K. Koch, Pharmazie **3**, 35 (1948).

Frangulae cortex   (Ph. Eur. 2), Frangula bark (*BAN*; BP 1988, BHP 1/1990)

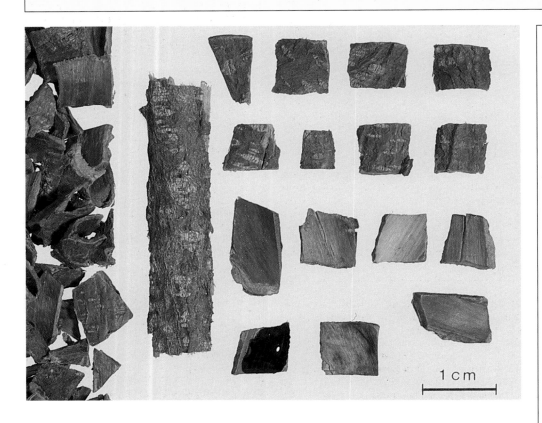

Fig. 1: Frangula bark

Description: The drug consists of the dried bark of the stems and branches. It comprises quills, double quills, or flats of varying lengths and not more than 2 mm thick. The cut drug consists of flat or slightly inwardly curved pieces. The outer surface is brownish red to greyish brown, shiny to matt, smooth to finely fissured, and has numerous horizontally elongated, whitish lenticels. On careful scraping, a red-coloured tissue is exposed. The inner surface is orange-yellow to brownish and distinctly striated longitudinally. The fracture is irregular, granular on the outside and short and finely fibrous on the inside (Fig. 3). With a drop of 6N ammonia solution, the inner surface takes on a red colour (Bornträger reaction).

Odour: Characteristic.

Taste: Mucilaginous and sweetish, somewhat bitter and astringent.

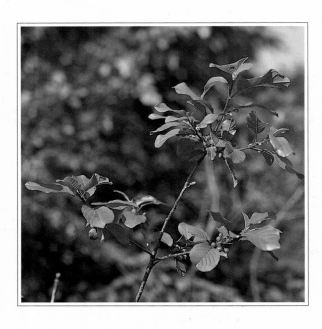

Fig. 2: *Rhamnus frangula* L.

Shrubs or (less often) small trees with alternate, entire, ovate leaves. Small, inconspicuous flowers in axillary cymes. Unripe fruits green to red, ripe fruits black. Bark with whitish, horizontal lenticels.

DAB 10: Faulbaumrinde
ÖAB: Cortex Frangulae
Ph. Helv. VII: Frangulae cortex
St.Zul. 9399.99.99

Plant source: *Rhamnus frangula* L. (syn. *Frangula alnus* J. S. MILLER), alder buckthorn (Rhamnaceae).

Synonyms: Cortex Rhamni frangulae, Cortex Alni nigri (Lat.), Buckthorn bark, Frangula, Black alder bark (Engl.), Faulbaumrinde, Gelbholzrinde, Zweckenbaumrinde (Ger.), Écorce de bourdaine, Écorce de frangule, Écorce d'aune noir (Fr.).

Origin: Native in Europe, the Mediterranean region, and north-west Asia. The drug comes from wild or "semi-wild" tended trees in lowland forest; it is imported from the former USSR, former Yugoslavia, and Poland.

Constituents: Above all, anthraquinone glycosides, especially glucofrangulins A and B (bis-glycosides with glucose and rhamnose (= A) and apiose (= B)) and frangulins A and B (monoglycosides containing only apiose); further, frangulaemodin 8-*O*-glucoside. In the fresh bark, the glucofrangulins occur mainly in the genuine reduced anthrone and dianthrone glycoside forms (es-

pecially frangula-emodin anthrone as rhamnoside/glucoside). On storage (for at least 1 year) or artificial ageing (e.g. by heating the drug in a stream of air) they are converted to the oxidized forms; at the same time, the glucofrangulins are partly decomposed to the frangulins or frangula-emodin 8-*O*-glucoside and to the aglycone frangula-emodin. The drug also contains physcion and chrysophanol in both free and monoglycosidic forms. In addition, there are the steam-volatile 2-acetyl-1,8-dihydronaphthalene and its 8-*O*-glucoside. Tannins, as well as small amounts of peptide alkaloids (frangulanin, franganin), are likewise present. The occurrence of bitter substances and saponins is disputed [1, 2].

Indications: As a laxative acting on the large intestine, in constipation and all complaints in which an easy defaecation with soft stool is desired, e.g. anal fissures, haemorrhoids, and after rectal operations; the drug takes effect 6–8 hours after administration. Regarding the mechanism of action: The transport forms of the anthracene glycosides reach the large intestine and are there hydrolysed by bacteria or enzymes present in the body (?) and reduced to the active anthrones or anthranols. In this form they inhibit the absorption of water and electrolytes through blockade of the Na^+/K^+-ATPase present in the intestinal epithelium. In addition, the secretion of water into the lumen of the intestine is increased through a rise in the permeability of the tight junc-

tions. This stimulates peristalsis and transport of the food mass is accelerated [1].

Side effects: Like other stimulant/irritant laxatives, frangulae cortex should not be used for long periods of time. It is contraindicated during pregnancy and lactation, and in ileus of whatever origin. Chronic use or abuse leads to loss of electrolytes, especially K^+, which can bring about muscular weakness and may thus give rise to constipation. This can also potentiate the effects of cardiac glycosides. The loss of K^+ is also increased by saluretics. However, unlike aloes, serious irritation does not spread to the pelvic region. Anthraquinone glycosides and the corresponding drugs are not suitable for rapidly emptying the intestinal tract, such as may be necessary in cases of poisoning, for example. It should also be noted that only aged drug (see above) is permitted, since the anthrones in the fresh bark strongly irritate the mucous membranes of the stomach and may thus cause vomiting, colic, and bloody diarrhoea [cf. 1].

Making the tea: Boiling water is poured over 2 g of the finely chopped drug and after 10 min. passed through a tea strainer. The use of cold water (12 hours at room temperature) is sometimes recommended.
1 Teaspoon = ca. 2.4 g.

Phytomedicines: Many stimulant/irritant laxatives, in the form of teas, mixed teas, dry extracts for infusions, cold macerates, as well as solid and liquid formulations.

	R¹	R²
Glucofrangulin A	α-L-Rhamnose	β-D-Glucose
Glucofrangulin B	β-D-Apiose	β-D-Glucose
Frangulin A	α-L-Rhamnose	H
Frangulin B	β-D-Apiose	H
Frangula-emodin	H	H
Physcion	CH₃	H
Chrysophanol	At C(6) H instead of OH	

Frangula-emodin anthrone

Extract from the German Commission E monograph (BAnz no. 228, dated 05.12.1984)

Uses

Complaints in which an easy defaecation with a soft stool is desirable, e.g. anal fissures, haemorrhoids, and after rectal-anal operations. Constipation.

Contraindications

Ileus of whatever origin; during pregnancy and lactation, only after consultation with a doctor.

Side effects

None known.
Chronic use or abuse may lead to loss of electrolytes, especially potassium; deposition of pigment in the intestinal mucosa (melanosis coli).
In the fresh state the drug contains anthrones, and it must therefore be stored for at least 1 year or artificially aged by heating in a stream of air.
When not used as prescribed, e.g. when used as the fresh drug, severe vomiting possibly accompanied by griping may occur.

Interactions

None known.
On chronic use or abuse, the resulting loss of potassium may potentiate the effect of cardiotonic glycosides.

Dosage

Unless otherwise prescribed: average daily dose, 20–180 mg hydroxyanthracene derivatives.

Mode of administration

Chopped or powdered drug, drug extracts for infusions, decoctions, cold macerates, or elixirs. Liquid and solid formulations exclusively for oral use.

Duration of use

Anthraquinone-containing laxatives should not be taken for long periods of time.

Effects

The substances bring about an active secretion of electrolytes and water into the lumen of the intestine, and they inhibit the absorption of electrolytes and water in the large intestine. The resulting increase in the volume of the bowel contents raises the intraluminal pressure, thereby stimulating peristalsis.

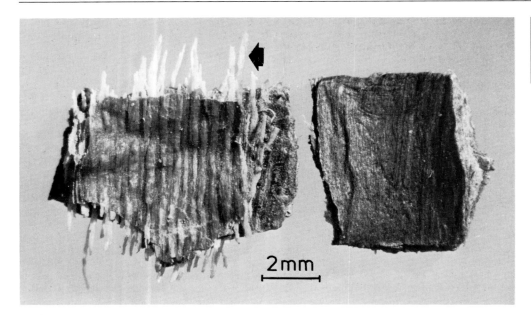

2mm

Fig. 3: Finely striated inner surface of *Rhamnus frangula* bark (right). Long fibrous fracture (arrow) of the bark from *Rhamnus alpinus* subsp. *fallax* (left)

Regulatory status (UK): General Sales List – Schedule 1, Table A.

Authentication: Macro- (see: Description) and microscopically, following the Ph. Eur. 2, BP 1988, etc.; see also [1, 4]. The powder is coloured red with alkali hydroxide solutions; stone cells must be absent – difference with *Rhamni purshiani* cortex.

The Ph. Eur. 2 (BP 1988, etc.) TLC test of purity requires examination for anthrones by spraying the TLC plate with *p*-nitrosodimethylaniline (0.1% in pyridine. Caution – carcinogenic! [1]):

Test solution: 0.5 g powdered drug heated to boiling with 5 ml 70% ethanol, cooled, centrifuged, and the supernatant decanted off; solution to be used within 30 min.

Reference solution: 20 mg barbaloin (aloin) dissolved in 10 ml 70% ethanol.

Loadings: 10 µl of each solution, as 2-cm bands on silica gel G.

Solvent system: ethyl acetate + methanol + water (100 + 17 + 10), 10 cm run.

Detection and Evaluation: after drying, within 5 min. sprayed with 0.1% nitrosodimethylaniline in pyridine. Test solution: **no** greyish blue zones visible (azomethine formation, indicating the presence of inadmissible amounts of anthrones).
Oversprayed with 5% potassium hydroxide in 50 % ethanol and heated for 15 min. at 100–105 °C. Reference solution: at Rf 0.4–0.5, the reddish brown barbaloin zone. Test solution: several red zones, those at Rf 0.25–0.35, belonging to the glucofragulins, being the most important; **no** red zone at Rf 0.1–0.15.

In UV 365 nm light. Test solution: **no** intense yellow (*R. purshianus* bark, due to the cascarosides and aloins) or blue (*R. catharticus* bark, due to naphthalide glycosides) fluorescent zones [cf. 3].

Tests for adulteration with the bark of *Rhamnus alpinus* subsp. *fallax* with the help of the Tauböck test according to the DAB 7 are only clearcut when the fallax bark is present on its own. The flavonol glycoside xanthorhamnin present in it forms a stable, ether-soluble complex with borax-oxalic acid which fluoresces green in daylight. According to [3], the presence of small amounts of admixed fallax bark can be established by the TLC detection of the xanthorhamnin – in the presence of this substance, after spraying the plate with diphenylboryloxyethylamine a yellow zone is formed.

Quantitative standards: Ph. Eur. 2: *Glucofrangulins*, not less than 6.0% calculated as glucofrangulin A (M_r 578.5). *Foreign matter*, not more than 1%. *Sulphated ash*, not more than 8.0%.

BHP 1/1990: Frangula bark complies with the requirements of the Ph. Eur. 2 or BP 1988 monographs.

Note: Frangulae cortex is the subject of an ESCOP proposed harmonized European monograph.

Wording of the package insert, from the German Standard Licence:

5.1 Uses

Constipation; all complaints in which a gentle emptying of the bowels with a soft stool is desired, e.g. when anal fissures or haemorrhoids are present, and after rectal-anal operations.

5.2 Contraindications

Preparations of frangula bark are not to be used in cases of occlusion of the intestines or during pregnancy and lactation.

5.3 Side effects

When used as prescribed, none known.
With frequent and prolonged use or with overdosage, there may be an increased loss of water and salts, especially potassium salts. Moreover, pigment may be deposited in the mucous membranes of the intestines (melanosis coli).

5.4 Interactions with other remedies

Because of the increased loss of potassium, the effects of cardiotonic glycosides may be potentiated.

5.5 Dosage and Mode of administration

Hot water (ca. 150 ml) is poured over about half a teaspoonful of **Frangula bark** and after 10–15 min. passed through a tea strainer.
Unless otherwise prescribed, a cupful of the freshly prepared tea is drunk in the morning and/or before going to bed.

5.6 Duration of use

Frangula bark tea should only be taken for a few days. For longer use, a doctor should be consulted.

Warning: To enable the bowels to regain their normal function, care should be taken to ensure that the diet contains sufficient roughage, that there is an adequate water intake, and that as much exercise as possible is taken.

5.7 Note

Store protected from light and moisture.

Adulteration: Occasionally, bark from *Rhamnus alpinus* subsp. *fallax* (BOISS.) MAIRE et PETITM. (syn. *Oreoherzogia fallax* (BOISS.) W. VENT), *R. catharticus* L. (buckthorn), *R. purshianus* DC. (cascara), *Prunus padus* L. (bird cherry), and *Alnus glutinosa* GAERTN. (alder) is found. Often, they are recognizable by their different external characters – some have stone cells or large single crystals and some may not contain any anthracene derivatives, so that their detection offers no difficulties (see also: Authentication).

Storage: Protected from moisture and light. Before use, the drug must be "aged" (artificially or by storage for at least 1 year; see: Authentication).

Literature:
[1] Kommentar DAB 10.
[2] H.W. Rauwald (Univ. Frankfurt), personal communication.
[3] H.W. Rauwald and H. Miething, Dtsch. Apoth. Ztg. **125**, 101 (1985).
[4] B.P. Jackson and D.W. Snowdon, Atlas of microscopy of medicinal plants, culinary herbs and spices, Belhaven Press, London, 1990, p. 102.

Fucus   Bladderwrack (BHP 1/1990)

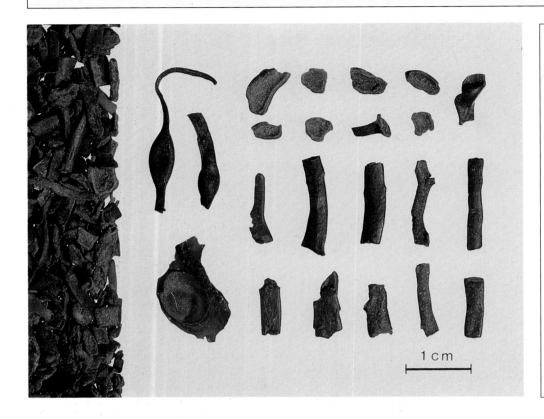

1 cm

Fig. 1: Bladderwrack

Description: The drug consists of flat, cartilaginous, ribbon-like fragments of brownish black to greenish black thallus, with an entire margin and often bifurcately branched. The air bladders, paired in *Fucus vesiculosus* and single in *Ascophyllum nodosum* (centre, left), are not always easily recognized in the cut drug. The drug derived from *Fucus vesiculosus* is finely verrucose at the thickened end of the thallus, owing to the presence of numerous conceptacles. In *Ascophyllum nodosum*, however, the conceptacles break off very easily and are therefore usually absent from the drug.

Odour: Characteristic (seaweed-like), fishy.

Taste: Mucilaginous and salty.

Fig. 2: *Fucus vesiculosus* L.

A brown alga with a regularly bifurcate thallus up to 1 m in length, the individual branches having a distinct midrib (difference with *Ascophyllum nodosum*) and generally paired air bladders.

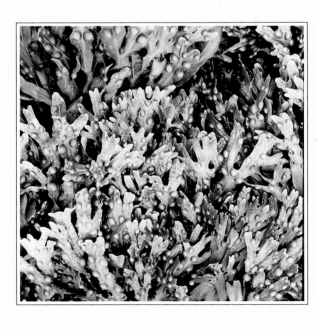

DAB 10: Tang[1]

Plant source: *Fucus vesiculosus* L., bladderwrack, and/or *Ascophyllum nodosum* LE JOLIS, knotted wrack (Fucaceae, Phaeophyceae).

Synonyms: Fucus thallus (Lat.), Seawrack, Kelpware, Black-tang, Rockweed (Engl.), Tang, Höckertang (Ger.), Varech vésiculeux (Fr.).

Origin: *Fucus vesiculosus* is a very frequent brown alga found on the rocky coasts of the Atlantic and Pacific Oceans. Together with *Ascophyllum nodosum*, it occurs in Europe along the coasts of the North Sea and the western part of the Baltic Sea. The drug is harvested partly with drag nets and imported from France, Ireland, or the United States.

Constituents: Iodine in the form of inorganic salts and bound to proteins (and to some

---

[1] The Monograph will be deleted from DAB 10 up to 1994 (2. Suppl.).

Extract from the German Commission E monograph (BAnz no. 101, dated 01.06.1990)

Uses

Bladderwrack preparations are used in thyroid disorders, obesity, overweight, arteriosclerosis, and digestive disorders, as well as for "cleansing the blood".

Risks

Preparations with a daily dose up to 150 µg iodine, none known.
Above 150 µg iodine/day, there is a danger of inducing and aggravating hyperthyroidism. In rare cases, idiosyncratic reactions may develop and become generalized.

Evaluation

Since the efficacy of a dosage below 150 µg iodine/day has not been substantiated for the conditions listed, therapeutic use of the drug cannot be advocated. In view of the risks, the therapeutic use of doses above 150 µg iodine/day cannot be defended on the grounds of lack of activity.

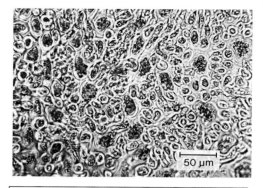

Fig. 3: Transverse section through the midrib of *Fucus vesiculosus*

extent also lipids) [1] and as a component of iodo-amino acids, e.g. di-iodotyrosine ("iodogorgoic acid"). In addition, the drug also contains mucilaginous polysaccharides, such as alginic acid, fucoidin, and laminarin, as well as polyphenols with antibiotic activity [2]. Very small amounts of abscisic acid are present in both commercial preparations and freeze-dried samples of *Ascophyllum nodosum* [3]. The lipid compositions of *F. vesiculosus* and *A. nodosum* are complex but very similar, with the glycosyldiacylglycerides constituting as much as 50% of the total lipids; small (less than 10%), though significant, amounts of phosphatidylethanolamine, as well as phosphatidylcholine, are also present; the major acyl chain is eicosapentaenoate and there is also a high proportion of arachidonate [4].

Indications: Formerly, for iodine therapy in thyroid deficiency, but owing to the variable iodine content and the varying absorption conditions for bound and unbound iodine the drug is now obsolete. Nowadays, Fucus is occasionally promoted as a "fat-removing

and slimming" cure (especially in *folk medicine*). By supplying iodine, there is supposed to be an increased production of thyroid hormones, resulting in increased metabolism and removal of depot fats. Although "slimming cures" based on influencing thyroid activity must be strongly discouraged because of possible side effects, the drug is still being included as a component in some herbal teas and prepared remedies. The external use in "slimming baths", etc. – which is regularly and repeatedly extolled – is also complete nonsense.

Side effects: On prolonged and uncontrolled use, iodine idiosyncrasy, as well as hyperthyroidism or thyrotoxicosis, are possible. Symptoms arising from an over-active thyroid are, e.g., palpitations, restlessness, insomnia, etc.

Making the tea: Not very usual and not recommended.

Herbal preparations: About a dozen ready-made herbal mixtures, mostly teas for slimming or removing of fat, but there are others for other indications.

Phytomedicines: Fucus is included in various preparations for the same indications, as

well as in prepared remedies for other indications. Cf. the remark under: Indications. Some UK products containing Fucus or its extract are: Gerard House Kelp Tablets and Potter's Boldo Aid to Slimming Tablets, and Potter's Malted Kelp Tablets.

Authentication: Macro- (see: Description) and microscopically, following the BHP 1/1990 or DAB 10; see also [1]. The lines of thickened cells which run alongside each other in the midrib are characteristic of *Fucus* (Fig. 3).
Determination of the iodine content is carried out iodometrically, with the protein-bound iodine being determined separately after precipitation of the protein with trichloracetic acid. The BHP 1/1990 TLC test of identity examines the amino acids of a methanol extract, with L-methionine as reference compound.

Quantitative standards: DAB 10: *Total iodine*, not less than 0.05%. *Protein-bound iodine*, not less than 0.02%. *Foreign (vegetable and/or mineral) matter*, not more than 2%. *Loss on drying*, not more than 15.0%. *Ash*, not more than 20.0%.
BHP 1/1990: *Water-soluble extractive*, not less than 15%. *Foreign matter*, not more than 2%. *Total ash*, not more than 22%. *HCl-insoluble ash*, not more than 4%.
Note: In the BHP 2/1993, *Ascophyllum* will be a separate monograph.

Adulteration: *Fucus serratus* is considered an adulterant, but was admitted in the former AB-DDR. Ref. [1] gives details of its polymorphism and varieties; the margin of the thallus is serrate.

Literature:
[1] E. Stahl, H.G. Menßen, K. Staesche, and H. Bachmann, Dtsch. Apoth. Ztg. **115**, 1893 (1975); *ibid.*, **116**, 51 (1976).
[2] K.W. Gombitza, H.W. Rauwald, and G. Eckhardt, Phytochemistry **14**, 1403 (1975).
[3] G.L. Beyer and S.S. Dougherty, Phytochemistry **27**, 1521 (1988).
[4] A.L. Jones and J.L. Harwood, Phytochemistry **31**, 3397 (1992).

Fumariae herba   (DAB 10), Fumitory (BHP 1/1990)

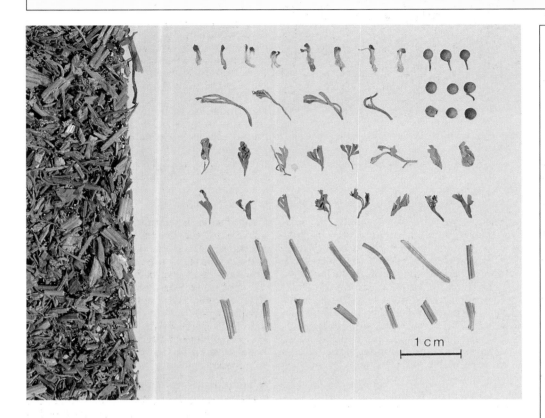

Fig. 1: Fumitory

<u>Description</u>: The grey to bluish green drug contains numerous fragments of the 2-pinnatisect leaves (2nd to 4th rows from above) and hollow, angular pieces of stem (the bottom two rows). The pale to dark violet shrivelled flowers with a dark purple or brown fleck at the tip (top row) are characteristic. The spherical achenes (at the top, right) are brownish green and contain a small brown seed.

<u>Taste</u>: Somewhat bitter and slightly salty.

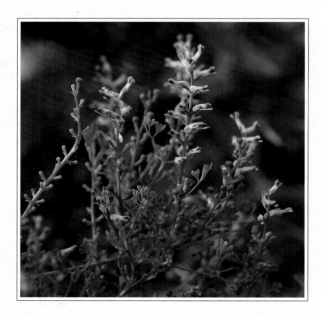

Fig. 2: *Fumaria officinalis* L.

An annual herb, up to 30 cm in height. Leaves bluish green, somewhat pruinous, pinnatisect. Flowers in racemes, corolla pink, with dark red tip, upper petal slightly spurred.

Plant source: *Fumaria officinalis* L., common fumitory (Fumariaceae).

Synonyms: Erdrauchkraut, Ackerrautenkraut (Ger.), Herbe de fumeterre (Fr.).

Origin: Native in Europe and Asia, growing along roadsides or on wasteland. The drug is imported from eastern European countries.

Constituents: Ca. 1% alkaloids [1, 2], about 30 of which are known structurally – they are benzylisoquinoline derivatives in the widest sense, e.g. protopine (= fumarine), fumariline, sinactine, etc. There are also flavonoids, plant acids, especially fumaric acid, mucilage, and choline.

Indications: Fumitory is used as a cholagogue; protopine not only promotes the secretion of bile, but is also said to reduce pathologically raised secretion of bile (so-called amphicholeretic action). In *folk medicine*, the drug is also ascribed diuretic and laxative properties, as well as a favourable effect on skin complaints [3]. This may be due to the fumaric acid, which nowadays, as a synthetic substance, is a component of several remedies for psoriasis.

Making the tea: Boiling water is poured over 2–3 g of the drug and after 10 min. strained. For biliary disorders, a cupful of the tea is drunk warm before meals.
1 Teaspoon = ca. 1.6 g.

Extract from the German Commission E monograph (BAnz no. 173, dated 18.09.1986)

Uses

Cramp-like complaints in the biliary and gastrointestinal tracts.

Contraindications

None known.

Interactions with other remedies

None known.

Dosage

Unless otherwise prescribed: average daily dose, 6 g drug; preparations correspondingly.

Mode of administration

Chopped drug and its galenical preparations for internal use.

Effects

Its mild spasmolytic effect on the upper part of the gastrointestinal tract is sufficiently well established.

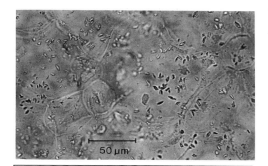

Fig. 3: Crystal layer of the upper leaf epidermis

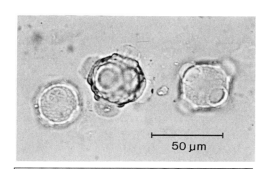

Fig. 4: Spherical pollen grains with six large pores

Herbal preparations: Fumitory is present in a few prepared herbal mixtures for a variety of indications.

Phytomedicines: The monovalent preparation Oddibil®-Filmtabletten contains an extract made from the whole flowering plant, including the roots. Cholongal®-Tropfen (drops), -Saft (juice) are polyvalent preparations.

Authentication: Macro- (see: Description) and microscopically; see also the BHP 1/

Wording of the package insert, from the German Standard Licence

6.1 Uses

Spastic biliary complaints and constipation.

6.2 Dosage and Mode of administration

Boiling water (ca. 150 ml) is poured over ca. 1–2 teaspoonfuls (2–4 g) of **Fumitory** and after 10 min. passed through a tea strainer.
Unless otherwise prescribed, the still warm, freshly prepared, infusion is drunk half-an-hour before meals.

6.3 Duration of use

Preparations of fumitory may, if required, be taken over a period of several weeks.

6.4 Note

Store protected from light and moisture.

1990. The stomata on the upper and lower surfaces of the leaves are broadly oval in shape. In places, the occurrence of characteristic crystals in the cells of the upper leaf epidermis is widespread (Fig. 3). The spherical pollen grains have six large pores, through which the contents protrude like a hood (Fig. 4).

The BHP 1/1990 TLC test of identity provides a flavonoid profile, while the St.Zul. specifies the following TLC examination for alkaloids:

Test solution: 1.0 g powdered drug refluxed with 10 ml methanol for 2 min., filtered, the filtrate taken to dryness, and the residue dissolved in 0.2 ml dichloromethane.

Reference solution: 10.0 mg noscapine (narcotine) hydrochloride dissolved in 5 ml methanol.

Loadings: 15 µl test solution and 10 µl reference solution, as 2-cm bands on silica gel GF_{254}.

Solvent system: dichloromethane + cyclohexane + diethylamine (7 + 1 + 1), 12 cm run.

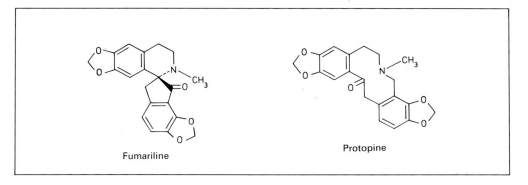

Fumariline

Protopine

Detection and Evaluation: in UV 365 nm light. Test solution: at Rf 0.7–0.8, two red fluorescent zones, appearing green in daylight; at Rf ca. 0.7 a yellow fluorescent zone and at Rf ca. 0.6 a blue fluorescent zone.

In UV 254 nm light. Reference solution: at Rf ca. 0.7, the noscapine quenching zone. Test solution: at about the same Rf, the quenching zone of the main alkaloid protopine; below it, three other weak quenching zones.

Sprayed with dilute Dragendorff reagent. Test and Reference solutions: the noscapine and protopine zones coloured orange. Test solution: additional, fainter zones at Rf 0.4, 0.5, 0.6; near the starting line, several narrow, greyish brown and green zones.

Quantitative standards: DAB 10: *Total alkaloid*, not less than 0.4% calculated as protopine (M_r 353.4). *Foreign matter*, not more than 2%. *Loss on drying*, not more than 10%. *Ash*, not more than 16.0%.

BHP 1/1990: *Water-soluble extractive*, not less than 20%. *Foreign matter*, not more than 2%. *Total ash*, not more than 16%. *HCl-insoluble ash*, not more than 5%.

Adulteration: The very similar *Fumaria* species which occur in the same localities and which are hardly distinguishable from the plant that supplies the drug, viz *F. vaillantii* LOISEL., fewflowered fumitory, or *F. schleicheri* SOY.-WILL., are only occasionally found in commerce.

Literature:

[1] Z.H. Mardirossian et al., Phytochemistry **22**, 759 (1983).

[2] P. Forgacs et al., Plantes Méd. Phytothérap. **20**, 64 (1986).

[3] H. Kreitmair, Pharmazie **4**, 242 (1949).

Galangae rhizoma   Galanga, Alpinia (BHP 1983)

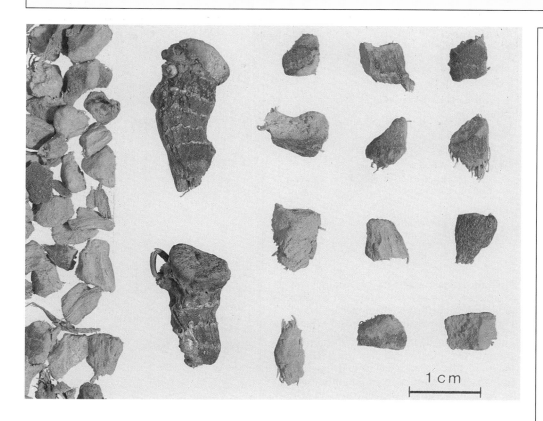

Fig. 1: Galanga

<u>Description:</u> The drug consists of cylindrical, 1–2 cm thick, pieces of reddish brown rhizome, which sometimes have the remains of the stems at the end. The white, irregular, horizontal rings, which originate from the scales of the rhizome, are characteristic. On the underside, there are root scars and occasional roots. The fracture is fibrous.

<u>Odour:</u> Characteristic, aromatic.

<u>Taste:</u> Spicy and pungent.

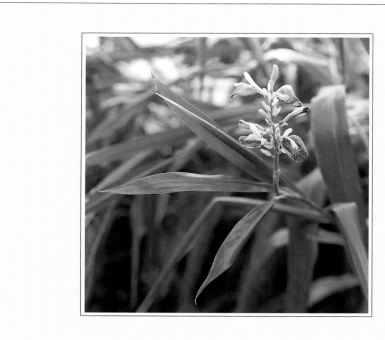

Fig. 2: *Alpinia officinarum* HANCE

An East Asian rhizomatous shrub with linear-lanceolate leaves up to 30 cm long. Racemose inflorescence 50–150 cm in height, corolla trilobate and tubular below.

DAB 6: Rhizoma Galangae
Ph. Helv. VII: Galangae rhizoma

Plant source: *Alpinia officinarum* HANCE (Zingiberaceae).

Synonyms: Galanga, Galangal or Colic or East Indian root, Chinese ginger (Engl.), Galgantwurzel (Ger.), Rhizome de galanga (Fr.).

Origin: From plantations in southern China, Thailand, and India.

Constituents: 0.5% to more than 1% essential oil, comprising mainly sesquiterpene hydrocarbons and alcohols, together with small amounts of eugenol; so-called pungent substances, a very complex mixture of compounds that are not volatile in steam (formerly known as galangol) which consists of various diarylheptanoids, in addition to gingerols (phenyl alkyl ketones); flavonoids, especially quercetin and kaempferol derivatives; sterols and sterol glycosides.

Indications: Principally as a stomachic and tonic in loss of appetite and "weak digestion".
The diarylheptanoids have been thoroughly investigated in recent years; they all bring about distinct inhibition of prostaglandin biosynthesis [1, 2], but so far no therapeutic use has been made of this. The phenyl alkyl ketones have a similar action [3].

Making the tea: Boiling water is poured over 0.5–1.0 g of the finely cut or coarsely powdered drug, allowed to draw for 5–10 min. in a covered vessel, and then passed through a tea strainer. A cupful is taken half-an-hour before each meal.
1 Teaspoon = ca. 2 g.

Herbal preparations: None. The drug is a component of so-called "Swedish bitters"; see the note under: Aloe capensis.

Extract from the German Commission E monograph
(BAnz no. 173, dated 18.09.1986)

Uses
Dyspeptic complaints. Lack of appetite.

Contraindications
None known.

Side effects
None known.

Interactions with other remedies
None known.

Dosage
Daily dose: tincture (Erg. B. 6), 2–4 g; drug, 2–4 g.

Mode of administration
Crushed or powdered drug, and other galenical preparations for internal use.

Effects
Spasmolytic, antiphlogistic (inhibition of prostaglandin synthesis), antibacterial.

Phytomedicines: Extracts of galanga are a component of a several prepared remedies, such as Klosterfrau Melissengeist®, etc. The drug is now little used in the UK.

Authentication: Macro- (see: Description) and microscopically; see also the BHP 1983. The very thick cortex has only a few collateral vascular bundles; on the other hand, they are numerous in the central stele, where they are surrounded by a yellow fibrous sheath. The club-shaped, slightly curved, 20–40 μm long, somewhat flattened starch grains are highly characteristic of the drug (the BHP 1983 is evidently in error on this point).
The following is a suitable TLC test of identity:

Test solution: oil obtained by the procedure for the determination of the essential-oil content (but without the use of xylene) is carefully removed and diluted 1:100 with toluene.

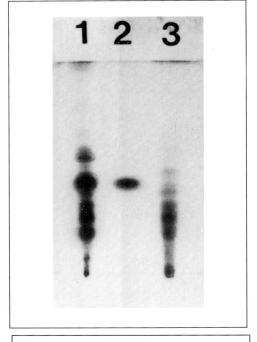

Fig. 3: TLC on 4 × 8 cm silica-gel foil

1: Genuine galanga
2: Cineole (reference substance)
3: Adulterant

For details, see the text

Reference solution: 5 mg cineole dissolved in 5 ml methanol.

Loadings: 2 μl test solution and 2 μl reference solution, on silica gel.

Solvent system: toluene + ethyl acetate (95 + 5), 5 cm run.

Detection: after complete evaporation of the solvent, sprayed with anisaldehyde reagent and heated for 3 min. at 100–105 °C.

Evaluation: in daylight. Reference solution: at Rf ca. 0.4, the bluish violet cineole spot. Test solution: with genuine galanga, an intense violet-coloured spot at the same Rf value; directly above it, a greyish green zone – absent with adulterants; only a very faint violet-coloured zone near the Rf of cineole with adulterants (Fig. 3).

Quantitative standards: Ph. Helv. VII: *Volatile oil*, not less than 0.5%. *Foreign matter*, not more than 1% (mainly leaves and primary roots). *Sulphated ash*, not more than 6.5%.

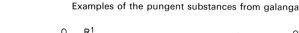

Examples of the pungent substances from galanga

Diarylheptanoids

[8]-Gingerol
(Phenyl alkyl ketone)

R^1 } = O R^1 —H R^1 —H
R^2 R^2 —OCH$_3$ R^2 —OH

BHP 1983: *Volatile oil*, 0.5–1.0%. *Foreign organic matter*, not more than 2%. *Acid-soluble ash*, not more than 3%.

Adulteration: Adulteration with the rhizomes of *Kaempferia galanga* L. and a number of other *Alpinia* species can be recognized macroscopically, since they are up to 4 cm thick, have a very pale-coloured central stele, and have scarcely any aromatic odour. However, the presence of some *Alpinia* species can only be established through their TLC behaviour (see: Authentication).

Storage: Cool and protected from light, but not in plastic containers.

Literature:
[1] F. Kiuchi, M. Shibura, and U. Sankawa, Chem. Pharm. Bull. **30**, 2279 (1982); C.A. **97**, 150626 (1982).
[2] H. Itokawa, M. Morita, and S. Mihashi, Chem. Pharm. Bull. **29**, 2383 (1981); C.A. **95**, 183902 (1981).
[3] F. Kiuchi, M. Shibura, U. Sankawa, Chem. Pharm. Bull. **30**, 754 (1982); C.A. **97**, 98204 (1982).

Galegae herba   Galega (BHP 1983), Goat's-rue herb

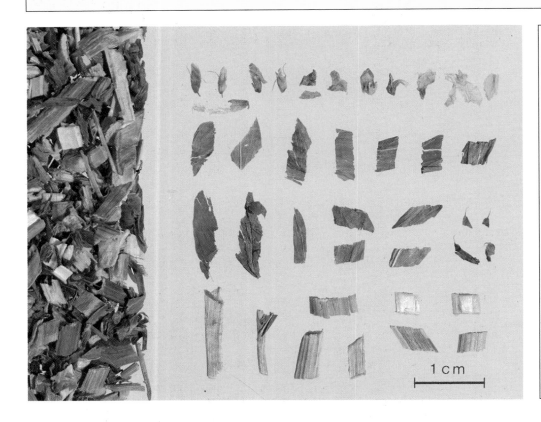

Fig. 1: Goat's-rue herb

<u>Description</u>: **The drug consists mainly of fragments of the up to 4 cm long pale green leaflets. The midrib is prominent on the under surface, while the lateral nerves are at an acute angle and give the leaf the appearance of being almost parallel-nerved; the tip of the leaflet ends in a mucro (Fig. 3). The whitish yellow or violet-blue papilionaceous flowers are rare, but when present are a good diagnostic feature (Fig. 1, uppermost row); pieces of the longitudinally grooved stem are likewise rare.**

Fig. 2: *Galega officinalis* L.

A perennial herb up to more than 1 m in height with imparipinnate leaves. White or light blue papilionaceous flowers in dense racemes.

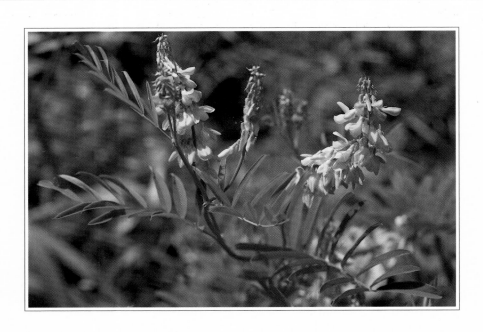

Erg. B. 6: Herba Galegae

Plant source: *Galega officinalis* L., goat's-rue (Fabaceae).

Synonyms: Herba Rutae caprariae (Lat.), French lilac herb (Engl.), Geißrautenkraut, Ziegenraute (Ger.), Herbe de galéga (Fr.).

Origin: In central, southern, and eastern Europe, and also cultivated to some extent. The drug is imported from Bulgaria, Poland, and Hungary.

Constituents: As a "glucokinin", the guanidine derivative galegine (isoamyleneguanidine) is present in all parts, with up to 0.5% in the seeds; in addition, hydroxygalegine and peganine; flavonoids (flowers), tannins, saponins in small amounts; ubiquitous substances [1]. Chromium salts (see: Indications).

Indications: Use is now almost entirely confined to *folk medicine*. Because of its galegine content, the drug is considered as

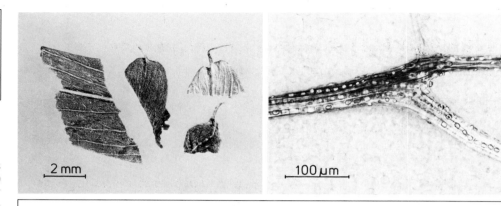

H₂N—C(=NH)—NH—CH₂—CH=C(CH₃)₂

Galegine

Fig. 3: Fragments of the leaflets, showing the prominent midrib (left) and small curved mucro (right)

Fig. 4: Rows of calcium oxalate prisms following a vascular bundle (far right)

an "antidiabetic". Older work (cf. [1]) has shown that galegine and other (synthetic) guanidine derivatives reduce blood-sugar levels. In 1974, a Russian group demonstrated that in healthy and alloxan-diabetic rabbits aqueous and alcoholic extracts of goat's rue had a hypoglycaemic effect, while the glycogen level in the liver and myocardium rose [2]. Even so, use of the drug is not to be recommended, because of the uncertain activity. With high doses of the drug, there is a danger of intoxication, such as was observed with the older guanidine derivatives (Synthalin). Most preparations of the biguanidine derivatives that were developed in the 1950s have also been withdrawn from the market [3].

More recently, the chromium salt content (ca. 3.7 ppm) has been implicated in a possible antidiabetic effect [4]. It is known that rats fed on a chromium-free diet show symptoms of diabetes mellitus II, which can be treated by administration of the so-called glucose tolerance factor – a low molecular weight chromium(III) complex.

Goat's-rue is also recommended in veterinary medicine for stimulating milk secretion.

Making the tea: Boiling water is poured over 2 g of the finely chopped drug and after 10 min. passed through a tea strainer.
1 Teaspoon = ca. 1.3 g.

Phytomedicines: The drug is a component of various prepared antidiabetic remedies, e.g. Antidiabeticum Hanosan (tablets), etc.

Authentication: Apart from the macroscopically recognizable characteristic nervature, the microscopy of the leaflets offers further means of identification. The epidermal cells of the upper surface are polygonal, those of the lower are surface wavy-walled, and both surfaces have stomata. Pubescence is sparse, but particularly at the leaf margin there are thick-walled trichomes (with thickened basal cells and thin-walled, short interstitial cells). Rows of calcium oxalate prisms accompany the nerves (Fig. 4). See further, the BHP 1983.

Quantitative standard: Erg. B. 6: *Ash*, not more than 10%.
BHP 1983: *Total ash*, not more than 10%.

Adulteration: In practice, rarely observed.

Literature:
[1] Hager, vol. **4**, p. 1082 (1973).
[2] D.Z. Shukyurov, D.Ya. Guseinov, and P.A. Yuzbashinskaya, Dokl. Akad. Nauk. Azer. SSR **30**, 58 (1974); Chem. Abstr. **82**, 106392 (1975).
[3] Lj. Kraus and G. Reher, Dtsch. Apoth. Ztg. **122**, 2357 (1982).
[4] A. Müller, E. Diemann, and P. Sassenberg, Naturwissenschaften **75**, 155 (1988).

Galeopsidis herba   Hemp-nettle herb

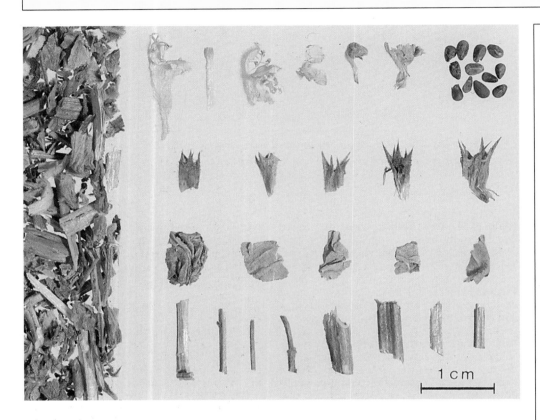

Fig. 1: Hemp-nettle herb

Description: Among the plant parts found in the drug are blunt, 4-angled, softly pubescent, branched purple-tinged pieces of stem; they have a wide pith and they are not thickened below the nodes. There are also yellowish green, slightly wrinkled leaves with a soft, velvety pubescence, and coarsely serrate margin; the pinnate nervature is prominent on the lower surface. Flowers are likewise present and consist mainly of the light yellow, tubular and campanulate calices with a glandular pubescence and, as a notable feature, their five mucronate teeth (2nd row); the usually much shrivelled, large petals are yellowish and they have a sulphur-yellow fleck on the lower lip. Often, fruits and brown nutlets marked with black spots are also present.

Odour: Very faint, characteristic.

Taste: Bitter and slightly salty.

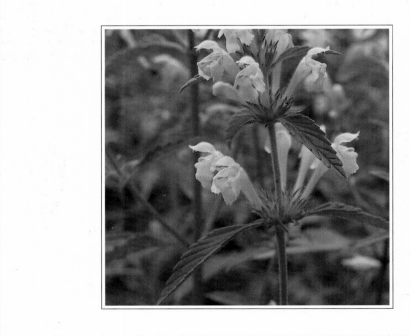

Fig. 2: *Galeopsis segetum* Neck.

A herbaceous annual, up to 50 cm in height, with a 4-angled, finely pubescent stem. Leaves with a short petiole and serrate margin. Flowers in false whorls, light yellow and with a lower lip having two hollow, tooth-like protuberances.

Erg. B. 6: Herba Galeopsidis

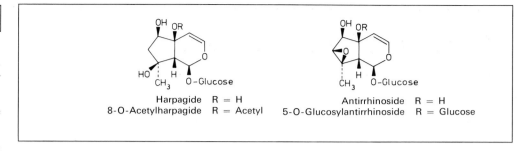

Harpagide   R = H
8-O-Acetylharpagide   R = Acetyl

Antirrhinoside   R = H
5-O-Glucosylantirrhinoside   R = Glucose

Plant source: *Galeopsis segetum* NECK. (syn. *Galeopsis ochroleuca* LAM.), downy hemp-nettle (Lamiaceae).

Synonyms: Hohlzahnkraut, Spanischer Tee (Ger.), Herbe de galéopside (Fr.).

Origin: In central and southern Europe on sandy ground. The drug is obtained from the wild (Hungary, Poland).

Constituents: Ca. 5% Lamiaceae tannin; 0.6–1% silica, a part of which is in the form of soluble silicates; flavonoids, the main ones being the 8-hydroxyflavones hypolaet-in 4′-methyl ether 7-(2″-allosyl)glucoside mono- and acetylated [1]; iridoids [2], especially harpagide, 8-*O*-acetylharpagide, antirrhinoside and its 5-*O*-glucoside.

Indications: As an astringent.
In *folk medicine,* like other silicate-containing plants, it is given for lung complaints (see also: Pulmonariae herba); however, there are no pharmacological or clinical findings which support this use. The same is true regarding its recommended application in folk medicine as a diuretic.

Making the tea: Boiling water is poured over 2 g of the finely chopped drug, or the drug is put into cold water which is brought to the boil, and after 5 min. strained. For bronchial complaints, as a (modest) remedy a cupful of the tea, if desired sweetened with honey, is drunk several times a day.
1 Teaspoon = ca. 1 g.

Herbal preparations: Instant teas containing extracts of the drug.

Phytomedicines: A few prepared remedies containing extracts of the drug, e.g. Tussi-florin® (drops), etc.

Authentication: Macro- (see: Description) and microscopically. Particularly characteristic are the infrequent glandular trichomes on the leaves (and more especially on the sepals); these have a long, multicellular stalk and a bowl-shaped head made up of 16–32 cells containing small single crystals or cluster crystals of calcium oxalate (Figs. 3 and 4). Glandular trichomes with a unicellular stalk and a head of 2–4-cells are more abundant. There are also numerous long, pointed, covering trichomes which arise from a spherical basal cell (Fig. 3). The small nuts are distinctly punctate (Fig. 5).
The following TLC procedure is a suitable test of identity:

Test solution: 1 g powdered drug refluxed with 10 ml methanol for ca. 10 min., filtered, the filtrate taken to dryness, and the residue dissolved in 20 ml methanol.

Reference solution: 10 mg rutin, 5 mg hyperoside, and 10 mg quercetin dissolved in 10 ml methanol.

Loadings: 4 µl of the test solution, as a band, and 1 µl of the reference solution, on silica gel.

Solvent system: ethyl acetate + anhydrous formic acid + water (88 + 6 + 6), 5 cm run.

Detection: after complete evaporation of the solvent in a current of hot air, sprayed with 1% methanolic diphenylboryloxyethylamine and then with 5% ethanolic polyethyleneglycol 400.

Evaluation: in UV 365 nm light. Reference solution: rutin spot situated in the lower third, the hyperoside spot about halfway, and the quercetin spot just below the front; all three with orange fluorescence. Test solution: at the same height as hyperoside, an intense orange-yellow fluorescent main zone; directly below it, a faint greenish fluorescent zone and just above it a weak orange fluorescent zone; immediately below the solvent front, the intense red fluorescent chlorophyll zone and below it a yellowish fluorescent spot; in the lower third, about three faint yellowish orange fluorescent zones and on the starting line a faint blue fluorescent zone (Fig. 6).

Quantitative standard: Erg. B. 6: *Ash*, not more than 12%.

Adulteration: Very often with other *Galeopsis* species, especially *G. tetrahit* L., common hemp-nettle, which has a very bristly stem and smaller, pinkish red or white flowers, and *G. speciosa* MILL., large-flowered hemp-nettle, which also has a bristly stem, and a violet spot on the lower lip of the corolla. Unlike *G. segetum* of the subgenus *Ladanum*, members of which only have 8-hydroxy-flavones, the above two species belong to the subgenus *Galeopsis*, which is characterized by the accumulation of the 7-*O*-β-D-glu-

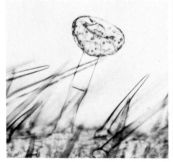
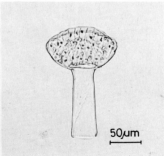
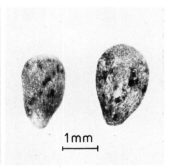

50 µm   1 mm

Figs. 3 and 4: Glandular trichomes, with a multicellular stalk and bowl-shaped head, and covering trichomes, from the leaves of *Galeopsis segetum*

Fig. 5: Brown punctate nuts

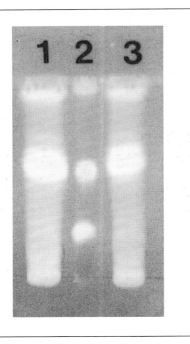

Fig. 6: TLC on 4 × 8 cm silica-gel foil

1 and 3: Hemp-nettle herb (from different origins)
2: Reference solution

For details, see text

curonides of luteolin, apigenin, and scutellarein and *p*-coumaroyl glucosides of apigenin and luteolin [2]. Reverse phase chromatography affords an effective means of differentiating the two groups of species. Other adulterants mentioned in the literature are very rarely met with in the commercial drug.

Literature:
[1] F.A. Tomás-Barberán et al., Phytochemistry **30**, 3311 (1991).
[2] U. Junod-Busch, Thesis, ETH Zürich 1976.

Galii veri herba   Lady's bedstraw herb

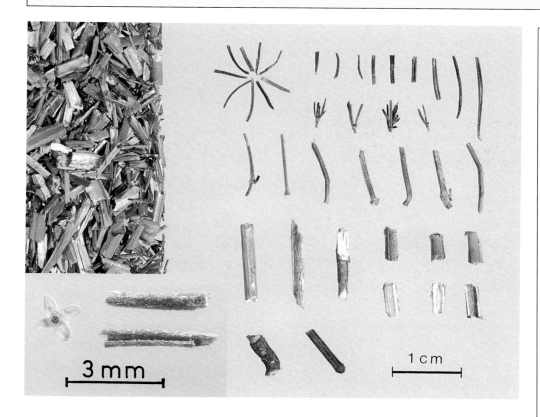

3 mm

1 cm

Fig. 1: Lady's bedstraw herb

<u>Description</u>: The drug consists chiefly of thin, roundish pieces of stem with (usually 4) prominent longitudinal lines; the pieces are often branched. There are also narrow and linear, mucronate leaves with an involute margin and with the lower surface covered with short, soft hairs; in the drug, there are occasional fragments of stem showing the whorled arrangement of the leaves (upper row). The very small, yellow flowers have flat wheel-shaped corollas (Fig. 3), but are not very numerous.

<u>Taste</u>: Somewhat bitter.

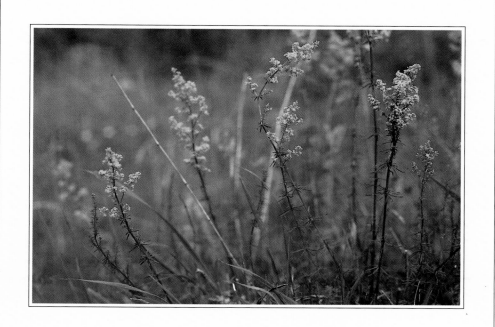

Fig. 2: *Galium verum* L.

A ca. 50 cm tall perennial with a 4-angled stem and whorls of linear leaves. In contrast to many other *Galium* species, golden yellow flowers; these only 2–3 mm in diameter, funnel-shaped, 4-lobed, without a calyx, and grouped in many-flowered panicles.

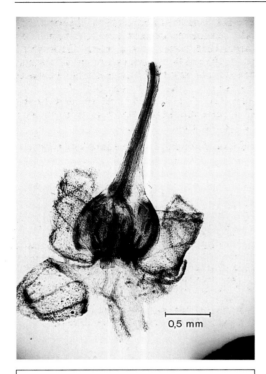

Fig. 3: *Galium verum* **flowers with raphides in the relatively large ovary**

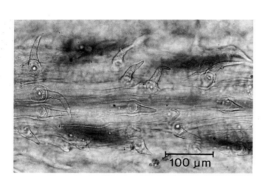

Fig. 5: **Narrow, linear leaf with translucent raphides**

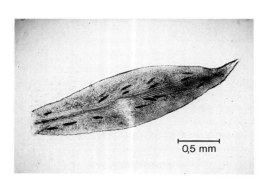

Fig. 4: **Prickly trichomes at the involute leaf margin**

Plant source: *Galium verum* L., lady's bedstraw (Rubiaceae).

Synonyms: Yellow bedstraw, Cheese rennet (Engl.), Gelbes Labkraut, Echtes Labkraut (Ger.), Sommité fleurie de caille-lait jaune (Fr.).

Origin: Distributed widely in Europe, and also occurring in North Africa and Asia. The drug is imported from eastern European countries,

Constituents: Ca. 2% flavonoids [1, 2], especially quercetin glycosides (isorutin, palustroside, cynaroside, etc.). The drug contains small amounts of iridoid glycosides, e.g. asperuloside, monotropein, scandoside, geniposidic acid, etc. [3, 4].

Indications: Only used in *folk medicine*, as a diuretic, rarely also as a diaphoretic and spasmolytic, and externally for injuries and damage to the skin. There are as yet no relevant investigations substantiating the uses indicated.
In Scotland, the drug is still in use as a dye [5].
Note: In UK herbal practice, it is Galii aparinis herba, clivers (cleavers) or goosegrass or hairif, that is used – as a diuretic and mild astringent; see the BHP 1983 and 1/1990.

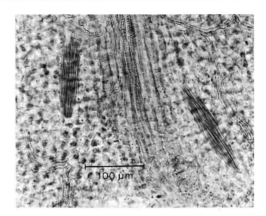

Fig. 6: **Bundles of raphides in the leaf**

Making the tea: Boiling water is poured over 3–4 g of the finely cut drug (two heaped teaspoons) and after 10 min. passed through a tea strainer. The drug can also be placed in cold water and then boiled. As a mild diuretic, two or three cupfuls a day are drunk.
1 Teaspoon = ca. 1.7 g.

Fig. 7: **TLC on 4 × 8 cm silica-gel foil**

1 and 3: Lady's bedstraw herb (different origins)
2: Reference substances

For details, see the text

Herbal preparations and **Phytomedicines:** Not on the market.

Note: In the UK, clivers, as the herb or extract, is a component of herbal teas and phyto- medicines for the relief of pain and rheumatic pain and against psoriasis, e.g. Gerard House Buchu Compound Tablets; Potter's Kas-bah Herb, Sciargo Herb (tea bags), Tabritis (tablets), and Psorasolv Ointment; and Seven Seas Rheumatic Pain Tablets; etc.

Authentication: Macro- (see: Description) and microscopically. The leaves have prickly trichomes at the margin (Fig. 4) and on the lower surface there are numerous bristles up to 100 μm long. The raphides in the leaves are also very characteristic (Figs. 5 and 6).

Note: For the authentication of Galii asparinis herba, see the BHP 1/1990.

A suitable TLC identity test is as follows:

Test solution: 1 g powdered drug refluxed for ca. 10 min. with 10 ml methanol, filtered, and the filtrate taken to dryness, and the residue dissolved in 2.0 ml methanol.

Reference solution: 10 mg rutin, 10 mg quercetin, and 5 mg hyperoside dissolved in 10 ml methanol.

Loadings: 3 μl test solution as a band and 1 μl reference solution, on silica gel.

Solvent system: ethyl acetate + anhydrous formic acid + water (88 + 6 + 6), 5 cm run.

Detection: after drying in a current of hot air, sprayed with 1% methanolic diphenylboryloxyethylamine and then with a 5% ethanolic polyethyleneglycol 400.

Evaluation: in UV 365 nm light. Reference solution: rutin in the lower third, hyperoside about the middle, and quercetin below the solvent front; all three as orange-yellow fluorescent spots. Test solution: orange fluorescent zones at the same level as the rutin and hyperoside spots; in the Rf range between hyperoside and quercetin, a blue fluorescent zone (just above that of hyperoside), two orange fluorescent zones, a faint blue fluorescent zone, and a green fluorescent zone; the red fluorescent chlorophyll zone at the solvent front and immediately below it an orange fluorescent zone (Fig. 7).

The BHP 1/1990 TLC test of identity for Galii aparinis herba provides a fingerprint chromatogram.

Adulteration: In practice, does not occur.

Literature:
[1] J. Raynaud and H. Mnajed, C.R. Acad. Sci., Ser. D **274**, 1746 (1972).
[2] M.I. Borisov, V.V. Belikov und T.I. Isakova, Rastit. Resur. **11**, 351 (1975); C.A. **83**, 190343 (1975).
[3] D. Corrigan, R.F. Timoney and D.M.X. Donnelly, Phytochemistry **17**, 1131 (1978).
[4] K. Böjthe-Horvath et al., Phytochemistry **21**, 2917 (1982).
[5] S. Grierson, D.G. Duff and R.S. Sinclair, J. Soc. Dyers Colour. **101**, 220 (1985); C.A. **104**, 52053 (1986).

Gei urbani rhizoma   Avens root

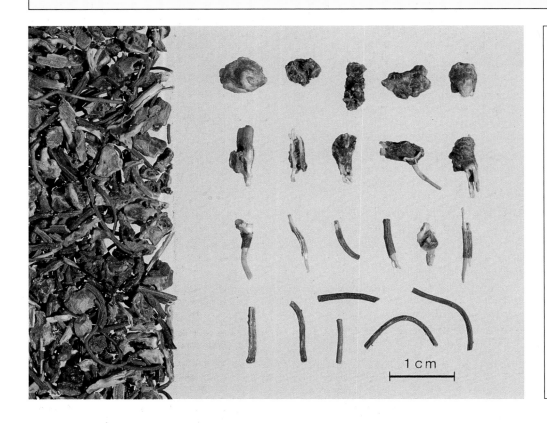

Fig. 1: Avens root

<u>Description</u>: The rhizomes with attached roots are gathered in spring. They are up to finger thickness, 3–7 cm long, and often have several crowns bearing numerous remains of stems and petioles; the rhizomes are slightly thicker at the top and taper into the main root. On the outer surface, they have light and dark brown regions, and they are ringed with small scales and surrounded with somewhat lighter-coloured roots, the thickness of a straw and ca. 5 cm or more in length. When fresh, inside they are pale flesh-coloured or violet with a yellow outline; when dried, they are fairly dark brown, hard, and brittle.

<u>Odour</u>: Faintly of cloves (eugenol); but distinctly so, especially when the fresh drug is powdered.

<u>Taste</u>: Astringent, slightly bitter.

Fig. 2: *Geum urbanum* L.

A ca. 60 cm tall herb bearing characteristic pinnate leaves, often with a very large, lobed, terminal leaflet. Numerous reddish styles (part of a coenocarpous gynoecium) lengthening considerably after anthesis and, unlike other *Geum* species, ending in a hook.

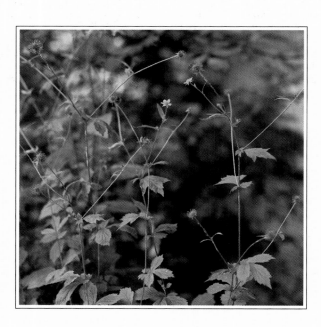

Plant source: *Geum urbanum* L., wood avens (Rosaceae).

Synonyms: Herb Bennet, Colewort, Geum (Engl.), Nelkenwurz, Benediktenwurz (Ger.), Racine de Benoîte, Herbe de Saint-Benoît (Fr.).

Origin: In humid, deciduous woods and fields throughout Eurasia. The drug is collected in the wild and imported from eastern and south-eastern Europe, including former Yugoslavia.

Constituents: 12–28% tannins, especially gallotannins, but also gallic, ellagic, caffeic, chlorogenic, and protocatechuic acids, (+)-catechin [1–3], free sugars (including saccharose, glucose, fructose, vicianose), and glycosides [4, 5]; these last are almost entirely gein (= geoside) with eugenol as aglycone and vicianose (α-L-arabinosido-(1→6)-D-glucose) as the sugar component. The primary glycoside is largely hydrolysed during the drying process to free eugenol. The drug also contains 0.3% essential oil, which according to [8] consists of up to 80% eugenol;

newer gas-chromatographic analyses [7a] indicate that the proportion of eugenol varies between 50 and 89%, averaging ca. 67%, a figure also indicated in older studies [8, 9]. Further, there are oxygenated monoterpenes, among which *cis*-myrtanal, *trans*-myrtanal, and *trans*-myrtanol have been detected [7b].

Whether sesquiterpenes of the germacranolide type which are present in the herb, also occur in the roots and rhizomes [9], has not yet been established.

Indications: Used exclusively in *folk medicine* as an antidiarrhoeal and astringent for inflamed mucous membranes and gums (gargle for the mouth and throat), for chilblains and haemorrhoids (like Tormentillae rhizoma, Ratanhiae radix, and Quercus cortex, which could all be readily replaced by avens rhizome). Occasionally, the drug is also given as a tonic and bitter stomachic. In homoeopathy, it is recommended for excessive sweating.

Note: The BHP 1983 monograph prescribes the herb, rather than the rhizome, primarily for its antidiarrhoeal, antihaemorrhagic, and febrifugal properties.

Side effects: When used in the normal way, none are to be expected.

Making the tea: Boiling water is poured over $^1/_2$–1 teaspoon of the coarsely powdered drug, left to draw in a closed vessel for 10 min., and then strained. For mild cases of diarrhoea, a cupful is drunk lukewarm several times a day.

As an astringent, for mouthwashes, a teaspoonful of the coarsely powdered drug is placed in cold water, boiled for a short period, kept hot for 10 min., and then passed through a tea strainer.

1 Teaspoon = ca. 3.6 g.

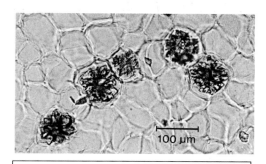

Fig. 3: Relatively large cluster crystals of calcium oxalate from the pith of the rhizome

Phytomedicines: Various mixed herbal teas contain, among other things, avens root – nerve, cardiotonic, bronchial, and diabetic teas. Extracts of the drug are found in some tonics and roborants. These uses have no scientific basis and they should be discouraged (particularly the tea for diabetics).

Authentication: Macro- (see: Description) and microscopically, following [10]. The cortical parenchyma as seen in the transverse section of the *rhizome* has beaded and pitted thickened cells, some of which have clusters of calcium oxalate crystals. In the xylem, in addition to very short-celled, perpendicular and horizontal vessels, there are fibres and an unusually regularly arranged parenchyma. The pith also has large clusters of calcium oxalate crystals (Fig. 3). The transverse section of the *root* shows a narrow primary and a very regular secondary cortex inside the periderm, an easily recognized cambium, and very broad medullary rays. The inner part of the xylem consists, in the case of older roots, of one or several connecting rings of vessels and fibres. Oxalate clusters

are absent. Idioblasts with a yellowish brown or violet content are characteristic of both rhizome and root.

Quantitative standard: *Tannin content*, not less than 15% (gravimetrically [11], 21 authentic samples of the drug have been shown to contain 15–20% total tannin [12]).

For the authentication of Gei urbani herba, see the BHP 1983.

Adulteration: Occasionally with underground parts of *Geum rivale* L., water avens (Gei aquaticae radix); they contain ca. 15% tannins [1, 3], but only 0.0015% essential oil [8], and are used in *folk medicine* in the same way as avens root.

Storage: Protected from light and moisture; if possible, for not more than one year, since the tannins are degraded to inactive products.

Literature:
[1] D. Murko and Z. Devetak, Glas. Hem. Tehnol. Bosne Hercegovine **16**, 113 (1968).
[2] F. Gstirner and H. Widenmann, Sci. Pharm. **32**, 98 (1964).
[3] Z. Kh. Khabibow and Kh.Kh. Khalmatov, Mater. Yubileinioi Resp. Naunchn., Konf. Farm., Posvyashsch. 50-Letiyu Obraz. SSSR 68 (1972).
[4] M. Pšenák et. al., Česk. Farm. **14**, 397 (1965).
[5] M. Pšenák et. al., Planta Med. **22**, 93 (1972).
[6] Em. Bourquelot and H. Hérissey, Compt. rend. l'Acad. des sciences **140**, 870 (1905). H. Hérissey, J. Cheymol, Compt. rend. l'Acad. des sciences **180**, 384 (1925); **181**, 565 (1925); **183**, 1307 (1926).
[7a] C. Vollmann (Univ. Würzburg), personal communication (1987).
[7b] C. Vollmann, W. Schultze and K.-H. Kubeczka, Pharm. Weekbl., Sci. Ed. **9**, 247 (1987).
[8] R. Hegnauer, Pharm. Weekbld. **88**, 385 (1953).
[9] E. Tyihák, I. Pályi and V. Pályi, Naturwissenschaften **52**, 209 (1965).
[10] W. Schier, personal communication 1988.
[11] E. Stahl und W. Schild, Pharmazeutische Biologie 4., Drogenanalyse, G. Fischer Verlag Stuttgart-New York 1981, Seite 307.
[12] F.-C. Czygan, unpublished work (1987).

Genistae herba   Dyer's greenweed herb

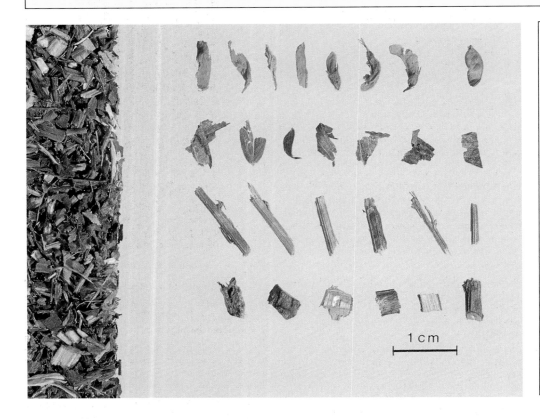

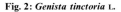

1 cm

Fig. 1: Dyer's greenweed herb

<u>Description:</u> The shrivelled, yellow to yellow-brown papilionaceous flowers (upper row) are a conspicuous feature. The elliptic to lanceolate leaves are glabrous and often ciliate at the margin; the midrib is particularly prominent on the lower surface of the leaf. The pieces of stem are 1–3 mm thick, with coarse longitudinal grooves and glabrous or with very fine appressed hairs. Occasionally, the flat, glabrous pods are also present (upper row, right).

<u>Odour:</u> Very faintly spicy.

<u>Taste:</u> Mildly bitter and astringent.

Fig. 2: *Genista tinctoria* L.

An up to 80 cm tall undershrub with green, thornless branches. Leaves lanceolate, flowers yellow, up to 15 mm long, and arranged in racemes.

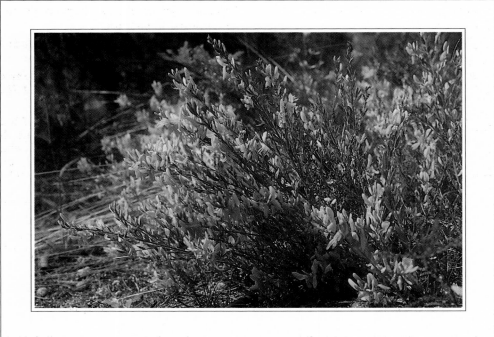

St. Zul. 1489.99.99

Plant origin: *Genista tinctoria* L., dyer's greenweed (Fabaceae).

Synonyms: Greenweed, Dyer's weed or broom (Engl.), Färberginsterkraut (Ger.), Genêt de teinturies (Fr.).

Origin: The plant is an undershrub found throughout Central Europe; it is also cultivated to some extent. Drug imports come mainly from former Yugoslavia.

Constituents: 0.5 to more than 3% flavonoids, particularly derivatives of luteolin [1], along with isoflavones such as genistin and genistein (this last name is not to be confused with that of the quinolizidine alkaloid (−)-α-isosparteine). The drug contains 0.3–0.8% alkaloids, chiefly of the sparteine-type (tetracyclic quinolizidines), the principal ones being *N*-methylcytisine and anagyrine; isosparteine, lupanine, tinctorine, rhombifoline, and traces of cytisine

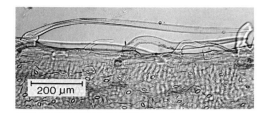

Fig. 3: Appressed trichomes at the leaf margin

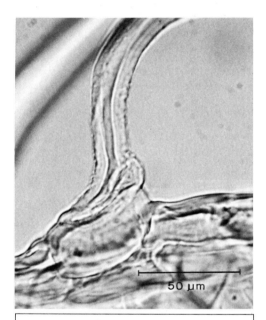

Fig. 4: The base of the trichomes shown in Fig. 3, comprising two small cells

(localized in the seeds) have also been detected [2]. The drug contains some tannin, proteins partly of the lectin-type (in the seeds), and traces of an essential oil which has not been further investigated.

Indications: In *folk medicine*, it is used primarily as a diuretic (see the Standard Licence) and also as a laxative. Again, but only in *folk medicine*, it is applied in rheumatic complaints and gout.

Making the tea: Boiling water is poured over 1–2 g of the finely chopped drug (one teaspoonful), allowed to stand for 10 min., and then strained. As a diuretic, one to three cups a day are drunk. The drug can also be put into cold water, which can then be

6.1   Uses
To increase the amount of urine and in supportive treatment of complaints requiring an increased urine output (gravel, prevention of urinary calculi).

6.2   Contraindications
Dyer's greenweed preparations should not be used when there is high blood pressure.

6.3   Side effects
Warning: Exceeding the stated dosage may give rise to diarrhoea.

6.4   Dosage and Mode of administration
Boiling water (ca. 150 ml) is poured over one small teaspoonful (1–2 g) of **Dyer's greenweed herb** and after 10 min. passed through a tea strainer.
Unless otherwise prescribed, a cup of the freshly prepared infusion is drunk up to three times a day.

6.5   Note
Store protected from light and moisture.

brought to the boil. Owing to possible side effects (diarrhoea), other diuretics such as birch leaves, herniary, or dandelion are to be preferred.
1 Teaspoon = ca. 1.2 g.

Phytomedicines: Dyer's weed is present in several prepared herbal teas (Bladder and Kidney teas).

Authentication: The epidermal cells of the leaves contain mucilage and this makes them conspicuous, when observed under the microscope, because of their greater refraction of light.
Trichomes only occur at the leaf margin; they are normally tricellular with the terminal cell long and narrowing to a point (Figs. 3 and 4). The epidermis of the petals is papillose and the cuticle is striated. In microscopical preparations, numerous round, triporate pollen grains, diameter ca. 35 μm, can be seen.
The following TLC procedure is a suitable identity test:

Test solution: 1 g powdered drug refluxed for 10 min. with 20 ml ethanol, cooled and

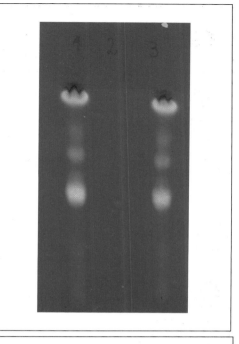

Fig. 5: TLC on 4 × 8 cm silica-gel foil

1 and 3: Dyer's greenweed herb (different origins)
2: Hyperoside (reference substance)

For details, see the text

filtered, the filtrate taken to dryness, and the residue dissolved in 5 ml methanol.

Reference solution: 5 mg hyperoside dissolved in 10 ml methanol.

Loadings: 2 μl test solution and 1 μl reference solution, on silica-gel GF$_{254}$ foil.

Solvent system: upper phase of: ethyl acetate + conc. formic acid + water (67 + 7 + 26), 5 cm run.

Detection: after drying in a current of hot air, sprayed with 1% methanolic diphenylboryloxyethylamine and oversprayed with 5% ethanolic polyethylene glycol 400, followed by heating for a few min. at 100–105 °C.

Luteolin

N-Methylcytisine

Anagyrine

Evaluation: in UV 365 nm light. Reference solution: about half way up, hyperoside as an orange fluorescent zone. Test solution: directly above the hyperoside zone, a bright yellow fluorescent zone and above that several green to yellowish green fluorescent zones; immediately below the solvent front, an intense yellow fluorescent ozone; additional faint fluorescent zones possibly also present (Fig. 5).

Quantitative standards: St.Zul. 1489.99.99: *Flavonoids*, not less than 0.5% calculated as hyperoside. *Foreign matter*, not more than 1.0%. *Loss on drying*, not more than 0.6%. *Sulphated ash*, not more than 6.0%.

Adulteration: Occurs occasionally, with broom tops (Scoparii herba, q.v.). The stem fragments of this plant have five distinct, light green, protruding ridges; the trichomes of the leaves are tricellular, up to 600 µm long, and tortuous.

Storage: Protected from light and kept dry.

Literature:
[1] A. Ulubelen et al., Lloydia **34**, 258 (1971).
[2] V. Hrochova and H. Sitaniova, Farm. Obz. **51**, 131 (1982); C.A. **96**, 159373 (1982).

Gentianae radix

(Ph. Eur. 2, etc.), Gentian (*BAN*; BP 1988, BHP 1/1990)

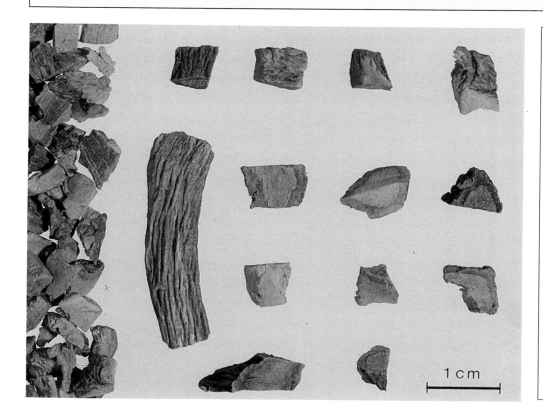

Fig. 1: Gentian

Description: The drug consists of the brownish, reddish brown, or deep brown roots, which are up to several centimetres thick and often fragments of the rhizome, which is transversely wrinkled on the surface; the roots are longitudinally grooved. In the transverse section of the broken drug, there is a relatively narrow bark (with a coarsely wrinkled cork) and a distinct ring of cambium delimiting the xylem (Fig. 4).

Odour: Weak and peculiarly sweetish, reminiscent of dried figs.

Taste: At first sweetish, then persistently and intensely bitter.

Fig. 2: *Gentiana lutea* L.

An up to more than 1 m tall perennial, herbaceous mountain plant. Opposite, oval, bluish green, robust leaves. Axillary flowers with 5, rarely more, yellow petals.

Fig. 3: *Gentiana lutea* L., flowers

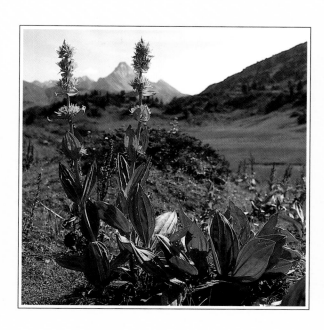

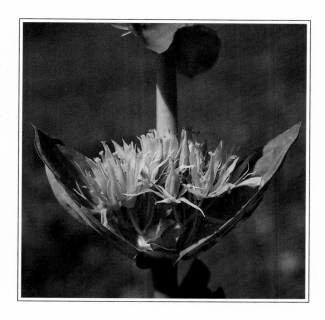

DAB 10: Enzianwurzel
ÖAB: Radix Gentianae
Ph. Helv. VII: Gentianae Radix
St. Zul. 9199.99.99

Plant source: *Gentiana lutea* L., yellow gentian (Gentianaceae).

Synonyms: Gentiana, (Yellow) gentian root (Engl.), Enzianwurzel, Bitterwurz, Fieberwurzel (Ger.), Racine de gentiane (Fr.).

Origin: France, Spain, the Balkans (where the roots are obtained from wild plants). There are small-scale plantations in France and Germany (where the plant is fully protected).

Constituents: Seco-iridoid bitter substances, including 2–3% gentiopicroside (gentiopicrin), the main component, and swertiamarin and sweroside. Although present to the extent of only 0.049–0.084%, in market samples [6], because of its very high bitterness value (58,000,000) the acylglycoside amarogentin is the essential component.
Other constituents: xanthone derivatives (gentisin, isogentisin, gentioside, etc.) [7]; the darker internal colour of the dried European root as compared with the dried Japanese product, may be due to greater hydrolysis of the colourless glycosides to the yellow xanthones during the drying process [7]. Besides saccharose and the trisaccharide gentianose, there is the bitter-tasting gentiobiose (5–8%) [8]; also present are phyto-

Gentiopicroside
(= Gentiopicrin)

Amarogentin

sterols and pectins, or similar gel-forming substances, which may be responsible for the considerable swelling that the drug undergoes when moistened. The alkaloids that have been described in the literature, e.g. gentianine, are probably artefacts arising during work-up. The small amount of essential oil obtained on distillation has a complex composition [4, 5]. Starch is absent.

Indications: A strong bitter (Amarum purum) for stimulating the appetite and also as a roborant and tonic. By stimulating the taste buds and influencing especially the encephalic phase of the secretion, the drug brings about reflex promotion of gastric-juice and saliva production [1]; it also has a cholagogic effect.

Making the tea: Boiling water is poured over 1–2 g of the finely cut or coarsely powdered drug and after 5 min. passed through a tea strainer; the drug can also be put into cold water, which can then boiled for a brief period. A cold extract (macerate, but at least 8–10 hours) can also be made.
1 Teaspoon = ca. 3.5 g.

Herbal preparations: Gentian root is contained in many (stomach) teas and extracts of it are found in instant teas, e.g. Dr. Klinger's Bergischer Kräutertee, Magentee, etc.

Phytomedicines: Chiefly in numerous prepared gastrointestinal remedies, as the powdered drug or extract, tincture, percolate, etc., e.g. Aciphyt® (drops), Gastricard® (tablets, drops), Ventrodigest® (tablets), etc., but also in the cholagogues or roborants and tonics. Homoeopathic dilutions of gentian root are also present in more than a dozen preparations.
Among the UK multi-ingredient products containing gentian root and/or extracts of it are: Lanes Kalms Tablets, Potter's Appetiser, Indigestion, and Stomach Mixtures; Seven Seas Nerve Tablets; Effico® contains compound gentian infusion.

Regulatory status (UK): General Sales List – Schedule 1, Table A.

Authentication: Macro- (see: Description) and microscopically, following the Ph. Eur. 2, BP 1988. In the powdered drug, there are only a few fragments of tortuous vessels with reticulate and scalariform thickening; colourless parenchyma occasionally with very small needles of calcium oxalate and droplets of oil is also present. See also [9]. Testing for the absence of starch with iodine solution can be done on the powder or by spotting the cut drug with the reagent.
The TLC test of identity given in the Ph. Eur. 2, BP 1988, etc., is as follows:

Test solution: 2.00 g powdered drug stirred mechanically for 20 min. with 50.0 ml methanol, filtered avoiding losses by evaporation; 25.0 ml taken to dryness under reduced pressure, not above 50 °C; residue dissolved in a little methanol to give finally 5.0 ml solution; a sediment may be present.

Reference solution: 50 mg phenazone dissolved in methanol and made up to 10.0 ml.

Loadings: 50 µl test solution and 10 µl reference solution, as 3-cm bands on silica gel GF$_{254}$.

Solvent system: water + chloroform + acetone (2 + 30 + 70), 15 cm run.

Detection and **Evaluation:** in UV 254 nm light. Test solution: quenching zones in the lower and also upper parts; the amarogentin zone at about the middle, at more or less the same level as the (marked) reference phenazone zone.
Sprayed with freshly prepared 0.2% Fast Red salt B solution and stood for 10 min. Test solution: amarogentin zone, orange and turning red on exposure to ammonia fumes; other zones visible in the upper and lower regions; a usually intense zone with

Fig. 4: Transverse surface of *Gentiana lutea* root with a dark cambium line and porous, parenchyma- rich xylem

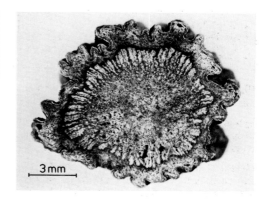

3 mm

---

the same colour as the amarogentin zone in the upper part; violet zones immediately above the amarogentin zone (presence of other *Gentiana* species).
About the TLC of gentian root (from different plant sources), see below and also [2]. Quantitative determination of the amarogentin content can be found in [3]. Low amounts of extractive and low bitterness values suggest fermented roots (for the preparation of spirits) and hence a pharmaceutically inferior drug.
On microsublimation, gentian root (and the root from other species as well) affords yellowish crystals (gentisin) which are coloured yellow by potassium hydroxide.
It has been suggested that TLC of gentiobiose and gentianose could be a useful additional parameter for characterizing gentian root [8].

Quantitative standards: Ph. Eur. 2, BP 1988, etc.: *Total extractive*, not less than 33%. *Bitterness value*, not less than 10,000. *Sulphated ash*, not more than 5.0%.
BHP 1/1990: Gentian and Powdered Gentian is required to comply with the relevant monographs in the Ph. Eur. 2 and BP 1988.

Adulteration: The Ph. Eur. 2, BP 1988, etc., do not permit the roots of other *Gentiana* species, but these cannot be recognized macro- or microscopically. TLC detection of additional acyl- glycosides – amaropanin and amaroswerin – point to the occurrence of such admixture [2, 3, 10]. As already mentioned, gentian root contains little or no starch, so that the roots of other plants are mostly detectable by the occurrence of a positive iodine reaction. Occasional adulteration with *Rumex alpinus* L., monk's rhubarb (Polygonaceae), can be recognized on microsublimation: the sublimate is coloured red with potassium hydroxide (Bornträger reaction).

Literature:
[1] W. Schmid, Planta Med. **14** (Suppl.), 34 (1966).
[2] H. Wagner and K. Vasirian, Dtsch. Apoth. Ztg. **114**, 1245 (1974).
[3] H. Wagner and K. Münzing-Vasirian, Dtsch. Apoth. Ztg. **115**, 1233 (1975).
[4] F. Chialva, C. Fratini, and A. Martelli, Z. Lebensm. Unters. Forsch. **182**, 212 (1986).
[5] H. Glasl, Habilitations-Schrift, Hamburg, 1977.
[6] A. Krupinska et. al., Sci. Pharm. **59**, 135 (1991).
[7] T. Hayashi and T. Yamagishi, Phytochemistry **27**, 3696 (1988).
[8] M. Buffa et al., Acta Pharm. Jugoslav. **41**, 67 (1991).
[9] B.P. Jackson and D.W. Snowdon, Atlas of microscopy of medicinal plants, culinary herbs and spices, Belhaven Press, London, 1990, p. 108.
[10] H. Wagner, S. Bladt, and E.M. Zgainski, Plant drug analysis, Springer-Verlag, Berlin, Heidelberg, New York, Tokyo, 1984, p. 136.

Ginseng radix   (DAB 10), Ginseng (BHP 1/1990), Ginseng root

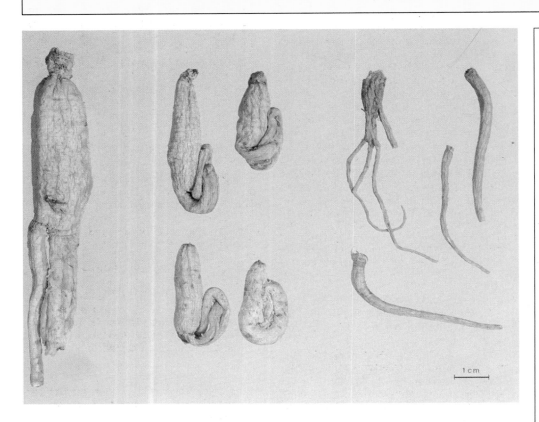

Fig. 1: Ginseng

There are several commercial varieties, including Korean ginseng, which is the most highly valued, followed by Chinese, Japanese, and American ginseng (this last variety comes mostly from *Panax quinquefolius*). Among the varieties of Korean ginseng, there are the white variety (official in the DAB 10, ÖAB, and Ph. Helv. VII), the roots of which after harvesting and washing are immediately dried, and the red variety, which is official in Japan and which are cartilaginous, translucent, and reddish as a result of the roots being first scalded for $1^1/_2$-4 hours and then dried. The illustration shows white ginseng – the commercial forms "curved" (centre) and "slender tails" (right; not official!).

Description: The cylindrical roots are transversely rugose in the upper part, from the middle sometimes repeatedly divided, and they taper towards the bottom. Often, the roots still bear the remains of the stem like a crown. The light yellow to light brown bark contains scattered small orange-red resin glands. Internally, the root is white to yellowish, cartilaginous, and brittle.

Odour: Faint and pleasant.

Taste: At first bitter, then sweet and mucilaginous.

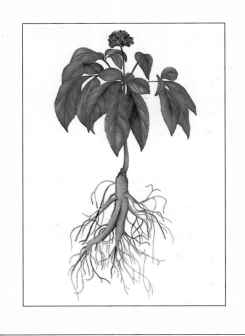

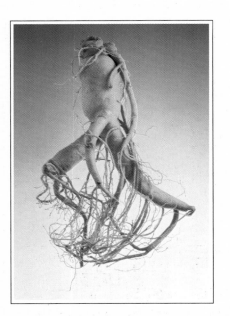

Fig. 2: *Panax ginseng* C.A. MEYER

An up to 80 cm tall herb with palmate, verticillate leaves. Flowers small and grouped 15–20 in umbels.

Fig. 3: *Panax ginseng* C.A. MEYER, tap root and lateral roots

DAB 10: Ginsengwurzel
ÖAB: Radix Ginseng
Ph. Helv. VII: Ginseng radix

Plant source: *Panax ginseng* C.A. MEYER (syn. *Panax schinseng* NEES), ginseng (Araliaceae).

Synonyms: Panax, Korean ginseng (Engl.), Ginsengwurzel, Kraftwurzel (Ger.), Racine de ginseng (Fr.).

Origin: Native to the montane forests of eastern Asia. Cultivated in China, Japan, former USSR, and Korea. The drug is imported principally from Korea, China, and Japan; the root of *Panax quinquefolius* L. is imported from the United States (but it is not official).

Constituents: 2–3% Ginsenosides (triterpene saponins), of which ginsenosides Rg_1, Rc, Rd, Rb_1, Rb_2, and Rb_0 are quantitatively the most important (Russian investigators use the designations panaxosides A–F); ca. 0.05% essential oil (limonene, terpineol, citral, polyacetylenes); ubiquitous substances such as sugars, starch, etc.
More recently, a series of poly-acetylenes, the ginsenoynes A-K, some of which are acetylated, has been isolated [14].

Indications: Ginseng derives from East Asian medicine, where the drug has been used for thousands of years as a tonic (and presumably also as an aphrodisiac); it should therefore not be judged by the criteria of modern rational therapeutics. This drug is not a therapeutic agent for the treatment of particular illnesses, but rather a prophylactic which heightens in an unspecific way (details of which have only now been investigated scientifically) the resistance of the organism to various environmental influences and stimuli and/or reduces the disposition or susceptibility to illness [1].
Nowadays, the "active principles" are considered to be the ginsenosides, some of which have been examined pharmacologically in detail, so that a very extensive literature is now available; but other ginseng constituents also have pharmacological activity. Interestingly, some of the ginsenosides have opposing activities, e.g. ginsenoside Rg_1 raises the blood pressure and is a central stimulant, while ginsenoside Rb_1 lowers the blood pressure and is a central depressant. The standardization of ginseng preparations is therefore of particular significance.
Ginseng is an adaptogen, i.e. it is a substance that is able to improve the ability of an organism to adapt to differing external or internal disturbances [2].
The immunostimulant action of ginseng extracts has been repeatedly confirmed in animal experiments [3–5]. Various groups of workers have described in detail the enhancement of RNA and protein biosynthesis after administration of ginseng extracts [6, 7].
Also worth noting is the effect on carbohydrate and lipid metabolism; there are results from both animal experiments and clinical studies [8, 9].
Clinical work has demonstrated that ginseng affects human performance and ability to react in a positive way, though it has to be realized that the effect does not take place immediately (in Chinese medicine, ginseng has been, and is, taken over rather long periods of time).
Good reviews are in [10, 11, 15].

Side effects: Relatively rare and only with high doses and/or use over very long periods of time. They include sleeplessness, nervousness, diarrhoea (particularly in the morning), menopausal bleeding, and hypertony [12]. See also [16].

Making the tea: Boiling water is poured over 3 g of the finely chopped drug, covered and allowed to draw for 5–10 min., and then passed through a tea strainer. The infusion is taken one to three times a day for a period of three to four weeks. Many manufacturers recommend taking the cut drug as such and chewing it.
1 Teaspoon = ca. 3.5 g.

Herbal preparations: The drug is offered in the form of an instant tea (and in 3 g tea bags).

Phytomedicines: The powdered drug (in some cases with a standardized ginsenoside content) or extracts as prepared geriatric remedies, e.g. Geriatric Pharmaton® (capsules), etc., and roborants and tonics, e.g. Ginsana® Ginseng, Kumsan Ginseng Much, etc.
Among the products available on the UK market are [15]: Blackmore's Ginseng Tablets, Vitalia Gerimax Tablets, Booker Healthcrafts Korean Ginseng Tablets, Herbal Laboratories Herbal Korean Ginseng Tablets, Larkhall Naturtabs Red Panax Ginseng, Unichem Pharmaton Capsules,

Extract from the German Commission E monograph (BAnz no. 11, dated 17. 01. 1991)

Uses
As a tonic to combat feelings of lassitude and debility, lack of energy and ability to concentrate, and during convalescence.

Contraindications
None known.

Side effects
None known.

Interactions with other remedies
None known.

Dosage
Unless otherwise prescribed: daily dose, 1–2 g drug; preparations correspondingly.

Mode of administration
Comminuted drug for infusions, powdered drug and galenical formulations for internal use.

Duration of use
As a rule, up to 3 months.

Effects
In various stress models, e.g. the immobilization test and the cold test, the resistance of rodents is increased.

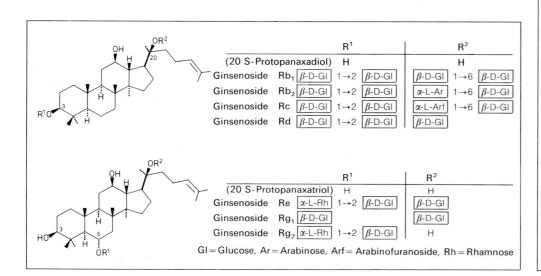

		R¹			R²		
(20 S-Protopanaxadiol)		H			H		
Ginsenoside Rb₁	β-D-Gl	1→2	β-D-Gl	β-D-Gl	1→6	β-D-Gl	
Ginsenoside Rb₂	β-D-Gl	1→2	β-D-Gl	α-L-Ar	1→6	β-D-Gl	
Ginsenoside Rc	β-D-Gl	1→2	β-D-Gl	α-L-Arf	1→6	β-D-Gl	
Ginsenoside Rd	β-D-Gl	1→2	β-D-Gl	β-D-Gl			

		R¹		R²	
(20 S-Protopanaxatriol)		H		H	
Ginsenoside Re	α-L-Rh	1→2	β-D-Gl	β-D-Gl	
Ginsenoside Rg₁	β-D-Gl			β-D-Gl	
Ginsenoside Rg₂	α-L-Rh	1→2	β-D-Gl	H	

Gl = Glucose, Ar = Arabinose, Arf = Arabinofuranoside, Rh = Rhamnose

Power Ginseng GX 2500 Extract Capsules, English Grains Red Kooga Capsules and Tablets, Boots Second Nature Korean Ginseng Tablets, etc.

Authentication: Macroscopically, authentication is not possible with complete certainty, since the appearance of the commercial products varies considerably. Microscopical features include the occurrence of large secretory canals (only in the bark) containing a brownish yellow resin, whose size diminishes towards the inside; near the cambium, they form an almost continuous ring. Two- to four-seriate, to some extent tortuous medullary rays traverse the rather spongy parenchyma, the cells of which contain calcium-oxalate clusters and single crystals. There is abundant starch consisting of simple and aggregate grains. See also the BHP 1/1990. Microscopic examination does not allow the differentiation of *Panax ginseng* from *P. quinquefolius* [13]. However, the following TLC procedure, which is similar to that to that given in the DAB 10, can be used for this purpose:

Test solution: 1 g powdered drug refluxed with 10 ml 70% aqueous methanol for 15 min., cooled, and filtered.

Reference solution: 5 mg aescin, 5 mg amygdalin, and 25 mg arbutin, dissolved in 10 ml methanol.

Loadings: 5 µl test solution and 3 µl, as band, on silica-gel.

Solvent system: upper phase of: ethyl acetate + butanol + water (25 + 100 + 50), 6 cm run.

Detection: after drying in a current of hot air, sprayed with anisaldehyde reagent and heated at 105–110 °C for 2–3 min.

Evaluation: in daylight. Reference solution: aescin as a blue to blue-violet zone at Rf ca. 0.3, amygdalin as a greyish green zone at Rf ca. 0.5, and arbutin as a brown zone at Rf ca. 0.8. Test solution: greyish blue to greyish violet zones of the ginsenosides Rg_1 (Rf ca. 0.7) and Re (Rf ca. 0.55), between the arbutin and amygdalin reference zones, and Rb_1, at the same Rf as the reference aescin zone but not sharply separated from other ginsenosides (Fig. 4).
The following optimized HPTLC procedure enables various ginsengs, including red (steamed) and white (dried naturally), American, and sanchi (notoginseng), to be distinguished [17]:

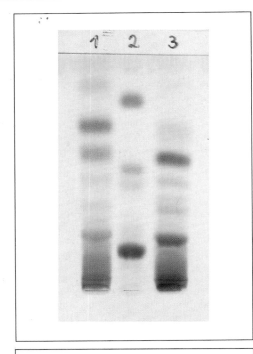

Fig. 4: TLC on 4 × 8 cm silica-gel foil

1: Official ginseng root
2: Reference substances
3: American ginseng (*Panax quinquefolius*)

For details, see the text

Test solution: 1 g powdered drug refluxed with 40 ml chloroform and the solution discarded; then refluxed for 1 h with 50 ml methanol and solution passed through a basic alumina column (15 g; 1 cm ∅), followed by elution with 50% methanol; hydrophilic components removed from the eluate with butan-1-ol and the solution taken to dryness in a vacuum desiccator over phosphorus(V) oxide; residue (ca. 8 mg) dissolved in 0.1 ml methanol (= crude ginsenosides); American ginseng and sanchi, 4 mg residue dissolved in 0.1 ml methanol.

Solvent system: lower phase of chloroform (no ethanol present) + ethyl acetate + methanol + water (15 + 40 + 22 + 10) after standing overnight at 8–10 °C, 7 cm run on silica gel $60F_{254}$ at 26–28 °C for best results..

Detection: dipped in 5% ethanolic sulphuric acid for 2 sec., followed by heating at 105 °C for 1 min.; then dipped for 2 sec. in liquid paraffin + hexane (1 + 1) to stabilize the fluorescence for more than 24 h.

Evaluation: in UV 366 nm light. 19 zones divided into 4 groups: A (ginsenosides Ra, Rb_1, Rb_2, Rb_3), B (Rc, Re, Rd), C (Rg_1, Rf, F11, F2, Rg_2), and D (6 minor ginsenosides). <u>Macro-fingerprints</u> (based on densitometric measurements): ginseng (group A > B ≳ C > D) pattern more complex than that of American ginseng (group A ≥ B > > C > > > D) and much more complex than that of notoginseng (sanchi); in red ginseng more minor ginsenosides (group D) than in white ginseng.
The clean-up stage causes some loss of ginsenosides, but the resulting extract gives better chromatograms.

Quantatitive standards: <u>DAB 10:</u> *Ginsenosides*, not less than 1.5% calculated as ginsenoside Rg_1. *Foreign matter*, not more than 2%. *Loss on drying*, not more than 12%. *Ash*, not more than 8.0%. *HCl-insoluble ash*, not more than 1.0%.
<u>ÖAB:</u> 69–71% *ethanol extractive*, not less than 14%. *Ash*, not more than 4%.
<u>Ph. Helv. VII:</u> *Total ginsenosides*, not less than 2.0% calculated as ginsenoside Rg_1 (M_r 800.0). *Sulphated ash*, not more than 12.0%.
<u>BHP 1/1990:</u> 70% *Ethanol extractive*, not less than 20%. *Foreign matter*, not more than 2%. *Loss on drying*, not more than 10%. *Total ash*, not more than 8%. *HCl-insoluble ash*, not more than 2%.

Literature:
[1] U. Sonnenborn, Dtsch. Apoth. Ztg. **127**, 433 (1987).
[2] F.Z. Merson, Adaptation, stress and prophylaxis, Springer, Berlin – Heidelberg – New York – Tokyo, 1984.
[3] Y.-H. Jie, S. Cammisuli, and M. Baggiolini, Agents Actions **15**, 386 (1984).
[4] V K. Singh, S.S. Agarwal, and B.M. Gupta, Planta Med. **50**, 462 (1984).
[5] V.K. Singh et al., Planta Med. **47**, 234 (1983).
[6] Z.-Q. Lu and J.F. Dice, Biochem. Biophys. Res. Commun. **126**, 636 (1985).
[7] M. Iijima and T. Higashi, Chem. Pharm. Bull. **27**, 2130 (1979).
[8] A.A. Qureshi et al., Lipids **20**, 817 (1985).
[9] M. Yamamoto and A. Kumagai, Planta Med. **45**, 149 (1982).
[10] E. Sprecher, Apoth. Journal **9**, Heft 5, 52 (1987).
[11] Ch. Chinna, Österr. Apoth. Ztg. **37**, 1022 (1983).
[12] E. Röder, Dtsch. Apoth. Ztg. **122**, 2083 (1983).
[13] L. Langhammer, Pharm. Ztg. **127**, 2187 (1982).
[14] K. Hirakura et al., Phytochemistry **30**, 3327, 4053 (1991); idem., *ibid.* **31**, 899 (1992).
[15] C.A. Baldwin, L.A. Anderson, and J.D. Phillipson, Pharm. J. **237**, 583 (1986).
[16] P.F. D'Arcy, Adverse Drug React. Toxicol. Rev. **10**, 189 (1991).
[17] P.-S. Xie and Y.-Z. Yan, J. High Resol. Chromatogr. **10**, 607 (1987).

Graminis flos   Grass flowers

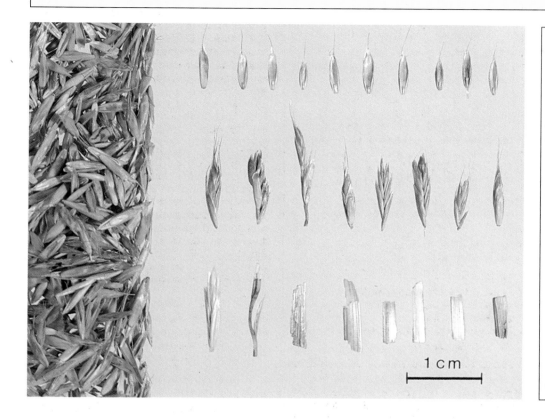

1 cm

Fig. 1: Grass flowers

This drug is a by-product of haymaking and varies greatly in appearance, depending on the origin. Fig. 1 shows the inflorescences and flowers, as well as stems, of various grasses (*Elymus repens* (L.) GOULD, *Lolium perenne* L., etc.), which are typical of the drug.

Description: The material consists essentially of yellowish green or reddish glumes, as well as flowers and flower parts, of various grasses, as well as numerous parallel-nerved stem and leaf fragments. In addition, flowers of clover species (*Trifolium* spp.) are often present in the drug as much shrivelled whitish yellow-brown flowers.

Odour: Faint, of coumarin.

Taste: Somewhat bitter.

Fig. 2: *Elymus repens* (L.) GOULD, etc.

Typical fresh grass with narrow, linear leaves and up to 15 cm long spikes. Dense distichous, multiflowered spikelets.

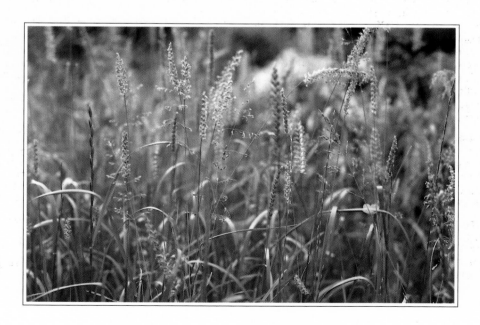

Plant sources: These cannot be precisely indicated, since the drug is obtained by sieving hay from farms and hence can vary widely in composition. Mostly, however, *Anthoxantum odoratum* L., sweet vernal-grass, *Elymus repens* (L.) GOULD (syn. *Agropyron repens* (L.) P. BEAUV.), common couch, *Lolium perenne* L., perennial rye-grass, *Bromus hordeaceus* L., lop grass, *Festuca pratensis* HUDS., meadow fescue, *Phleum* spp., cat's-tails, timothy, *Alopecurus* spp., foxtails, *Dactylis* spp., cock's-foot, etc. (all Poaceae), are present in the drug; for recent investigations see [4].

Origin: In Central Europe, the drug is obtained by passing hay through several sieves to get rid of the larger stem fragments and then dust, sand, and soil are removed, until finally a product consisting predominantly of flower parts is left. The drug is not imported.

Constituents: Quite inadequately known. Apart from ubiquitous substances (flavonoids, plant acids, sugar, starch, protein), tannins and essential oil can be de-

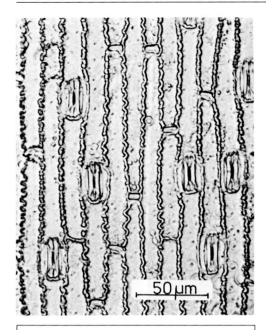

Fig. 3: Typical graminaceous (poaceous) epidermis with wavy cell walls and dumbbell-shaped guard cells

*Extract from the German Commission E monograph
(BAnz no. 85, dated 05. 05. 1988)*

Uses

For topical heat treatment of degenerative rheumatic conditions.

Contraindications

Open wounds, acute rheumatic attacks, acute inflammation.

Side effects

Allergic skin reactions are possible in very rare cases.

Interactions with other remedies

None known.

Dosage and Mode of administration

Unless otherwise prescribed: Externally, once or twice a day as a hot fomentation. The warm (ca. 42°) bag with the hay flowers in it is placed directly on the part to be treated, covered over, and left for 40–50 min.
For hygienic reasons, the contents of the bag should only be used once.

Effects

Increases the local blood circulation. Affects internal organs through cutaneous visceral reflexes.

known and the use is purely empirical; medically, a mild sedative effect is ascribed to coumarins and furanocoumarins [1].

Side effects: The possibility of allergic reactions (hayfever!) should be borne in mind.

Making the tea (Use): For a grass-flower bath, 3–4 l boiling water is poured over about 500 g of the drug, boiled for about 1 min., allowed to draw for about 30 min., strained, and the infusion added to a normal bath (38 °C); the bath should not be longer than 15 min. and it should be followed by an hour's rest in bed [2].
For inhalation, 5–10 g drug to 1 l boiling water is used.
1 Tablespoon = ca. 2.3 g.

Authentication: It has to be ensured that the material contains an appropriately high proportion of grass flowers. Prominent on microscopical examination are the wavy cell walls and the dumb-bell-shaped guard cells of the stomata at the ends of the epidermal cells (Fig. 3). For the detailed microscopy of powdered *Lolium perenne*, common or perennial rye-grass, see [3].

Adulteration: In practice, rarely happens.

tected in trace amounts; coumarins and furanocoumarins are also present.

Indications: The drug is used exclusively in *folk medicine* for preparing baths to allevi-ate the pain of rheumatic conditions, lumbago, chilblains, and in neurasthenia. Occasionally, and again in *folk medicine*, the drug is also used for inhalations in catarrhal conditions. In no case is the active principle

Literature:
[1] H.H. Froehlich and W. Müller-Limmroth, Münch. Med. Wochenschr. **118**, 317 (1976).
[2] M. Pahlow, Dtsch. Apoth. Ztg. **128**, 564 (1988).
[3] B.P. Jackson and D.W. Snowdon, Atlas of microscopy of medicinal plants, culinary herbs and spices, Belhaven Press, London, 1990, p. 112
[4] R. Länger and W. Kubelka, Sci. Pharm. **61**, 65 (1993).

Graminis rhizoma   (DAB 10), Couch-grass root, Agropyron (BHP 1983)

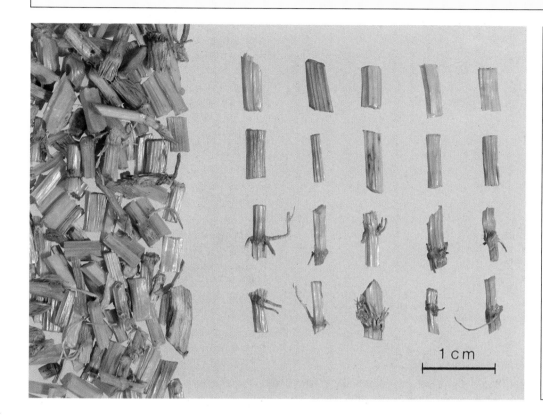

1 cm

Fig. 1: Couch-grass root

<u>Description:</u> The drug consists of rhizomes, roots, and short pieces of stems. The shiny, pale straw-yellow, hollow pieces of rhizome and stem are longitudinally grooved and 2–3 mm thick. At the unthickened nodes, there are whitish to brownish, short fibre-like cataphylls and very thin roots.

<u>Taste:</u> Bland, slightly sweetish.

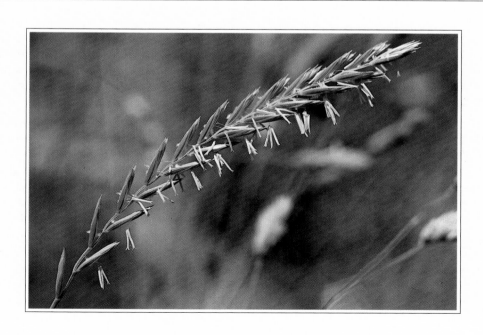

Fig. 2: *Elymus repens* (L.) GOULD

A grass, up to 1.5 m tall, spreading by means of long underground stolons. Spikes up to 15 cm long with compact, many-flowered distichous spikelets.

**DAB 10: Queckenwurzelstock
Ph. Helv. VI: Rhizoma graminis
St. Zul. 1169.99.99**

Plant source: *Elymus repens* (L.) GOULD (syn. *Agropyron repens* (L.) P. BEAUV., *Triticum repens* L.), common couch (Poaceae).

Synonyms: Triticum (Lat.), Scutch, Twitch, Dog grass (Engl.), Queckenwurzelstock (Ger.), Rhizome de petit chiendent, Chiendent officinal (Fr.).

Origin: A widely distributed weed throughout the northern hemisphere. Drug imports come from Romania, Hungary, former Yugoslavia, and Albania.

Constituents: 3–8% Triticin, a polysaccharide related to inulin, which on hydrolysis yields fructose; ca. 10% mucilage; possibly saponins (detectable haemolytic activity); 2–3% sugar alcohols (mannitol, inositol); 0.01–0.05% essential oil with polyacetylenes (agropyrene), carvone, etc.; small amounts of vanilloside (vanillin monoglucoside), vanillin, and phenolcarboxylic acids [1]; sili-

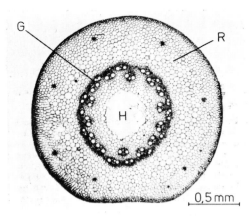

Fig. 3: Transverse section through the (swollen) rhizome of *Elymus repens*. R = cortical parenchyma, G = ring of vascular bundles of the central stele, H = hollow pith

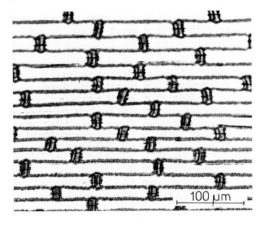

Fig. 4: Epidermis of the stem with alternating long and short cells (surface view)

6.1 Uses

To increase the amount of urine in catarrh of the urinary tract; to supplement treatment in catarrh of the upper respiratory tract.

6.2 Dosage and Mode of administration

Ca. 2–3 teaspoonfuls (ca. 5–10 g) of **Couch-grass root** is infused with ca. 150 ml boiling water and after 10 min. passed through a tea strainer.
Unless otherwise prescribed, a cupful of the freshly prepared infusion is drunk up to four times a day.

6.3 Note

Store protected from moisture.

cic acid and silicates. Lectins found in the seedlings and leaves may also be present in the rhizome.

Indications: The drug is used, on the one hand, as a diuretic in cases of bladder catarrh and bladder and kidney stones and, on the other hand, as a cough remedy to alleviate irritation in bronchial catarrh, based on medical and *folk-medicinal* experience. Other uses in *folk medicine* are for gout, rheumatic disorders, and chronic skin conditions. Extracts of the drug are a dietary component for diabetics. Pharmacological and clinical investigations are lacking.

Making the tea: Boiling water is poured over 5–20 g of the finely chopped drug and after 5–10 min. passed through a tea strainer; it is also recommended to put the drug into cold water and slowly bring it to the boil.
1 Teaspoon = ca. 1.5 g.

Herbal preparations and **Phytomedicines:** The drug and extracts made from it are present in a few prepared diuretics, cholagogues, and in dietary supplements (not rated as drugs).
Among the multi-component U.K. products containing couch grass are: Gerard House Herbal Powder no. 8 and Potter's Kas-bah Herb and Potter's Antitis Tablets.

Regulatory status (UK): General Sales List – Schedule 1, Table A (under: *Agropyron*).

Authentication: Macro- (see: Description) and microscopically. See also the BHP 1983. The rhizome can be easily cut after allowing it to swell in water and it furnishes a characteristic transverse section (Fig. 3) in which the cortical parenchyma, central stele, and hollow pith can all be recognized. The endodermis is formed of U-shaped, thickened and pitted cells, the walls of which are distinctly stratified. In surface view, the epidermis of the stem fragments shows wavy-walled, alternating long and short cells (Fig. 4). Starch is absent. Addition of α-naphtholsulphonic acid to fragments of the drug produces a reddish violet colour (triticin).

Quantitative standards: DAB 10: *Ash*, not more than 8%.
Ph. Helv. VI:
BHP 1983: *Total ash*, not more than 5%.
Acid-insoluble ash, not more than 3%.

Adulteration: The principal adulterant is the rhizome of *Cynodon dactylon* (L.) PERS., Bermuda grass (Poaceae), known as Rhizoma Graminis italici; since it contains starch, its detection is simple: transverse sections with iodine solution are stained blue-black. Rhizomes of *Imperata cylindrica* (L.) RAEUSCH., alang-alang or lalang (Poaceae), have also been noted as an adulterant; they can be recognized by the 2–3 cm long internodes with very fine longitudinal corrugations.

Literature:
[1] D.C. Whitehead, H. Dibb, and R.D. Hartley, Soil Biol. Biochem. **15**, 133 (1986).

Extract from the German Commission E monograph (BAnz no. 22a, dated 01. 02. 1990)

Uses
For irrigation therapy in inflammatory disorders of the urinary tract and in the prevention of renal gravel.

Contraindications
None known.
Warning: No irrigation therapy in cases of oedema resulting from cardiac or renal insufficieny.

Side effects
None known.

Interactions with other remedies
None known.

Dosage
Unless otherwise prescribed: daily dose, 6–9 g drug; preparations correspondingly.

Mode of administration
Chopped drug for infusions and other galenical preparations for internal use.
Warning: An adequate fluid intake must be ensured during irrigation therapy.

Effects
The essential oil is antimicrobial.

Hamamelidis cortex   Witch hazel bark

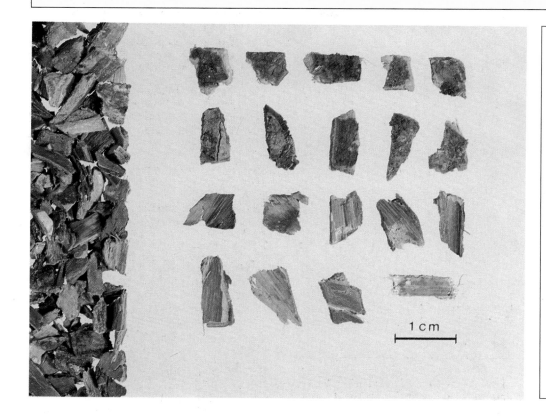

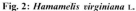

1 cm

Fig. 1: Witch hazel bark

<u>Description</u>: **The pieces of dried bark are from the trunk and branches; they are of different lengths, channelled, less often quilled or in strips, and up to 3 cm wide and 2 mm thick. The cinnamon-brown or reddish brown outer surface has a thin, whitish or greyish brown cork with numerous lenticels. The yellowish brown to reddish brown inner surface is longitudinally striated. The fracture is splintery and fibrous.**

<u>Taste</u>: **Strongly astringent and bitter.**

Fig. 2: *Hamamelis virginiana* L.

A branch with flowers. For the description, see Hamamelidis folium, Fig. 2, p. 245.

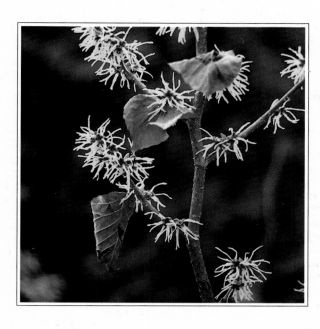

DAC 1986: Hamamelisrinde
St. Zul. 9799.99.99

Plant source: *Hamamelis virginiana* L., witch hazel (Hamamelidaceae).

Synonyms: Hamamelis bark (Engl.), Hamamelisrinde, Virginische Zaubernuß-rinde (Ger.), Ecorce d'hamamélis de virginie, Ecorce de noisetier de la sorcière (Fr.).

Origin: See, Hamamelidis folium.

Constituents: Up to 10% tannins (a mixture of hamamelitannin = digalloylhamamelose and catechols), free gallic acid, monogalloyl-hamamelose [1–5]; soft fats and waxes [1]; essential oil smelling of eugenol and with a sesquiterpene as the main component [6]; saponins (?) [7].

Indications: See Hamamelidis folium.

Side effects: See Hamamelidis folium.

Making the tea: Ca. 2 g of the finely chopped or coarsely powdered drug in cold water is brought to the boil, kept boiling for

10–15 min., and then strained while still hot.
In cases of diarrhoea, a cupful up to three
times a day, but the infusion should not be
taken over a prolonged period of time.
For inflammation of the gums or the mucous membranes of the mouth, the infusion
can be used several times a day as a mouthwash or gargle.
1 Teaspoon = ca. 2.5 g.

Phytomedicines: See, Hamamelidis folium.
The number of preparations made from
hamamelis bark is even greater than that
made from the leaves.

Regulatory status (UK): General Sales List –
Schedule 1, Table B (external use only).

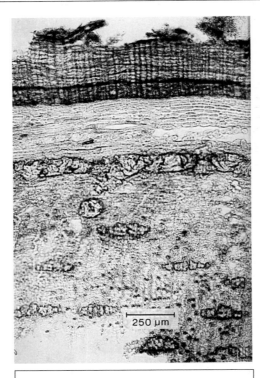

**Fig. 3: Witch hazel bark, transverse section; numer-
ous rows of cork cells, narrow primary cortex, ring of
stone cells, secondary cortex with medullary rays,
groups of fibres, and cluster crystals of calcium oxalate**

Authentication: Macro- (see: Description);
microscopically according to the DAC 1986
(Fig. 3); see also the BHP 1983. According
to the DAC 1986, pieces of bark with adher-
ing fragments of yellowish white wood
(xylem) must not be used. In the powdered
drug, attention should be paid to the groups
of small and the groups of larger, greatly
thickened, distinctly striated and pitted
stone cells (Fig. 4), a few of which have a
wider lumen with a brown content or a crystal. The microscopy of powdered Witch
hazel bark is also dealt with in [8].
The DAC 1986 has a TLC examination for
tannins, as well as a procedure for the quantitative estimation of the gallotannins (cal-

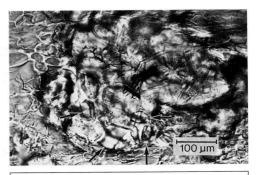

**Fig. 4: A group of stone cells in witch hazel bark. Cells
with striated walls, distinctly pitted, and sometimes
containing a crystal (arrow)**

culated as gallic acid) by the method using
casein/folin reagent.

Quantitative standards: DAC 1986: *Tannins*,
not less than 9.0% precipitable with hide
powder. *Foreign matter*, not more than 2%.
Loss on drying, not more than 12%. *Ash*, not
more than 7.0%.
BHP 1983: *Total ash*, not more than 5%.
Acid-insoluble ash, not more than 1.5%.

Adulteration: Rarely happens. Occasionally,
hamamelis bark is "substituted" by that of
the hazel, *Corylus avellana* L. Anatomically,
the two barks differ in the thickness of the
cork cambium, which in *Hamamelis* comprises 10–12 and in *Corylus* fewer rows. The
cells of the cork cambium are thinner-walled
in *Hamamelis* and not as flat as in *Corylus*.

Storage: Protected from light and moisture.

Literature:
[1] F. Grüttner, Arch. Pharm. **236**, 278 (1898).
[2] K. Freudenberg and F. Blümel, Liebigs Ann. Chem.
    440, 45 (1924).
[3] R. Ganday, Pharm. J. **156**, 73 (1946).
[4] F. Loebich, Thesis, Heidelberg (1964).
[5] H. Friedrich and N. Krüger, Planta Med. **25**, 138
    (1974).
[6] H.A.D. Jowett and F.L. Pyman, Pharm. J. **91**, 129
    (1913).
[7] Hager, vol. **5**, 12 (1976); vol. **5**, 372 (1993).
[8] B.P. Jackson and D.W. Snowdon, Atlas of microscopy
    of medicinal plants, culinary herbs and spices, Bel-
    haven Press, London, 1990, p. 246.

Hamamelidis folium   Witch hazel leaf

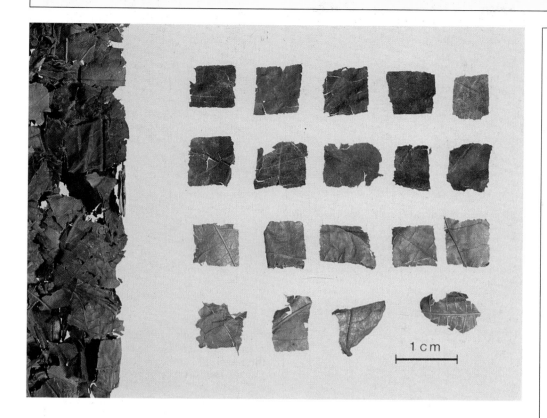

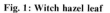
1 cm

Fig. 1: Witch hazel leaf

<u>Description</u>: The thin, somewhat leathery, pliable leaves and fragments of leaves have an entire or jagged and undulate margin. The upper surface is dark green and the lower surface light greyish green and shiny. A prominent midrib and distinct lateral nerves are joined by a series of fine nerves at right angles. Only the lower surface is pubescent, in the angles of the nerves. Numerous punctiform protuberances can be seen with a hand lens.

<u>Taste</u>: Weakly astringent.

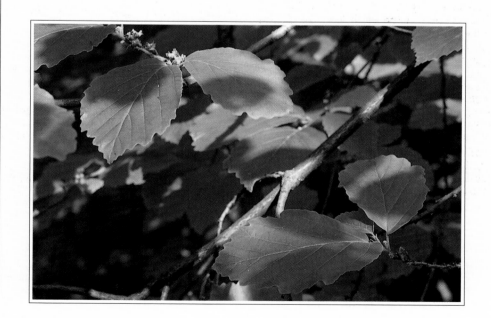

Fig. 2: *Hamamelis virginiana* L.

An up to 7 m tall shrub with broadly ovate leaves. Small yellow flowers with long corolla tips, first appearing in the autumn.

DAC 1986: Hamamelisblätter
Ph. Helv. VII: Hamamelidis folium
St. Zul. 9699.99.99

Plant source: *Hamamelis virginiana* L., witch hazel (Hamamelidaceae).

Synonyms: Hamamelis leaf (Engl.), Hamamelisblätter, Virginische Zaubernußblätter, Hexenhaselblätter (Ger.), Feuilles d'hamamélis, Feuilles du noisetier de la sorcière (Fr.).

Origin: Native to eastern North America (New Brunswick, Quebec to Minnesota, south to Florida, Louisiana, and Texas); in Europe, the plant is cultivated to a limited extent. Imports come from North America.

Constituents: 3–10% Tannins (a mixture of gallotannins, condensed catechins, and procyanidins), free gallic acid and hamamelose; choline; saponins (?); resins (?) [1–3]. According to [3], the leaves do not contain hamamelitannin (=digalloylhamamelose); various flavone glycosides (with myricetin, quercetin, and kaempferol as aglycones) [4]. 0.01–0.50% Essential oil [5, 6], comprising up to ca. 40% alcohols, up to ca. 15% esters, and up to 25% carbonyl compounds (*n*-hex-2-en-1-al, acetaldehyde, α- and β-ionone, 6-methylhepta-3,5-dien-2-one), and safrole [6]. – The "hamamelin" reported in the literature for witch hazel leaf [e.g. 3] is a preparation obtained by precipitating a concentrated alcoholic extract of the powdered leaves with water.

Indications: In the form of an infusion, as an astringent in supportive therapy for acute diarrhoea (and dysentery) in school children and adults. As a gargle in inflammation of the mouth and throat, especially when accompanied by inflammation of the gums. In *folk medicine*, the drug is used additionally in menorrhagia and dysmenorrhoea as a haemostyptic, and there are similar uses in homoeopathy: in haemorrhage, varicose veins, haemorrhoids, meno- and metrorrhagia, dysmenorrhoea, and haemoptysis. Total extracts, such as hamamelis extracts or distillates from flowering branches freshly collected in the late autumn ("hazeline", witchhazel water), dry extracts of the leaves ("green hamamelin") and bark ("brown hamamelin") [3] are applied in the form of infusions, ointments, or suppositories, far more often than teas made from the leaves or bark. Therapeutically, they are used for their astringent [7], antiseptic [8], and haemostatic [5] properties, and especially for their ability to increase blood-vessel tonus [8, 9], properties which have been demonstrated in animal experiments. Hence their use against haemorrhoids, varicose veins

(varicose ulcers of the tibia), local inflammation of the mucous membranes with swelling, and superficial skin damage, e.g. fissures and cracks; it is also used in face lotions.

Side effects: In susceptible patients, occasionally irritation of the stomach may occur. In rare cases, witch hazel tannins may cause liver damage.

Making the tea: Boiling water is poured over 1–2 g of the finely chopped drug, allowed to stand for 10 min., and strained. For mild diarrhoea, a cupful two or three times a day, but not for a prolonged period.
For inflammation of the mucous membranes of the mouth, the infusion can be used as a mouthwash or gargle several times a day.
1 Teaspoon = ca. 0.5 g (cf. the St.Zul.).

Herbal preparations: Witch hazel leaf and bark are present in a few haemorrhoid teas and antiphlebitis remedies.

Phytomedicines: Witch hazel preparations (from the leaves, bark, flowering branches) are found on their own or together with other drugs from the Rote Liste® under Skin Preparations, e.g. Hametum-Extrakt; wound preparations, e.g. Hamasana, Hametum-Salbe (ointment); haemorrhoid preparations, e.g. Hametum-Suppositorien (suppositories), Anisan-Suppositorien and -Salbe; phlebitis remedies, often together with aescin or extracts of horse chestnut, e.g. Aescuven-Dragees, Cycloven-Tropfen, Venotrulan-Tropfen (drops).
Among the available UK products are Potter's Adiantine, Potter's Varicose Ointment, and Arkopharma Phytovarix capsules; one of the better known US preparation is Tucks®.

Regulatory status (UK): General Sales List – Schedule 1, Table B (external use only).

Authentication: Macro- (see: Description) and microscopically according to the DAC 1986; see also the BHP 1983. The yellowish brown, unevenly thickened, stellate covering trichomes (Fig. 3), which are located on the larger leaf nerves, and the scattered, thick-walled, at most slightly branched, occasionally irregular, lignified stone cells (idioblasts), present in the mesophyll and often extending from the upper to the lower epidermis (Fig. 4), are particularly diagnostic. For the microscopy of powdered witch hazel leaf, see [11].
The DAC 1986 includes TLC examination of tannins. A method for the quantitative determination of the tannins and free gallic acid in spray-dried hamamelis-leaf extracts is given in [10]; it is based on densitometric estimation after TLC separation of the components. Possible methods for examining the volatile constituents of witch hazel leaf and its preparations obtained by steam distillation are discussed in [11]. They are based on the quantitative determination of the essential oil and TLC of the 2,4-dinitrophenylhydrazones of some of the carbonyl compounds; the DAC 1986 also uses this method.

Quantitative standards: DAC 1986: *Tannins*, not less than 5.0% precipitable with hide powder. *Foreign matter*, not more than 7% woody parts and not more than 2% other foreign matter. *Loss on drying*, 9.0%. *Ash*, not more than 7.0%.
Ph. Helv. VII: *Tannins*, not less than 5.5%. *Foreign matter*, not more than 7% woody branches; other foreign matter, not more than 2% (hazel leaves; see: Adulteration, below). *Sulphated ash*, not more than 8.0%.
BHP 1983: *Foreign organic matter*, not more than 2%. *Content of stalks*, not more than

6.1 Uses

In supportive therapy for acute, non-specific diarrhoea in school children and adults. Inflammation of the gums and mucous membranes of the mouth.

6.2 Side effects

In susceptible patients, occasionally stomach upsets may ensue after taking preparations of witch hazel leaf. The leaf contains tannins which in rare cases may cause liver damage.

6.3 Dosage and Mode of administration

Boiling water (ca. 150 ml) is poured over a teaspoonful (2–3 g) of **Witch hazel leaf** and after about 10 min. passed through a tea strainer.

Unless otherwise prescribed, a cup of the freshly prepared infusion is drunk two or three times a day between meals.

For inflammation of the gums and mucous membranes of the mouth, the infusion is used as a mouthwash several times a day.

6.4 Duration of use

If the diarrhoea persists for more than 3 or 4 days, a doctor should be consulted.

6.5 Note

Store protected from light and moisture.

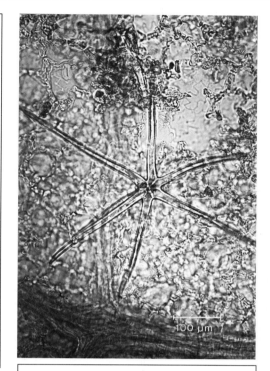

Fig. 3: Stellate trichome from the lower epidermis of a witch hazel leaf

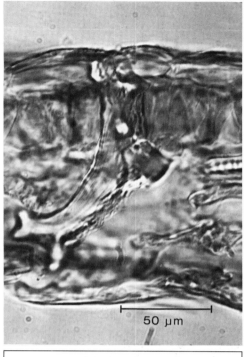

Fig. 4: Transverse section of a leaf with an irregular, slightly branched stone cell (idioblast) extending from the upper to the lower epidermis

3%. *Total ash*, not more than 7%. *Acid-insoluble ash*, not more than 0.04%.

Adulteration: Occasionally, by hazel leaves (Coryli folium, from *Corylus avellana* L.). The distinguishing characters are: the cordate, symmetrical lamina, the doubly serrate margin, the acuminate tip of the otherwise roundish leaf, the larger number of lateral nerves branching off from the midrib (8–10 on each half of the leaf), the pubescence which comprises unicellular trichomes on the lamina and petiole, small multicellular glandular trichomes on the nerves, and glandular trichomes with multicellular stem and head on the petiole. In the mesophyll of *Corylus* there are occasional rosettes of calcium oxalate crystals, but the slightly branched and lignified stone cells (idioblasts) characteristic of witch hazel leaf are absent.

Storage: Store away from light and moisture. When used as a herbal drug, witch hazel leaf should not be older than a year (loss of essential oil; conversion of the tannins to inactive phlobaphenes).

Literature:

[1] R. Ganday, Pharm. J. **156**, 73 (1946).
[2] H. Friedrich and N. Krüger, Planta Med. **26**, 327 (1974).
[3] Hager, vol. **5**, p. 9 (1976); vol. **5**, p. 376 (1993).
[4] K. Egger and H. Reznik, Planta **57**, 239 (1961).
[5] H. Neugebauer, Pharmazie **3**, 313 (1948).
[6] W. Messerschmidt, Arzneimittel.Forsch. **18**, 161 (1968).
[7] E. Keeser et al., Naunyn-Schmiedebergs Arch. Exper. Pathol. Pharmakol. **180**, 557 (1936).
[8] P. Bernard et al., J. Pharm. Belg. **27**, 505 (1972).
[9] P. Bernard, Plantes Méd. Phytothérap. **11** (no. spécial) (1977).
[10] M. Vanhaelen and R. Vanhaelen-Fastre, J. Chromatogr. **281**, 263 (1983).
[11] W. Messerschmidt, Dtsch, Apoth. Ztg. **111**, 299 (1971).
[12] B.P. Jackson and D.W. Snowdon, Atlas of microscopy of medicinal plants, culinary herbs and spices, Belhaven Press, London, 1990, p. 248.

Harpagophyti radix   (DAB 10), Devil's claw (BHP 1990)

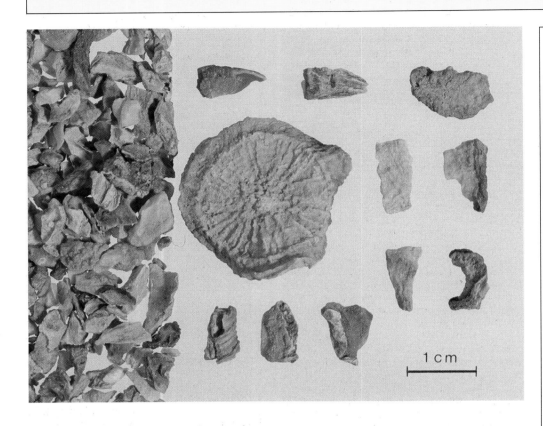

Fig. 1: Devil's claw

<u>Description:</u> The drug consists of the secondary storage roots (tubers of the lateral roots). The whole drug consists of cylindrical or tuberous, also often spindle-shaped, organs, up to 25 cm in length and up to 6 cm in diameter, which may weigh up to 500 g. They are covered by a yellowish grey to light rust-coloured, occasionally also medium brown, smooth periderm. Directly after harvesting, they are cut into slices which are then often reduced to sections, and mostly dried on the spot. The cut drug is very hard and its fracture is short, with the broken surface cartilaginous and light grey to whitish. Nowadays, devil's-claw root is mostly sold in small pieces or as a coarse powder [1, 2].

<u>Taste:</u> Very bitter.

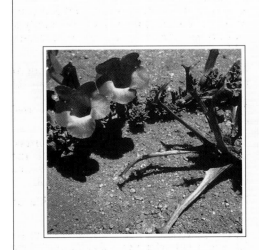
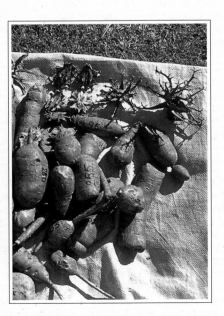

Fig. 2: *Harpagophytum procumbens* DC. ex MEISSN.

A plant with up to 1.5 m long branches lying flat on the ground. Opposite to alternate, petiolate and lobed leaves. Single, axillary, gloxinia-like, reddish violet flowers, ca. 5 cm in diameter. Woody fruits, ca. 15 cm fruits in diameter and covered with hook-shaped projections (hence the name). See Fig. 3, below.

Fig. 3: *Harpagophytum procumbens* DC. ex MEISSN.

Secondary storage roots, up to 6 cm thick and 20 cm long, and covered with a light-coloured to reddish brown cork; occurring within a circle up to 1.5 m in diameter and at a depth of 0.3–1.0 m. Lateral roots often forming more than one such storage organ.

Harpagoside: R = trans-Cinnamoyl
Harpagide: R = H

Procumbide

DAB 10: Teufelskrallenwurzel

Plant source: *Harpagophytum procumbens* DC. ex MEISSN. and *H. zeyheri* DECNE., devil's claw (Pedaliaceae).

Synonyms: Radix (Tubera) harpagophyti (Lat.), Grapple plant (Engl.), Teufelskralle, Trampelklette, Südafrikanische Teufelskrallenwurzel (Ger.), Tubercule de griffe du diable (Fr.).

Origin: Native to the Kalahari savannas of southern Africa and Namibia; it is collected in the wild and imported, and was first introduced into Europe by O.H. Volk in 1953.

Constituents: The secondary storage roots of both species [3] contain a range of iridoids and phenolic glycosides, mainly 0.1–2.0% of the iridoid glycoside harpagoside, a cinnamic-acid ester [4]; further, procumbide and its 6'-*O*-*p*-coumaroyl ester [13], harpagide (possibly a degradation product of harpagoside), and free cinnamic acid [4]; phenolic glycosides, including acteoside and isoacteoside, are also present [13]. The water-soluble extractive, which contains stachyose, raffinose, saccharose, glucose, etc. [5], may form as much as 70% of the dry weight of the drug; the bitterness value, determined by the DAB 10 method, ranges from 5,000 to 12,000 [4]. *n*-Alkanes, sterols, fats, and waxes, among other things, have also been detected in *H. procumbens*.

Indications: Clinical and pharmacological studies are scarce. Slight analgesic, antiphlogistic, and anti-arthritic effects of the whole extract have been demonstrated in animal experiments (e.g. in white rats with formaldehyde-induced arthritis [6]; cf. [7]).

More recent work with the aqueous extract (containing chiefly harpagoside) showed significant dose-dependent antiinflammatory and analgesic effects (carrageenan-induced oedema in rats and the writhing test in mice); harpagoside is not implicated in the anti-inflammatory action; but, along with other constituents, it does appear to be involved in the peripheral analgesic properties. However, loss of activity after treatment with 0.1N hydrochloric acid (as in the stomach) suggests the necessity of formulating appropriate galenical preparations to protect the active principles [14].

Beneficial results have been reported in the treatment of rheumatic conditions with subcutaneous lateral and medial injections of drug extracts on both sides of the knee joint [9]; it is, however, pointed out that it should not be used on its own, but rather as a supportive measure [15].

The bitter iridoids are certainly responsible for the use of the drug as a stomachic. Thus, in the book by R. F. Weiß it is indicated that a decoct of *Harpagophytum* is one of the strongest bitter tonics known [10]. Further investigations [11] have shown that drinking *Harpagophytum* tea over a period of several days – like Radix Gentianae – because of the bitter substances present (especially harpagoside), leads to a distinct improvement in the symptoms of disorders of the upper part of the small intestine which are accompanied by disturbances of choleresis and cholekinesis. A similar improvement brought about by the tea is noted in the reduction of the slightly raised serum bilirubin levels that are experienced in the hepatic cholestasis which often accompanies disorders of the small intestine and pancreas. The local enteritis in duodenal diverticulitis has also been successfully treated with the tea. – In *South African folk medicine*, the drug is used in digestive disorders as a bitter tonic, in blood disorders, as a febrifuge (doctrine of signatures, because it is bitter?), as an analgesic, and in complaints during pregnancy. A recent review concludes that because the drug is very bitter it is a good stomachic and stimulates the appetite and is therefore useful in dyspeptic complaints [15].

In Europe, the *folk medicinal* indications are: digestive complaints, arthritic, liver, bile, kidney, and bladder complaints, allergies, and general manifestations of ageing, but its use for these conditions, and the repeatedly mentioned use as an antidiabetic, have no clinical or scientific foundation [15]. – Reviews of research on devil's claw root, especially on the medicinal uses of the drug, are to be found in [2a, 2b]. For a summary of the pharmacology and toxicology of the drug, see [2a, 2b, 8, 15].

Extract from the German Commission E monograph (BAnz no. 43, dated 02. 03. 1989)

Uses
Lack of appetite, dyspeptic complaints; in supportive therapy for degenerative disorders of the locomotor system.

Contraindications
Gastric and duodenal ulcers.
With gallstones, to be used only after consultation with a doctor.

Side effects
None known.

Interactions with other remedies
None known.

Dosage
Unless otherwise prescribed, daily dose: for loss of appetite 1.5 g and preparations with an equivalent bitterness value; otherwise, 4.5 g drug and preparations correspondingly.

Mode of administration
Comminuted drug for infusions and other formulations for internal use.

Effects
Appetite-stimulating, choleretic, antiphlogistic, weakly analgesic.

Making the tea: Boiling water (ca. 300 ml) is poured over ca. 4.5 g of the finely chopped or coarsely powdered drug and allowed to stand at room temperature for 8 hours before being strained; the infusion is drunk in three portions in the course of the day.
1 Teaspoon = ca. 4.5 g.

Herbal preparations: The drug is marketed by several firms, usually under the name Teufelskrallen-Tee or Harpago-Tee.

Phytomedicines: In the form of powdered drug or extracts, devil's-claw root is a component of prepared remedies for a variety of indications and is available as capsules, tablets, tinctures, ointments, etc.

Authentication: Macro- (see: Description), microscopically, following [1]; see also the BHP 1/1990.
The following TLC procedure may be used as a test of identity [4]:

Test solution: 0.1 g powdered drug warmed with 10 ml methanol on the water-bath and filtered; 5 ml filtrate taken to dryness and the residue dissolved in 1 ml methanol.

Reference solution: 1 mg harpagoside in 1 ml methanol.

Loadings: 10 and 20 µl test solution and 10, 20, and 40 µl reference solution, as 1.5 cm bands on silica gel GF$_{254}$.

Solvent system: chloroform + methanol (90 + 30), 15 cm run in a saturated tank.

Detection and **Evaluation:** after drying, in UV 254 nm light. Test solution: greyish quenching bands on a yellowish green fluorescent layer. Then sprayed with 1% dimethylaminobenzaldehyde in 2N hydrochloric acid, followed by heating at 105 °C for 15 min. Test solution: iridoids as bluish grey bands, with harpagoside at Rf ca. 0.5. The TLC examination required by the BHP 1990 makes use of the solvent system: ethyl acetate + methanol + water (77 + 15 + 8), with rutin as the reference substance and vanillin/sulphuric acid as the spray. A coloured illustration of the chromatogram is given in [16]; this reference also illustrates a chromatogram run in: ethyl acetate + formic acid + glacial acetic acid + water (100 + 11 + 11 + 26), and then sprayed with anisaldehyde/sulphuric acid reagent; neohesperidin is the reference compound used.

A simpler spot test for *Harpagophytum* roots is as follows [12]: Parts of the parenchyma of the primary and secondary storage roots are stained green with phloroglucinol/hydrochloric acid. This test can also be carried out on the powdered drug; see the BHP 1/1990. Differentiation of the primary and secondary storage roots on the basis of their harpagoside content requires previous accurate quantitative analysis of this iridoid [4]. For the microscopical differentiation, see [1].

Quantitative standards: DAB 10: *Harpagoside,* not less than 1.0%. *Foreign matter,* not more than 2%. *Loss on drying,* not more than 10.0%. *Ash,* not more than 8.0%.
Ph. Helv. VII: *Harpagoside,* not less than 1.2% (M_r 494.5).
BHP 1/1990: *Water-soluble extractive,* not less than 50%. *Foreign matter,* not more than 2%. *Total ash,* not more than 22%. *HCl-insoluble ash,* not more than 2%.

Adulteration: Occasionally with the harpagoside-poor primary roots, extracted secondary roots, and intensely bitter-tasting roots of other African plants, e.g. *Elephantorrhiza* sp. (Mimosaceae) and *Acanthosicyos naudinianus* (SOND.) C. JEFFREY (Cucurbitaceae).

Storage: Protected from moisture in well-closed containers.

Literature:
[1] O.H. Volk, Dtsch. Apoth. Ztg. **104**, 573 (1964).
[2a] F.-C. Czygan, Z. Phytotherap. **8**, 17 (1987).
[2b] M. Vanhaelen, Phytotherapy **16**, 19 (1985).
[3] F.-C. Czygan and A. Krüger, Planta Med. **31**, 305 (1977).
[4] F.-C. Czygan, A. Krüger, W. Schier, and O. H. Volk, Dtsch. Apoth. Ztg. **117**, 1431 (1977). Here, further literature, including that relating to P. Tunmann's group (Würzburg), who were the first to study the phytochemistry of *Harpagophytum procumbens* in detail.
[5] K.H. Ziller and G. Franz, Planta Med. **37**, 340 (1979).
[6] B. Zorn, Z. Rheumaforsch. **17**, 135 (1958).
[7] O. Eichler and C. Koch, Arzneimittel.Forsch. **20**, 107 (1970).
[8] A. Erdös, R. Fontaine, H. Friehe, R. Durand, and Th. Pöppinghaus, Planta Med. **34**, 97 (1978).
[9] S. Schmidt, Therapiewoche **13**, 1072 (1972).
[10] R.F. Weiß, Herbal Medicine, Arcanum, Gothenburg, and Beaconsfield Publishers, Beaconsfield, 1988.
[11] W. Zimmermann, 33. Dtsch. Kongr. für ärztl. Fortbildung, Berlin, 1984.
[12] W. Schier and H. Bauersfeld, Dtsch. Apoth. Ztg. **113**, 795 (1973).
[13] J.F.W. Burger, E.V. Brandt, and D. Ferreira, Phytochemistry **26**, 1453 (1987).
[14] M.-C. Lanhers et al., Planta Med. **58**, 117 (1992).
[15] R. Jaspersen-Schib, Dtsch. Apoth. Ztg. **130**, 71 (1990).
[16] H. Wagner, S. Bladt, and E.M. Zgainski, Plant drug analysis, Springer-Verlag, Berlin, Heidelberg, New York, Tokyo, 1984, pp. 132–133.

Hederae folium   Ivy leaf

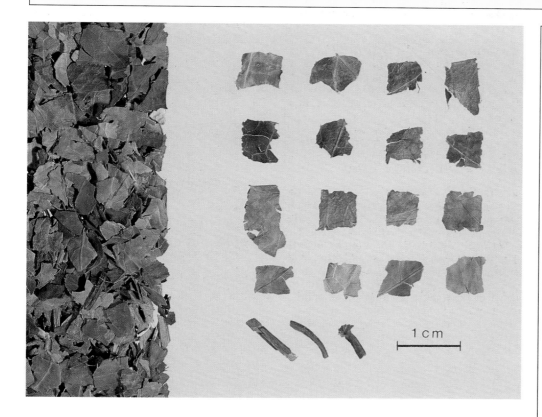

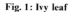

1 cm

Fig. 1: Ivy leaf

<u>Description</u>: The 3–5-lobed leaves, with more or less triangular lobes, collected between spring and early summer from the non-flowering shoots in the lower reaches of the evergreen woody plant are the part used as the drug. The 4–10 cm long and equally wide, dark green, shiny leaves are cordate at the base; they are firm and leathery, with a white, fan-like nervature which is easily recognized in the cut drug on the lower surface. Young leaves are pubescent, older ones glabrous. Occasionally, the ovate-rhombic to lanceolate leaves with a long acumen and an entire margin, which are found on the flowering shoots from the upper part of the plant, are collected along with the rest; the dark green petiole is mostly round and longitudinally grooved.

<u>Odour</u>: Faint, characteristic, and somewhat musty.

<u>Taste</u>: Bland, mucilaginous, somewhat bitter, and slightly irritating.

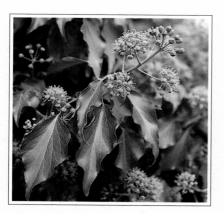

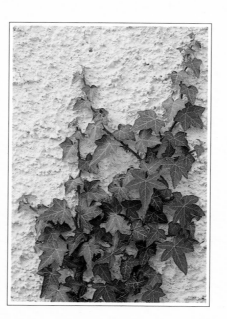

Fig. 2: *Hedera helix* L., flowering branch

For the description, see Fig. 3; flowers pale green; fruit green when unripe, blue-black when ripe.

Fig. 3: *Hedera helix* L.

A climbing plant with evergreen leaves, up to 20 m in height. Dimorphous leaves: on non-flowering branches, 3–5-lobed with a white fan-like nervature; on branches with flowers, rhombic to lanceolate (Fig. 2).

Plant source: *Hedera helix* L., ivy (Araliaceae).

Synonyms: Folia Hederae helicis (Lat.), Woodbind (Engl.), Efeublätter, Totenranke (Ger.), Lierre commun (Fr.).

Origin: Native in western, central, and southern Europe, occurring scattered in the north and east, and in the Mediterranean region. The drug is imported from eastern European countries.

Constituents: Ca. 2.5–6% saponins, comprising the hederagenin glycosides hederacoside C (the main component, up to ca. 5%) and α-hederin (= helixin) (ratio 18 : 1 to 13 : 1) and the oleanolic-acid glycosides hederacoside B and β-hederin, as well as a saponin which differs from hederacoside C only in the absence of the rhamnose at C-3 [1]; the flavonol glycosides rutin and kaempferol 3-rutinoside; traces of the alkaloid emetine; the polyacetylenes falcarinone and falcarinol; the sterols stigmasterol, sitosterol, cholesterol, campesterol, α-spinasterol, and 5α-stigma-7-en-3β-ol; scopolin, chlorogenic acid, caffeic acid, the sesquiterpene hydro- carbons germacrene, β-elemene, and elixin [1–5].

Indications: As an expectorant, secretolytic (saponins), and antispasmodic in whooping cough, spastic bronchitis, and chronic

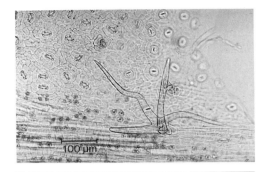

Fig. 4: Lower epidermis of a young leaf showing a stellate trichome, stomata, and clusters of calcium oxalate

catarrh. Whether the small amounts of emetine present are involved in the secretolytic action has yet to be clarified. The substances responsible for the spasmolytic effects that have been demonstrated with leaf extracts *in vitro* [3] are still unknown. In *folk medicine*, ivy leaf is also used for arthritis, rheumatism, and scrofula, and decoctions are applied externally against parasitic conditions (lice, scabies, pyodermias) and to sores and burns. The hedera saponins are antimycotic, antibacterial, an-

thelmintic, and antiprotozoic [3–6]. The polyacetylenes falcarinone and falcarinol are also antimycotic [7], and the latter substance has been shown to have antibacterial, analgesic, and sedative effects as well [8].

Side effects: Fresh ivy leaves and the leaf sap can cause allergic contact dermatitis [9–11]. Falcarinol has been identified as an allergen [4].

Making the tea: Rarely done. Boiling water is poured over ca. 0.5 g of the drug, allowed to stand for 10 min., then strained. For coughs, catarrh, and colds, a cupful (if desired, sweetened with honey) is drunk one to three times a day.
1 Teaspoon = ca. 0.8 g.

Phytomedicines: Nowadays, the drug itself is an infrequent component present in a few cough and bronchial teas, including Bad Heilbrunner Husten- and Bronchial-Tee. Extracts are chiefly used, in prepared remedies such as Prospan®, Hedelix® and Bronchoforton®.

Authentication: Macro- (see: Description) and microscopically. The upper epidermis has a thick cuticle, lacks stomata, and in surface view the cells are seen to have stout and strongly sinuate walls. The lower epidermis has numerous anomocytic stomata (a few may be anisocytic instead) and in surface view the cell have white, sinuate to angular walls; near the stomata there are faint cuticular striations and occasional stellate

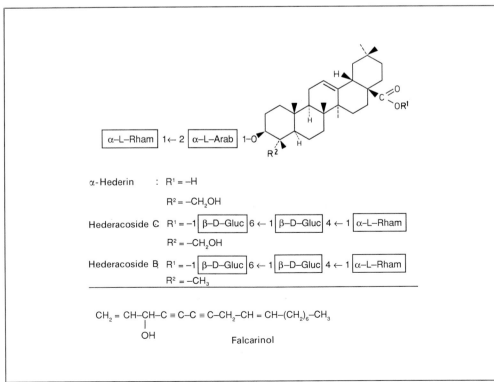

α-Hederin : R^1 = –H

R^2 = –CH$_2$OH

Hederacoside C R^1 = –1 β–D–Gluc 6 ← 1 β–D–Gluc 4 ← 1 α–L–Rham

R^2 = –CH$_2$OH

Hederacoside B R^1 = –1 β–D–Gluc 6 ← 1 β–D–Gluc 4 ← 1 α–L–Rham

R^2 = –CH$_3$

$$CH_2 = CH–CH–C \equiv C–C \equiv C–CH_2–CH = CH–(CH_2)_6–CH_3$$
OH

Falcarinol

trichomes are present (Fig. 4). A cross section of the leaf shows 2 (1–3) rows of palisade cells and a very porous spongy parenchyma; in both layers there are clusters of calcium oxalate crystals, ca. 40 μm in diameter, and a few mucilage cells.

Proof of identity can also be established by TLC examination of the saponins using the method given in [12] or [13]; the latter method is as follows:

Test solution: 2 g powdered drug refluxed with 10 ml 70% ethanol, filtered, and the clear filtrate evaporated to 5 ml.

Reference solution: 0.1% *β*-hederin in methanol.

Loadings: 25–40 μl test solution and 10 μl reference solution, as bands on silica-gel GF$_{254}$.

Solvent system: chloroform + methanol + water (64 + 50 + 10), 15 cm run.

Detection: vanillin/phosphoric acid reagent (1 g vanillin in 100 ml 50% acid, or 2 parts 24% acid to 8 parts 2% ethanolic vanillic acid), followed by heating at 100 °C for 10 min.

Evaluation: in daylight. Test solution: violet or blue-black zones – hederin at Rf ca. 0.75 and hederacoside mixture at Rf ca. 0.4–0.6; see coloured illustration of the chromatogram in [13].

HPLC analysis is also possible [1].

Adulteration: Scarcely ever occurs.

Literature:

[1] H. Wagner and Reger, Dtsch. Apoth. Ztg. **126**, 2613 (1986).

[2] J. Reymond and J. Reymond, Plantes Méd. Phytothérap. **16**, 318 (1982).

[3] H. Mayer, A. Pfandl, A. Grigorieff, and I. Zickner, Pharm. Ztg. **132**, 2673 (1987).

[4] P.M. Boll and L. Hansen, Phytochemistry **26**, 2955 (1987).

[5] J.R. Hillman, B.A. Knights, and R. Mehail, Lipids **10**, 542 (1975).

[6] J.M. Gasquet, C. Maillard, G. Balansard, and P. Timon-David, Planta Med. **51**, 205 (1985).

[7] L. Hansen and P.M. Boll, Phytochemistry **25**, 285 (1986).

[8] S. Tanaka and Y. Ikeshiro, Arzneimittel.Forsch. **27**, 2039 (1977).

[9] J. Boyle and R.M.H. Harman, Contact Derm. **12**, 111 (1985).

[10] G. Hahn and M. Hahn, Österr. Apoth. Ztg. **36**, 954 (1982).

[11] C.D. Calnan, Contact Derm. **7**, 124 (1981).

[12] Kommentar DAB 7 – DDR, Akademie Verlag, Berlin, 1969.

[13] H. Wagner, S. Bladt, and E.M. Zgainski, Plant drug analysis, Springer-Verlag, Berlin, Heidelberg, New York, Tokyo, 1984, p. 242.

Helenii rhizoma
Elecampane (BHP 1/1990)

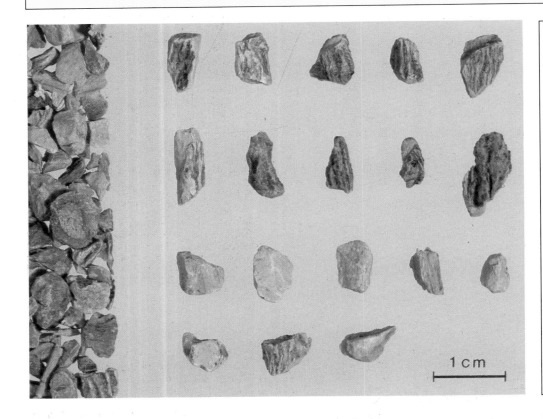

1 cm

Fig. 1: Elecampane

Description: Elecampane consists of the broken roots, rhizomes, and lateral roots obtained from 2–3 year old cultivated plants. The drug is usually supplied as greyish brown, hard, and horny pieces which are longitudinally wrinkled on the outside and which have a short and fibrous fracture showing a dark brown cambium line and glistening because of the presence of numerous resin cells.

Odour: Characteristically aromatic.

Taste: Spicy and bitter.

Fig. 2: *Inula helenium* L.

A herb up to 2.5 m in height with broadly lanceolate, irregularly toothed leaves. Flowering heads up to 7 cm in diameter, with numerous very narrow ligulate florets and many small tubular florets.

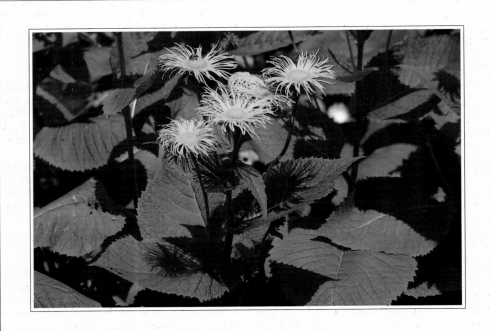

Erg. B. 6: Rhizoma Helenii

Plant source: *Inula helenium* L., elecampane (Asteraceae).

Synonyms: Rhizoma Helenii, Radix Inulae, Radix Enulae (Lat.), Elecampane root, Inula, Scabwort (Engl.), Alantwurzelstock (Ger.), Rhizome d'aunée (Fr.).

Origin: Indigenous in southern and eastern Europe; naturalized in central Europe, the Near East, and North America. The drug is derived from cultivated plants and present-day imports come mainly from China, the former USSR, and Bulgaria, and also the USA.

Constituents: Sesquiterpene lactones (bitter substances): the eudesmanolides alantolactone, isoalantolactone, 11,13-dihydroalantolactone, 4,5-dihydro-5,6-dehydroalantolactone (= 1-desoxy-8-*epi*-ivangustin), and others, and also germacrene D-lactone. The mixture of alanto-lactones is also known as helenin or elecampane camphor. Ca. 1–3%

Alantolactone

Isoalantolactone

Germacrene-D-lactone

8,9-Epoxy-10-isobutyryloxy-thymol isobutyrate

Dammaranedienol

Extract from the German Commission E monograph (BAnz No. 85, dated 05. 05. 1988)

Uses

Elecampane preparations are used for complaints and problems affecting the respiratory and gastrointestinal tracts, as well as the kidneys and lower urinary tract.
The activity of the drug in the areas indicated has not been fully established.

Risks

The sesquiterpene lactones present in elecampane (the main component is alantolactone) irritate the mucous membranes. They are sensitizing and cause allergic contact dermatitis. Alantolactone is bound as a hapten to the proteins of the skin: the adduct induces hypersensitivity to alantolactone and other compounds with a α-methylene-γ-lactone (cross-reaction).
Large amounts of the drug lead to vomiting, diarrhoea, cramps, and symptoms of paralysis.

Evaluation

Since the activity of the drug and its preparations in the areas indicated has not been adequately substantiated, in view of the risks of an allergy its therapeutic use cannot be justified.

essential oil containing alantolactone and its degradation products (alantol, alantic acid) as principal components, along with sesquiterpene hydrocarbons (including β-elemene). Polyacetylenes, aliphatic hydrocarbons (including nonacosane), 8,9-epoxy-10-isobutyryloxythymol isobutyrate. Triterpenes: friedelin, dammaranedienol and its acetate. Sterols: β-sitosterol and its glucoside, stigmasterol. Up to 44% inulin, together with various degradation products.

Indications: Antiseptic expectorant in bronchial catarrh, whooping cough (and irritating cough), and bronchitis. In *folk medicine*, the drug, which is grouped with the bitter aromatics, is further used as a stomachic, carminative, and cholagogue (among other things, the action of the bitter substances), as well as a diuretic, anthelmintic, and in menstrual complaints. Externally (as bandages) in exanthema and other skin conditions, especially as an antiseptic.

The secretolytic, choleretic, and diuretic actions of the drug have been confirmed experimentally and clinically [1, 2]. The active substances are alantolactone, isoalantolactone, and the other sesquiterpene lactones. They have an exomethylene group on the γ-lactone ring, which is an important structural feature in bringing about various pharmacological effects. Compounds of this kind have antiphlogistic and antibiotic actions [3, 4]. Alantolactone and isoalantolactone have been shown, both *in vitro* and *in vivo*, to have antifungal [5, 6] and antitumour [7] activity. The minimum inhibitory concentration for human pathogenic fungi (*Epidermophyton, Trichophyton* species) is about 15–35 µg/ml.

Alantolactone increases the tonus of the rabbit small intestine at a dilution of 1:800,000 and it completely paralyses its spontaneous contractions at a dilution of 1:100,000. As with other sesquiterpene lactones, an increase in uterine tonus cannot be excluded. No vermicidal (worm-killing) activity against porcine ascarides has been demonstrated, although a vermifugal (worm-repelling) action was found in cats dosed with 0.15–0.20 g alantolactone mixture.

Side effects: The alantolactones irritate the mucous membranes. They sensitize and bring about allergic contact dermatitis [e.g. 8, 9]. It has been shown experimentally that alantolactone is bound to the proteins of the skin as a hapten and also that the alantolactone-skin protein adduct can induce hypersensitivity to alantolactone and other α-methylene-γ-lactone systems (cross-reaction) [10]. Alantolactone (1 mg/ml) exhibits toxic effects in *in-vitro* leucocyte cultures [11]. Large doses of the drug lead to vomit-

ing, diarrhoea, cramps, and symptoms of paralysis. About the biological and pharmacological effects of sesquiterpene lactones, see [12–14].

Making the tea: Boiling water is poured over 1 g of the coarsely powdered drug and after 10–15 min. passed through a tea strainer. As an expectorant, a cupful, if desired sweetened with honey, is drunk three or four times a day.
1 Teaspoon = ca. 4 g.

Phytomedicines: Elecampane or its extracts are incorporated into prepared antitussives and expectorants, cholagogues and biliary remedies, diuretics, arthritis remedies, laxatives, gastrointestinal remedies, roborants and tonics, and alteratives.
Among the UK multi-ingredient products containing elecampane extract are Potter's Vegetable Cough Remover and Potter's Horehound and Aniseed Cough Mixture (both liquids).

Regulatory status (UK): General Sales List – Schedule 1, Table A.

Authentication: Macro- (see: Description) and microscopically; see also the BHP 1/1990 monograph, which in addition describes the powdered drug. The absence of starch is diagnostic (asteraceous drugs). In cross-section, numerous oval to round resin glands, up to 200 μm in diameter and often containing needle crystals of alantolactone, can be seen in the cortex, medullary rays, and pith. Inulin masses are present in the parenchyma cells (histochemical detection with 1-naphthol/sulphuric acid reagent).

The following TLC examination can provide further support for the identification:

Test solution: 25 g drug placed in the apparatus for the determination of essential oils, with 0.5 ml xylene in the graduated side tube, and distilled with 250 ml water for ca. 2 h; essential oil-containing xylene solution carefully removed and diluted with a further 0.5 ml xylene.

Reference solution: 10 mg thymol dissolved in 10 ml methanol.

Loadings: 1 μl test solution and 5 μl reference solution, on silica gel.

Solvent system: toluene + ethyl acetate (97 + 3), 5 cm run.

Detection: sprayed with 5% ethanolic sulphuric acid and then 1% ethanolic vanillin, followed by heating for 3–5 min. at 105 °C.

Evaluation: in daylight immediately after heating. Reference solution: thymol as a red zone just below the middle. Test solution: an intense reddish violet to bluish violet zone in the same region; slightly below it, two violet zones and sometimes also a reddish violet one; above the main zone, two fainter violet zones; directly below the solvent front, a more intense violet zone (Fig. 3).

Another TLC identification procedure is to be found in the BHP 1/1990.

Quantitative standards: Erg. B. 6: *Volatile oil*, not less than 1.8%. *Ash*, not more than 6%.

BHP 1/1990: *Water-soluble extractive*, not less than 27%. *Foreign matter*, not more than 2%. *Loss on drying*, not more than

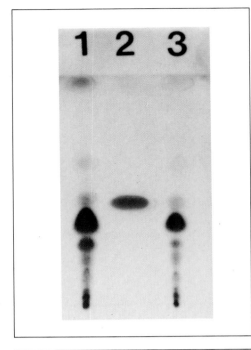

Fig. 3: TLC on 4 × 8 cm silica-gel foil

1 and 3: Elecampane root (of different origins)

2: Thymol (reference substance)

For details, see the text

14%. *Total ash*, not more than 8%. *HCl-insoluble ash*, not more than 1%.

Adulteration: Very rare. Belladonna roots – a dangerous admixture – are sometimes encountered, but are easily recognized by the lack of resin glands and the presence of cells with crystal sand.

TLC offers a good means of detection in doubtful cases:

Test solution: 1 g powdered drug briefly boiled with 10 ml methanol, solution cooled, and filtered.

Loading: 40 μl, as a 15 mm band on a 10 × 20 cm silica-gel plate, 10 cm run.

Solvent system: chloroform + ethanol (98 + 2).

Detection: after evaporation of the solvent, sprayed with 10% potassium hydroxide solution.

Evaluation: in UV 365 nm light. Test solution: when belladonna root is present, an intense bluish green fluorescent band is observed at Rf ca. 0.2; it should not be present in the case of elecampane.

Admixture of 0.5% belladonna root can be detected by this procedure.

Storage: Cool and protected from light and moisture, but **not** in plastic containers.

Literature:

[1] E. Schneider and H. Harms, Hippokrates **11**, 1061 (1940).
[2] H. Schindler, Arzneimittel.Forsch. **4**, 516 (1954).
[3] K.H. Lee, T. Ikuba, R.Y. Wu, and T.A. Geissman, Phytochemistry **16**, 1177 (1977).
[4] I.H. Hall et al., J. Pharm. Sci. **68**, 537 (1979).
[5] W. Olechnowicz-Stepien and S. Stepien, Diss. Pharm. **15**, 17 (1963).
[6] A.K. Picman, Biochem. Syst. Ecol. **11**, 183 (1983).
[7] H.J. Woerdenbag et al., Planta Med. **52**, 112 (1986).
[8] J.C. Mitchell, B. Fritig, B. Singh, and C.H.N. Towers, J. Invest. Derm. **54**, 233 (1970).
[9] J.L. Stampf, C. Benezra, H. Geleick, K. H. Schulz, and B. Hausen, Contact Dermatitis **8**, 16 (1982).
[10] G. Dupuis, C. Benezra, G. Schlewer, and J.-L. Stampf, Mol. Immunol. **17**, 1045 (1980).
[11] G. Dupuis and J. Brisson, Chem. Biol. Interactions **15**, 205 (1976).
[12] A.K. Picman, Biochem. Syst. Ecol. **14**, 255 (1986).
[13] G. Willuhn, Dtsch. Apoth. Ztg. **127**, 2511 (1987).
[14] B.M. Hausen, in: P.A.G.M. de Smet, K. Keller, R. Hänsel, and R.F. Chandler, Adverse effects of herbal drugs, Springer-Verlag, Berlin – Heidelberg – New York, 1992, vol. 1, p. 227.

Helichrysi flos   Helichrysum flower

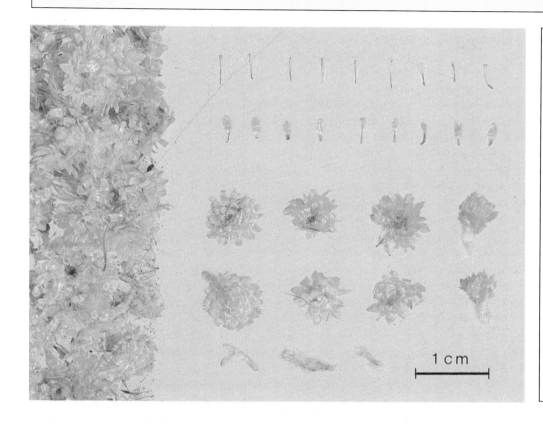

Fig. 1: Helichrysum flower

<u>Description:</u> The drug consists of the yellow flower-heads collected before opening which are borne on woolly pubescent peduncles and several of which are tangled together to give the appearance of false umbels. The straw-like, shiny, lemon-yellow, imbricate, and somewhat spreading involucral bracts enclosing the orange-yellow tubular (and very small ligulate) florets are characteristic. The latter are inconspicuous, since they have not opened; they have a light yellow pappus.

<u>Taste:</u> Slightly bitter, and spicy and aromatic.

Fig. 2: *Helichrysum arenarium* (L.) MOENCH

A ca. 20 cm tall perennial with conspicuous white, tomentose, lanceolate leaves. Small flower-heads arranged in cymes, comprising yellow tubular florets and bearing membranaceous involucral bracts.

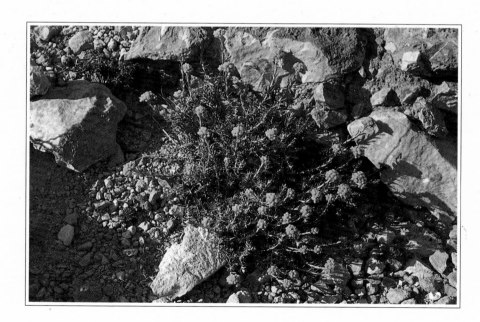

Ph. Helv. VII: Helichrysi flos
St. Zul. 1649.99.99 (Ruhrkrautblüten)

Plant source: *Helichrysum arenarium* (L.) MOENCH (Asteraceae).

Synonyms: Stoechados flos, Flores Gnaphalii arenarii (Lat.), Everlasting, Yellow chaste weed (Engl.), Katzenpfötchenblüten, Harnblumen (Ger.), Fleur de pied de chat (Fr.).

Origin: Native in central, eastern, and southern Europe. The drug is presumed to come entirely from collections made in the wild. The main suppliers are the former USSR, Poland, and Turkey.

Constituents: Flavonoids: ca. 0.4% isosalipurposide (a chalcone, responsible for the yellow colour of the involucral bracts), naringenin and its 5-*O*-diglucoside, the C(2) diastereoisomeric naringenin 5-*O*-glucosides helichrysin A and B (B = salipurposide), kaempferol glucosides, apigenin and its 7-*O*-glucoside, luteolin 7-*O*-glucoside, quercetin 3-*O*-glucoside, 3,5-dihydroxy-6,7,8-trime-

Fig. 3: Long, slender covering trichomes from the peduncle

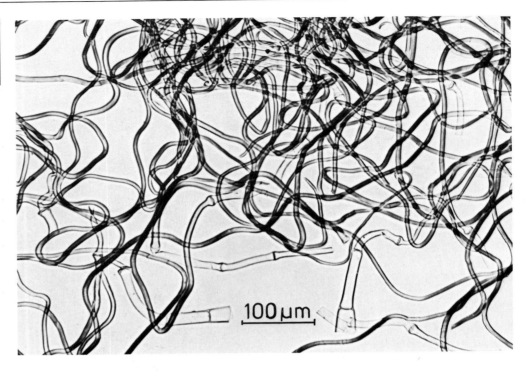

100 µm

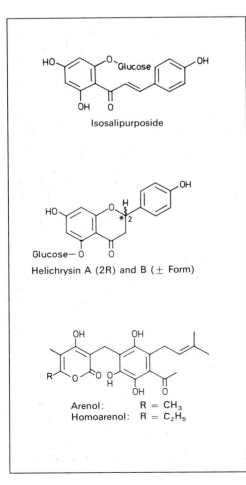

Isosalipurposide

Helichrysin A (2R) and B (± Form)

Glucose—O

Arenol: R = CH₃
Homoarenol: R = C₂H₅

thoxyflavone [1], etc. Ca. 0.05% essential oil; phthalides; small amounts of scopoletin, umbelliferone, and aesculetin [2]; the yellow-coloured pyranone derivatives arenol and homoarenol; a so far unidentified complex of antibiotic substances known as arenarin – bearing on this is the isolation from the aerial parts of other *Helichrysum* species, including *H. stoechas* (L.) MOENCH (see: Adulteration), of a group of phloroglucinol and acetophenone derivatives which appear to be related to arenol and which have activity against both gram positive and gram negative bacteria, as well as fungi [5]; bitter substances – these latter may be sesquiterpene lactones, typical asteraceous bitter substances which have already been detected in other species of *Helichrysum* (xanthanolides and guaianolides); campesterol and β-sitosterol glucuronic acid; tannins.

Indications: Helichrysum flower is often included simply to improve the appearance of various industrially-prepared herbal teas. Experimentally, a mild choleretic and spasmolytic effect (flavonoids?) has been observed in dogs [3]. The drug is therefore used as an adjuvant in the treatment of chronic cholecystitis and cramp-like gall-bladder disorders. In *folk medicine,* the drug is also employed as a diuretic.
The flowers contain antibacterial constituents (arenarin) [4] which are also said to promote gastric and pancreatic secretions; this may be due to the effect of the bitter substances (possibly sesquiterpene lactones).

Making the tea: Boiling water is poured over 1 g of the finely chopped drug and after 5–10 min. passed through a tea strainer.
1 Teaspoon = ca. 0.4 g.

Phytomedicines: As already mentioned, the drug is a frequent component of herbal mixtures, added simply to enhance the appearance. Extracts of the drug are included in some cholagogues, e.g. Aristochol® (drops).

Authentication: Careful macro- and microscopic examination is usually enough to identify and, at the same time, to exclude the presence of other *Helichrysum* species (see: Adulteration), which are used to some extent in the Mediterranean region as drugs. Good diagnostic features are the long, slender covering trichomes on the peduncle (Fig. 3), the unicellular club-shaped glandular trichomes on the ovary (Fig. 4), and the pappus hairs (Fig. 5).
A suitable TLC method for the identification is as follows:

Test solution: 1 g powdered drug refluxed with 20 ml methanol for 15 min. and, after cooling, filtered.

Reference solution: 5 mg each of quercetin, hyperoside, and rutin dissolved in 10 ml methanol.

Loadings: 3 µl test solution and 2 µ reference solution, as bands on silica gel.

Solvent system: ethyl acetate + anhydrous formic acid + water (88 + 6 + 6), 5 cm run.

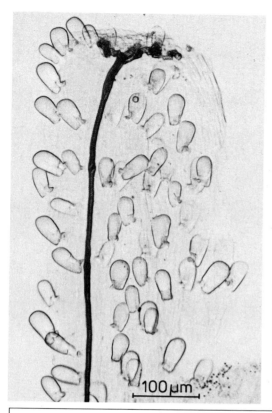

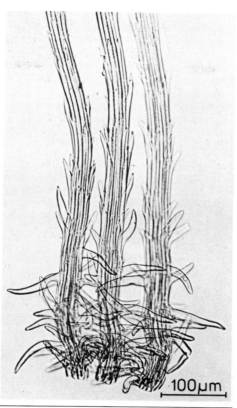

Fig. 4: Wall of the ovary with club-shaped glandular trichomes

Fig. 5: At the base, downy and fused pappus hairs

Extract from the German Commission E monograph (BAnz no. 122, dated 06. 07. 1988)

Uses

Dyspeptic disorders.

Contraindications

Occlusion of the biliary duct. When gall-stones are present, only after consultation with a doctor.

Side effects

None known.

Interactions with other remedies

None known.

Dosage

Unless otherwise prescribed: average daily dose, 3 g drug; preparations correspondingly.

Mode of administration

Comminuted drug for infusions and other galenical preparations for internal use.

Effects

Mildly choleretic.

Detection: after complete evaporation of the solvent in a stream of hot air, sprayed with a 0.5% solution of Fast Blue salt B and then with 10% methanolic potassium hydroxide.

Evaluation: in daylight. Reference substances: as reddish brown zones at Rf ca. 0.15 (rutin), ca. 0.40 (hyperoside), and ca. 0.90 (quercetin). Test solution: genuine drug – a zone (absent in adulterants) with an Rf in between those of hyperoside and quercetin, yellow before spraying and intense reddish brown after spraying; below it, two other reddish brown zones; when adulterated with other *Helichrysum* species, an entirely *different* picture – in particular, absence of the reddish brown spots mentioned above (Fig. 6).

The St.Zul. method chromatographs a methanol extract on silica gel HF$_{254}$ in the solvent system: ethyl acetate + anhydrous formic acid + water (83+6+6), with quercetin and apigenin monoglucoside as the reference substances; after spraying with 1% methanolic diboryloxyethylamine, the plate is evaluated in daylight.

In [6], the procedure indicated makes use of the solvent system: ethyl acetate + formic acid + glacial acetic acid + water (100+11+11+27), followed by spraying with 1% methanolic diboryloxyethylamine and overspraying with 5% ethanolic polyethylene glycol 400, and examination under UV 365 nm light; this reference includes a coloured illustration of the chromatogram obtained.

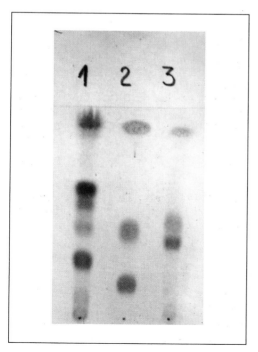

Fig. 6: TLC on 4 × 8 cm silica-gel foil

1: Helichrysum flower
2: Reference substances
3: Adulterant

For details, see the text

Quantitative standards: St.Zul. 1649.99.99: *Flavonoids*, not less than 0.5% calculated as quercetin. *Foreign matter*, not more than 2%; absence of flower-heads of *H. angustifolium* DC. and *H. stoechas* (see: Authentication). *Loss on drying*, not more than 10.0%. *Ash*, not more than 7.0%.

Ph. Helv. VII: *Foreign matter*, not more than 2%; absence of flower-heads of *H. italicum* (ROTH) GUSS. and *H. stoechas*. *Sulphated ash*, not more than 8.5%.

Adulteration: Occasionally, with the flower-heads of *H. stoechas* and *H. angustifolium*. Both these species have brownish yellow flowers (the genuine drug is bright yellow) and a more or less complete ring of ligulate florets (which in the genuine drug are very small). For their detection by means of TLC, see: Authentication.

Literature:
[1] A. H. Meriçli, B. Damadyan, and B. Çubukçu, Sci Pharm. **54**, 363 (1986).
[2] A.I. Derkach, N.F. Komissarenko, and V.T. Chernobai, Chem. Nat. Comp. **6**, 722 (1986).
[3] A. Szadowska, Acta Polon. Pharm. **19**, 465 (1962); C.A. **61**, 1136 (1964).
[4] K.G. Bel'tyukowa, Mikrobiol. Zh. (Kiev) **30**, 390 (1968); C.A. **70**, 35049 (1969).
[5] F. Tomás-Barberan, E. Iniesta-Sanmartín, F. Tomás-Lorente, and A. Rumbero, Phytochemistry **29**, 1093 (1990).
[6] H. Wagner, S. Bladt, and E.M. Zgainski, Plant drug analysis, Springer-Verlag, Berlin, Heidelberg, New York, Tokyo, 1984, p. 174.

Hennae folium Henna leaf

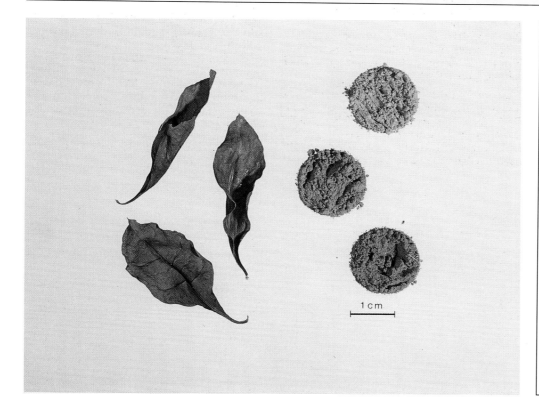

Fig. 1: Henna leaf

Commercially, the drug is encountered almost exclusively in the powdered form, sometimes mixed with other colorant drugs (see: Indications). The illustration shows (right) samples of readily available commercial powders with the following designations: "neutral" (top), "red-colouring" (middle), and "black" (bottom).
The leaf drug itself consists of 2–4 cm long, glabrous, entire, somewhat crumpled leaves with pinnate venation. The ovate-lanceolate lamina ends in a small mucro.

<u>Taste</u>: Not characteristic, somewhat astringent and bitter.

Plant source: *Lawsonia inermis* L. (syn. *L. inermis forma alba* LAM.), henna (Lythraceae).

Synonyms: Lawsoniae folium, Folia hennae (Lat.), Hennablätter, Ägyptisches Färbekraut (Ger.), Feuilles d'Henné (Fr.).

Origin: Presumably native in the Mediterranean region, the Near East, and India; it is cultivated throughout the Orient and is imported from India and Egypt.

Constituents: 1,4-Naphthoquinone-type pigments, including 1% lawsone (2-hydroxy-1,4-naphthoquinone); hydroxylated naphthalene derivatives, e.g. 4-glucosyloxy-1,2-dihydroxy- and 1,4-diglucosyloxy-2-hydroxynaphthalene; coumarins, xanthones, flavonoids, 5–10% tannins and some free gallic acid; small amounts of sterols, e.g. sitosterol. See [7].

Indications: In Europe, the plant is not used medicinally. In *folk medicine,* it is utilized as a diuretic and astringent: externally, against eczema, scabies, mycoses, and sores, and in-ternally, against amoebic dysentery and gastrointestinal ulcers. Henna is included in face lotions and hair rinses; and since ancient times it has been a hair and nail dye [1]. Because of its lawsone content, in Central Europe and the US, henna is nowadays applied especially as a hair dye. The powdered leaves are applied in the form of a paste, and on prolonged contact the hair acquires a strong and lasting colour. Hot water is used to prepare the paste. Sometimes, the addition of sour milk or lemon juice, or of red wine, is recommended in order to intensify the effect and to obtain a bronze tint. To optimize the colour and fix the dye, moist heat is required for the development of the colour. It is best to apply the paste hot and then wrap the head in towels. Henna on its own dyes normal brownish hair red, white hair light blond, ash-blond hair medium red, and chestnut-brown hair mahogany red. Dark brown hair acquires a red sheen. Henna does not dye black hair. Fairly weak henna preparations give a reddish shimmering effect to blond hair. In many cases, to obtain natural hair tints, a mixture of henna and indigo leaves (*Indigo tinctoria* L.) is applied. The blue colour of the indigo neutralizes the red colour of the natural henna and, depending on the amount and the time of contact, natural blond, brown, and deep black colours are produced [after 2, q.v. for recipes].

Phytomedicines: As a component of many hair-care products. A "neutral" or "non-colouring" henna is also available on the market. It is supposed to keep the natural colour of the hair and to make it shiny. "Neutral" henna should be tested for its "non-colouring" properties before use (see: Authentication).
About the adverse reaction arising from the addition of so-called "black powder", *p*-phenylene-diamine (*p*-diaminobenzene), to henna in order to speed up the dyeing process, see [5].

Authentication: Microscopically: The epidermal cells are polygonal and domed (bulliform). The nervature is pinnate and finely

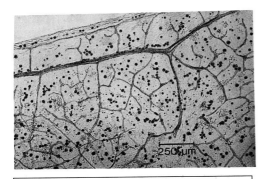

Fig. 2: The mesophyll of henna leaf, showing the pinnate, finely branched venation and numerous calcium-oxalate clusters of varying sizes

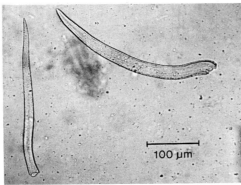

Fig. 4: Unicellular, thick-walled trichomes with a warty cuticle, from "neutral" and "black" henna powder

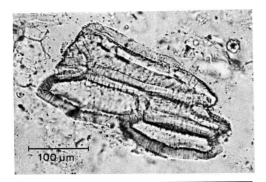

Fig. 3: Stone cells from the fruit wall (infrequent)

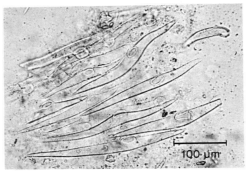

Fig. 5: T-shaped trichomes, from "black" henna powder

firm Caesar & Loretz (Hilden, Rhineland) recommends a simple test for the dyeing power: 5 g henna powder is stirred with 25 ml distilled water and then carefully brought to the boil. A strip of agar-agar is dipped halfway into the hot slurry and after 10 min. removed and washed well under the cold tap. The strip should be dyed a distinct reddish orange colour.

Reference [4] gives the following TLC method for the separation of lawsone, which can also be adapted for its photometric quantitative determination (by elution and measurement of the red colour produced with saturated sodium carbonate solution):

Test solution: an acidified sodium-carbonate extract of the leaves shaken with chloroform, the organic extract concentrated.

Stationary phase: silica gel G + aluminium oxide G $(1+1)$.

Solvent system: ethyl acetate + methanol + 5N ammonia solution $(60+15+5)$.

Evaluation: Reference solution: lawsone at Rf ca. 0.56.

Adulteration: Occasionally with senna leaves. These can be recognized by the characteristic trichomes, the isobilateral structure of the leaf, and the presence of a crystal sheath (see: Sennae folium).

Literature:
[1] Hager, vol. **5**, p. 468 (1976).
[2] Berger, vol. **2**, p. 158 (1950).
[3] M. Wellendorf, Arch. Pharm. Chem. **113**, 756, 800 (1956).
[4] M.S. Karawya, S.M. Abdel Wahhab, and A.Y. Zaki, Lloydia **32**, 76 (1969).
[5] P.F. D'Arcy, Adverse Drug React. Toxicol. Rev. **10**, 189 (1991).
[6] B.P. Jackson and D.W. Snowdon, Atlas of microscopy of medicinal plants, culinary herbs and spices, Belhaven Press, London, 1990, pp. 118–119.
[7] Y. Takeda and M.O. Fatope, J. Nat. Prod. **51**, 725 (1988).

branched, and the mesophyll contains numerous clusters of calcium oxalate of varying greatly in size (Fig. 2). There are occasional stone cells from the fruit wall (Fig. 3).

"Black" and "neutral" henna powders have unicellular, thick-walled trichomes (Fig. 4) and in "black" henna powder there are also T-shaped trichomes (Fig. 5). See also [6]. The

Herniariae herba   Rupturewort

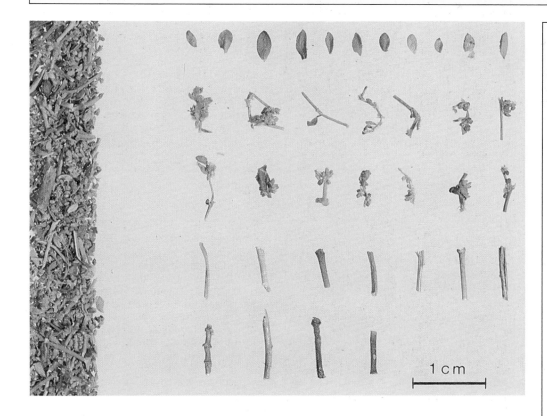

Fig. 1: Rupturewort

Description: All parts of the plants are very small. The terete, up to 2 mm thick, much-branched stems bear obovate, almost sessile, up to 7 mm long, thickish stipules, which are sparsely ciliate and membranaceous. The small 5-merous flowers occur as axillary clusters; very small achenes surrounded by the calyx are also present. In *Herniaria hirsuta* the stem, leaves, and flowers are greyish green and very hairy, while in *H. glabra* they are light green and almost glabrous (Fig. 3).

Odour: Pleasant, reminiscent of coumarin.

Taste: Somewhat acrid.

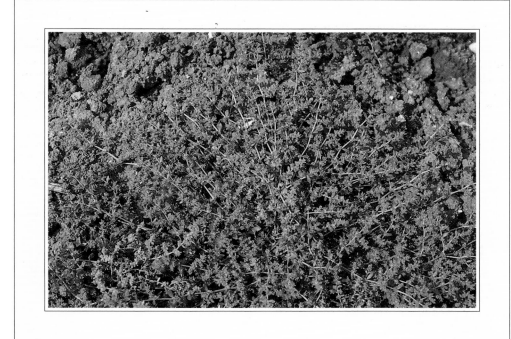

Fig. 2: *Herniaria glabra* L.

Bi- to perennial, mat-forming prostrate plants. All parts (leaves, flowers, fruit) very small.

DAC 1986: **Bruchkraut**
ÖAB: **Herba Herniariae**

Plant sources: *Herniaria glabra* L., smooth rupturewort, and *H. hirsuta* L., hairy rupturewort (Caryophyllaceae).

Synonyms: Herniary (Engl.), Bruchkraut, Harnkraut (Ger.), Herbe d'herniaire (Fr.).

Origin: *Herniaria glabra* occurs in temperate Europe and Asia, and *H. hirsuta* is found in the Mediterranean region, North Africa, and also in parts of Central Europe. The drug is mostly collected from the wild.

Constituents: 3–9% saponins, mainly derivatives of medicagenic acid, gypsogenic acid, and 16α-hydroxymedicagenic acid [1]; 0.2–1.2% flavonoids (isorhamnetin and quercetin derivatives); 0.1–0.4% coumarins (umbelliferone, herniarin, etc.); small amounts of tannin.

Indications: Based on the saponin and flavonoid content, as a diuretic; in chronic cystitis, urethritis, as well as bladder tenesmus [2]. Pharmacological data on the different constituents are lacking.

Making the tea: 1.5 g of the finely cut drug in cold water is boiled for a short time and strained after 5 min. As a diuretic, a cupful is drunk two or three times a day.
1 Teaspoon = ca. 1.4 g.

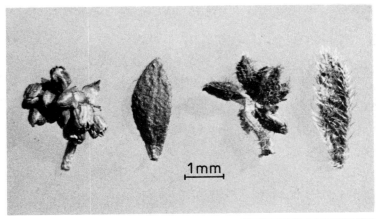

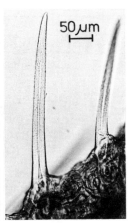

Fig. 3: Inflorescence and leaf of *Herniaria glabra* (left; glabrous) and *H. hirsuta* (right; very hairy)

Fig. 4: Unicellular trichomes with warty cuticle, from *H. hirsuta* (far right)

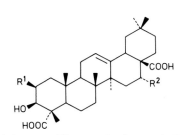

Aglycones of the saponins from rupturewort

	R¹	R²
Medicagenic acid	– OH	– H
Gypsogenic acid	– H	– H
16α-Hydroxymedicagenic acid	– OH	– OH

Herniarin   R = – CH₃
Umbelliferone R = – H

Extract from the German Commission E monograph
(BAnz no. 173, dated 18. 09. 1986)

Uses

Rupturewort is used for the treatment and alleviation of conditions and disorders involving the kidneys and urinary tract or the respiratory tract, and in neuritis and neural catarrh, in arthritis and rheumatism, and for "for purifying the blood".
Efficacy in the indicated areas of use has not been adequately substantiated.

Risks

None known.

Evaluation

Since the efficacy in the areas of use indicated has not been fully substantiated, therapeutic application of the drug cannot be recommended.

Effect

Weakly spasmolytic.

Phytomedicines: Some ready-made urological preparations, e.g. Dr. med. Bahnholzer's Herniol® (drops), Nephri-Dolan (drops), Nephrisol® (drops), Nieral® (dragees), Blasen- und Nierentee Stada® (bladder and kidney tea), Nephronorm®-Tee, Nieron®-Tee, etc.

Authentication: Macro- (see: Description) and microscopically. The epidermal cells of the leaves are wavy-walled; *Herniaria hirsuta*, especially, has unicellular, up to 250 µm long, thick-walled, pointed trichomes with a warty cuticle (Fig. 4), which at the leaf margin are curved like a sabre. The spongy parenchyma has cells containing cluster crystals of calcium oxalate up to 40 µm in diameter.

The sepals are very similar to the foliage leaves. The pollen grains are small, smooth, and they have three slit-like pores. In the stem, there are thickened fibres and oxalate clusters, and in the epidermis trichomes similar to those on the leaves.

If 1 g powdered drug is shaken vigorously with 15 ml water, a stable froth is formed. Microsublimation at 100 °C yields herniarin (m.p. 116–117 °C); and on dissolving the sublimate in water and adding a drop of dilute ammonia solution, a distinct blue fluorescence is observed under UV light. The following TLC method is a suitable means of identification:

Test solution: 1 g powdered drug extracted with 10 ml methanol at 60 °C for 5 min. and the still warm solution filtered.

Reference solution: 5 mg rutin and 10 mg chlorogenic acid dissolved in 5 ml methanol.

Loadings: 1 µl reference solution as a spot, 4 µl test solution as a band.

Solvent system: ethyl acetate + conc. formic acid + water (65 + 15 + 20), 6 cm run.

Detection: dried in a current of hot air, then sprayed with 1% methanolic diphenylboryloxyethylamine and oversprayed with 5% methanolic polyethyleneglycol 400, followed by brief heating at 100–105 °C.

Evaluation: in UV 365 nm light. Reference solution: rutin, a yellow-orange fluorescent zone at Rf ca. 0.5, with the chlorogenic-acid zone above it as a blue fluorescent zone. Test solution: at the same Rf as rutin an orange fluorescent zone and at the same Rf as chlorogenic acid a blue-green fluorescent zone; below the Rf of rutin, a faint yellow-

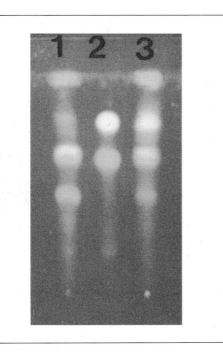

Fig. 5: TLC on 4 × 8 cm silica-gel foil

1: Rupturewort (*Herniaria hirsuta*)
2: Reference compounds
3: Rupturewort (*Herniaria glabra*)

For details, see the text

orange fluorescent zone in the case of *Herniaria glabra*, which is much more intense with *H. hirsuta*; additional fluorescent zones possibly present (Fig. 5).

Quantitative standards: <u>DAC 1986</u>: *Water-soluble extractive*, not less than 25.0%. *Foreign matter*, not more than 3%. *Loss on drying*, not more than 10.0%. *Ash*, not more than 10.0%.
<u>ÖAB</u>: *Haemolytic index*, not less than 1500. *Foreign matter*, not more than 2%. *Ash*, not more than 10.0%.

Adulteration: Rare.

Literature:
[1] G. Klein, J. Jurenitsch, and W. Kubelka, Sci. Pharm. **50**, 216 (1982).
[2] G. Vogel, Planta Med. **11**, 362 (1963).

Hibisci flos   (DAB 10), Red-sorrel flower

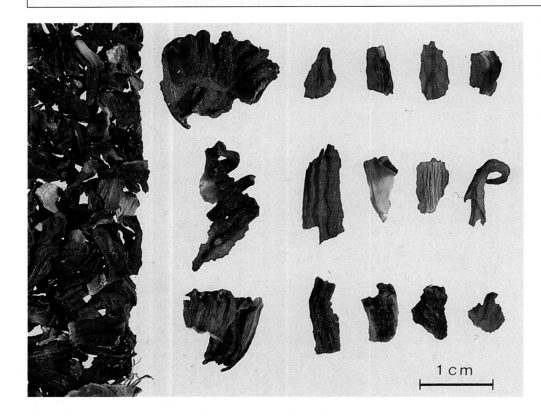

Fig. 1: Red-sorrel flower

Description: The drug consists of the dried calyx and epicalyx of *Hibiscus sabdariffa* collected during the fruiting period.

The calyx is usually ca. 2–3.5 cm long, with the lower half fused and urceolate and the upper half divided into five long, pointed apices that curve towards each other; these have a distinct and somewhat prominent midrib, with in the upper part of the calyx a thickish and darkish nectary, ca. 1 mm in diameter.

The epicalyx comprises 8–12 narrow, ca. 6–15 mm long, leaflets which are broader at the base and which are adnate to the base of the calyx. The calyx and epicalyx are fleshy, dry, rather brittle, and glossy light red to dark violet in colour, and paler at the base on the inside [1, 2].

Odour: Faint and characteristic.

Taste: Sourish.

Fig. 2: *Hibiscus sabdariffa* L.

An annual herbaceous plant with lobed leaves, growing to a height of 5 m. Flowers with a 5-lobed calyx and divided epicalyx, becoming red and fleshy after anthesis.

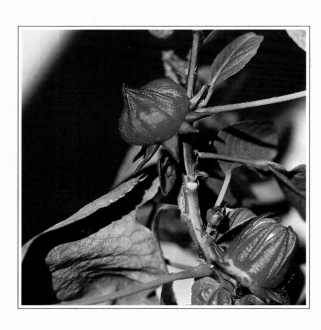

DAB 10: Hibiscusblüten

Plant origin: *Hibiscus sabdariffa* L. var. *ruber*, red sorrel (Malvaceae).

Synonyms: Jamaica sorrel, Roselle or Rozelle (Engl.), Hibiscusblüten, Sabdariff-Eibisch, Sudan-Tee (Ger.), Karkadé (Fr.).

Origin: Originally from Angola (?), but nowadays cultivated worldwide throughout the tropics; imports come especially from Sudan and Egypt, as well as Thailand, Mexico, and China.

Constituents: 15–30% plant acids, including citric, malic, and tartaric acids and (+)-*allo*-hydroxycitric acid lactone – so-called hibiscus acid – which is specific to the drug; these give drinks prepared from red sorrel a pleasant and refreshing acid taste. Ca. 1.5% anthocyans, among them delphinidin 3-sambubioside, delphinidin, cyanidin 3-sambubioside, colour the tea wine-red. In addition, flavone derivatives, such as gossypetin (= hexahydroxyflavone) 3-glucoside. Phyto-

Delphinidin 3-sambubioside
(=Delphinidin 3-xylosylglucoside)
(=Hibiscin)

Hibiscus acid
(=(+)-Allohydroxycitric
acid lactone)

Extract from the German Commission E monograph
(BAnz no. 22a, dated 01. 02. 1990)

Uses

Hibiscus flowers are used to stimulate the appetite, in chills, catarrh of the upper respiratory passages and of the stomach, to dissolve phlegm, as a gentle laxative, diuretic, and for disorders of the circulation. The efficacy of the drug in the conditions indicated has not been substantiated.

Risks

None known.

Evaluation

Since the efficacy of hibiscus flower in the indications listed has not been substantiated, therapeutic use cannot be recommended. However, there are no objections to its being used to enhance appearance and taste.

sterols [1]. In aqueous extracts, ca. 15% mucilage polysaccharides and 2% pectins; the neutral polysaccharides are composed of arabinans and arabinogalactans, while the main acidic fraction is pectin-like and contains a high proportion of galacturonic acid, as well as rhamnose, galactose, and arabinose, and small amounts of glucose, xylose, and mannose [3, 7, 8].

Indications: Principally as a caffeine-free refreshing drink. Taken in large amounts, because of the plant acids, which are difficult to absorb, red-sorrel tea acts as a mild laxative. In *African folk medicine*, the drug is ascribed, among other things, spasmolytic, antibacterial, cholagogic, diuretic, and anthelmintic properties. Aqueous extracts of hibiscus flowers are said to relax the muscles of the uterus and to lower the blood pressure [summary in 3]. Antiphlogistic and antioedema effects are attributed to an ointment containing hibiscus extract [4]. These actions may be associated with the mucilage content of the drug, and hence decoctions of red-sorrel flowers are also recommended for the treatment of weeping skin in allergic eczema.

The polysaccharide fractions have some immune-modulating activity [8].

Making the tea: Boiling water is poured over 1.5 g of the finely chopped drug and strained after 5–10 min.
1 Teaspoon = ca. 2.5 g.

Herbal preparations: The drug on its own, or in mixtures with hips, is available in tea bags and other forms (which make up about 20 % of the "herbal-tea" market).

Phytomedicines: These include tea bags obtainable from various manufacturers.

Authentication: Macro- (see: Description) and microscopically.
The DAB 10 gives the following TLC test of identity:

Test solution: 1.0 g powdered drug extracted by shaking with 6 ml of 25% hydrochloric acid + methanol (10 + 90) for 15 min.; filtrate = test solution.

Reference solution: 5 mg methylene blue in 10 ml methanol.

Loadings: 20 µl test solution and 10 µl reference solution, as 2 cm bands.

Mobile phase: water + anhydrous formic acid + 25% hydrochloric acid + butan-1-ol (6 + 12 + 12 + 70), 15 cm run.

Detection: after removal of the solvent, zones outlined, in diffuse daylight. Reference solution: Blue zone of methylene blue visible in daylight. Test solution: Halfway between the starting line and the methylene-blue zone, an intense red-violet zone and immediately above it a second, fainter, red zone; above the methylene-blue zone, one or two other reddish zones; near the starting line, possibly also a red zone.
Examination of the plant acids can be carried out according to [6] and their quantitative estimation according to the DAB 10.

Quantitative standards: <u>DAB 10</u>: *Plant acids*, not less than 13.5% calculated as citric acid. *Foreign matter*, not more than 2% fruit parts (red fruit stalks and parts of the 5-locular yellowish grey capsule, the wall of which consists of several layers of fibre groups running in different directions; flattened reniform seeds with a punctate surface). *Loss on drying*, not more than 10.0%. *Ash*, not more than 10.0%. *Colouring power*, 0.4 g powdered drug extracted with 100 ml water on the water-bath for 15 min. with occasional stirring should give a filtrate that is not less strongly coloured than a solution of 60 g cobalt(II) chloride dissolved in ca. 900 ml of a mixture of 25 ml 36% hydrochloric acid + 975 ml water and diluted to 1000.0 ml with this mixture – 1 ml of the final solution should contain 59.5 mg $CoCl_2 \cdot 6H_2O$.

Literature:
[1] Kommentar DAB 10.
[2] H.G. Menßen and K. Staesche, Dtsch. Apoth. Ztg. **114**, 1211 (1974).
[3] M. Franz and G. Franz, Z. Phytotherap. **9**, 63 (1988).
[4] A. Stirn, Z. Allgemeinmed. **54**, 616 (1975).
[5] R. Weiß, Phys. Med. **3**, 50 (1970).
[6] P. Pachaly, Dünnschichtchromatographie in der Apotheke, 2nd ed., Wissenschaftliche Verlagsgesellschaft m.b.H., Stuttgart, 1983.
[7] B.M. Müller and G. Franz, Dtsch. Apoth. Ztg. **130**, 329 (1990).
[8] B.M. Müller and G. Franz, Planta Med. **58**, 60 (1992).

Hippocastani cortex   Horse-chestnut bark

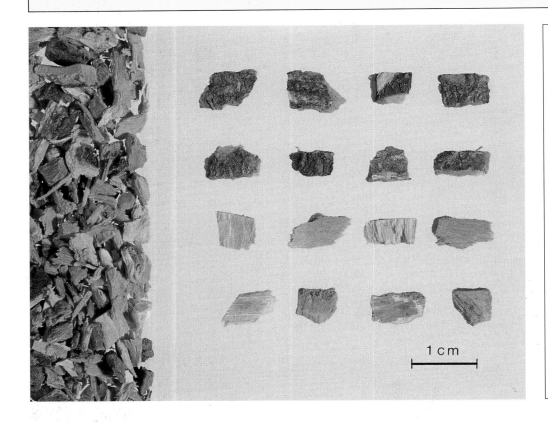

Fig. 1: Horse-chestnut bark

Description: The drug is obtained by decorticating 3- to 5-year old branches collected in the spring or autumn. It consists of 1–2 mm thick, channelled or quilled pieces or chips. The outer surface is copper-coloured, smooth and slightly shiny, and partly with round lenticels (young bark) or matt grey to blackish, rugose to cracked, with horizontal elongated lenticels and, sometimes, also a covering of lichens (older bark). The inner surface is smooth and yellowish brown. The fracture in the outer layers is granular and in the inner layers short and fibrous.

Odour: Very faint and somewhat musty.

Taste: Astringent and somewhat bitter.

1 cm

Fig. 2: *Aesculus hippocastanum* L.

Branches with flower buds, in spring. For the description of the plant, see: Hippocastani folium.

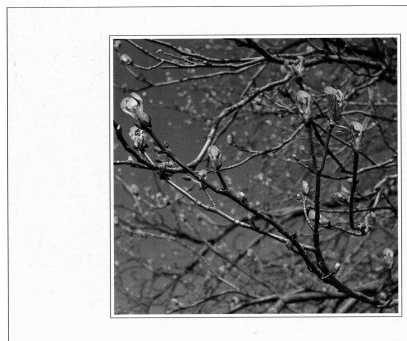

Plant source: *Aesculus hippocastanum* L., horse-chestnut (Hippocastanaceae).

Synonyms: Cortex castanae equinae (Lat.), Roßkastanienrinde, Vixirrinde (Ger.), Écorce de marronier d'Inde (Fr.).

Origin: Native in northern Greece, Iran, the Caucasus, and northern India. Cultivated and naturalized throughout Europe, reaching Great Britain and Scandinavia. The drug is mainly imported from Poland.

Constituents: The coumarin glycosides aesculin (ca. 3%), fraxin, and scopolin, as well as their aglycones aesculetin, fraxetin, and scopoletin; the flavonol glycoside quercitrin and its aglycone quercetin; the heterogeneous mixture of saponins aescin (diacylated protoaescigenin and barringtogenol C with a C(3) glucuronic-acid residue substituted at the 2′- or 4′-position with glucose, xylose, or galactose); allantoin, sterols, leucocyanidin, leucodelphinidin, catechol tannins, alkanes (homologous series from C_{15} to C_{30}).

Indications: The drug is now little used. It is employed in *folk medicine* as an astringent in diarrhoea and haemorrhoids. Externally, decocts are (rarely) used for sores and skin complaints (lupus). Formerly, the drug was considered to be a febrifuge and a substitute for cinchona bark in treating malaria. The bark is used industrially in tanning. Nowadays, the bark yields aesculin, which improves vascular resistance, reduces pathologically raised capillary-wall permeability, and, because of its ability to absorb skin-damaging UV radiation (UV-B), is added to suntan products. Aescin, which occurs in larger amounts in the seeds, has anti-exudative and oedema inhibiting properties [1, 2], and, among other things, is used against haemorrhoids. Ca. 5–10% is absorbed on peroral administration.

Side effects: Not known for the drug. In the skin test, a case of contact dermatitis with aesculin has been encountered [3].

Making the tea: Cold water is poured over half a teaspoonful of the finely chopped or coarsely powdered drug, boiled for a short period, and passed through a tea strainer. For diarrhoea, a cupful is drunk two or three times a day.
For dressings or as a bath additive: a handful of the finely chopped or coarsely powdered drug is added to one litre of water, boiled for a short time, and after 10 min. strained.
1 Teaspoon = ca. 2.5 g.

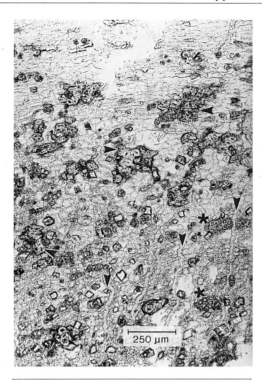

Fig. 3: **Transverse section through the secondary bark, showing groups of pholem fibres (*), stone cells (◀) and medullary rays (▼)**

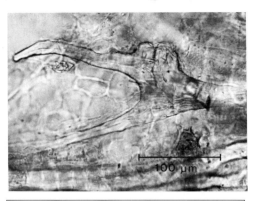

Fig. 4: **Irregularly branched stone cells**

Phytomedicines: A few, but only a few, mixed herbal haemorrhoidal and antiphlebitis teas contain horse-chestnut bark. Some of the phytomedicines mentioned under Hippocastani folium also contain bark extracts.

Authentication: Macro- (see: Description) and microscopically. Youngish bark has on-

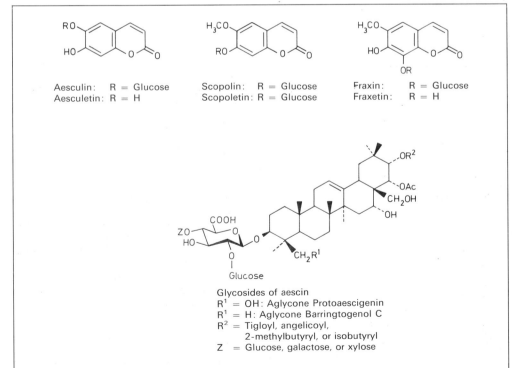

Aesculin: R = Glucose
Aesculetin: R = H

Scopolin: R = Glucose
Scopoletin: R = Glucose

Fraxin: R = Glucose
Fraxetin: R = H

Glycosides of aescin
R^1 = OH: Aglycone Protoaescigenin
R^1 = H: Aglycone Barringtogenol C
R^2 = Tigloyl, angelicoyl,
  2-methylbutyryl, or isobutyryl
Z = Glucose, galactose, or xylose

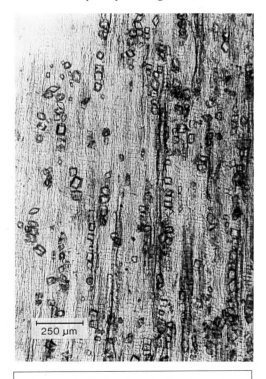

Fig. 5: **Longitudinal section, showing phloem fibres and large prisms of calcium oxalate**

ly a thin-walled cork. Later on, the layers of thin-walled cork alternate with layers of thickened cork cells. At the boundary between the primary and secondary phloem, there is a discontinuous ring of thickened fibres and stone cells. The secondary phloem has uniseriate medullary rays and, in its outer part, bundles of phloem fibres surrounded by stone cells (Fig. 3) and groups of irregular branched stone cells (Fig. 4); in the inner part of thicker barks, there are tangential bands of phloem fibres accompanied by septate fibres containing large rhombic crystals of calcium oxalate (Fig. 5). In the primary phloem, there are numerous calcium-oxalate clusters; these are rare in the inner parts of the bark.

The DAB 10 TLC test of identity for Hippocastani semen, which is presumably also applicable to other aescin-containing drugs, is as follows:

Test solution: 1.0 g powdered drug refluxed for 15 min. with 10 ml 70% ethanol, cooled, and filtered.

Reference solution: 10 mg aescin dissolved in 1.0 ml 70% ethanol.

Loadings: 20 µl test solution and 10 µl reference solution, as 2-cm bands on silica gel GF$_{254}$.

Solvent system: upper phase of: 98% acetic acid + water + butan-1-ol (10 + 40 + 50), 12 cm run.

Detection: quenching zones seen in UV 254 nm light marked, then sprayed with anisaldehyde reagent and heated for 5–10 min. at 100–105 °C.

Evaluation: in UV 254 nm light. Reference solution: the aescin quenching zone. Test solution: a distinct quenching zone at about the same level.

After spraying, in daylight. Reference solution: the bluish violet aescin zone. Test solution: a similar zone; above it, a series of narrower and fainter brown to brownish red zones; in the lower Rf region, a conspicuous brownish grey zone and somewhat below it a brown zone.

In [4], the solvent system advocated (it gives a higher Rf value for aescin) is: chloroform + methanol + water (64 + 50 + 10), and antimony(III) chloride, followed by heating for 5–6 min. at 100 °C, is used as detecting agent; the chromatogram is evaluated in daylight and in UV 365 nm light. Aescin appears at Rf ca. 0.5 as a broad zone, violet in daylight and with an intense greenish grey fluorescence in UV light; other zones in the Rf range 0.05–0.2, violet in daylight and black in UV light, are due to sugars.

Adulteration: Rarely occurs.

Literature:
[1] M. von Rothkopf and G. Vogel, Arzneimittel.Forsch. 26, 225 (1976).
[2] D. Longiave et al., Pharmacol. Res. Commun. 10, 145 (1978).
[3] J.S. Comaish and P.J. Kersey, Contact Dermatitis 6, 150 (1980).
[4] H. Wagner, S. Bladt, and E.M. Zgainski, Plant drug analysis, Springer-Verlag, Berlin, Heidelberg, New York, Tokyo, 1984, p. 242.

Hippocastani folium   Horse-chestnut leaf

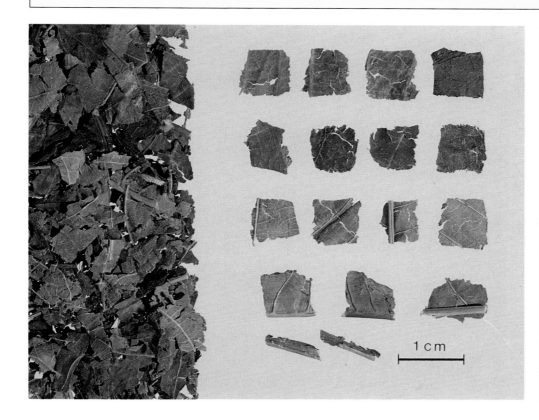

1 cm

Fig. 1: Horse-chestnut leaf

<u>Description</u>: The rather stiff leaf fragments, some of which show the crenate-serrate margin, have a dark greenish brown upper surface and a lighter lower surface. The 5–7 leaflets of the digitate leaves are pinnately nerved, with clearly parallel lateral nerves. Young leaves have a brownish red pubescence, while mature ones are glabrous. Fragments of the grooved petioles are also present.

<u>Taste</u>: Astringent and somewhat bitter.

Figs. 2 and 3: *Aesculus hippocastanum* L.

A ca. 25 m high tree with characteristically 5–7 digitate leaves and erect racemes of flowers with a yellow or reddish spot at the base of the white petals. Fruit a spiny capsule containing up to three shiny, reddish brown seeds with a light-coloured hilum.

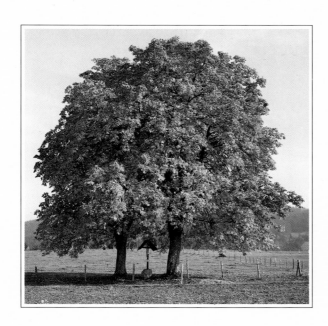

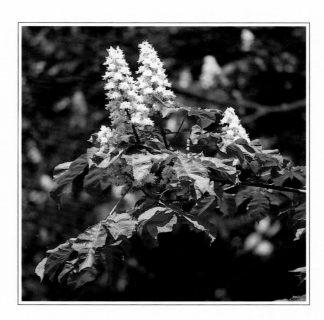

Plant source: *Aesculus hippocastanum* L., horse-chestnut (Hippocastanaceae).

Synonyms: Roßkastanienblätter (Ger.), Feuilles du marronier d'Inde, Châtaignier de cheval (Fr.).

Origin: Native in northern India, the Caucasus, Asia Minor, northern Greece, but now widespread in Europe through cultivation and naturalization. The drug is imported from eastern Europe.

Constituents: The coumarin glycosides aesculin, scopolin, and fraxin (for the structures, see Hippocastani cortex), the flavonol glycosides quercetin 3-rhamnoside, 3-rhamnosidoglucoside, 3-glucoside (= quercitrin, rutin, and isoquercitrin, respectively), and 3-arabinoside, as well as the corresponding four glycosides of kaempferol [1, 2]; tannins; traces of aescin [3, 4]; *cis,trans*-polyprenols; amino acids; fatty acids; sterols (sitosterol, stigmasterol, campesterol) [5]; leucoanthocyans.

Indications: In *folk medicine,* the drug is still occasionally given as a cough remedy. Like extracts of sweet chestnut leaves, extracts of horse-chestnut leaves are used in the treatment of coughs [1] and arthritis and rheumatism [5]. Appropriate active principles have not been identified. In combination with seed and bark extracts, horse-chestnut leaf extracts are a component of numerous antiphlebitis remedies.

Making the tea: Boiling water is poured over a teaspoon of the finely chopped drug, boiled for a short while, and after 5–10 min. passed through a tea strainer. In *folk medicine,* as a cough remedy, two or three cupfuls of the infusion are drunk a day.
1 Teaspoon = ca. 1 g.

Phytomedicines: The drug is a component of a few prepared antiphlebitis and haemorrhoid teas. A standardized leaf extract is present in Venoplant ampoules. Standardized extracts from various parts of the horse-chestnut (bark, seeds, leaves) are found in many galenical preparations for use, internally and externally, in treating "venous conditions" (in the broadest sense), e.g. Venostasin® (drops, ointment, suppositories, capsules), Vasoforte®, Aescorin® and together with other active ingredients, e.g. Amphodyn® retard, RR-plus® Dragees, Venopyrum®, etc.

Authentication: Macro- (see: Description) and microscopically. Among the diagnostic features are the spherical oil cells and calcium-oxalate clusters in the mesophyll (Fig. 4), the cuticular striations of the upper

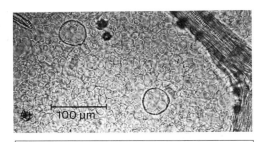

Fig. 4: Spherical oil cells and calcium-oxalate clusters in the mesophyll

epidermis, and occasional long, multicellular trichomes with a warty cuticle.

Adulteration: Occasional adulteration with Castaneae folium (sweet-chestnut leaf) has been observed. The adulterant can be readily distinguished by the deviating microscopical features.

Literature:
[1] Hager, vol. **1**, p. 11 (1969); vol **4**, p.112 (1992).
[2] M. Tissut, Phytochemistry **11**, 631 (1972).
[3] U. Fiedler, Dtsch. Apoth. Ztg. **94**, 889 (1954).
[4] Th. Kartnig, R. Herbst, and F.J. Graune, Planta Med. **13**, 39 (1965).
[5] C. Souleles and K. Vayas, Fitoterapia **57**, 201 (1986).

Hyperici herba   St. John's wort

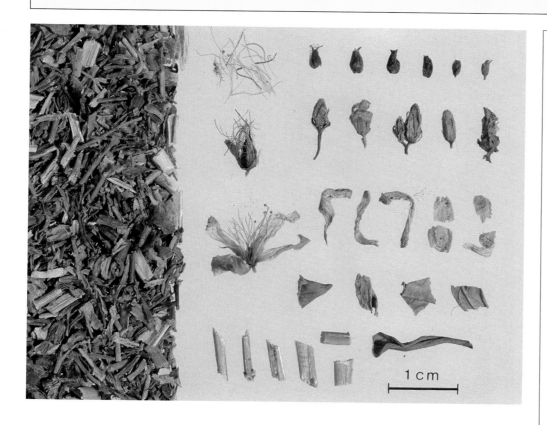

Fig. 1: St. John's wort

<u>Description:</u> The drug consists of the dried flowering tops. Particularly noteworthy are the yellow to yellowish brown flowers, which under certain circumstances are still present in cymes and whose petals are covered with numerous dark spots or streaks; the sepals are lanceolate, sharply pointed, and at the time of flowering twice as long as the ovary. The ca. 50–60 stamens of each flower are usually fused into three groups. The often shrivelled and folded pale green to brownish green, glabrous, ovate-elliptic leaves are up to 3.5 cm long, with an entire margin and clearly visible translucent dots. The yellowish green, round pieces of stem are hollow and often have two longitudinal ridges opposite each other (see also: Adulteration).

1 cm

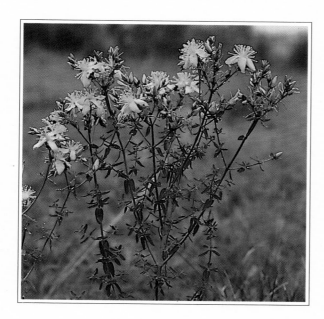

Fig. 2: *Hypericum perforatum* L.

A ca. 60 cm tall herbaceous plant having 5-merous yellow flowers with many and prominent, long stamens and opposite, translucently dotted leaves. Distinguished from other *Hypericum* species by a stem with two longitudinal ridges.

DAC 1986: Johanniskraut
St. Zul.: 1059.99.99

Plant source: *Hypericum perforatum* L., common or perforate St. John's wort (Hypericaceae, or Clusiaceae = Guttiferae).

Synonyms: Hypericum (Engl.), Johanniskraut, Blutkraut, Herrgottsblut, Walpurgiskraut, Hexenkraut (Ger.), Herbe de millepertuis (Fr.).

Origin: From the wild in Europe and western Asia. Imports come from Eastern Europe.

Constituents: 0.05–0.3% hypericin and hypericin-like substances, notably pseudohypericin [1], isohypericin, protohypericin, etc.; the northern European broad-leaved var. *perforatum* tends to have less of the hypericins than the southern Europe narrow-leaved var. *angustifolium* DC., the concentrations correlating well with the leaf oil-gland counts [1, 15, 16]. Flavonoids: especially hyperoside (= "hyperin") and rutin, as well as biflavones, particularly I3,II8-biapigenin (0.26%) [2, 16]. Among the antibiotic substances, up to 3% hyperforin [1, 16, 17], a phloroglucinol derivative structurally related to the bitter substances of hops. 0.05–0.3% Essential oil (*n*-alkanes, especially $C_{29}H_{60}$, also α-pinene and other monoterpenes). Up to more than 10% tannins. Small amounts of procyanidins [4].

Indications: For milder forms of neurotic depression, e.g. during the menopause and in nervous exhaustion; up to now, the hypericins have been considered the source of activity [5–8], but it must be realized that the biflavones (those from *Taxus baccata* are CNS-depressant) and hyperforin are involved in the sedative effect of the drug [1]. Hypericin is said to be a monoamineoxidase inhibitor [9].
In *folk medicine,* the drug is also employed as an antidiarrhoeal (tannin content), di-

Hypericin

*Extract from the German Commission
E monograph
(BAnz no. 228, dated 05. 12. 1984)*

Uses

Internally: psychogenic disturbances, depressive states, anxiety, and/or nervous excitement. Oily hypericum preparations for dyspeptic complaints.
Externally: oily hypericum preparations for the treatment and after-treatment of incised and contused wounds, myalgia, and first-degree burns.

Contraindications

None known.

Side effects

Photosensitization may develop, especially in people with fair skins.

Interactions

None known.

Dosage

Unless otherwise prescribed: average daily dose for internal use, 2–4 g drug or 0.2–1.0 mg total hypericin in other formulations.

Mode of administration

Chopped or powdered drug, liquid and solid preparations for oral use. Liquid and semi-solid preparations for external use. Preparations made with fixed oils for external and internal use.

Effects

There are numerous medical reports dealing with the drug and its preparations which indicate a mild antidepressive effect. Hypericin has been shown experimentally to be a monoamineoxidase inhibitor. Oily hypericum preparations have antiphlogistic activity.

uretic (flavonoid content), and against bed-wetting [10], rheumatism, and gout.
It is used in the form of Oleum hyperici (an extract made with olive, sunflower, or, best, wheatgerm oil [11]) for healing wounds and for burns [12, 13]. The oil does not contain hypericin, but lipophilic breakdown products that colour it red [17]; the activity of the oil is attributed rather to hyperforin [3].
For a wide-ranging review of the literature on St. John's wort, see [18].

Side effects: Hypericin is photosensitizing, which under certain circumstances may need to be taken into account with high doses (avoid sunray (UV) and solarium treatment). Though there are no reported cases of phototoxicity in human beings, there is the possibility of its arising during the (recently developed) application of high doses of hypericin against retroviruses [19].

Making the tea: Boiling water is poured over 2–4 g of the finely chopped drug and after 5–10 min. strained. Possible side effects on prolonged use must be considered.
1 Teaspoon = ca. 1.8 g.

Herbal teas: Tea bags of the drug (mostly containing 2 g) are available.

Phytomedicines: There are a few ready-made in the group psychomedicinal preparations, some with a standardized hypericin content, e.g. Hyperforat® (dragees, drops, ampoules), Jarsin® (dragees), Psychotonin® (tincture), Neurapas® (coated tablets), and urological preparations affecting micturition, e.g. Psychatrin® (drops), Inconturina® (drops), Rhoival® (dragees, drops).

Authentication: Macro- (see: Description) and microscopically. The scattered, large-spherical excretory glands in the mesophyll of the leaves are a noteworthy feature (Figs. 3 and 4); they often take up more than half the thickness of the leaf and they are filled with a strongly refracting drops. Near the leaf margin, there are blackish, hypericin-containing secretory glands. The yellowish petals have numerous ca. 200 µm wide hypericin glands; these are also found at the top of the connective of the stamens. The pollen grains are ca. 25 µm in diameter and are roundish to three-sided and smooth.
The following TLC method is a suitable identification test:

Test solution: 0.4 g powdered drug first exhaustively extracted (soxhlet) with chloroform; marc then dried and exhaustively extracted with acetone; solution concentrated under reduced pressure and the residue taken up in 10 ml methanol.

Reference solution: 5 mg hypericin dissolved in 5 ml methanol.

Loadings: 10 µl test solution and 5 µl, both as bands.

Solvent system: toluene + ethyl acetate + anhydrous formic acid (50 + 40 + 10), 5 cm run.

Detection: plate dried in a current of hot air and observed under UV 366 nm light, then sprayed with pyridine + acetone (10 + 90).

Evaluation: in UV 366 nm light. Reference solution: hypericin at Rf > 0.5, as a red fluorescent band. Test solution: two red fluorescent bands at about the same Rf value (hypericin and pseudohypericin).
After spraying with pyridine + acetone, the fluorescence is considerably enhanced.
A more comprehensive TLC examination [17], for: (a) hypericin, pseudohypericin, and their lipophilic derivatives, (b) the lipophilic hyperforin derivatives, and (c) the flavonoids, can be achieved by separation in the solvent system: heptane + acetone + *tert.*-butyl methyl ether + 85% formic acid (35 + 35 + 33 + 2) and detection: (a) in UV 254 nm light, as quenching zones or, after

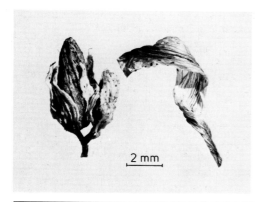

Fig. 3: Flower bud (left) and petal (right), showing blackish red dots (hypericin idioblasts)

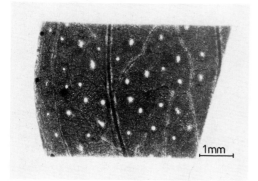

Fig. 4: Leaf with translucent (*perforatum*) excretory glands

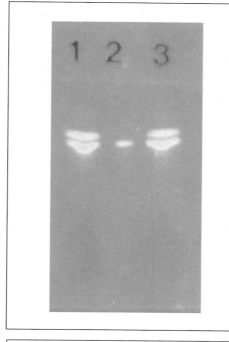

Fig. 5: TLC on 4 × 8 cm silica-gel foil

1 and 3: St. John's wort (different sources)
2: Hypericin (reference compound)

For details, see the text

spraying with 0.5% aq. Fast Blue salt, as yellow zones, (b) in UV 366 nm light, as orange-red fluorescent zones, and (c) heating at 100 °C for 10 min. and spraying with 1% methanolic diphenylboryloxyethylamine, followed by 5% methanolic Macrogol 400, yielding fluorescent zones (dark yellow, biapigenin; orange, quercetin; green, xanthones).

Quantitative standards: <u>DAC 1986</u>: *Dianthrones of the hypericin group*, not less than 0.04% calculated as hypericin (M_r 504.5). *Foreign matter*, not more than 2%. *Loss on drying*, not more than 10%. *Ash*, not more than 5.0%.
<u>BHP 1983</u>: *Total ash*, not more than 8%. *Acid-insoluble ash*, not more than 2.5%.

Adulteration: Relatively frequent, with other *Hypericum* species. These can be recognized especially by the pieces of stem: *H. maculatum* CRANTZ, imperforate St. John's wort (the most frequent adulterant), has a 4-angled stem and *H. montanum* L., pale or mountain St. John's wort, has a round stem. The leaves of *H. barbatum* JACQ. are not or only very sparsely dotted.
A detailed discussion of the *Hypericum* species which could be present as adulterants, including the TLC examination (with coloured illustration), is given in [14].

Literature:
[1] J. Hölzl and E. Ostrowski, Dtsch. Apoth. Ztg. **127**, 1227 (1987).
[2] R. Berghöfer and J. Hölzl, Planta Med. **53**, 216 (1987).
[3] A.I. Gurevich et al., Antibiotiki **6**, 510 (1971); C.A. **75**, 95625 (1971).
[4] J. Hölzl and H. Münker, Acta Agron. **34** (Suppl.), 52 (1985).
[5] K.W.O. Daniel, Erfahrungsheilkunde **18**, 229 (1969).
[6] M. Pahlow, Naturheilpraxis **26**, 350 (1982).
[7] H.-G. Siedentopf and K.-H. Bauer, Z. Angew. Phytotherap. **2**, 215 (1981).
[8] J. Hoffmann and E.D. Kühl, Z. Allgem. Med. **55**, 776 (1981).
[9] O. Suzuki et al. Planta Med. **50**, 273 (1984).
[10] A. Haselhuber, H. Kleinachmidt, and S. Knust von Wedel, Hippokrates **40**, 105 (1969).
[11] A. Fröhlich, Präparative Pharmazie **1**, 40, 59 (1965).
[12] J. Klosa, Heilkunde **65**, 333 (1952).
[13] P. Mutschler, Arzt und Patient **63**, 6 (1950).
[14] R. Berghöfer and J. Hölzl, Dtsch. Apoth. Ztg. **126**, 2569 (1986).
[15] I.A. Southwell and M.H. Campbell, Phytochemistry **30**, 475 (1991).
[16] J. Hölzl and E. Ostrowski, Dtsch. Apoth. Ztg. **127**, 127 (1987).
[17] P. Maisenbacher and K.-A. Kovar, Planta Med. **58**, 351 (1992).
[18] C. Hobbs, Herbal Gram no. **18/19**, 24 (1989).
[19] S. Stock and J. Hölzl, Med. Mo. Pharm. **14**, 304 (1991).

Wording of the package insert, from the German Standard Licence

6.1   Uses
In supportive treatment for nervous excitement and disturbances of sleep.

6.2   Contraindications
St.John's-wort preparations should not be used in cases of known photosenstivity.

6.3   Side effects
Occasionally, particularly with fair-skinned people, photosensitivity may arise. This appears as sunburn-like inflammation of those parts of the skin exposed to fairly strong sunshine.

6.4   Dosage and Mode of administration
1–2 Teaspoonfuls of **St. John's wort** are infused with boiling water (ca. 150 ml) and after about 10 min., passed through a tea strainer.
Unless otherwise prescribed, one or two cups of the freshly prepared tea are drunk regularly morning and evening.

6.5   Duration of use
Normally, to obtain an effect, use over a period of several weeks or months is required.

6.6   Note
Store away from light and moisture.

Ipecacuanhae radix
(DAB 10, Ph. Eur. 2), Ipecacuanha
(*BAN*; BP 1988, BHP 1/1990), Ipecac (*USAN*),

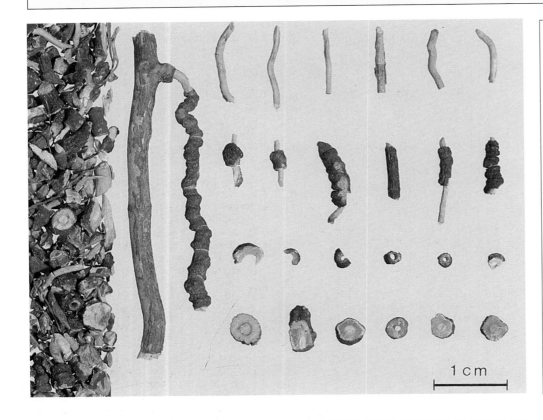

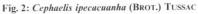

1 cm

Fig. 1: Ipecacuanha root

<u>Description:</u> The dark reddish brown to greyish brown roots are 4–5 mm (*Cephaelis ipecacuanha*) or 6–10 mm (*Cephaelis acuminata*) thick and show characteristic closely spaced circular or semi-circular swellings which make them appear knobbly and ringed. The whitish grey bark is fairly easily removed from the solid yellowish wood.

<u>Odour:</u> Faint and somewhat musty.

<u>Taste:</u> Bitter and somewhat pungent.

Fig. 2: *Cephaelis ipecacuanha* (Brot.) Tussac

A low shrub, up to 40 cm in height, in the undergrowth of the tropical rain and cloud forests of South America. Stem becoming woody near the ground. Leaves up to 7 cm long, oblong, with an entire margin. Bisexual flowers in hemispherical clusters.

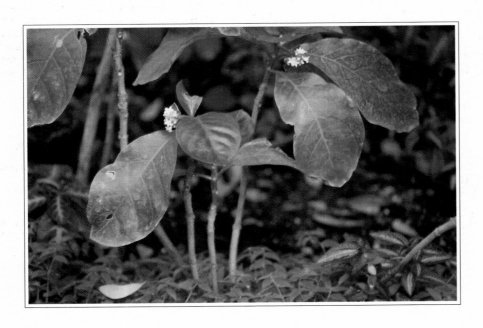

DAB 10: Ipecacuanhawurzel
ÖAB: Radix Ipecacuanhae
Ph. Helv. VII: Ipecacuanhae radix

Plant sources: *Cephaelis ipecacuanha* (Brot.) Tussac, Rio, Matto Grosso, Minas, or Brazilian ipecacuanha, and *Cephaelis acuminata* H.Karst., Cartagena, Panama, Costa Rica, or Nicaragua ipecacuanha (Rubiaceae).

Synonyms: Ipecacuanha or Ipecac root (Engl.), Ipecacuanhawurzel, Brechwurzel (Ger.), Racine d'ipécacuanha (Fr.).

Origin: Principally from Brazil (collected in the wild), and to a smaller extent from Central American countries such as Costa Rica and Nicaragua.

Constituents: 1.8–4% Alkaloids, especially emetine and cephaeline, their 1′,2′-dehydro-derivatives psychotrine, *O*-methylpsychotrine, and other minor alkaloids; the ratio emetine : cephaeline is 2 : 1 to 3 : 1 for

Emetine   R = —CH₃
Cephaeline   R = —H

the Rio drug and 1 : 1 to 3 : 2 for the Cartagena drug. Contrary to older reports, saponins are absent, and the supposed "ipecacuanhin", "ipecacuanhic acid", and "saponin of ipecac" are crude mixtures of ipecoside, a tetrahydroisoquinoline monoterpenoid glucoside, and sucrose [1]; other such N-containing glucosides are present and also the iridoids sweroside and 7-dehydrologanin [4].

Indications: Owing to its alkaloid content, as an expectorant with a strong secretolytic action. Emetine and cephaeline have about the same expectorant activity [2] and their toxicity is very similar; hence, the former preference for the emetine-richer Rio drug (cephaeline was believed to be particularly toxic) was not justified [2].

Ipecacuanha, in the form of infusions or as tincture, is used in chronic bronchitis or in the initial stages of acute bronchitis which is accompanied by a relatively dry cough with moderate and thick mucus, but not by a mild cough with an abundant thin discharge. The action arises from irritation of the mucous membrane of the stomach, which brings about a reflex stimulation of the ascending branch of the parasympathetic division of the autonomic nerve system, coupled with viscosity).

Dover's powder – a mixture of 10 parts ipecacuanha, 10 parts opium, and 80 parts lactose – is widely used as an expectorant which at the same time has a soothing effect on the irritation of the throat; however, the addictive and narcotic effects must be borne in mind.

In higher doses (0.5–2 g), ipecacuanha acts as an emetic. For example, in Switzerland Sirupus emeticus (Ph. Helv. VII: 0.11% alkaloid, emetic dose for adults 40 ml, for school children 25–40 ml, for 2–5-year old children 20–25 ml, and 1-year old infants 12 ml) is used to bring about vomiting in children who have swallowed poisonous berries. Cf. the Paediatric Ipecacuanha Emetic Mixture BP (also in the BNF; emetic dose for adults 30 ml, older children 15 ml, for 1/2- 11/2-year old infants 10 ml), which is equivalent in strength to Ipecac Syrup USP. Reports that the drug or its preparations should no longer be used as an emetic have been contradicted by the medical profession [3].

Emetine itself has amoebicidal activity and can be given against the vegetative forms of *Entamoeba histolytica*, the causative agent in amoebic dysentery.

Side effects: Owing to the general irritant effect on skin and mucous membranes, care should be taken in handling the drug; floating dust from the drug can lead to inflammation of the eyes and inhaling it can cause asthmatic attacks in susceptible people. Prolonged use should be avoided owing the danger of sensitization.

Larger amounts of the drug (and of its preparations), i.e. about 10 times the therapeutic dose, are strongly emetic; the symptoms of intoxication that have been observed are bloody diarrhoea, spasms, and even shock and coma.

Making the tea: Not recommended, since it must be measured very precisely! It is better to take 0.5 g of the tincture (ca. 27 drops) with a fluid (tea or milk) or 10 ml of a 0.5% infusion.

Phytomedicines: Only a few antitussive and expectorant preparations.
The multi-ingredient preparations available in the UK include: Alophen, Aperient Dellipsoids D9, Bronchial Dellipsoids D15, Linituss, Pectomed, Phenergan Compound Expectorant, Tussifans, Unitussin, etc.
The drug is also a component of Potter's Vegetable Cough Remover (liquid).

Regulatory status (UK): General Sales List – Schedule 1, Table A.

Authentication: Macro- and microscopically, following the Ph. Eur. 2, BP 1988, etc. Among the diagnostic features are the presence of compound starch grains, as well as the oxalate raphides of the bark and the very regular xylem. The detailed microscopy of the powdered drug is set out in [5]. The TLC procedure given in the Ph. Eur. 2, BP 1988, etc. enables the Rio drug to be distinguished from the Cartagena drug.

Quantitative standards: Ph. Eur. 2, etc.: *Total alkaloid*, not less than 2.0% calculated as emetine (M_r 480.7). *Foreign matter*, not more than 1.0%. *Sulphated ash*, not more than 6.0%. *Acid-insoluble ash*, not more than 3.0%.
USP XXII: *Ether-soluble alkaloids*, not less than 2%, with emetine and cephaeline together not less than 90% of the total ether-soluble alkaloids. (Powdered ipecac is adjusted to contain not less than 1.9% and not more than 2.1% ether-soluble alkaloids of ipecac.)
BHP 1/1990: Material of ipecacuanha must comply with the requirements of the Ph. Eur. 2 for Ipecacuanha radix and of the BP 1988 for Ipecacuanha or Powdered Ipecacuanha.

Adulteration: has occasionally been observed in the drug trade. So-called Radix Ipecacuanhae amylaceae, the root of *Richardsonia scabra* (L.) A.ST.HIL., which is very similar to genuine ipecacuanha root in external appearance, should not be forgotten. However, it has larger and more clearly layered (striated) starch grains; moreover, in the xylem, medullary rays and vessels, as well as calcium-oxalate clusters, can be recognized. The drug does not contain any emetine. "Black ipecacuanha root" (Radix Ipecacuanhae nigrae or Ipecacuanha glycyphloea) has been identified several times as an adulterant. It is the root of *Cephaelis emetica* PERS. and is similar to Cartagena ipecacuanha, but it has no starch and only ca. 0.03% alkaloid.

Literature:
[1] K. Schneider, J. Jurenitsch, and K. Jentzsch, Sci. Pharm. **54**, 339 (1986).
[2] E.M. Body and L.M. Knight, J. Pharm. Pharmacol. **16**, 118 (1964).
[3] K. Schneider, Österr. Apoth. Ztg. **41**, 1017 (1987).
[4] A. Itoh, T. Tanahashi, and N. Nagakura, Phytochemistry **30**, 3117 (1991).
[5] B.P. Jackson and D.W. Snowdon, Atlas of microscopy of medicinal plants, culinary herbs and spices, Belhaven Press, London, 1990, p. 132.

Iridis rhizoma   Iris florentina (BHP 1983), Orris root

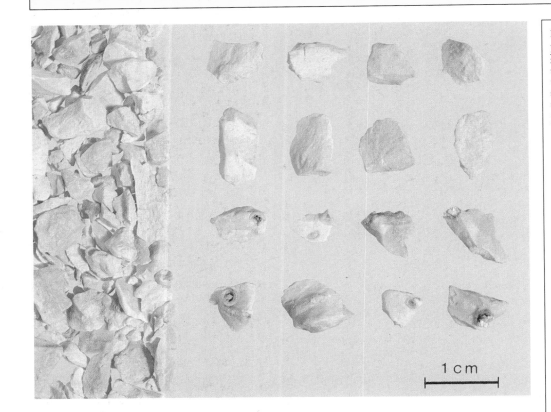

Fig. 1: Orris root

Description: The peeled, white to yellowish white rhizome, which consists of flattened, compressed sections, is mostly 3–4 cm wide and ca. 10 cm long. On the upper surface there are indistinct annular leaf scars and on the flatter lower surface root scars can be seen. The fairly short fracture reveals a white bark and a yellowish, peripheral, clearly punctate central stele. The cut drug consists of pale white to yellowish white, irregular pieces, which quite often have root scars, with fairly smooth broken surfaces (Fig. 3).

Odour: Like violets.

Taste: Slightly bitter and somewhat pungent.

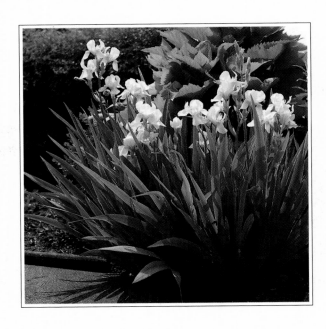

Fig. 2: *Iris* sp. L.

Rhizome with ca. 80 cm long ensiform, basal leaves overtopped by by a stem bearing several flowers having three outer deflexed ('falls') and three inner erect ('standards') perianth segments and three petaloid, broadened style branches ('crests'), each surrounding one stamen and an inferior ovary. Colour of the flowers dependent on the plant source.

DAB 6: Rhizoma Iridis

Plant sources: *Iris germanica* L., garden iris or common German flag, *I. germanica* L. var. *florentina* DYKES (syn. *I. florentina* auct.), Florentine orris, and *I. pallida* LAM., Dalmatian iris (Iridaceae).

Synonyms: Orris, Florentine orris (Engl.), Veilchenwurzel, Iriswurzel (Ger.), Racine de violette, Rhizome d'iris (Fr.).

Origin: Native in the Mediterranean region, cultivated to some extent in Germany. The drug is imported from Morocco and Italy.

Constituents: Ca. 0.2% essential oil containing irone (10–20% of the oil) which smells like violets; the principal compounds are α-, β-, and γ-irone, and other stereoisomers (neo-α-, iso-α-, neo-iso-α-, neo-β-, neo-γ-, iso-γ-, and neo-iso-γ-irone) are also present [1, 2]. In addition, the essential oil contains myristic acid, aromatic aldehydes and ketones, sesquiterpenes, and naphthalene. In the drug, there are also flavonoids and more especially isoflavones (irilone, irisolone, irigenin, tectoridin, homotectoridin, etc.) [3, 4]. The first bicyclic and monocyclic triterpenes to be found in nature were isolated from Iridis rhizoma, viz α- and δ- and iridogermanal [2, 5]. *C*-Glucosylxanthones have also been detected in the drug.

Indications: The drug is mainly used in _folk medicine_ as an expectorant and demulcent for colds, catarrh, etc. Several flavonoids from orris root, in particular the isoflavone irigenin, have been reported to inhibit cAMP phosphodiesterase [6].
Turned pieces were, and to some extent still are, given to teething infants to chew on; this is to be discouraged on hygienic grounds, since the wet drug is a good breeding ground for microorganisms.
To a small extent, the drug is still employed as a corrective in various preparations in the food and cosmetic industries and as an aroma component of fine liqueurs and other alcoholic drinks.

Making the tea: The drug is only used in herbal mixtures.

Phytomedicines: The drug is present in several cough teas and bronchial teas. Extracts are used in prepared antitussive remedies, e.g. Bronchitussin® (tablets), etc.

Authentication: Macro- (see: Description) and microscopically. See also the BHP 1983. The starch grains with a horseshoe-shaped hilum (Fig. 4) and fairly large whole or bro-

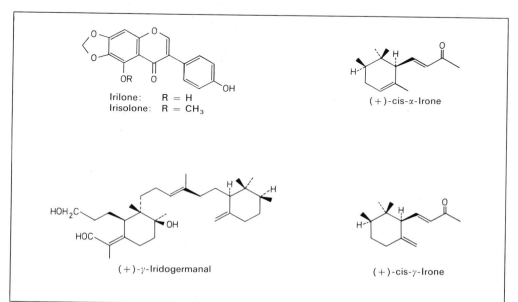

Irilone: R = H
Irisolone: R = CH₃

(+)-cis-α-Irone

(+)-γ-Iridogermanal

(+)-cis-γ-Irone

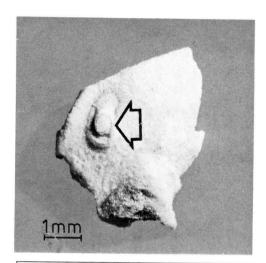

Fig. 3: Fragment of the rhizome, showing a lateral root (arrow)

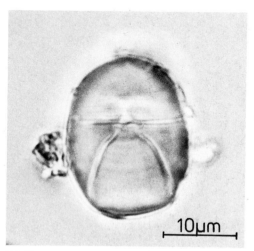

Fig. 4: Typical starch granule with horseshoe-shaped hilum

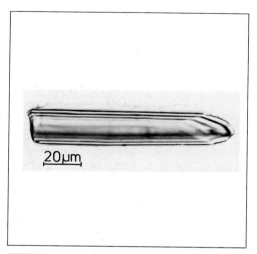

Fig. 5: Large elongated prism of calcium oxalate showing the chisel-shaped end

ken, much elongated prisms of calcium oxalate with oblique or chisel-shaped ends (Fig. 5) are highly characteristic features. The parenchyma is pitted and non-lignified, and stone cells are absent. The microscopy of the powdered drug is detailed in [7].

The following TLC procedure is a suitable identification test:

Test solution: the xylene/essential oil mixture obtained from 50 g drug in determining the essential-oil content using 0.5 ml xylene is carefully collected and a further 0.5 ml xylene added to it.

Reference solution: 20 µl anisaldehyde dissolved in 10 ml methanol.

Loadings: 2 µl each of the test and reference solutions, as bands on silica gel.

Solvent system: toluene + ethyl acetate (97 + 3), 5 cm run.

Detection: after complete removal of the solvent, examined first under UV 254 nm light and then sprayed with a 1% vanillin in ethanol/sulphuric acid (4 + 1) and heated for 1–3 min. at 105 °C.

Evaluation: in UV 254 nm light. Reference solution: anisaldehyde, a strong quenching

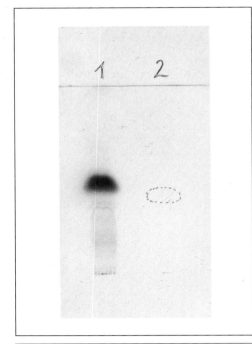

Fig. 6: TLC on 4 × 8 cm silica-gel foil

1: Orris root
2: Anisaldehyde (reference substance)

For details, see the text

zone (to be marked) in the middle Rf range. After spraying and heating. Test solution: at about the same Rf or just above it, an intense blue-green zone; slightly below, a violet, a grey and two bright red zones (Fig. 6).

Quantitative standard: DAB 6: *Ash*, not more than 5%.

Adulteration: Rarely occurs in practice. It should be detected on microscopical examination.

Storage: With this drug, the exclusion of light and moisture is particularly important, since it otherwise rapidly turns yellow (if necessary, re-dry without using heat).

Literature:
[1] P. Fusi and M. Bosetto Fusi, Fitoterapia **48**, 51 (1977).
[2] W. Krick, F.J. Marner, and L. Jaenicke, Helv. Chim. Acta **67**, 318 (1984).
[3] K.L. Dhar and A.K. Kalla, Phytochemistry **11**, 3097 (1972); *ibid.*, **12**, 734 (1973).
[4] A.A. Ali et al., Phytochemistry **22**, 2061 (1983).
[5] F.K. Marner, W. Krick, B. Gellrich, L. Jaenicke, and W. Winter, J. Org. Chem. **47**, 2531 (1982).
[6] R. Nikaido, T. Ohmoto, U. Sankawa, T. Hamanaka, and K. Totsuka, Planta Med. **46**, 162 (1982).
[7] B.P. Jackson and D.W. Snowdon, Atlas of microscopy of medicinal plants, culinary herbs and spices, Belhaven Press, London, 1990, pp. 172–173.

Juglandis folium   Walnut leaf

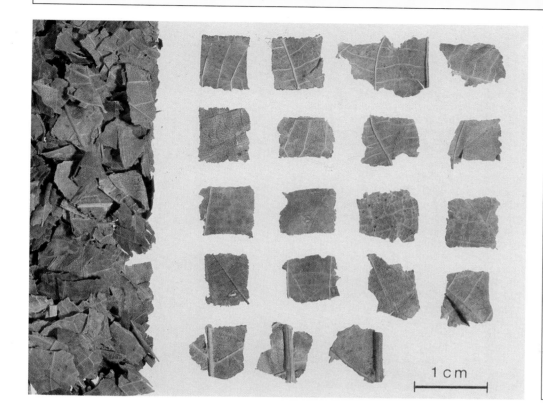

Fig. 1: Walnut leaf

Description: The drug consists of the entire-margined leaflets freed from the rachis. When cut, the drug comprises brittle, fairly stiff, glabrous leaf fragments which are more or less brownish green on both surfaces. In the angles of the nerves on the lower surface, small tufts of fine hairs can be seen with a hand lens (Fig. 3). The venation on the lower surface is characteristic: the second order lateral veins (tertiary veins) branch off at right angles to the first order lateral veins (secondary veins) which in turn branch off from the reddish brown main vein (Fig. 4), thus producing a characteristic, more or less rectangular tesselation; within the fields, there is a dense, but not prominent, reticulate venation.

Odour: Faintly aromatic.

Taste: Astringent, somewhat bitter and harsh.

Fig. 2: *Juglans regia* L.

A 10–25 m tall tree bearing ca. 25 cm wide, first reddish and later green, imparipinnate leaves made up of 7–9 elliptic, entire leaflets. Male flowers hanging in long, green catkins, female ones grouped in twos or threes. Drupe surrounded by a smooth, green (later brown), fleshy shell (it is not a nut!).

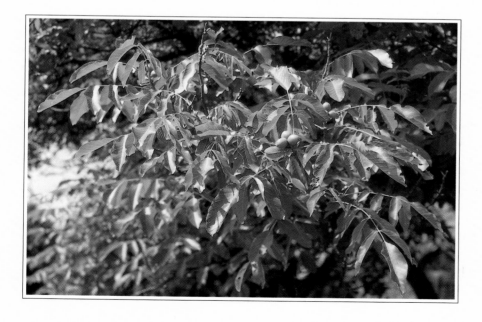

DAB 6: Folia Juglandis

Plant source: *Juglans regia* L., walnut (Juglandaceae).

Synonyms: Walnußblätter (Ger.), Feuilles de noyer (Fr.).

Origin: Native in south-eastern Europe, Asia Minor, and as far as northern India, China, and Central Asia. Cultivated throughout Europe, North Africa, North America, and East Asia. Imports of the drug come from Eastern Europe.

Constituents: Ca. 10% tannin (ellagitannins). Juglone (= 5-hydroxy-1,4-naphthoquinone), and hydrojuglone almost entirely in the form of the monoglucoside [1]; juglone is unstable and readily polymerizes to brown and black pigments; it is therefore present only in traces in older leaves and in the drug. Related compounds, including a series of volatile 1,4-naphthoquinones like plumbagin, β-hydroplumbagin, and others are present in other parts of the plant (stem bark, fruit husks) [10, 11]; whether such sub-

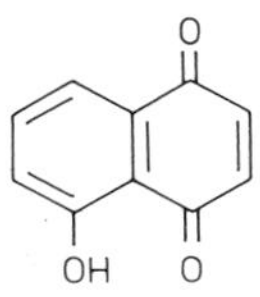

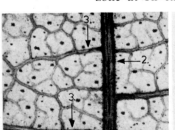

Juglone

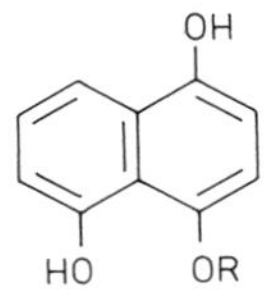

Hydrojuglone: R = H
Hydrojuglone glucoside: R = Glucose

*Extract from the German Commission
E monograph
(BAnz no. 101, dated 01.06.1990)*

Uses
External use: mild, superficial inflammation of the skin; excessive sweating, e.g. of the hands and feet.

Contraindications
None known.

Side effects
None known.

Interactions with other remedies
None known.

Dosage
Unless otherwise prescribed: for poultices and hip-baths, 2–3 g drug to 100 ml water; preparations correspondingly.

Mode of administration
Comminuted drug for infusions and other galenical preparations for external use.

Effects
Astringent.

stances also occur in the leaves still has to be determined. Flavonoids: quercetin, hyperoside, quercitrin, etc. Gallic, caffeic, and neo-chlorogenic acids. Ca. 0.01–0.03% essential oil, with germacrene D as the main component [2]. Walnut leaf contains a notable amount of ascorbic acid, viz 0.85–1.0% [3].

Indications: Based on its tannin content, as an astringent. It is mainly used externally (baths, rinses, dressings) for skin conditions such as acne, eczema, scrophula, pyodermia, and ulcers. The drug is also employed internally as an adjuvant for the conditions indicated and as an antidiarrhoeal.
In *folk medicine,* it is given for gastrointestinal catarrh, as an anthelmintic, and as a so-called "blood-purifying" agent.
Juglone [4] and the essential oil [5] are antifungal. There are indications that, on i.p. administration in mice, the isolated constituent juglone has an inhibitory effect on tumours, e.g. the Ehrlich ascites tumour [6, 7].

Making the tea: 1.5 g of the finely chopped drug is put into cold water, heated to boiling, and after 3–5 min. passed through a tea strainer. Internally as an adjuvant (see: Indications) for skin conditions, a cupful of the tea is drunk one to three times a day. For dressings and lotions, a decoction of 5 g drug in 200 ml water is used.
1 Teaspoon = ca. 0.9 g.

Phytomedicines: Walnut leaf or extracts from it are present, mostly as adjuvants, in only a few prepared alteratives, analgesics and antirheumatics, cholagogues, gastrointestinal remedies, roborants and tonics, etc.

Authentication: Macro- (see: Description) and microscopically. Stomata with four subsidiary cells are found only in the lower epidermis. In the angles between the main veins and the first-order lateral veins, there are unicellular trichomes which are united in groups of three to five (Fig. 5). On both surfaces, there are glandular trichomes with uni- or bi-(less often quadri-)cellular stalks and bi- or quadri-(less often multi-)cellular heads, similar to those found in Lamiaceae (Labiatae). The spongy parenchyma has colourless cells with large calcium-oxalate clusters (Fig. 4).
Since the drug is relatively rich in flavonoids, identification of the drug through their TLC separation is also possible. A description of the method with a coloured illustration of the chromatogram is to be found in [8]; see also [9]. The procedure is the same as that for Althaeae radix (q.v.);

Evaluation: in UV 365 nm light. Test solution: a yellowish green fluorescent zone at Rf 0.95; an orange fluorescent quercitrin zone at Rf ca. 0.8; an orange fluorescent

zone above the orange fluorescent hyperoside zone at Rf 0.6; an intense bluish white fluorescent zone at Rf ca. 0.55 (neochlorogenic acid?). Rutin and chlorogenic acid absent.

Quantitative standard: DAB 6: *Ash*, not more than 10%.

Adulteration: In practice, does not occur.

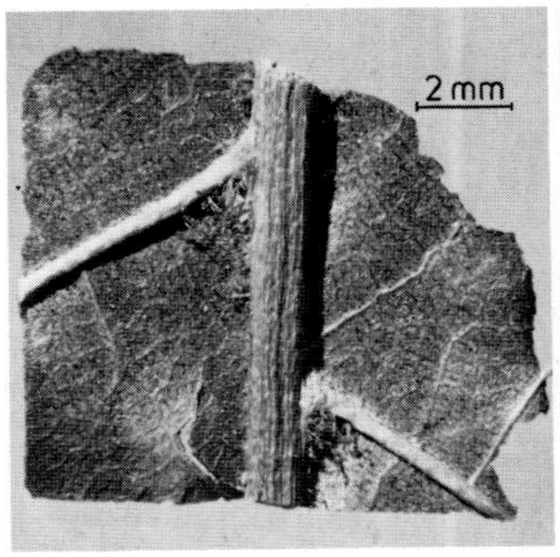

Literature:
[1] E. Wojcik, Farm. Polon. **40**, 523 (1984); C.A. **103**, 3761 (1985).
[2] R.G. Buttery et al., J. Agric. Food Chem. **34**, 820 (1986).
[3] E. Jones and R.E. Hughes, Phytochemistry **23**, 2366 (1984).
[4] V.L. Aizenberg, A.V. Gvozdov, and F.A. Lisinger, Tr. Kishinev Sel'skokhoz. Inst. (72), 88 (1971); C.A. **78**, 106417 (1973), via: Zh. Biol. Khim. **1972**, Abstr. no. 16F20.
[5] A. Nahrstedt, U. Vetter, and F.J. Hammerschmidt, Planta Med. **42**, 313 (1981).
[6] U.C. Bhargava and B.A. Westfall, J. Pharm. Sci. **57**, 1674 (1968).
[7] T.A. Okada, E. Roberts, and F. Brodie, Proc. Soc. Exptl. Biol. Med. **126**, 583 (1967).
[8] H. Wagner, S. Bladt, and E.M. Zgainski, Plant drug analysis, Springer-Verlag, Berlin, Heidelberg, New York, Tokyo, 1984, p. 182.
[9] P. Rohdewald, G. Rücker, and K.-W. Glombitza, Apothekengerechte Prüfvorschriften, Deutscher Apotheker-Verlag, Stuttgart, 1986, p. 1051.
[10] R.G. Binder, M.E. Benson, and R.A. Flath, Phytochemistry **28**, 2799 (1989).
[11] S.K. Talapatra, B. Karmacharya, S.C. De, and B. Talapatra, Phytochemistry **27**, 3929 (1988).

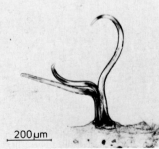

Fig. 3: Tufts of fine hairs in the angles between the secondary veins and the midrib (lower leaf surface)

Fig. 4: The tertiary veins (3) run at right angles to the secondary veins (2). Further, numerous clusters of calcium-oxalate crystals in the mesophyll

Fig. 5: United, unicellular, thick-walled trichomes

Juniperi fructus   (DAB 10), Juniper berry

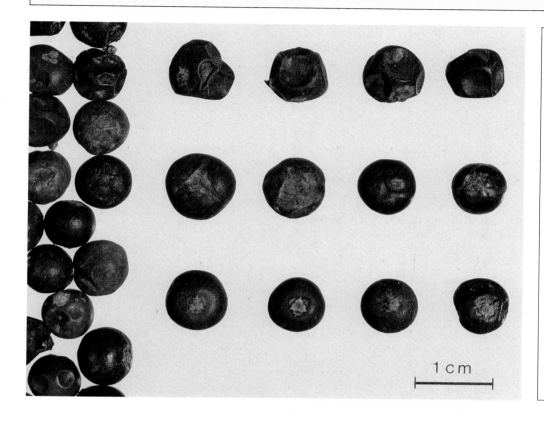

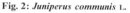
1 cm

Fig. 1: Juniper berry

Description: The drug consists of the ripe, carefully dried, berry-like fruits, which are globose, violet to black-brown, often bluish pruinose, and up to 10 mm in diameter. At the apex, there is a triradiate mark and depression which indicate the sutures of the three scales. Quite often, the remains of the peduncle can be seen at the base of the fruit. Inside, embedded in a sticky fruit flesh, there are usually three, very hard, oblong, triangular seeds (Fig. 3).

Odour: Characteristically spicy.

Taste: Sweet, aromatic and spicy.

Fig. 2: *Juniperus communis* L.

Male and female flowers both dull yellow. Berry-like cones (fruits), with a characteristic triradiate mark arising from fusion of the three uppermost scales, developing on the female plant. Fruits green in the first year after fertilization, becoming blue-black and pruinose in the second year.

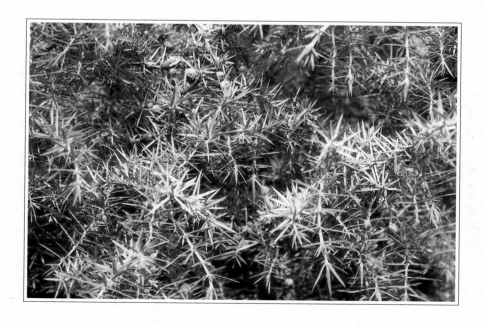

DAB 10: Wacholderbeeren
ÖAB: Fructus Juniperi
Ph. Helv. VII: Iuniperi fructus (Pseudofructus iuniperi)
St. Zul. 1369.99.99

Plant source: *Juniperus communis* L., juniper (Cupressaceae).

Synonyms: Baccae juniperi, Galbuli juniperi (Lat.), Wacholderbeeren (Ger.), Juniperus, Juniper berries or fruit (Engl.), Baies de genièvre (Fr.).

Origin: Native in Europe, northern Asia, and North America (in Germany and Austria under partial or complete protection). The drug is imported from former Yugoslavia, Italy, Albania and other countries. The trade names often relate to the quality and not to the origin: "Italian" drug refers particularly to large, selected berries that do not necessarily have to have come from Italy.

Constituents: 0.5–2.0% essential oil with more than 70 isolated components; monoterpenes are the main components:

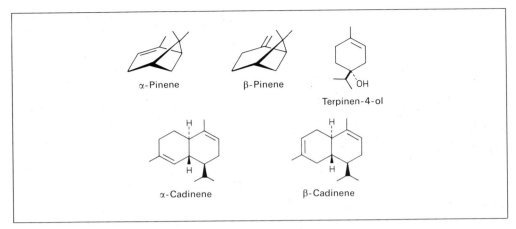

α-Pinene   β-Pinene   Terpinen-4-ol

α-Cadinene   β-Cadinene

16.5–80% α- and β-pinene, 0.2–50% sabinene, 1–12% limonene; up to 5% terpinen-4-ol, α-terpineol, borneol, geraniol, etc.; and sesquiterpenes (including the cadinenes) often present only in traces; also, phenols and esters. The qualitative and quantitative composition of the essential oil depends on the origin and on the ripeness of the berries, e.g. often the 1,4-cineole mentioned in the literature is absent [1, 2, 8]. Further, ca. 30% invert sugar (glucose + fructose), 3–5% catechol tannins, flavonoids, and leucoanthocyanidins [1].

Indications: As a diuretic and urinary antiseptic (which is disputed; see below). At any rate, only water diuresis takes place (the loss of sodium ions is slight). This is considered to be due particularly to the content of terpinen-4-ol, which in contrast to other terpenes is said not to irritate the tissues; it is certain, however, that other terpenes (especially pinene) are also involved in the diuresis, since the irritant action of these substances on the kidneys is evident from hyperaemia of the glomeruli, which stimulates the activity of the secretory epithelium [1, 3, 4]. The use of juniper berries as a diuretic is much disputed, because the diuresis is brought about by irritation (which under certain circumstances may be toxic) of the kidneys. This is the reason for not including this indication in the Standard Licence (q.v.). In *folk medicine*, the drug is used as a stomachic, carminative, and as an aromatic in dyspeptic complaints (this is the only indication given in the Standard Licence). In *veterinary medicine*, the drug is also used as a diuretic, to stimulate feeding and as a component of "crop powders" [5].
Large amounts of the drug are used as a spice and in the manufacture of spirits (gin) and liqueurs [5].

Side effects: On prolonged use and with overdoses (urine smelling of violets), there may be renal irritation, gastrointestinal upsets, haematuria, and symptoms of central stimulation. Owing to this cellular stimulation and irritation, the drug is contraindicated in inflammatory kidney disorders and during pregnancy (in the later stages, uterine contractions may be initiated) [1, 4, 6].

Making the tea: Boiling water (ca. 150 ml) is poured over ca. 2 g of the freshly crushed berries and after 10 min. strained.
1 Teaspoon = ca. 3 g.

Warning: Not to be used in nephritis; on prolonged use, watch out for side effects!

Herbal teas: Juniper-berry dry extracts are present in some diuretics and urological instant teas, e.g. Harntee® 400, NB-Tee Siegfried®, etc.

Phytomedicines: The drug and extracts prepared from it are contained in several prepared diuretic remedies, often in combination with other diuretic drugs (Betulae folium – birch leaves, Equiseti herba – horsetail herb, Petroselini fructus – parsley fruit, Ononidis radix – restharrow root, etc.).

Note: In the Ph. Helv. VII, there are two juniper preparations: (a) Wacholderöl (Iuniperi aetheroleum) (juniper oil), which is obtained from the berries of *J. communis* by steam distillation and preserved with a small amount of a suitable antioxidant. (b) Wacholdergeist (juniper spirit), the composition of which is: 0.5 g juniper oil, 66.3 g ethanol containing 0.1% camphor, and 33.2 g purified water.

Regulatory status (UK): General Sales List – Schedule 1, Table A.

Authentication: Macro- (see: Description) and microscopically, following the DAB 10. See also the BHP 1983. The presence of the large, lignified idioblasts (Fig. 4) should be noted; they are unbranched, in contrast to those of other *Juniperus* species; see: Adulteration.
The TLC test of identity given in the DAB 10 (cf. [7]) is as follows:

Test solution: 0.5 g crushed drug shaken with 5 ml dichloromethane for 2–3 min. and the solution filtered over ca. 2 g anhydrous sodium sulphate – the filtrate to be used immediately.

Reference solution: 10 µl cineole and 4.0 mg guaiazulene dissolved in 10 ml dichloromethane.

Loadings: 20 µl test solution and 10 µl reference solution, as 2-cm bands on silica gel G.

Solvent system: dichloromethane, 10 cm run.

Detection: sprayed with anisaldehyde reagent and observed while heated at 100–105 °C for 5–10 min.

Extract from the German Commission E monograph (BAnz no. 228, dated 05. 12. 1984)

Uses
Dyspeptic complaints.

Contraindications
Pregnancy and inflammation of the kidneys.

Side effects
On prolonged use or with an overdose, kidney damage may result.

Interactions
None known.

Dosage
Unless otherwise prescribed: daily dose, 2 g up to a maximum of 10 g, of the dried juniper fruit, corresponding to 20 mg to 100 mg of the essential oil.

Mode of administration
Whole, crushed, or powdered drug for infusions and decoctions, alcoholic extracts, and in wine. Essential oil.

Note
Combinations with other plant drugs in bladder and kidney teas and similar preparations may be helpful.

Effects
In animal experiments, an increase in urinary output has been demonstrated, as well as a direct action on the contraction of smooth muscle.

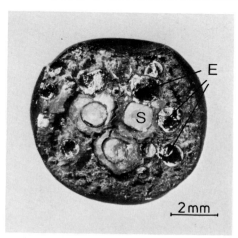

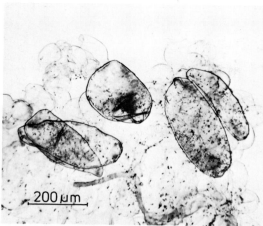

Fig. 3: Cut-open fruit (berry) of *Juniperus communis* with three hard seeds (S) and several oil glands (E) in the brown, mealy and sticky fruit flesh

Fig. 4: Large, lignified idioblasts in the fruit flesh

Evaluation: Reference solution: brown to greyish violet cineole zone in the lower third and the orange-brown guaiazulene zone slightly below the solvent front. Test solution: slightly below the level of the cineole zone of the reference solution, a broad irregular reddish violet zone (diterpene acids); an intense reddish violet zone at the same height as the guaiazulene zone of the reference solution (mono- and sesquiterpene hydrocarbons); between these two zones, usually four, fainter reddish or bluish violet zones.

Quantitative standards: DAB 10: *Volatile oil*, not less than 1.0%. *Foreign matter*, not more than 5% unripe or discoloured fruit and not more than 2% other foreign matter. *Loss on drying*, not more than 15.0%. *Ash*, not more than 4.0%.

ÖAB: *Volatile oil*, not less than 1.0% Ph. Helv. VII: *Volatile oil*, not less than 1.0%. *Foreign matter*, immature or otherwise coloured berries not more than 5%; see also: Adulteration (below). *Water content*, not more than 12.0%. *Sulphated ash*, not more than 6.0%.
The crushed drug has to be used for determining the essential-oil content.

Adulteration: This occasionally happens with the fruit of other *Juniperus* species. *J. phoenicea* L. and *J. oxycedrus* L. (including subsp. *macrocarpa* (SIBTH. et SMITH) BALL) have fruit differing in size and colour. The fruit of *J. sabina* L., savin, has 3 or 4 (less often 1 or 2) scales and large, lignified, branched idioblasts in the mesocarp.

Storage: It is recommended to keep supplies of dried juniper berries for herbal teas over a suitable desiccant in well-closed containers made of glass or metal (but not plastic) as protection from light. When required, they are rubbed through a sieve. Mixtures with these comminuted berries are distinguished by their homogeneity from those which for convenience have been prepared from "somewhat crushed" fruit [5]. The very high loss of essential oil after the fruits are broken up or crushed is the reason why the DAB 10 indicates that the powder must not be kept for longer than 24 hours.

Wording of the package insert, from the German Standard Licence

6.1 Uses

Dyspeptic complaints such as belching, heartburn, and a feeling of distension.

6.2 Contraindications

Juniper-berry should not be taken during pregnancy or if renal inflammation (nephritis, pyelitis) is present.

6.3 Side effects

On prolonged use or with overdoses, renal damage may occur, evident from renal pain with an increased urge to urinate, pain during urination, and the presence of blood and protein in the urine (haematuria and albuminuria).

6.4 Dosage and Mode of administration

About one teaspoonful (2–3 g) of **Juniper berry** is crushed, boiling water (ca. 150 ml) poured over them, and after about 10 min. passed through a tea strainer. Unless otherwise prescribed, a cupful of the tea is drunk three or four times a day.

6.5 Duration of use

Juniper-berry tea should be taken for longer than 4 weeks without consulting a doctor.

6.6 Note

Store protected from light and moisture.

Literature:
[1] Kommentar DAB 10.
[2] V. Formácek and K.-H. Kubeczka, Essential oil analysis by capillary gas chromatography and carbon-13 NMR spectroscopy, Wiley, Chichester, 1982.
[3] G. Harnischfeger and H. Stolze, Bewährte Pflanzendrogen in Wissenschaft und Medizin, Notamed, Bad Homburg/Melsungen, 1983.
[4] R. Hänsel and H. Haas, Therapie mit Phytopharmaka, Springer, Berlin, 1984.
[5] Hager, vol. **5**, p. 333 (1976); vol. **5**, p. 571 (1993).
[6] H. Braun and D. Frohne, Heilpflanzenlexikon für Ärzte und Apotheker, Gustav Fischer, Stuttgart – New York, 1987.
[7] P. Pachaly, Dünnschichtchromatographie in der Apotheke, 2nd ed., Wissenschaftliche Verlagsgesellschaft m.b.H., Stuttgart, 1983.
[8] G. Vernin et al., Phytochemistry **27**, 1061 (1988).

Juniperi lignum   Juniper wood

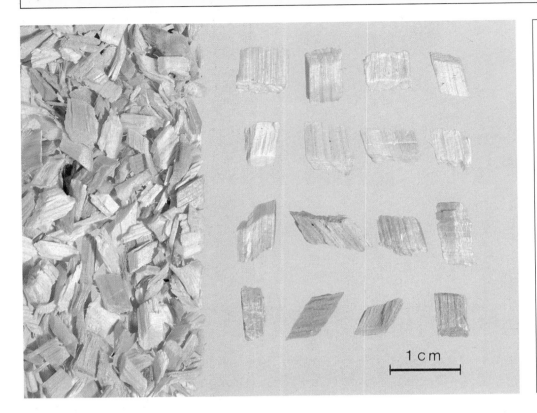

1 cm

Fig. 1: Juniper wood

<u>Description:</u> **The drug consists of the trunk, branch, and root wood. The material comprises yellowish white, pale yellowish brown, to reddish yellow pieces of wood, often in the form of chips, with easily removed remnants of the thin bark. The pieces are fibrous, easily split, and brittle. In transverse sections the annual rings are clearly recognizable, while in radial longitudinal sections the medullary rays are visible as fine striations.**

<u>Odour:</u> **On warming, aromatic and pleasant.**

<u>Taste:</u> **Aromatic and spicy.**

Fig. 2: *Juniperus communis* L.

An evergreen bush or tree up to 6 m in height, with ca. 1.5 cm long, sharply-pointed, needle-like leaves arranged in threes and having a broad, light-coloured stripe on the upper surface. Dioecious plants growing on moors and in stony and rocky soil in heaths and mountains.

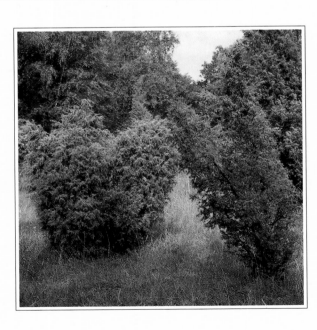

Erg. B. 6: Lignum Juniperi

Plant source: *Juniperus communis* L., juniper (Cupressaceae).

Synonyms: See under, Juniperi fructus; Wacholderholz (Ger.), Bois de genièvre (Fr.).

Origin: See under, Juniperi fructus.

Constituents: Unusual diterpenes (including sugiol, xanthoperol, communic acid), sesquiterpenes (among them thujopsene, pygmaein), and other terpenes in the wood; longifolene and other terpenes in the bark. Further, tannins (gallocatechins), lignans (including podophyllotoxin), and stigmasterol [1, 2].

Indications: In *folk medicine* as a diuretic and diaphoretic; as a so-called "blood-purifying remedy", for skin conditions, arthritis, and rheumatism. For fumigation, the material is often coloured (see [3]).

Making the tea: Boiling water is poured over ca. 3 g of the finely chopped drug, kept

Sugiol

Xanthoperol

trans-Communic acid

Thujopsene

Pygmaein

Podophyllotoxin

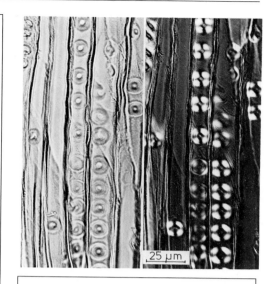

Fig. 3: Tracheids with bordered pits, under ordinary illumination (left) and under crossed polaroids (right)

on the boil for 5 min., allowed to draw for 10 min., and then strained.
1 Teaspoon = ca. 2 g.

Phytomedicines: The drug is a component of only a few prepared diuretics, "rheumatism teas", and "blood-purifying teas".

Authentication: Macro- (see: Description) and microscopically, according to Erg. B. 6. The wood has tracheids with bordered pits (Fig. 3) and xylem parenchyma, but no fibres and vessels.

The colour of an aqueous drug extract is not changed on addition of iron(III) chloride solution.

Adulteration: Hardly ever occurs; adulteration with or admixture of wood from deciduous trees is readily detected by the presence of vessels.

Quantitative standard: <u>Erg. B. 6</u>: *Vessels and fibres of hard woods*, must be absent. *Ash*, not more than 7%.

Storage: Protected from light and moisture in metal or glass (but not plastic) containers.

Literature:
[1] H.T. Erdmann and T. Norin, Fortschr. Chem. Naturstoffe **24**, 207 (1966).
[2] G. Harnischfeger and H. Stolze, Bewährte Pflanzendrogen in Wissenschaft und Medizin, Notamed, Bad Homburg/Melsungen, 1983.
Refs. [1] and [2] cite mainly the work of J.B. Bredenberg and co-workers who have made a particular study of the constituents of Lignum juniperi.
[3] Hager, vol. **5**, p. 337 (1976); vol. **5**, p. 576 (1993).

Lamii albi flos
Lamii albi herba

White deadnettle flower

White deadnettle

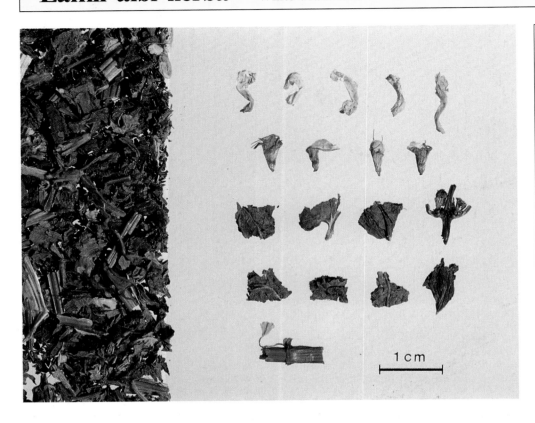

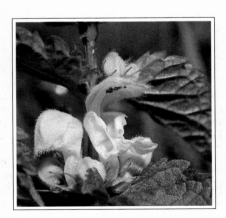

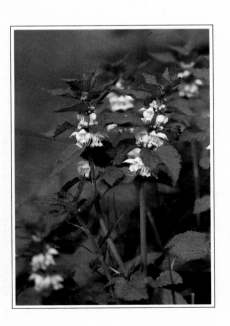

Fig. 1: White deadnettle flower

<u>Description:</u> The flower drug consists of the dried petals with attached stamens. It is made up of yellowish white, wrinkled and compressed, 10–15 mm long, two-lipped corollas curved in the shape of an S. The strongly arched upper lip distinctly is pubescent, especially towards the tip, while the lower lip is three-lobed with the lateral lobes ending in a long tooth. The four stamens (the two upper ones of which are shorter) are fused as far as the throat of the corolla.

<u>Odour:</u> Very faint.

<u>Taste:</u> Hardly bitter.

White deadnettle (herb)

<u>Description:</u> The drug consists of the aerial parts harvested during the flowering period and rapidly dried. The much crumpled leaf fragments have a coarsely dentate margin, with the upper surface a deep green and the lower surface lighter; both surfaces are pubescent. In addition, the lower surfaces shows a fine, reticulate venation. The 4-angled pieces of stem are hollow. The flowers are as described above.

<u>Odour:</u> Very faint.

<u>Taste:</u> Slightly bitter.

Figs. 2 and 3: *Lamium album* L.

A 50 cm tall pubescent herb with creeping and branched rhizomes, erect stems, and petiolate, cordate leaves with a dentate margin. Whorls of white axillary flowers with a ca. 2-cm long corolla and a 5-toothed calyx.

Erg. B. 6: Flores Lamii albi
St. Zul. 1359.99.99 (Weißes Taubnesselkraut)

Synonyms: Archangel (Engl.), Weiße Taubnesselblüten, Weißes Taubnesselkraut (Ger.), Fleurs d'ortie blanche, Fleurs de lamier blanc (Fr.).

Origin: Native and widespread in Europe and Asia. The drug is imported from former Czechoslovakia, Poland, and the former USSR.

Constituents: Both the herb and the flower drugs have been very inadequately studied. The occurrence of triterpenoid saponins [1], phenol-carboxylic acids [2], flavonoids [3], and mucilage has been reported, without any exact structural proofs. Only the iridoid glycoside present in the herb, lamalbide, has been well studied [4, 5]. Very probably, the drug contains tannins and presumably also the betaine stachydrine, rosmarinic acid and similar compounds, and traces of essential oil.

Indications: The drug is used only in *folk medicine* as an expectorant in respiratory complaints, for dissolving phlegm in catarrhal conditions, and also against flatulence and gastrointestinal complaints (see St.Zul.).

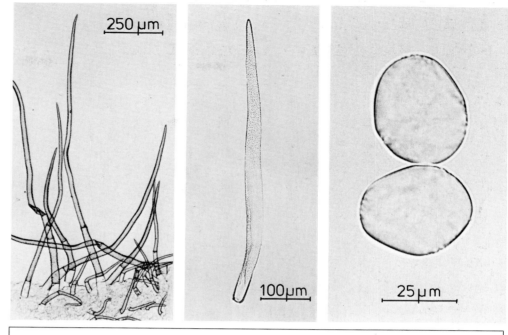

Fig. 4: **Multicellular trichomes (basal cell often without a warty cuticle), from the petals**

Fig. 5: **Tubular trichome with punctate cuticle, from the anthers**

Fig. 6: **Potato-shaped pollen grains (tricolpate)**

It is also employed in *folk medicine* for menopausal disorders, leucorrhoea, and urogenital disorders. Poultices made with the boiled-up drug are applied to swellings of the skin, bruises, varicose veins, and arthritic swellings. It is also a so-called "blood-cleansing" agent.

In animal experiments, the triterpenes of this drug have exhibited a clear-cut anti-inflammatory effect, but the diuretic effect (accompanied by definite kaliuresis) is less distinct; on i.v. administration, the saponins exhibit a dose-related hypotensive action [1].

Lamalbide

Making the tea: Boiling water is poured over ca. 1 g of the finely chopped drug and after 5 min. passed through a tea strainer. As an expectorant, a cupful, sweetened with honey, is drunk several times a day.
1 Teaspoon = ca. 0.5 g.

Herbal preparations: The herb is rarely, the flowers are occasionally, included as a component in nervine and sedative teas (also in tea bags), bronchial teas, and in herbal cures.

Phytomedicines: The drug is present in only a few prepared remedies.

Authentication: Macro- (see: Description) and microscopically, following the Erg. B. 6. The petals have various types of trichomes, mostly with a warty cuticle and mostly with a smooth basal cell (Fig. 4). The trichomes of the anthers are up to 800 µm long, unicellular, and finely punctate (Fig. 5). The pollen grains are round or elliptic, smooth, ca. 30 µm in diameter, and tricolpate (Fig. 6). The following TLC procedure (slightly modified from the St.Zul.) is a suitable identification test:

Test solution: 3 g powdered drug shaken for ca. 15 min. with 30 ml water; the filtrate

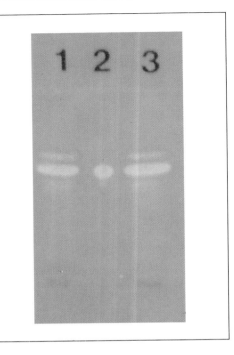

**Fig. 7: TLC on 4×8 cm silica-gel foil
Evaluation in UV 366 light**

1 and 3: White deadnettle herb (different origins)
2: Caffeic acid (reference compound)

shaken twice with 2×25 ml ethyl acetate; the combined organic phases, after filtration through anhydrous sodium sulphate, as the test solution.

Reference solution: 50 mg caffeic acid dissolved in 10 ml methanol.

Loadings: 5 µl test solution and 2 µl reference solution, both as 2-cm bands on silica gel GF_{254}.

Solvent system: toluene + ethyl formate + anhydrous formic acid (50 + 40 + 10), 5 cm run.

Detection: after drying the chromatogram in a current of hot air, examined in UV 254 and 366 nm light and then sprayed with a 10.5% iron(III) chloride solution and evaluated in daylight.

Evaluation: in UV 254 nm light. Reference solution: caffeic acid, as a quenching band at Rf ca. 0.6. Test solution: a quenching band at the same Rf; slightly above it a more intense zone and below it several other quenching zones. In UV 366 nm light. Reference solution: caffeic acid, intense blue fluorescence. Test solution: intense blue fluorescent zones at the same Rf and above it; also some weaker fluorescent zones below it (Fig. 7).
After spraying. Reference solution: caffeic-acid zone, greyish blue. Test solution: greyish blue zones at the same Rf and slightly above and in the region below (Fig. 8).

Quantitative standards: St.Zul. 1359.99.99: *Foreign matter*, not more than 5% of flattened pieces of stem; leaves with unicellular, and some multicellular, trichomes containing silica in their walls and with epidermal cells containing warty cystoliths must not be present. *Loss on drying*, not more than 10%. *Ash*, not more than 16%. *Acid-insoluble ash*, not more than 1%.

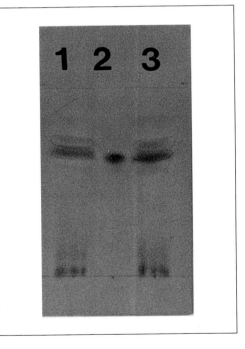

**Fig. 8: TLC on 4×8 cm silica-gel foil
Evaluation after spraying, see also fig. 7**

For details, see the text

Wording of the package insert, from the German Standard Licence:

6.1   Uses

As supportive treatment for gastrointestinal upsets, such as irritation of the mucous membranes of the stomach, a feeling of distension, and flatulence.

6.2   Dosage and Mode of administration

Hot water (ca. 150 ml) is poured over 3–4 teaspoonfuls (3–4 g) of **White deadnettle (herb)** and after 10–15 min. passed through a tea strainer.
Unless otherwise prescribed, a cupful of the freshly prepared infusion is drunk warm several times a day between meals.

6.3   Note

Store protected from light and moisture.

Adulteration: In practice, rarely happens. Flowers of various *Lonicera* species have pinkish red petals.

Literature

[1] M. Kory et al., Clujul Med. **55**, 156 (1982); C.A. **98**, 46480 (1983).

[2] J. Gora et al., Acta Polon. Pharm. **40**, 389 (1983); C.A. **100**, 135882 (1984).

[3] M. Tamas, V. Hodisan, and E. Muica, Clujul Med. **51**, 266 (1978); C.A. **90**, 83647 (1979).

[4] C.H. Brieskorn and R. Ahlborn, Tetrahedron Lett. (41), 4037 (1973).

[5] P. Eigtved, S.R. Jensen, and B.J. Nielsen, Acta Chem. Scand. Ser. **B 28**, 85 (1974).

Lavandulae flos   Lavandula (BHP 1983), Lavender

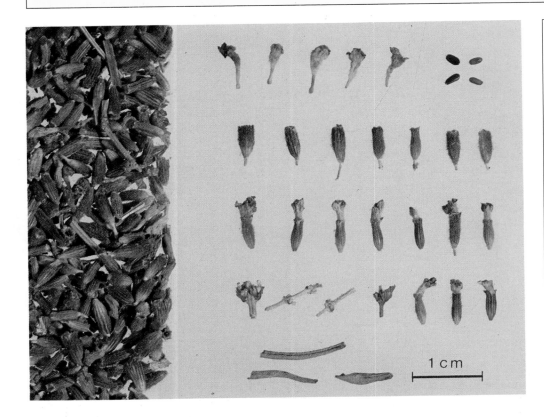

Description: To obtain the drug, the inflorescences, consisting of flowers arranged in false whorls, are stripped before flowering is finished and dried. Because the petals readily fall off during the drying process, the drug consists mainly of the tubular-ovoid, ribbed, bluish grey calices; these have five teeth, four of which are short, while the fifth one forms an oval or cordate projecting lip. The petals, which in the drug are much crumpled, are fused into a tube with a lower lip consisting of three small lobes and an upper lip comprising two larger erect lobes; the colour varies from deep bluish grey to a discoloured brown. Inside the corolla, there are four stamens and the superior ovary.

Odour: Intense, with a pleasant and aromatic scent.

Taste: Bitter.

Figs. 2 and 3: *Lavandula angustifolia* MILL.

A ca. 50 cm tall shrub with narrow lanceolate leaves initially are densely pubescent, later becoming glabrous. Flowers on long peduncles and in dense whorls forming a false spike. Leaves of spike lavender, *L. latifolia* MEDIK. (syn. *L. spica* DC.), somewhat broader and densely pubescent.

DAC 1986: Lavendelblüten
St. Zul. 8999.99.99

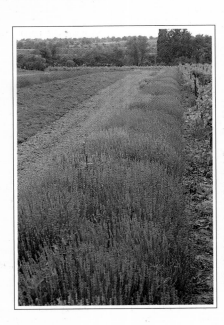

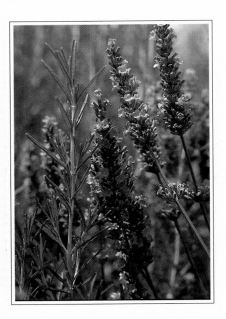

Plant source: *Lavandula angustifolia* MILL. subsp. *angustifolia* (syn. *L. officinalis* CHAIX, *L. vera* DC.), lavender (Lamiaceae).

Synonyms: Flores spicae (Lat.), Lavender, Garden or English Lavender (Engl.), Lavendelblüten (Ger.), Fleurs de lavande (Fr.).

Origin: Native in the Mediterranean region and grown there on a large scale. The drug is imported from France, former Yugoslavia, Bulgaria, and Spain.

Constituents: 1–3% essential oil, containing mainly monoterpenes (Lavandulae aetheroleum, DAB 10), the most important component of which is linaloyl acetate (30–55%), also linalool (20–35%), β-ocimene, cineole, and camphor, and also the sesquiterpene caryophyllene oxide; tannins (5–10%), probably derivatives of rosmarinic acid; coumarin; flavonoids; phytosterols.

Indications: The drug is applied as a mild sedative in excitement, nervous exhaustion, disturbances of sleep, and is frequently included as a component of calming teas. The drug is also used as a cholagogue, without, however, being able to pinpoint particular constituents of the drug as active principles for this, or its sedative, action. In *folk medicine,* the drug is also employed as a spasmolytic, carminative, stomachic, and diuretic. Lavender baths are still often prepared for the treatment of wounds and as a mild stimulant for the skin, and so also are herbal cushions as an aid to sleeping.

Making the tea: Boiling water is poured over 1.5 g lavender, covered and allowed to stand for 5–10 min., and then strained. 1 Teaspoon = ca. 0.8 g.

Phytomedicines: The drug and extract are components of some prepared sedatives, e.g. Sedatruw®, Nervoflux®, Beruhigungstee (calming tea) Salus® Nerven-Schlaf-Tee, etc., cholagogues such as Chol-Truw®, etc., and tonics.

Authentication: Macro- (see: Description) and microscopically, following the DAC 1986. There are several microscopical characters that are diagnostic for lavender; these include the branched trichomes of the sepals and petals, i.e. branched multicellular trichomes with a warty cuticle (Fig. 4), the long, papillose glandular trichomes with rounded terminal cells (Fig. 5) on the inside of the petals; the peculiar pollen grains with six pores and six bands on the exine (Fig. 6) are typical of the Lamiaceae.

The DAC 1986 has the following TLC test of identity:

Test solution: 0.5 g powdered drug boiled briefly with 5 ml dichloromethane, filtered, taken to dryness, and the residue dissolved in 0.5 ml ethyl acetate.

Reference solution: 0.01 ml linalool and 0.01 ml linaloyl acetate in 10 ml methanol and 2 ml of this solution made up to 10 ml with methanol.

Loadings: 20 µl test solution and 10 µl reference solution, as bands on silica gel 60.

Solvent system: dichloromethane, 10 cm run; then 5 min. drying; again, 10 cm run.

Detection: after drying, sprayed with anisaldehyde reagent, then heated at 100–105 °C.

Evaluation: in daylight. Reference and Test solutions: in the middle one-third, each showing two dark coloured zones with the same Rf values. Test solution: several minor zones also present.

Quantitative standards: DAC 1986: *Volatile oil*, not less than 1.3%. *Foreign matter*, entirely greyish brown or grey flowers not more than 10%; leaves and stems, not more than 5%; other foreign matter, not more than 1%. *Loss on drying*, not more than 12%. *Ash*, not more than 7.0%.

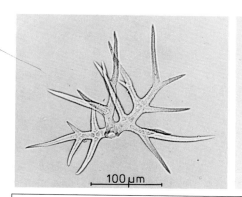
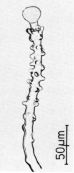
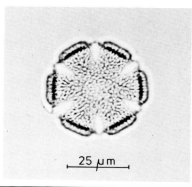

100 µm   50 µm   25 µm

Fig. 4: Branched trichome

Fig. 5: Glandular trichome from the ovary

Fig. 6: Hexacolpate pollen grain

Wording of the package insert, from the German Standard Licence

7.1 Uses

In complaints such as restlessness, sleeplessness, lack of appetite, and functional disorders of the upper abdomen (nervous irritable stomach, meteorism, and nervous disorders of the intestines).

7.2 Dosage and Mode of administration

Hot water (ca. 150 ml) is poured over 1–2 teaspoonfuls of **Lavender** and after 10 min. passed through a tea strainer.

Unless otherwise prescribed, a cupful of the freshly prepared tea is drunk several times a day, especially at night before going to sleep.

7.3 Note

Store away from light and moisture.

Extract from the German Commission E monograph (BAnz no. 228, dated 05. 12. 1984)

Uses

Internally: in health disorders such as restlessness, difficulties in sleeping, functional disorders of the upper abdomen (irritable stomach of nervous origin, Roehm-Held syndrome, meteorism, intestinal disorders of nervous origin).

In balneotherapy: for the treatment of functional disorders of the circulation.

Contraindications

None known.

Side effects

None known.

Interactions

None known.

Dosage

Unless otherwise prescribed:
Internally: as a tea, 1–2 teaspoonfuls of drug per cup; as lavender oil, 1–4 drops (ca. 20–80 mg), e.g. on a piece of cube sugar.
Externally: as a bath additive, 20–100 g drug to 20 l water.

Note

Combinations with other sedative and/or carminative drugs may be helpful.

Effects

Used internally: calming and antiflatulent.
Adequate pharmacological studies on man and animals have not yet been carried out.

BHP 1983: *Total ash*, not more than 8%. *Acid-insoluble ash*, not more than 2%.

Adulteration: Occurs with flowers of closely related species, especially *Lavandula hybrida*, a cross between *L. angustifolia* MILLER and *L. latifolia* MEDIKUS, which are used to obtain lavandin oil.

In practice, the recognition of such adulteration is possible only by accurate analysis of the essential oil, in which a higher cineole and lower linaloyl acetate content is found [1]. The DAB 10 TLC method of examination given under Lavandulae aetheroleum is as follows:

Test solution: 20 µl oil dissolved in 1.0 ml toluene.

Reference solution: 10 µl each of linalool and linalyl acetate dissolved in 1.0 ml toluene.

Loadings: 10 µl of each solution, as 2-cm bands on silica gel G.

Solvent system: dichloromethane, 2 × 10 cm run with 5 min. drying in between.

Detection: sprayed with anisaldehyde reagent and observed while being heated at 100–105 °C for 5–10 min.

Evaluation: in daylight. Reference solution: the violet linalool zone in the lower half and the violet linalyl acetate zone slightly above the middle. Test solution: zones of similar colour and intensity of colour at about the same Rf values; below the linalool zone, a further 2, and usually 4–5, greenish brown or reddish violet zone, a greenish brown zone directly below the linalool zone being the most intense; above the linalool zone and near the solvent front, further reddish violet zones; the brownish violet cineole zone sometimes observed between the linalool zone and the red caryophyllene oxide zone above it should only be faintly visible (lavandin oil).

Storage: Protected from light, in closed containers (not made of plastic).

Literature:
[1] Kommentar DAB 10.

Levistici radix   (DAB 10), Lovage

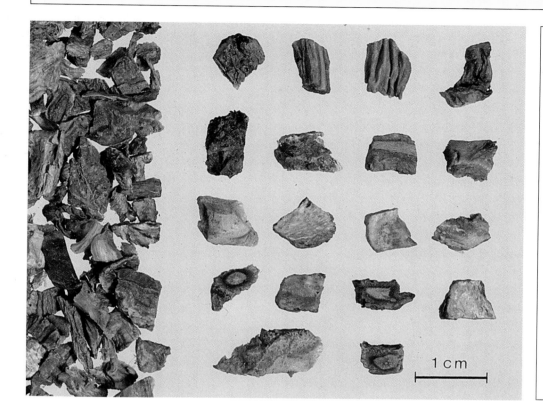

1 cm

Fig. 1: Lovage

<u>Description:</u> The material consists of wax-like and soft, yellow to dark reddish brown pieces of root and rhizome, which often have transverse rings. Examination of the transverse section shows a very porous and broad, spongy, externally whitish and towards the inside yellow to reddish brown cortex with oil ducts (ca. 70–150 µm) which are visible as tiny brown, often glistening, points; the narrow xylem is lemon-yellow and radially striate. The fragments of rhizome exhibit a pith. The fracture is short.

<u>Odour:</u> Characteristic, aromatic, reminiscent of seasoning for soups ("Maggi").

<u>Taste:</u> Sweetish and spicy, then slightly bitter.

Fig. 2: *Levisticum officinale* KOCH

An umbelliferous plant, up to 2 m in height, bearing large 2- to 3-pinnate leaves with broad, coarsely serrate segments. Small yellow flowers in double umbels bearing distinct bracts and bracteoles.

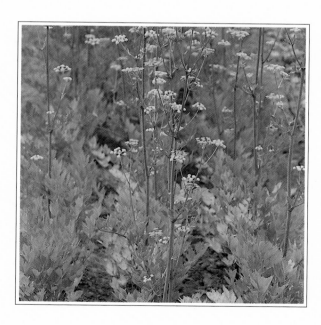

DAB 10: Liebstöckelwurzel
ÖAB: Radix Levistici
Ph. Helv. VII: Levistici radix
St. Zul. 1569.99.99

Plant source: *Levisticum officinale* KOCH (syn. *Ligusticum levisticum* L.), lovage (Apiaceae).

Synonyms: Radix Ligustici, Radix Laserpitii germanici (Lat.), Levisticum (Engl.), Liebstöckelwurzel, Maggiwurzel, Sauerkrautwurz, Gichtstockwurzel (Ger.), Racine de livèche (Fr).

Origin: Originally native in western Asia, the Orient, and southern Europe. It has been cultivated for thousands of years in Europe and later in North America where it has become to some extent naturalized. The drug comes exclusively from cultivated plants. The principal suppliers are Poland, the eastern part of Germany, Holland, and some of the Balkan states.

Constituents: Ca. 0.2–1.7%, but mostly 0.6–1.0%, essential oil, with up to 70% alkyl-

3-Butylphthalide

Ligusticum lactone

Senkyunolide
(= Sedanenolide)

Ligustilide

(+)-Falcarindiol

Extract from the German Commission E monograph
(*BAnz no. 101, dated* 01. 06. 90)

Uses

For irrigation therapy in inflammation of the urinary tract and in the prevention of renal gravel.

Contraindications

Lovage preparations should not be used in cases of acute inflammation of the renal parenchyma or impaired kidney function.

Side effects

None known.

Interactions with other remedies

None known.

Dosage

Unless otherwise prescribed: daily dose, 4–8 g drug; preparations correspondingly.

Mode of administration

Comminuted drug and other galenical preparations for internal use.
Irrigation therapy: an abundant fluid intake must be assured.

Warning

With prolonged use of lovage, UV irradiation and sun-bathing must be avoided.

Effects

The ligustilide-containing essential oil is spasmolytic.

phthalides as the characteristic odoriferous components of the drug: 3-butylphthalide (32%), *cis*- and *trans*-butylidenephthalide (= ligusticum lactone), *cis*- and *trans*-ligustilide (24%), 3-butyl-4,5-dihydrophthalide (= senkyunolide = sedanenolide), and Diels-Alder dimers (angeolide) derived from (*Z*)- and (*E*)-ligustilide and other dimers (levistolide A and B) [1]; α- and β-pinene, pentacyclohexadiene, α- and β-phellandrene, and α- and γ-terpinene, camphene, myrcene, etc.; coumarins: coumarin, umbelliferone, bergapten, psoralen; β-sitosterol O-β-D-glucoside; ferulic and caffeic acids, benzoic acid, angelic and isovaleric acids, and other volatile acids; and the poly-acetylene (+)-falcarindiol (0.06% in the fresh root) [1].

Indications: As a diuretic, especially with oedema, e.g. of the feet. The diuretic action is derived mainly from the essential oil present, the effect of which has been demonstrated in animal experiments on cats and mice; there is only a modest increase in the amount of urine produced and there is also a rise in the chloride and total nitrogen excreted [10]. Use of the drug is contraindicated in inflammatory renal conditions, because of the local irritant effect of the essential oil.
In *folk medicine*, the drug is also utilized as a stomachic and carminative; as with other phthalide-containing drugs, such as celery, the action is due to a reflex increase in the secretion of saliva and gastric juice brought about by the specific aroma and mild bitter taste [10]. Lovage is further used as an emmenagogue, and to dissolve phlegm in catarrhal conditions of the respiratory passages. Butylidenephthalide and ligustilide have been shown to have a spasmolytic action; butylphthalide and sedanenolide have a sedative effect [2, 10]. Lovage root is included in spice extracts, liqueurs, and (bitter) spirits.

Side effects: Furocoumarins may give rise to photodermatoses [3, 4]. However, there is no fear of phototoxic, photomutagenic, and photocarcinogenic effects on therapeutic use of the drug, especially as a tea, among other things because of the poor water-solubility of the furocoumarins [5].
The amount of the toxic, fungicidal, and antibacterial falcarindiol in the drug is so small that it can be ignored. Unlike the falcarinol occurring in ivy leaves, it does not cause contact allergies [6].

Making the tea: Boiling water is poured over 1.5–3.0 g of the finely cut drug, covered, allowed to stand for 10–15 min., and then strained. As a diuretic, a cup of the tea is drunk two or three times a day; as a stomachic, a cup of the tea is taken half-an-hour before meals.
1 Teaspoon = ca. 3 g.

Phytomedicines: The drug is a component of combination preparations which are urological, diuretic, and cardiac remedies.

Authentication: Macro- and microscopically, following the DAC 1986. See also the BHP 1983. Adulteration with other umbelliferous roots can be established simply through the characteristic odour.
In the DAC 1986 TLC examination of the essential oil, ligustilide is the main spot on the chromatogram:

Test solution: 1.0 g powdered drug boiled for 1/2 min. with 10 ml methanol, cooled, and filtered; the filtrate made up to 10 ml with methanol.

Reference solution: none.

Loadings: 20 μl, as a band on silica gel 60F$_{254}$.

Solvent system: diethyl ether + 12% acetic acid + toluene (50 + 50 + 50), 15 cm run.

Detection and **Evaluation:** after evaporation of the solvent, in UV 365 nm light. Test solution: in lower half, a brownish and three light or dark blue zones; in the upper half, a bright fluorescent main zone.
Sprayed with 26% ammonium hydroxide solution + methanol (20 + 80), followed by examination in UV 365 nm light. Test solution: zones more intensely fluorescent and the main zone (ligustilide) with an intense greenish blue fluorescence.
The TLC examination of the coumarins is discussed in [7–9] with illustrations of the chromatograms.

If the TLC examination is carried out as described under Angelicae radix, under UV 366 nm light the reference compound umbelliferone appears at Rf ca. 0.4 as an intense blue fluorescent zone, while in the chromatogram of lovage there is a large, intense greenish blue fluorescent zone at Rf ca. 0.8 which is not present in such adulterants as Angelicae radix, Pimpinellae radix, Pastinaceae radix, etc.; see Fig. 3 in the monograph on Angelicae radix (p. 72).

Quantitative standards: DAC 1986: *Volatile oil*, not less than 0.35%. *Water-soluble extractive*, not less than 45.0%. *Foreign matter*, not more than 5% stem fragments; other foreign matter, not more than 2%. *Loss on drying*, not more than 12%. *Ash*, not more than 8.0%. *Acid-insoluble ash*, not more than 1.0%.
ÖAB: *Volatile oil*, not less than 0.5%. *Foreign matter*, not more than 5% stem fragments. *Ash*, not more than 8.0%.
Ph. Helv. VII: *Volatile oil*, not less than 0.30%. *Foreign matter*, not more than 3%. *Sulphated ash*, not more than 7.0%.
BHP 1983: *Total ash*, not more than 8%.

Adulteration: Especially in the cut drug, admixture or adulteration with Angelicae radix is not uncommon. It can be detected by the TLC examination indicated above under: Authentication.

Storage: Protected from light in well-closed containers (not made of plastic – essential oil). The drug is readily attacked by insects.

Literature:

[1] M. Cichy, V. Wray, and G. Höfele, Liebigs Ann. Chem. **1987**, 397.
[2] M.J.M. Gijbels, J.J.C. Scheffer, and A. Baerheim Svendsen, Rivista Italiana E.P.P.O.S. **61**, 335 (1979).
[3] J. Buchnicek, Planta Med. **21**, 89 (1972).
[4] K.W. Glombitza, Dtsch. Apoth. Ztg. **112**, 1593 (1972).
[5] O. Schimmer, Planta Med. **47**, 79 (1983).
[6] L. Hansen, O. Hammershoy, and P.M. Boll, Contact Derm. **14**, 91 (1986).
[7] L. Hörhammer, H. Wagner, and D. Kraemer-Heydweiler, Dtsch. Apoth. Ztg. **106**, 267 (1966).
[8] O.-B. Genius, Dtsch. Apoth. Ztg. **121**, 386 (1981).
[9] H. Wagner, S. Bladt, and E.M. Zgainski, Plant drug analysis, Springer-Verlag, Berlin, Heidelberg, New York, Tokyo, 1984, p. 154.
[10] C. Vollmann, Z. Phytotherap. **9**, 128 (1988).

Lini semen (DAB 10, Ph. Eur. 2, etc.), Linseed (*BAN*; BP 1988), Linum (BHP 1983)

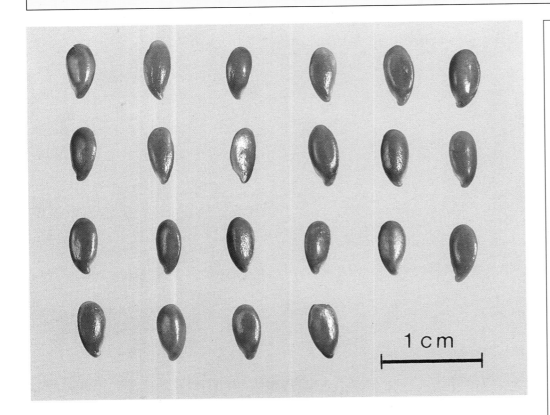

Fig. 1: Linseed

<u>Description:</u> **Mostly glossy brown to reddish brown, flattened, ovoid seeds, 4–6 mm long, 2–3 mm wide, and 0.75–1.5 mm thick. They are broadly rounded at one end and conically pointed at the other, where they are generally drawn out into a small, laterally bent beak. On examination with a hand lens, the micropyle and hilum can be seen in the concave side of the beak; the hilum is recognizable as a pale-coloured dimple, from which the raphe runs as a paler-coloured striation towards the other end of the seed. With a hand lens, the smooth testa is seen to be irregularly and minutely pitted. When the seeds are placed in water, a thick coating of mucilage forms.**

<u>Taste:</u> **Mild and oily, and on chewing mucilaginous.**

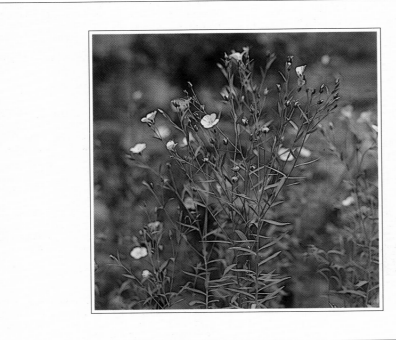

Fig. 2: *Linum usitatissimum* L.

An up to ca. 1 m tall, slender annual, with light blue, 5-part corollas, only opening in sunshine; numerous narrow, linear, 3-nerved, glabrous leaves; light brown capsules containing several seeds.

DAB 10: Leinsamen
ÖAB: Semen Lini
Ph. Helv. VII: Lini Semen
St. Zul. 1099.99.99

Plant source: *Linum usitatissimum* L., flax (Linaceae).

Synonyms: Flaxseed (Engl.), Leinsamen (Ger.), Grain de lin (Fr.).

Origin: One of the oldest cultivated plants, and grown worldwide in many varieties and forms for its fibre and oil, as well as for the seeds used in pharmacy. The most important suppliers are Morocco, Argentina, and Turkey.

Constituents Ca. 3–6% mucilage, localized in the epidermis of the testa, which can be separated into a neutral and two acidic components that after hydrolysis afford galactose (8–12%), arabinose (9–12%), rhamnose (13–29%), xylose (25–27%), and galacturonic and mannuronic acids (ca. 30%), and, according to other data, also fucose and glucuronic acid; ca. 30–45% fixed oil, principally triglycerides of linolenic, linoleic, and oleic acids; ca. 25% protein; ca. 0.7% phosphatides; sterols and triterpenes: cholesterol, campesterol, stigmasterol, sitosterol, Δ^5- avenasterol, cycloartenol, etc.; 0.1–1.5% cyanogenic glycosides, especially the diglycosides linustatin and neolinustatin [1, 2], as well as the monoglycosides linamarin and lotaustralin.

Indications: Linseed, whole or crushed, is a mildly active bulk-forming laxative. The effect is due to the mucilage localized in the epidermis and to the fibre (cellulose) of the testa. Peristalsis is stimulated through an increase in the volume of the contents of the bowel, especially of the colon; and movement of the contents is facilitated by the mucilage, which acts as a lubricant and improves the consistency of the stools. Because of the considerable energy content (nutritional value: ca. 1960 kJ or 470 kcal per 100 g), *with overweight people only the whole seeds should be used* – except for the swelling of the mucilage in the testa, they remain intact in the bowel and lubricating action of the fixed oil plays no part.

In *folk medicine*, the seeds are employed as fairly dilute decoctions (1 tablespoonful of seeds to a cup, or ca. 30–50 g seeds to a litre) for their demulcent properties in catarrhal complaints and acute or chronic gastritis. Externally, the powdered seeds (linseed meal) or the press cake remaining after expression of the oil (Placenta Seminis lini, also used as cattle food) are used as an emollient in poultices for boils, carbuncles, festering sores, and other skin afflictions. *When taken internally, linseed must be accompanied by plenty of fluids*, otherwise flatulence may occur. The drug is, of course, contraindicated in cases of intestinal obstruction.

Side effects: Toxic effects, alleged especially in the lay press and supposedly arising from the liberation of hydrocyanic acid from the cyanogenic glycosides, need not be feared even on prolonged use and have never been observed [3–6]. Theoretically, under optimal conditions (very finely ground seeds, pH value between 4 and 6, hydrolysis time 4 hours, etc.), from 100 g linseed the enzyme linamarase may liberate up to 50 mg hydrocyanic acid, which is enough to bring about symptoms of poisoning. However, under the acid conditions in the stomach, the linamarase (linase) is partly inactivated and even with moderate acidity less than 1% of the cyanogenic glycosides is hydrolysed (at pH 6, ca. 75–84%). The fairly long hydrolysis time of 4 hours is also required *in vivo* [4, 6, 7]. The hydrocyanic acid liberated during this period of time is rendered harmless through a rapidly acting detoxification mechanism in the body. A minor part is exhaled and eliminated via the urine and faeces, while the major part is metabolized with the help of the enzyme rhodanase, which is able to convert 30–60 mg HCN per hour into the relatively non-toxic thiocyanate. Thus, a relatively slow rate of formation is opposed by a relatively fast rate of elimination. Even with doses of 150–300 g of ground linseed, no symptoms of poisoning were observed in volunteers [3]. Single doses of up to 100 g linseed do not cause any significant rise in blood hydrocyanic acid and thiocyanate levels [5]. On taking 15 g linseed

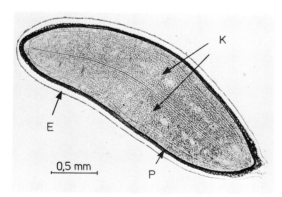
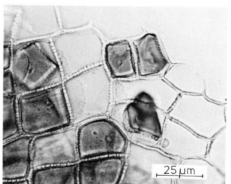

Fig. 3: Section through a seed (E = Mucilage-containing epidermis, P = Pigment layer, C = Cotyledons)
Fig. 4: Polygonal cells with plate-like masses of pigment

three times daily, after 3–4 weeks raised thiocyanate levels in blood and urine were observed – values which correspond to those noted with heavy smoking. These findings mean that no deleterious effects on health are to be expected [5].

Linseed can accumulate cadmium. Following the WHO guidelines concerning heavy metal accumulation, the German Ministry of Health has fixed the permissible level at 0.3 mg/kg [8].

Making the tea: Not applicable. When used as a laxative, 10 g whole (or freshly crushed – see: Indications) seeds should be taken with plenty of fluids during meals; in cases of bowel inflammation, preswelling of the seeds is recommended. To prepare a demulcent for use in cases of catarrh or gastritis, 5–10 g (whole) linseed is allowed to stand in cold water for 20–30 min., after which the liquid is poured off.
1 Teaspoon = ca. 4 g, 1 tablespoon = ca. 10 g.

Phytomedicines: A few ready-made gastrointestinal remedies, e.g. Linusit® and Linusit® Gold (an introduced yellow-coloured cultivar), and laxatives, e.g. Salus® Abführ-Tee, etc. The press cake from linseed-oil production (Placenta Seminis lini) is also used to make such preparations.

Regulatory status (UK): General Sales List – Schedule 1, Table A.

Authentication: The macroscopic, microscopic, and sensory characters given in the Ph. Eur. 2 (BP 1988) are fully adequate for determining the identity and quality. A detailed account of the diagnostic microscopical features is to be found in [9]; see also the BHP 1983.
In cross-section, the epidermis of the testa and the pigment layer can be clearly seen, as well as the two large cotyledons (Fig. 3); the pigment layer is characteristic (Fig. 4).

Quantitative standards: Ph. Eur. 2, BP 1988, etc.: *Swelling index*, not less than 4 for the whole drug and not less than 4.5 for the powdered drug. *Smell and Taste*, the drug must not smell or taste rancid. *Foreign matter*, not more than 1.5%. *Sulphated ash*, not more than 6.0%.

Adulteration: Very rare. Nevertheless, possible contamination with foreign plant matter should be checked.

Storage: The whole drug should be stored in a well-closed container and protected from light. According to the DAB 10, the comminuted seeds should not be stored for longer than 24 hours. There is no such limitation in the Ph. Eur. 2 (BP 1988), and the storage requirement is the same as for the whole drug.

Literature:

[1] C.R. Smith, D. Weisleder and R.W. Miller, J. Org. Chem. **45**, 507 (1980).
[2] H. Schilcher and M. Wilkens-Sauter, Fette, Seifen, Anstrichm. **88**, 287 (1986).
[3] C. Härtling, Dtsch. Apoth. Ztg. **109**, 1025 (1960).
[4] H. Schilcher, Pharmaz. Ztg. **127**, 2178 (1982).
[5] DAZ-aktuell, Dtsch. Apoth. Ztg. **123**, 876 (1983).
[6] H. Schilcher, Dtsch. Ärzteblatt **76**, 955 (1979).
[7] H. Schilcher, V. Schulz and A. Nissler, Z. Phytother. **7**, 113 (1986).
[8] Bundesgesundheitsblatt **30**, 11, 397 (1987), see. Dtsch. Apoth. Ztg. **128**, 145 (1988).
[9] B.P. Jackson and D.W. Snowdon, Atlas of microscopy of medicinal plants, culinary herbs and spices, Belhaven Press, London, 1990, p. 142.

Liquiritiae radix

Liquorice (Ph. Eur. 2; *BAN*, BP 1988),
Liquorice root (BHP 1/1990), Glycyrrhiza (*USAN*)

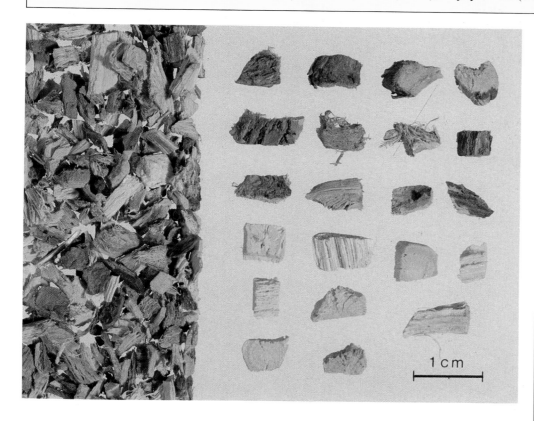

Fig. 1: Liquorice

Description: The drug consists of the dried, unpeeled (Ph. Eur. 2, BP 1988, DAB 10, Ph. Helv. VII) and/or peeled roots and stolons. In the cut condition, the drug is characterized by more or less cylindrical, roughly fibrous, distinctly lemon-yellow pieces which can be readily split longitudinally. The unpeeled drug includes small pieces with wrinkled, grey to brownish shreds of cork.

Odour: Faint, but chraracteristic.

Taste: Very sweet and mildly aromatic.

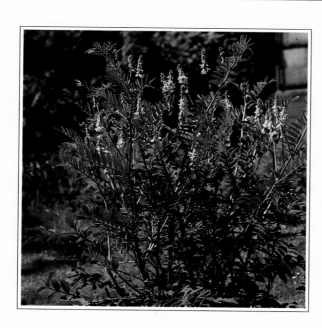

Fig. 2: *Glycyrrhiza glabra* L.

A shrub attaining a height of 1 m or more and bearing imparipinnate (3–7 pairs) leaves covered with sticky glandular trichomes. Erect, axillary, flowering racemes with pale lilac papilionaceous flowers.

DAB 10: Süßholzwurzel
ÖAB: Radix Liquiritiae
Ph. Helv. VII: Liquiritiae radix
St. Zul. 1309.99.99

Plant source: *Glycyrrhiza glabra* L., liquorice (Fabaceae).

Synonyms: Radix glycyrrhizae, Rhizoma Glycyrrhizae nativum (Lat.), Liquorice or Sweet root (Engl.), Süßholzwurzel, Spanisches or Russisches Süßholz, Lakritzenwurzel (Ger.), Réglisse officinale, Racine de réglisse, Bois doux, Racine douce (Fr.).

Origin: In several varieties, native in the Mediterranean region, central to southern Russia, and Asia Minor to Iran. The drug comes from plantations and is imported from the former USSR, Iran, Turkey, and China.

Constituents: 2–15% triterpenoid saponins, particularly glycyrrhizin (ammonium and calcium salts of glycyrrhizinic acid) and 24-hydroxyglycyrrhizin, which taste 50 and 100 time as sweet as sucrose, respectively. On hydrolysis, glycyrrhizinic acid affords diglucuronic acid and the aglycone glycyrrhetinic acid. There are, in addition, many other triterpenoid saponins, some of whose aglycones are known, e.g. glabranin A and B (both with glycyrrhetic acid as aglycone), glycyrrhetol, glabrolide, isoglabrolide, etc. Triterpenes, sterols: β-amyrin, onocerin, sitosterol, stigmasterol.

More than 30 flavonoids and isoflavonoids, including liquiritigenin, its 4′-*O*-glucoside (= liquiritin) and 4′-*O*-apiosyl-β1→2-glucoside, and the chalcones isoliquiritigenin, its 4′-*O*- glucoside (= isoliquiritin), licuroside and neolicuroside (= isoliquiritigenin 4′- and 4-β-D-apiofuranosyl-2″-β-D glucopyranoside [27]), glabrol and its 3′-hydroxy derivative, the isoflavonoids neoliquiritin, hispaglabridin A and B, etc.; coumestanes; coumarins: herniarin, umbelliferone, etc.; licobenzofuran.

Indications: 1. As an expectorant with secretolytic and secretomotor actions for coughs and bronchial catarrh, also for inflammation of the upper respiratory tract. The active substances are the saponins, especially glycyrrhizinic acid, which also has bacteriostatic and antiviral activity [1]. The *Glycyrrhiza* saponins inhibit the growth of influenza A viruses in hen embryos [2]. The antiviral action is probably based on the induction and enhancement of interferon formation, which has been demonstrated experimentally for glycyrrhizin [3, 4]. The isoflavonoids hispaglabridin A and B and glabridin likewise have antimicrobial activity [5, 6], and so does licobenzofuran [7].

2. As an antiphlogistic and spasmolytic in gastritis and stomach ulcers, as well as in the prophylaxis of ulcers. The activity has been established with certainty, both experimentally and clinically, but full understanding of the activity has not yet been attained [8, 9]. Glycyrrhizinic acid and its aglycone glycyrrhetinic acid are an essential active component, whose antiphlogistic activity has been proved in many different models. They do not inhibit prostaglandin synthesis, but rather the movement of leucocytes towards the inflamed spot [10]. Glycyrrhizin inhibits the activity of phospholipase A [cited from 4] and the formation of prostaglandin E_2 in activated peritoneal macrophages [11]. After oral administration, glycyrrhizin is partially converted by the intestinal flora to its aglycone and to 3-dehydro-18β-glycyrrhetinic acid [12]. After i.v. injection, up to 80% of it is secreted from the liver into the bile and excreted, as part of an enterohepatic cycle [13]. Glycyrrhizin and its aglycone reduce the toxic action of tetrachloromethane on cultured hepatocytes, by functioning as antioxidants, via a mechanism that differs somewhat from that of vitamin E [15]. The two compounds are responsible for the mineralocorticoid effects of the drug, and there are connections between them and the adrenocortical hormones, since, among other things, these effects are only observed when there is still at least a little functional adrenal cortex. It has been shown with rat-liver preparations that both compounds have a strong inhibiting effect on the Δ^4-5β-reductase, which in human liver plays an important role in regulating cortisol and al-

Glabrol: R = H
3-Hydroxyglabrol :   R = OH

Liquiritigenin: R = H
Liquiritin: R = Glucose

Isoliquiritigenin: R = H
Isoliquiritin   R = Glucose

Hispaglabridin A

Glycyrrhizinic acid

dosterone metabolism [16]. The essential structural feature for this inhibitory effect is the 11-oxo function. Currently, it is thought that the action of glycyrrhizin and glycyrrhetin is based on inhibition of the Δ^4-5β-reductase activity, thereby retarding the metabolic excretion of corticosteroids and extending the biological half-life of cortisol and aldosterone. This leads to synergism between this hormone and both glycyrrhizin and glycyrrhetin. In Russia, liquorice preparations are used as an adjunct in long-term cortisone treatment, which enables the steroid dose, and hence the side effects, to be considerably reduced [17].

This indirect corticoid action, which is also utilized therapeutically in the form of the hemisuccinate ester of glycyrrhetinic acid (Carbenoxolone = Biogastrone®), is only part of the overall effect of the drug in treating gastritis and ulcers. Deglycyrrhinized extracts also have ulcer-protecting properties and are used in the treatment of stomach ulcers [review in 18]. Among other things, through a direct inhibitory effect on the cells (liberation of gastrin is not suppressed), they reduce gastric-juice secretion [19] and prevent or reduce acetylsalicylic acid-induced inflammation of mucous membranes [20, 21]. In the anti-ulcer activity, synergism between glycyrrhizinic acid and other components of the extract has been demonstrated [22]. Here, the effect is accompanied by a clear-cut, and desirable, spasmolytic action, brought about by some of the flavonoids of the drug, in particular by liquiritigenin, and more especially isoliquiritigenin, which inhibits the monoamine oxidase (MAO, EC_{50}: 17.3 mM) in rat-liver mitochondria *in vitro* [23].

3. Because of the intensely sweet taste, the drug is incorporated into medicines, foodstuffs, and condiments to enhance the taste. In laxative herbal teas, liquorice potentiates the action of anthraquinone drugs (raising the wettability of the bowel contents, owing to the high surfactant activity of glycyrrhizin), so that smaller doses of these latter are required.

Side effects: Owing to the mineralocorticoid activity of glycyrrhizin and glycyrrhetin, large doses (more than 50 g drug a day) taken over a prolonged period of time lead to hypokalaemia, hypernatraemia, oedema, hypertension, and cardiac disorders. In extreme cases, pseudo-aldosteronism with all its manifestations may develop [24]. The problems disappear in the course of a few days after stopping the drug. Preparations of liquorice should not be taken for longer than 6 weeks. During this time, care must be taken to ensure a potassium-rich diet with, e.g. bananas, dried apricots. When high

Extract from the German Commission E monograph (BAnz no. 90, dated 15. 05. 1985)

Uses

Catarrh in the upper respiratory tract, and stomach and duodenal ulcers.

Contraindications

Cholestatic liver disorders, liver cirrhosis, hypertonia, hypokalaemia, pregnancy.

Side effects

On prolonged use and with higher doses, mineralocorticoid effects may occur in the form of sodium and water retention and potassium loss, accompanied by hypertension, oedema, and hypokalaemia, and in rare cases myoglobinuria.

Interactions

Potassium loss may be increased in the presence of other drugs, e.g. thiazide and loop diuretics. With loss of potassium, sensitivity to digitalis glycosides increases.

Dosage

Unless otherwise prescribed: average daily dose, liquorice: ca. 5–15 g drug, corresponding to 200–800 mg glycyrrhin. Succus liquiritiae: 0.5–1 g for catarrh of the upper respiratory tract, and 1.5–3.0 g for stomach and duodenal ulcers; preparations correspondingly.

Mode of administration

Finely cut or powdered drug, dry extract for infusions. Decocts, fluid and solid formulations for oral use (Succus liquiritiae).

Duration of use

Not longer than 4–6 weeks, without consulting a doctor.

Note: There are no objections to use of the drug as a taste enhancer, up to a maximum daily dose of 100 mg glycyrrhizin.

Effects

According to controlled clinical studies, glycyrrhizinic acid and its aglycone accelerate the healing of stomach ulcers. Secretolytic and expectorant actions have been demonstrated in animal experiments. In the isolated rabbit ileum, a spasmolytic action has been observed at concentrations of 1 : 2500 to 1 : 5000.

blood pressure is present, as well as impaired cardiac and renal function, a doctor must be consulted before taking the drug for a longer period, which should not involve the simultaneous administration of spironolactone or amiloride. See also [28].

Making the tea: Boiling water (ca. 150 ml) is poured over 1–1.5 g of the finely chopped or coarsely powdered drug, or the drug can be put into cold water and boiled for a short time, and after 10–15 min. passed through a tea strainer. Not for prolonged use (see: Side effects).
1 Teaspoon = ca. 3 g.

Herbal preparations: The drug is also available in tea bags (2 g). Extracts of the drug are present in instant teas for various indications (bronchial teas, stomach teas, laxative teas).

Phytomedicines: Liquorice or extracts from it are to be found in many prepared bronchial remedies, gastrointestinal remedies, liver and bile remedies, and urological remedies, and in a few other preparations as a taste enhancer. Besides the chopped and powdered drug, among the other forms in which it is used are: the concentrated aqueous extract (= Succus Liquiritiae or liquorice), the fluid extract (= Liquiritiae extractum fluidum DAB 10, with not less

than 4.0% and not more than 6.0% glycyrrhizinic acid), deglycyrrhinized extracts, e.g. Caved S® (it and Rabro® are chewable tablets available in the UK), the isolated glycyrrhizinic acid and semi-synthetically modified glycyrrhetinic acid – Carbenoxolone, Biogastrone® (no longer marketed in Germany).

Regulatory status (UK): General Sales List – Schedule 1, Table A.

Authentication: Macro- (see: Description) and microscopically, following the Ph. Eur. 2, BP 1988, etc. The microscopy of the powdered drug is described and illustrated in [29]. The orange-yellow colour obtained with conc. sulphuric acid and the TLC detection of glycyrrhetinic acid, following the Ph. Eur. 2, etc., (figure in [25]) can be used as identity tests. TLC of the flavonoids can also be used as an identity ([26], includes coloured figure).

Quantitative standards: <u>Ph. Eur. 2, etc.</u>: *Glycyrrhizinic acid*, not less than 4.0%. *Water-soluble extractive*, not less than 20.0%. *Sulphated ash*, not more than 10.0%. *Acid-insoluble ash*, not more than 2.0%.

<u>BHP 1/1990</u>: Liquorice Root complies with the requirements of the Ph. Eur. 2 monograph on Liquiritiae radix and of the BP 1988 monographs on Liquorice or Powdered Liquorice, as appropriate.

Wording of the package insert, from the German Standard Licence:

5.1   Uses

For dissolving and facilitating the discharge of mucus in catarrh of the upper respiratory tract (bronchitis). For supportive treatment of cramp-like disorders in inflammation of the gastric mucosa (chronic gastritis).

5.2   Contraindications

Chronic hepatic inflammation, cirrhosis of the liver, high blood pressure, and potassium deficiency in the blood.

5.3   Side effects

When correctly used, not known.

Warning: On prolonged use or with larger doses of liquorice preparations, there may be an increased accumulation of water with some swelling, especially in the face and feet.
Sodium excretion is reduced and potassium excretion is increased. A rise in blood pressure is also possible.

5.4   Interactions with other remedies

When correctly used, not known.

Warning: Liquorice preparations should not given over a prolonged period concurrently with potassium-sparing diuretics, such as spironolactone, triamterene, or amiloride. Because of the increased loss of potassium, the action of cardiotonic drugs may be potentiated. Reduced sodium and water excretion may make adjustment of the dose of drugs for hypertension more difficult.

5.5   Dosage and Mode of administration

About one teaspoonful (2–4 g) of **Liquorice** is brewed with boiling water (ca. 150 ml), boiled for a further 5 min., and after cooling passed through a tea strainer. Unless otherwise prescribed, a cup of the infusion is drunk after each meal.

Duration of use

High doses of liquorice preparations should not be taken for longer than 4–6 weeks. During this time, a potassium-rich diet should be ensured with, e.g. bananas and dried apricots.

5.7   Note

Store protected from light and moisture.

Literature:

[1] R. Pompei, Riv. Farmacol. Ter. **10**, 281 (1979); C.A. **92**, 104967 (1980).
[2] V.A. Vichkanova and L.V. Goryunova, Tr. Vses. Nauch.-Issled. Inst. Lek. Rast. **14**, 204 (1971); C.A. **78**, 155107 (1973).
[3] Y. Hayashi et al., Yakuri to Chiryo **7**, 3861 (1979).
[4] M. Shinada et al., Proc. Soc. Exptl. Biol. Med. **181**, 205 (1986).
[5] L.A. Mitscher et al., Heterocycles **9**, 1533 (1978).
[6] L.A. Mitscher, Y.H. Park, and D. Clark, J. Nat. Prod. **43**, 259 (1980).
[7] X. Chang et al., Zhongcaoyao **12**, 530 (1981); C.A. **97**, 20701 (1982).
[8] J. Lutomski, Pharmazie in unserer Zeit **12**, 49 (1983).
[9] M.R. Gibson, Lloydia **41**, 348 (1978).
[10] F. Capasso et al., J. Pharm. Pharmacol. **35**, 332 (1983).
[11] K. Ohuchi et al., Prostaglandins Med. **7**, 457 (1981).
[12] M. Hattori et al., Planta Med. **48**, 38 (1983).
[13] T. Ichikawa et al., J. Pharm. Sci. **75**, 672 (1986).
[14] Y. Kiso, M. Tohkin, and H. Hikino, Planta Med. **42**, 222 (1983).
[15] Y. Kiso et al., Planta Med. **50**, 298 (1984).
[16] Y. Tamura et al., Arzneimit.-Forsch. **29**, 647 (1979).
[17] H. Müller-Dietz, Arzneipflanzen in der Sowjet Union, 3rd issue, Osteuropa-Institut, Berlin, 1966.
[18] R.N. Brodgen, T.M. Speight, and C.S. Avery, Drugs **8**, 330 (1974).
[19] R. Hakanson et al., Experientia **29**, 570 (1973).
[20] W.D.W. Rees et al., Scand. J. Gastroenterol. **14**, 605 (1979).
[21] A. Bennett et al., J. Pharm. Pharmacol. **32**, 151 (1980).
[22] S. Okabe et al., Oyo Yakuri **18**, 469 (1979); C.A. **92**, 157697 (1980).
[23] S. Tanaka, Y. Kuwai, and M. Tabata, Planta Med. **53**, 5 (1987).
[24] E. Röder, Dtsch. Apoth. Ztg. **122**, 2081 (1982).
[25] P. Pachaly, Dünnschichtchromatographie in der Apotheke, 2nd ed., Wissenschaftliche Verlagsgesellschaft, Stuttgart, 1982.
[26] H. Wagner, S. Bladt, and E.M. Zgainski, Plant drug analysis, Springer, Berlin – Heidelberg – New York – Tokyo, 1984, p.
[27] H. Miething and A. Speicher-Brinker, Arch. Pharm. (Weinheim) **322**, 141 (1989).
[28] P.F. D'Arcy, Adverse Drug React. Toxicol. Rev. **10**, 189 (1991).
[29] B.P. Jackson and D.W. Snowdon, Atlas of microscopy of medicinal plants, culinary herbs and spices, Belhaven Press, London, 1990, p. 144.

Lupuli strobulus   Lupuli glandula

(DAB 10), Hops (BHP 1/1990)

Hop grains

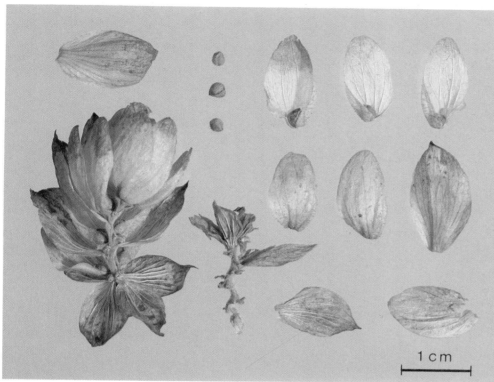

Fig. 1

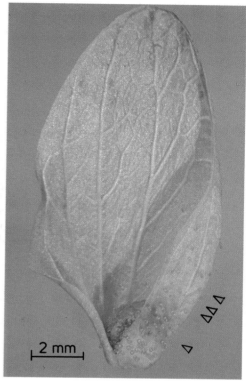

Fig. 2

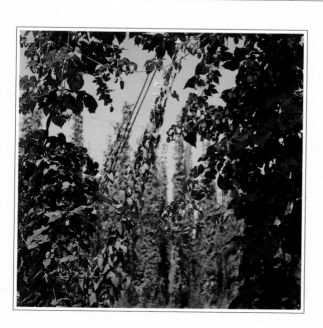

Fig. 1: Hops, Fig. 2: Hop grains

<u>Description:</u> Hops consist of the 2–4 cm long, yellowish green female inflorescence (the hop or 'cone' or strobile), which is built up from imbricated ovate bracts, in the axils of each of which are two female flowers, each one surrounded by a small oblique ovate bract. The leaf fragments of the drug clearly show the golden-yellow shining glandular trichomes (hop grains) (Fig. 2).

<u>Odour:</u> Intensely spicy.

<u>Taste:</u> Somewhat bitter and harsh.

Hop grains are the glandular trichomes obtained from the hops by sieving. They form a greenish yellow to orange-yellow sticky powder.

<u>Odour:</u> Characteristic, strongly spicy.

<u>Taste:</u> Spicy and bitter.

Fig. 3: *Humulus lupulus* L., female plants

A 3–6 m tall (in cultivation up to more than 10 m) plant twining to the right. Coarsely pubescent, long-petioled, deeply 3–7-lobed leaves, with a coarsely serrate margin. Female flowers in stalked cone-like spikes.

DAB 10: Hopfenzapfen
St. Zul.: 1029.99.99 (Hopfenzapfen)
ÖAB: Glandula Lupuli

Plant source: *Humulus lupulus* L., hop (Cannabaceae).

Synonyms: Humulus, Lupulus (Engl.), Hopfen, Hopfenzapfen, Hopfendrüsen (Ger.), Cônes d'houblon, Lupulin (Fr.).

Origin: Exclusively from cultivated female plants (which are multiplied vegetatively), grown in many parts of the temperate zones, including Western Europe, India, China, and the USA.

Constituents: Bitter substances (acylphloroglucides) present in the resin (15–30% in hops, 50–80% in hop grains), which is differentiated into the light-petroleum-insoluble part (hard resin) and the light-petroleum-soluble part (α- and β-soft resins). The most important component of the α-soft resin is the bitter substance humulone, while the β-soft resin contains mainly lupulone, another bitter substance. Many other bitter substances have been isolated in pure form. All the bitter substances are fairly labile compounds and on storage are slowly converted to components of the hard resin (mainly oxidation products). Essential oil (in hops 0.3–1%, in hop grains 1–3%), chiefly mono- and sesquiterpenes (myrcene, linalool, farnesene, caryophyllene, etc.; so far, more than 150 aroma substances have been identified). Tannins (2–4% in hops, little in hop grains) and flavonoids (kaempferol and quercetin mono- and diglycosides), including xanthohumol and other chalcones [6], which are biogenetically related to the flavonoids and which are specific to the drug. Small amounts of phenol-carboxylic acids (ferulic and chlorogenic acids, etc.) are present.

Indications: As a sedative, especially in the form of the extract combined with other sedative drugs, for restlessness, hyperexcitability, nervous insomnia, and stress states. The question of the sedative principles has not yet been clarified, but in 1980 R. Hänsel and co-workers were able to show that during storage autoxidation of humulone and lupulone splits off a C_5-alcohol, 2-methylbut-3-en-2-ol, which accumulates in the drug; after 2 years' storage, it was present to the extent of 0.15% [1] and in animal experiments it proved to have strong sedative activity [2]. The small amount of this alcohol present in hops is not sufficient to explain their sedative effect, but there are grounds for assuming that after oral intake of hops 2-methylbut-3-en-2-ol is formed from lupulone [3, 4].

Hops in the form of infusions are also used as a bitter and stomachic to stimulate the appetite and to increase gastric secretion.

In *folk medicine,* the drug is used in the form of an infusion to treat sores and skin injuries and internally for inflammation of the bladder.

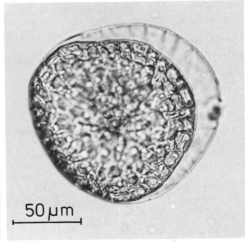

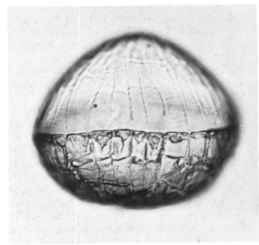

Fig. 4: Bowl-shaped, multicellular hop grain (glandular trichome) in side view (left) and top view (right)

Making the tea: Boiling water is poured over 0.5 g of the comminuted drug, covered, allowed to stand for 10–15 min., and then strained.

1 Teaspoon = ca. 0.4 g.

Herbal preparations: Dry extracts from hops or hop grains are contained in a few prepared sleep-inducing and sedative teas.

Phytomedicines: About 70 prepared sedative remedies contain hop extracts, e.g. Hovaletten®, Hova®-Zäpfchen, Nervenruh forte, Baldriparan®, Somnuvis®, Visinal®, Vivinox®-Beruhigungs-Dragees, and many others.

In the UK, Humulus is present in about 60 sedative preparations [7]. It is an ingredient in, e.g. Seven Seas Restful Night Tablets, Gerard 99 Tablets, Potter's Anased Pain Relief Tablets, and Potter's Newrelax, etc.

Regulatory status (UK): General Sales List – Schedule 1, Table A.

Authentication: On microscopical examination, the yellow hop grains can be recognized as glandular trichomes, 150–250 μm in diameter, the secretory cells of which form a single bowl-shaped layer, with the raised cuticle forming a dome; outlines of the secretory cells can be seen in the cuticle (Fig. 4). For a more detailed description, see the BHP 1/1990. The microscopical features of the powder are described in [8]. Old, degraded

---

Extract from the German Commission E monograph
(BAnz no. 228, dated 05.12.1984)

Uses
Health disorders such as restlessness, anxiety states, and insomnia.

Contraindications
None known.

Side effects
None known.

Interactions
None known.

Dosage
Unless otherwise prescribed: single dose of the drug, 0.5 g.

Mode of administration
Cut drug, drug powder, or powdered dried extract for infusions, decoctions, or other preparations. Liquid and solid formulations for internal use.

Note
Combinations with other sedative drugs may be advantageous.

Effects
Calming and sleep-inducing.

---

hops can be recognized by the intense smell of isovaleric acid; in contrast, good quality hops have a spicy smell.

It is important to test for copper, which may arise from fungicidal residues.

The following TLC identification test is modified from [5]:

Test solution: 1 g powdered hops extracted for 10 min. with 10 ml methanol in an ultrasonic bath and then filtered.

Reference solution: 3 mg curcumin and 2 mg *p*-aminoazobenzene dissolved in 10 ml methanol.

Loadings: 1 μl each of the test and reference solutions.

Mobile phase: cyclohexane + ethyl acetate + propionic acid (60 + 38 + 2), 5 cm run.

Solvent system: in UV 254 and 366 nm light and in daylight, then sprayed with 5% ethanolic sulphuric acid, followed by 1% ethanolic vanillin, and heated at 105 °C for 3–5 min.

Evaluation: immediately in daylight before spraying. Reference solution: curcumin, a yellow zone at Rf ca. 0.3; *p*-aminoazobenzene, an orange zone at Rf ca. 0.6. Test solution: a light yellow zone (xanthohumol) at about the same Rf value as curcumin and two to three yellowish zones (humulones and lupulones) slightly above the Rf of *p*-aminoazobenzene; see Fig. 5.

In UV 254 nm light. Test solution: xanthohumol, a brownish yellow zone at the same Rf as curcumin; the humulones, an intense quenching zone slightly above the Rf of the *p*-aminoazobenzene zone; the lupulones, somewhat higher, again as quenching zones (Fig. 6). In UV 366 nm light. Test solution: xanthohumol, a dark brown fluorescent zone; the humulones, yellow or yellow-green fluorescent zones; and the lupulones, pale blue fluorescent zones.

After spraying with vanillin/sulphuric acid and colours observed in daylight. Reference solution: curcumin yellow and *p*-aminoazobenzene orange-red. Test solution: xanthohumol yellowish orange, the humulones intense bluish grey, and the lupulones intense grey-blue (Fig. 7).

The DAB 10 TLC procedure chromatographs a 70% aqueous methanolic extract on silica gel GF$_{254}$ (15 cm run), together with the same reference compounds, in the solvent system: anhydrous formic acid + ethyl acetate + cyclohexane (2 + 38 + 60), followed by examination in UV 254 and 365 nm light and again after spraying with Folin reagent (sodium tungstate and molybdate in aqueous phosphoric/hydrochloric acid, with addition of lithium sulphate and

---

bromine – for details of the preparation, see DAB 10, Section VII.1.1).

The TLC method given in the St.Zul. deals with both the flavonoids and the phenolcarboxylic acids.

The BHP 1/1990 TLC identification test provides a fingerprint chromatogram.

Nowadays, mainly HPLC is used to analyse the bitter substances of hops.

Quantitative standards – Hops: DAB 10: 70% *Aqueous methanol extractive*, not less than 25%. *Odour*, the drug must not smell rancid. *Foreign matter*, not more than 1%; brown, discoloured drug must not be present. *Loss on drying*, not more than 8%. *Ash*, not more than 12%.

St.Zul. 1029.99.99: *Flavonoids*, 0.5% calculated as rutin. 70% *Aqueous methanol extractive*, not less than 25%. *Water-soluble extractive*, not less than 18%. *Foreign matter*, not more than 1%; brown, discoloured, and unpleasantly cheesy smelling drug is to be rejected. *Loss on drying*, not more than 8%. *Ash*, not more than 12%. *Copper*, not more than 400 ppm.

BHP 1990: *Water-soluble extractive*, not less than 18%. *Foreign matter*, not more than 2%. *Total ash*, not more than 10%. *HCl-insoluble ash*, not more than 5%.

– Glandula lupuli: ÖAB: *Ether-soluble extractive*, not less than 70.0%. *Condition*, old broken hop grains must not be discoloured and should not have more than a faint smell of valeric acid. *Foreign matter*, fragments of the fructification should not be visible under the microscope. *Ash*, not more than 10.0%.

Lupuli strobulus is the subject of a proposed ESCOP harmonized European monograph.

Adulteration: Rarely happens. Ripe fruits should not be present in hops.

Storage: Protected from light, under cool conditions, and for not longer than 1 year (according to, e.g. the ÖAB and Erg. B. 6, etc.).

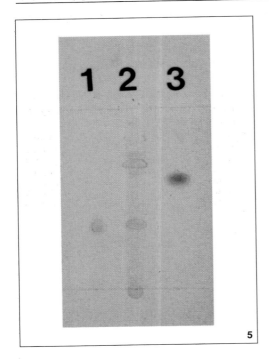

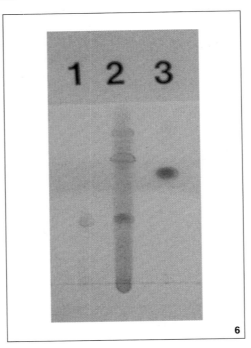

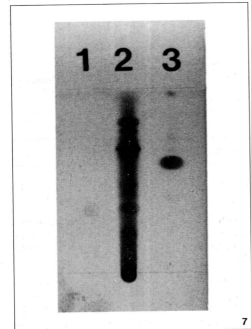

Literature:
[1] R. Wohlfart, G. Wurm, R. Hänsel and H. Schmidt, Arch. Pharm (Weinheim). **316**, 132 (1983).
[2] R. Wohlfart, R. Hänsel and H. Schmidt, Planta Med. **48**, 120 (1983).
[3] R. Hänsel, R. Wohlfart and H. Schmidt, Planta Med. **45**, 224 (1982).
[4] R. Wohlfart, Dtsch. Apoth. Ztg. **123**, 1637 (1983).
[5] R. Hänsel and J. Schulz, Dtsch. Apoth. Ztg. **126**, 2347 (1986).
[6] S. Song-San, S. Watanabe, and T. Saito, Phytochemistry **28**, 1776 (1989).
[7] J.D. Phillipson and L.A. Anderson, Pharm. J. **233**, 80, 111 (1984).
[8] B.P. Jackson and D.W. Snowdon, Atlas of microscopy of medicinal plants, culinary herbs and spices, Belhaven Press, London, 1990, p. 120.

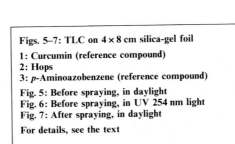

Figs. 5–7: TLC on 4 × 8 cm silica-gel foil

1: Curcumin (reference compound)
2: Hops
3: *p*-Aminoazobenzene (reference compound)

Fig. 5: Before spraying, in daylight
Fig. 6: Before spraying, in UV 254 nm light
Fig. 7: After spraying, in daylight

For details, see the text

Lycopodii herba   Lycopodium

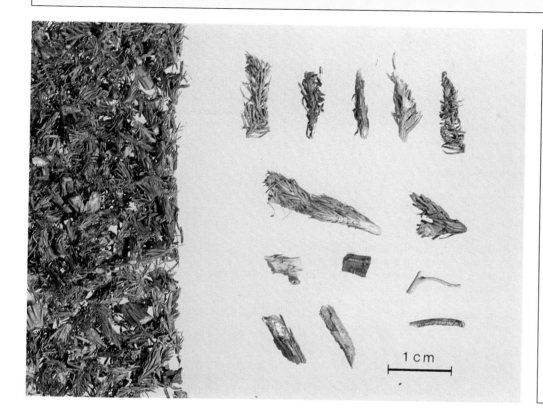

Fig. 1: Lycopodium (in the centre: the brown peduncle of a sporophyll, rarely met with in the drug)

Description: The slender round stems are densely covered with 3–5 mm long, pale yellowish green, pointed, stiff, sessile leaves. These have an entire margin and the end is drawn out into a white hair-like tip; they are arranged in dense whorls or in spirals (Fig. 3). In the whole drug, the stem is seen to be repeatedly forked. The cylindrical peduncles of the sporophylls are infrequent.

Taste: Bitter-sweet.

1 cm

Fig. 2: *Lycopodium clavatum* L.

Far-reaching, creeping stems, with ascending branches up to 30 cm in height, bearing imbricated leaves and with the sporangia mostly in pairs.

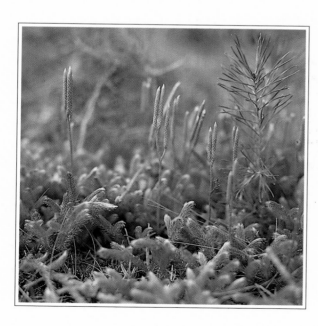

Erg. B. 6: Herba Lycopodii

Plant source: *Lycopodium clavatum* L., stag's-horn clubmoss (Lycopodiaceae).

Synonyms: Common or Running clubmoss, Running or Ground pine (Engl.), Bärlappkraut (Ger.), Herbe de lycopode (Fr.).

Origin: Widely distributed throughout the temperate and colder zones. In Germany, it is a protected plant. The drug is collected from the wild, especially in eastern European countries and China.

Constituents: Ca. 0.2% alkaloids, which belong to different heterocyclic ring systems. Over 100 alkaloids have been isolated from *Lycopodium* species, which belong to about 20 different skeletal types [1, 2]. The principal alkaloids of the drug are lycopodine and dihydrolycopodine; in addition, acetyldihydrolycopodine, lycodine, anhydrolycodoline, and lycodoline are also present. Small amounts of flavonoids (chrysoeriol, luteolin,

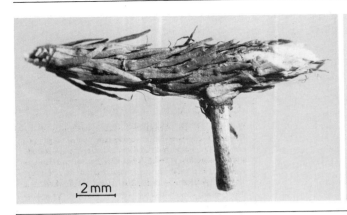

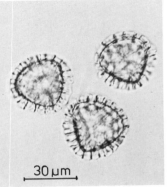

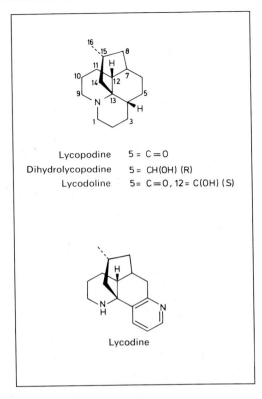

Lycopodine   5 = C=O
Dihydrolycopodine   5 = CH(OH) (R)
Lycodoline   5 = C=O, 12 = C(OH) (S)

Lycodine

Fig. 3: Fragment of *Lycopodium clavatum* stem with an attached sucker

Fig. 5: Typical *Lycopodium* spores, showing the multi-layered, reticulately thickened exospore

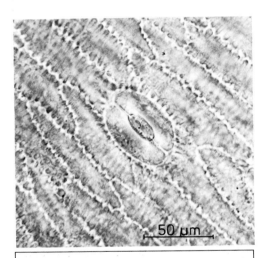

Fig. 4: Stoma and the "toothed" (sinuate) anticlinal walls of the epidermal cells of the lower surface

apigenin 4-glucoside, etc.), caffeic acid, and triterpenes have been found as well.

Indications: Almost exclusively in *folk medicine,* as a diuretic and for kidney and bladder complaints. It is not yet known to what the activity of the drug is due. Most of the alkaloids have been isolated in order to help in clarifying taxonomic relationships within the Lycopodiaceae. Pharmacological testing has demonstrated considerable toxicity, with the occurrence of emetic and strong laxative properties. In rodents, lycopine produces uterine contractions and stimulates peristalsis in the small intestine. Many of the alkaloids are also known to irritate mucous membranes and they may perhaps play a part, in addition to the flavonoids, in the diuretic action of the drug. In insects, Lycopodium extracts bring about a reduction in the carbohydrate content of the haemolymph [3].

Side effects: Especially on prolonged use, the irritant properties of the distinctly toxic alkaloids must be taken into account.

Making the tea: Boiling water is poured over 1.5 g of the finely cut drug and after 5–10 min. passed through a tea strainer. A cupful to be taken two to three times a day. **Warning:** Not to be used over a prolonged period of time. Watch out for side effects. 1 Teaspoon = ca. 1 g.

Phytomedicines: None.

Authentication: Macro- (see: Description) and microscopically. Diagnostic features include the "toothed" (sinuate), elongated epidermal cells (Fig. 4) and the stomata on the lower surface of the leaves. The spores are also characteristic – under the microscope, they are seen as rounded trigonal pyramids, ca. 30–35 μm in diameter, with a surface covered by a network of ridges forming 5- or 6-sided meshes (Fig. 5).

Quantitative standard: Erg. B. 6: *Ash,* not more than 4%.

Adulteration: Nowadays, this is no longer observed in the drug trade. Formerly, confusion with *Lycopodium annotinum* L., interrupted clubmoss, used to occur; this species does not have its leaves drawn out into a hair-like tip.

Literature:
[1] J.C. Braekman, I. Nyembo, and J.J. Symoens, Phytochemistry **19**, 803 (1980).
[2] R.V. Gerard and D.B. MacLean, Phytochemistry **25**, 1143 (1986).
[3] S. Mandal et al., Curr. Sci. **51**, 51 (1982); C.A. **97**, 179052 (1982).

Maidis stigma   Corn silk (BHP 1/1990)

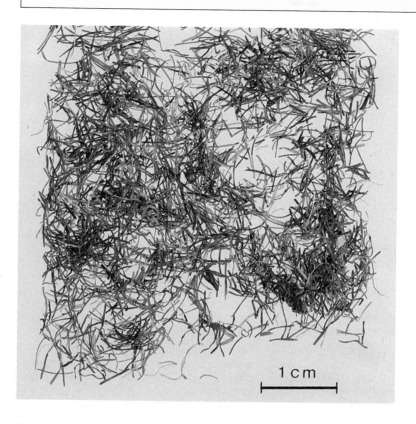

Fig. 1: Corn silk

<u>Description</u>: The drug consists of the stigmas of the female flowers harvested during the flowering period, but before fertilization, and rapidly dried in the shade. The pale yellowish or brownish stigmas are filamentous, ca. 0.1–0.2 mm thick, and up to 20 cm long. Viewed with a hand lens, they appear flattened and ribbon-like, or grooved and curled up, with spreading trichomes (Fig. 3).
In the cut form, the drug is made up of 5–10 mm long, filamentous, channelled pieces of stigma, pale yellowish or brownish red in colour.

<u>Odour</u>: Faint, characteristic.

<u>Taste</u>: Somewhat sweetish.

Fig. 2: *Zea mays* L.

A robust monoecious plant, up to 2.5 m in height, from Central America; halfway up the stem, female flowers in long cobs surrounded by glumes with projecting tuft of stigmas. Male flowers in terminal spikes.

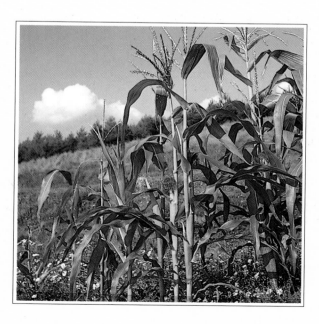

Erg. B. 6: Stigmata Maidis

Plant source: *Zea mays* L., maize (Poaceae).

Synonyms: Zea, Indian corn or Maize silk (Engl.), Maisgriffel (Ger.), Stigmates de maïs, Blé de Turquie (Fr.).

Origin: Native to Central America, but nowadays cultivated worldwide. The drug is imported from the former USSR, Bulgaria, Albania, and former Yugoslavia, and it is also obtained from the USA.

Constituents: Information on the constituents is only to be found in the older literature. The drug therefore needs renewed investigation. Ca. 2% fixed oil, ca. 0.1% essential oil (containing carvacrol and other terpenes); flavonoids (?); bitter substances (?); saponins (?); ca. 12% tannin-like polyphenols; reducing sugar; up to 0.85% alkaloid (?); mucilage (according to [1]); relatively rich in potassium salts [2].

Indications: As a diuretic, presumably on the basis of the relatively high potassium

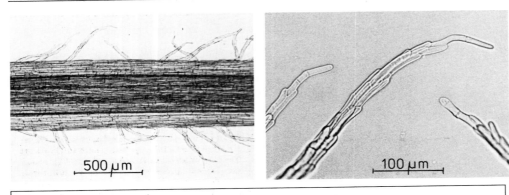

Fig. 3: Part of the filamentous stigma, showing the obliquely spreading trichomes

Fig. 4: Multicellular, multiseriate trichomes

content. In recently reported animal experiments, corn silk was found to have comparatively strong diuretic activity [3].

In *folk medicine*, it is additionally employed as a slimming cure and in cystitis, rheumatism, and arthritis.

There is no evidence for the antidiabetic action sometimes claimed in *folk medicine,* and its use for that purpose is to be rejected.

Its utilization by the Peruvian Indians as an intoxicant is supposed to be based on the presence of alkaloids of unknown composition, which, after being inhaled, cause psychic stimulation and, on prolonged use, vomiting, colic, and diarrhoea [1].

Making the tea: 0.5 g corn silk is put into cold water, which is boiled for a short while and after a few minutes strained. As a mild diuretic, a cup of the tea is drunk several times a day.

1 Teaspoon = ca. 0.5 g.

Phytomedicines: Extracts prepared from the drug are used in combination with other drug extracts as a diuretic (also in homoeopathy).

Among the UK products containing corn silk or its extracts are the liquid preparations Potter's Elixir of Damiana and Saw Palmetto and Potter's Protat.

Authentication: Macro- (see: Description) and microscopically. The obliquely spreading, 400–800 µm long, multicellular and multiseriate trichomes, some of which are bluntly toothed, are a characteristic feature (Fig. 4). For further detail, see the BHP 1/1990.

Addition of lead acetate solution to a 1:10 decoction affords a brownish precipitate. The BHP 1/1990 TLC identification test is as follows:

Test solution: 0.25 g powdered drug refluxed for 10–15 min. with 10 ml 60% aqueous methanol, cooled filtered, and the filtrate concentrated to ca. 1 ml.

Reference solution: 0.05% aescin in methanol.

Loadings: 20 µl of each solution, as 2-cm bands on silica gel.

Solvent system: chloroform + methanol + water (64 + 50 + 10), 15 cm run.

Detection: sprayed with freshly prepared anisaldehyde reagent (0.5 ml anisaldehyde mixed with 10 ml glacial acetic acid, 85 ml methanol, and 5 ml sulphuric acid, in that order), then heated at 105 °C for 5–10 min.

Evaluation: in daylight. Test solution: major bands relative to aescin at Rx 2.7 (deep purple), 2.6 (pale purple), 1.3 (broad yellow), 0.6 (brownish green).

Quantitative standards: BHP 1/1990: *Water-soluble extractive*, not less than 10%. *Foreign matter*, not more than 2%. *Total ash*, not more than 8%. *HCl-insoluble ash*, not more than 2%.

Adulteration: In practice, does not occur.

Literature:
[1] Hager, vol. **6**, p. 550 (1979).
[2] R. Hänsel and H. Haas, Therapie mit Phytopharmaka, Springer, Berlin – Heidelberg – New York, 1984.
[3] M. Rebuelta et al., Plantes Méd. Phytothérap. **21**, 267 (1987).

Malvae flos   Mallow flower

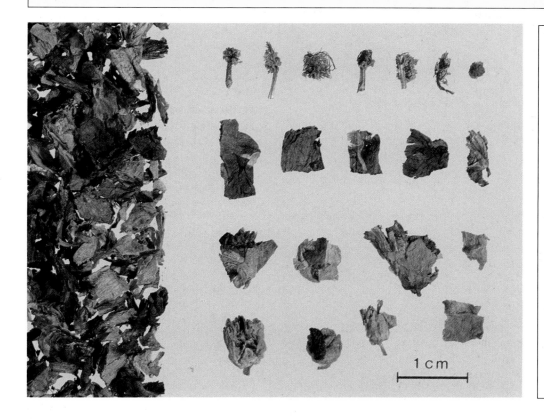

Fig. 1: Mallow flower

<u>Description:</u> The drug consists of the fused, foliaceous 5-part calyx together with the epicalyx of three lance-olate segments; all the sepals are pubescent. There are five pale violet or dark bluish violet (subsp. *mauritiana*) obovate petals, which are emarginate at the tip and which have a white beard at the base. The numerous stamens are fused to form a tube and the style has 10 thread-like, violet stigmas. Occasionally, the flattened, 10-locular ovaries are present.

<u>Taste:</u> Mucilaginous.

Note:

Flores Malvae arboreae come not from *Malva* species but from *Alcea rosea* L. (syn. *Althaea rosea* (L.) Cav.), the hollyhock, which is cultivated as a decorative plant; the drug comprises mostly double flowers. In the food trade, Mallow tea usually means Hibiscus flowers, Malvae flos (q.v.).

Fig. 2: *Malva sylvestris* subsp. *mauritiana*

For the description of the plant, see: Malvae folium. The subsp. *mauritiana* has dark bluish violet petals.

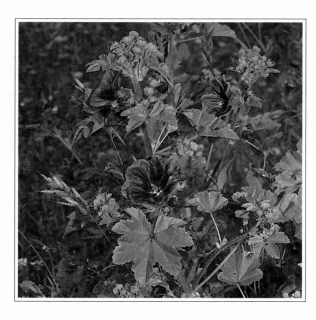

DAB 7: Malvenblüten
ÖAB: Flos Malvae
Ph. Helv. VII: Malvae flos

Plant source: *Malva sylvestris* L., common mallow, or also *M.sylvestris* subsp. *mauritiana* (L.) ASCH. et GRAEBN. (Malvaceae).

Synonyms: Malvenblüten, Käsepappel-blüten (Ger.), Fleurs de mauve (Fr.).

Origin: Native in Europe (subsp. *mauritiana* in southern Europe) and ranging towards Asia; the plant is cultivated to some extent. Imports of the drug come from Eastern Europe.

Constituents: More than 10% mucilage, which on hydrolysis affords galactose, arabinose, glucose, rhamnose, and galacturonic acid [1]. Small amounts of tannin. Less than 0.1% leucoanthocyanins, but ca. 7% (based on dry wt.) anthocyanins, about half of which is malvidin 3,5-diglucoside (malvin); delphinidin and malvidin 3-glucosides are also present [2]. For the rest, only ubiquitous substances have been detected.

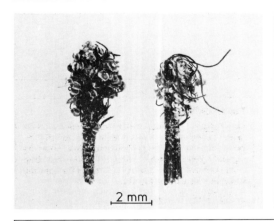

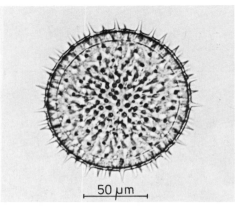

Fig. 3: Filaments of the anthers fused into a column

Fig. 4: Large pollen grain, showing the sharply spiny exine

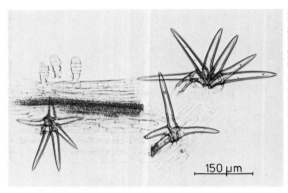

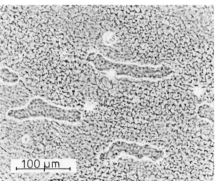

Fig. 5: Stellate trichomes and multicellular glandular trichomes

Fig. 6: Elongated mucilage idioblasts, from the petals

Indications: For the preparation of teas which are used for colds and against catarrh and inflammation of the mouth and throat; the drug also finds use as a mild astringent in gastroenteritis.

In *folk medicine*, it is employed internally for bladder complaints and externally in poultices for treating wounds and for baths in which to soak.

Because of the anthocyanin content, it is also used for colouring foodstuffs.

Making the tea: 1.5–2 g of the finely chopped drug is placed in cold water and boiled for a short time, or boiling water is poured over it, and after 10 min. strained.
1 Teaspoon = ca. 0.5 g.

Phytomedicines: The drug is a frequent component of herbal teas for treating coughs; while the concentration of anthocyanins is sufficient to give a therapeutic action, the amount of mucilage present at the dosages used may be too low to be effective [2].

Inclusion of Malvae flos in other teas is to enhance their appearance by imparting colour.

Authentication: Macro- (see: Description) and microscopically. Diagnostic features include: the column of fused anther filaments (Fig. 3), the glandular and stellate trichomes of the sepals (Fig. 5), the mucilage idioblasts of the petals (Fig. 6), and the very large, spiny pollen grains (Fig. 4).

Spores of the mould *Puccinia malvacearum* should only be present in small numbers (see: Malvae folium).

A TLC procedure for examining the anthocyanins is given in [4], which also has illustrations of the chromatograms obtained.

Quantitative standards: ÖAB: *Swelling index*, not less than 15 (see below). *Ash*, not more than 14.0%. *Acid-insoluble ash*, not more than 2.0%.

Ph. Helv. VII: *Swelling index*, not less than 20 (first moistened with ethanol). *Foreign matter*, not more than 2% peduncles and other foreign matter; discoloured flowers, not more than 10%; opened flowers with a diameter greater than 55 mm (*Lavatera thuringiaca* L.), absent. *Sulphated ash*, not more than 15%.

Experiments to determine the swelling volumes of different malvaceous herbal drugs have shown that, when converted to 1 g drug (as required by the pharmacopoeias), the swelling indexes can differ by as much as 115%, depending on the amount of drug taken for the determination. It is suggested that it would be more appropriate to give the swelling volume together with the amount of drug used, e.g. SwV = 15/0.1 g [3].

Adulteration: Almost never happens. Formerly, admixture with the flowers of other Malvaceae was sometimes observed.

Literature:
[1] G. Franz, Planta Med. **14**, 90 (1966).
[2] H. Pourrat, O. Texier, and C. Barthomeuf, Pharm. Acta Helv. **65**, 93 (1990).
[3] K. Schneider, V. Ullmann, and W. Kubelka, Dtsch. Apoth. Ztg. **130**, 2303 (1990).
[4] H. Wagner, S. Bladt, and E.M. Zgainski, Plant drug analysis, Springer, Berlin – Heidelberg – New York – Tokyo, 1984, p. 274.

Malvae folium   Mallow leaf

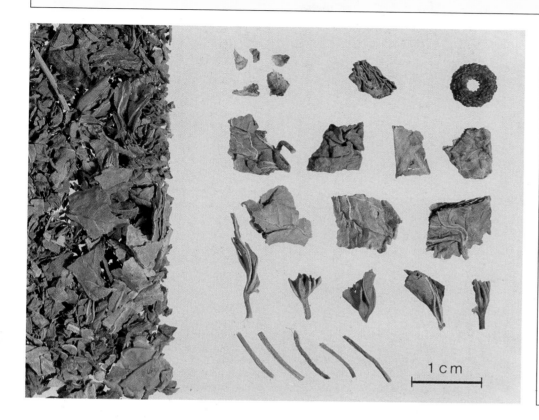

Fig. 1: Mallow leaf

Description: The material comsists of roundish, 3–7-lobed, long-petiolate leaves with a thin and slightly pubescent lamina having palmate venation and an irregularly jagged serrate margin. The chopped drug contains mostly square, much crushed leaf fragments, which are often stuck together.

Taste: Mucilaginous.

Fig. 2: *Malva sylvestris* L.

A shrub, up to 1 m in height, with characteristic 3–7-lobed and palmately nerved leaves; individual lobes rounded, with a jagged margin, and pubescent. 5-part, pink and violet-veined, malvaceous flowers with fused filaments (columna) and a calyx and epicalyx.

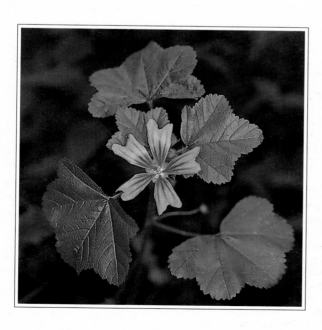

DAB 6, ÖAB: Folia Malvae
Ph. Helv. VII: Malvae folium
St. Zul. 1579.99.99

Plant sources: *Malva sylvestris* L., common mallow, *M. neglecta* WALLR., dwarf mallow (Malvaceae).

Synonyms: Blue mallow (Engl.), Malvenblätter (Ger.), Feuilles de mauve (Fr.).

Origin: Native in Europe, but introduced in other continents, and to some extent cultivated. The drug is imported from Bulgaria, Albania, and Morocco.

Constituents: Ca. 8% mucilage which on hydrolysis affords arabinose, glucose, rhamnose, galactose, and galacturonic acid; small amounts of tannin. The occurrence of flavonoid sulphates is noteworthy [1, 2]; several 8-hydroxyflavonoid glucuronides have been isolated as well, gossypetin 3-glucoside 8-glucuronide and hypolaetin 8-glucuronide being quantitatively the main ones [4].

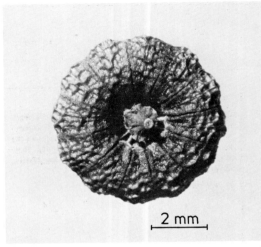

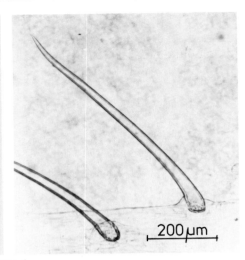

Fig. 3   Fig. 4

Fig. 3: Dehiscent fruit of *Malva neglecta*

Fig. 4: Large unicellular, bristly trichomes, found particularly on the veins of the leaves

Indications: Owing to its content of mucilage, the drug is used in the treatment of colds, catarrh of the upper respiratory tract, inflammation of the throat, and also as a mild astringent in angina or gastrointestinal inflammation.
In *folk medicine,* it is employed externally as a poultice for the treatment of wounds.

Making the tea: 3–5 g of the finely chopped drug is placed in cold water and boiled for a short time, or boiling water is poured over

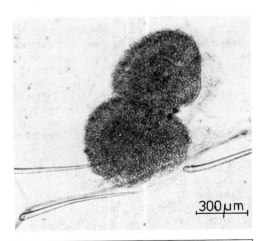

Fig. 5: Two sporangia of the rust *Puccinia malvacearum*

it, and after 5–10 min. passed through a tea strainer. Cold extracts (5–10 hours) are also recommended, but they should be boiled briefly before they are drunk. As a bronchial tea, a cupful, sweetened with honey, is drunk several times a day.
1 Teaspoon = ca. 1.8 g.

Phytomedicines: The drug is a component of a few mixed bronchial teas and the extract is present in some instant teas for the same indication.

Authentication: Macro- and microscopically [3]. The not very frequent 2–6-radiate stellate trichomes as well as a few single trichomes are characteristic (Fig. 4); both are relatively thick-walled and pointed. The upper **and** lower walls of the epidermal cells are sinuate. There are cluster crystals of calcium oxalate and mucilage cells in the mesophyll. Occasionally, the drug also contains fruits which have been gathered at the same time (Fig. 3).
Leaves that are heavily infected with the mould *Puccinia malvacearum,* recognizable by orange-red or brownish pustules, should be discarded. Microscopically, they can be recognized as spore masses (Fig. 5).

Quantitative standards: St.Zul. 1579.99.99: *Swelling index,* not less than 7. *Water-soluble extractive,* not less than 30%. *Foreign matter,* not more than 2%; proportion of leaves infected with the sporangium and spores of the rust *Puccinia malvacearum,* not more

than 5%; fruits and flowers, not more than 5%; stem, not more than occasional fragments. *Loss on drying,* not more than 10.0%. *Ash,* not more than 17.0%.
(The St.Zul. TLC identification test is merely a fingerprint chromatogram and is relatively unspecific.)
ÖAB: *swelling index,* not less than 8. *Foreign matter,* not more than 3%; only occasional spores of *Puccinia malvacearum* should be present. *Ash,* not more than 15.0%. *Acid-insoluble ash,* not more than 2.0%
Ph. Helv. VII: *Swelling index,* not less than 7. *Foreign matter,* not more than 8% (stems, buds, flowers, and other foreign matter); not more than 5% flowers with spores of *Puccinia malvacearum. Sulphated ash,* not more than 22%.

Adulteration: Not frequent. Confusion with marsh mallow leaves occurs. These have a velvety pubescence; under the microscope, numerous stellate trichomes can be seen; they have a woody and coarsely punctuate base, underneath which there are usually clusters crystals of calcium oxalate. Only the lower walls of the epidermal cells are sinuate.

Literature:
[1] A.M. Nawwar and J. Buddrus, Phytochemistry **20,** 2446 (1981).
[2] A.M. Nawwar, A.E. Elsherbainy, and M.A. El Ansary, Phytochemistry **16,** 145 (177).
[3] J. Saukel, Sci. Pharm. **50,** 37 (1982).
[4] M. Billter, B. Meier, and O. Sticher, Phytochemistry **30,** 987 (1991).

Marrubii herba   White horehound (BHP 1/1990)

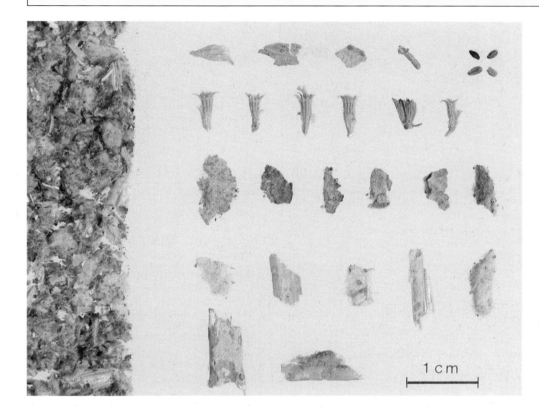

Fig. 1: White horehound

<u>Description:</u> The clumped and shrivelled leaf fragments are tomentose on the undersurface. The four-angled stem fragments bear downy hairs. Pieces of the flowers, especially of the tomentose sepals with their recurved, hooked teeth (Fig. 4), and occasional black triangular nutlets may also be present.

<u>Taste:</u> Bitter and somewhat acrid.

Fig. 2: *Marrubium vulgare* L.

30–60 cm tall, densely tomentose herbs. Leaves ovate with a crenate-serrate margin. Flowers numerous, in axillary whorls. Calyx with ten small recurved teeth.

ÖAB, Erg. B. 6: Herba Marrubii

Plant source: *Marrubium vulgare* L., white horehound (Lamiaceae = Labiatae).

Synonyms: Marrubium, Hoarhound (Engl.), Weißer Andorn, Andornkraut (Ger.), Marrube blanc, Herbe à la vierge (Fr.).

Origin: Long naturalized in parts of western, central, and northern Europe. The drug comes mostly from south-eastern Europe or Morocco.

Constituents: Diterpene bitter substances with the lactone marrubiin as main component (originating from premarrubiin ?), peregrinol, and vulgarol [1]; 14 flavonoids, including vitexin, as well as luteolin and apigenin and their 7-glucosides and 7-lactates, etc. [3]. Besides ubiquitous substances typical of the family, such as stachydrine and caffeic acid, there are also a small amount of essential oil and tannins.

Indications: As a bitter and choleretic in digestive and biliary complaints. The choleretic effect is ascribed to marrubiinic acid, which arises by opening of the lactone group in marrubiin [2]. It is also used as a mild expectorant for coughs.
In *folk medicine*, it is employed externally for skin lesions, sores, and wounds.

Making the tea: Boiling water is poured over 1.5 g of the finely cut drug and after 5–10 min. poured through a tea strainer. As

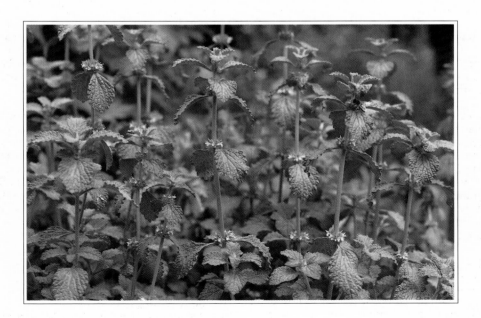

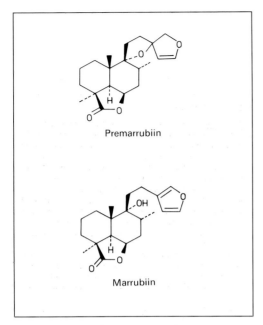

Premarrubiin

Marrubiin

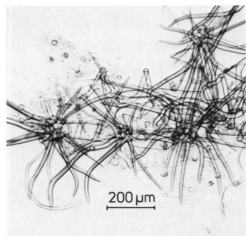

Fig. 3: Stellate trichomes from the undersurface of the leaf, often twisted together

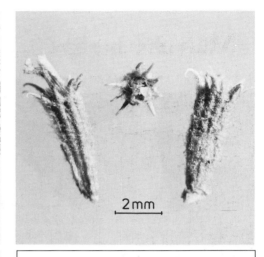

Fig. 4: Tomentose calices with recurved teeth, from *Marrubium vulgaris*

Extract from the German Commission E monograph (BAnz no. 22a, dated 01. 02. 1990)

Uses

Lack of appetite: dyspeptic complaints, such as a feeling of distention and flatulence; catarrh of the respiratory tract.

Contraindications

None known.

Side effects

None known.

Interactions with other remedies

None known.

Dosage

Unless otherwise prescribed: daily dose, 4.6 g drug or 2–6 tablespoonfuls of the expressed juice; preparations correspondingly.

Mode of administration

Comminuted drug, freshly expressed plant juice, and other galenical preparations for internal use.

Effects

Marrubic acid has a choleretic action.

a choleretic, a cupful is drunk before meals; as an expectorant, a cupful is taken several times a day.

1 Teaspoonful = ca. 1 g.

Phytomedicines: Only a few ready-made antitussives and expectorants. The drug is also a constituent of liver and bile teas, e.g. Species cholagogae (ÖAB).
Among the UK multi-ingredient products containing the drug and/or its extracts are: Heath & Heather Catarrh Tablets; Potter's Chest Mixture, Vegetable Cough Remover, and Horehound and Aniseed Cough Mixture (all liquid); Seven Seas Catarrh Tablets, etc.

Regulatory status (UK): General Sales List – Schedule 1, Table A.

Authentication: The leaves have characteristic stellate trichomes (Fig. 3) and the sepals

are tomentose and have shiny, recurved teeth (Fig. 4). The BHP 1/1990 gives detailed macroscopical and microscopical descriptions of the drug, as well as the following TLC identification test:

Test solution: 1 g powdered drug extracted with 20 ml on the water-bath for 10–15 min., filtered, and concentrated to ca. 5 ml.

Reference solution: 0.025% rutin in methanol.

Loadings: 20 μl of each solution, as 2-cm bands on silica gel.

Solvent system: ethyl acetate + anhydrous formic acid + glacial acetic acid + water (100 + 11 + 11 + 27), 15 cm run.

Detection: sprayed with 1% methanolic diphenylboryloxyethylamine, followed by 5% ethanolic polyethylene glycol 400.

Evaluation: in UV 366 nm light. Test solution: relative to rutin, bands at Rx 2.6 (blue), 1.7 and 1.4 (yellow), 1.0 (whitish blue).
The bitter substances can be examined chromatographically by the method described under Quassiae lignum (q.v.), using the solvent system: chloroform + methanol (95 + 5), and vanillin/sulphuric acid as detecting agent [4]:

Evaluation: Test solution: three conspicuous violet zones in the Rf range 0.5–0.9, that at Rf 0.8 being due to marrubiin and that at Rf 0.5 presumably to premarrubiin.

Quantitative standards: Erg. B. 6: *Ash*, not more than 15%.
ÖAB: *Bitterness value*, not less than 3000. *Foreign matter*, not more than 1%. *Ash*, not more than 12.0%. *Acid-insoluble ash*, not more than 1.5%.
BHP 1/1990: *Water-soluble extractive*, not less than 15%. *Foreign matter*, not more than 2%. *Total ash*, not more than 12%. *HCl-insoluble ash*, not more than 3%.

Adulteration: Seldom; perhaps with other *Marrubium* species, e.g. *M. incanum* DESR., which has leaves with a dense white tomentum.

Literature:
[1] D.P. Popa and G.S. Pasechnik, Khim. Prir. Soedin 11, 722 (1975); C.A. **84**, 150776 (1976).
[2] I. Krefči and R. Zadina, Planta med. 7, 1 (1959).
[3] M.A.M. Nawwar et al., Phytochemistry **28**, 3201 (1989).
[4] H. Wagner, S. Bladt, and E.M. Zgainski, Plant drug analysis, Springer-Verlag, Berlin, Heidelberg, New York, Tokyo, 1984, p. 134.

Mate folium   Paraguay tea, Maté leaf

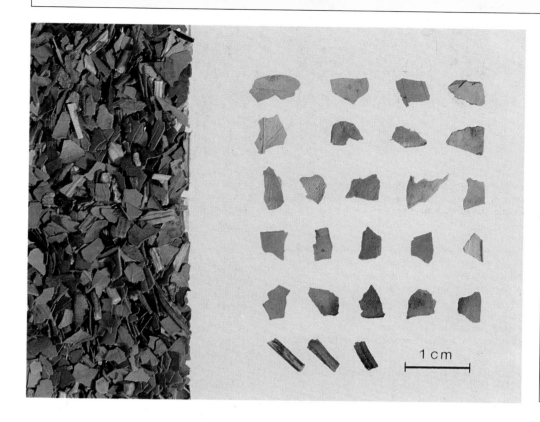

Fig. 1: Maté leaf

Description: The material consists of irregular, broken, glabrous, and stiff pieces of leaf, which are light green to brownish green (the green untreated drug is usual in South America, while the brown roasted leaves are available in Europe). The venation is clearly visible only on the lower surface; it is pinnate with a prominent midrib and arcuate lateral veins. Occasionally, on the lower surface, there are dark-coloured corky nodules. The sinuate, serrate leaf margin is not usually recognizable as such in the chopped drug. Occasional fragments of the stout, angular brown petioles are present.

The leaves, harvested from May to September, are briefly heated to inactivate the enzymes, thereby becoming dark in colour, then dried at 60°C, and finally powdered to different degrees depending on the market [2].

Odour: Faintly aromatic.

Taste: Astringent and somewhat smoky.

Fig. 2: *Ilex paraguariensis* A.St.Hil.

A small, evergreen tree or bush with alternate, ca. 15 cm long, leathery leaves having a sinuate, serrate margin and very small stipules. Monoecious, 4-partite, axillary white flowers; red spherical drupes ca. 7 mm in diameter.

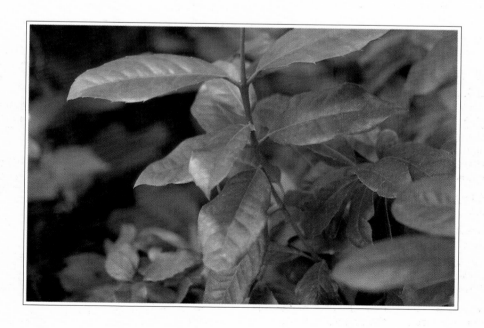

Erg. B. 6: Folia Mate

Plant source: *Ilex paraguariensis* A.St.Hil., maté (Aquifoliaceae).

Synonyms: Ilex, Jesuit's Brazil or St. Bartholomew's tea, Yerba maté, Hervea (Engl.), Mate (Ger.), Thé de Paraguay (Fr.).

Origin: An evergreen tree, maintained to some extent as a bush, growing in Brazil between latitudes 30° and 20° south and there also cultivated. The drug is exported (in 1988, more than 300 tonnes to Germany) from Brazil and partly also from Argentina and Paraguay [2].

Constituents: Varying amounts of caffeine (0.3–1.7%), part of which is combined with "tannins", and a little theobromine; 4–16% tannin-like substances which are mainly derivatives of phenol-carboxylic acids: condensation products of caffeic acid, 5-*O*-caffeoylquinic acid, and at least 10% chlorogenic acid (including isochlorogenic and neochlorogenic acids) [1]. An ursolic-acid derivative matesaponin 1 [3], a little essential oil, and (only in the fresh leaves?) a "resin fraction".

Indications: Based on its caffeine content, as a centrally acting stimulant (tonic, etc.) and as a diuretic. Since maté tea is greatly appreciated throughout much of South America as a "national drink", the people ascribe many other effects to it. It is thus not surprising that in Europe as well maté is praised as "the green gold of the Indios", as a "natural remedy and magic drink" and especially as "the ideal slimming remedy which facilitates losing weight in a natural way and stills the distressing feelings of hunger and thirst".

Making the tea: Hot water, just off the boil, is poured over ca. 1 teaspoon of maté and after 5–10 min. passed through a tea strainer. As with ordinary black tea, the stimulating effect of the briefly brewed tea is stronger and has a more pleasant taste, being less astringent, than tea which has been allowed to draw for a longer time: caffeine dissolves more rapidly than the tannins!
1 Teaspoon = ca. 2 g.
In South America, maté is prepared in the following way: In a roughly fist-size gourd (*cuja* or *cuia*), the same quantity of hot water, which is no longer boiling, is poured over the maté leaves. The drink is sucked up through a silver "straw" which has a sieve-like bottom end (*bombilla* or *bomba*), more water being added several times to the *cuja*. When *chimarrão* (a mixture of the powdered leaves and branches) is used, the characteristic taste is much stronger [2].

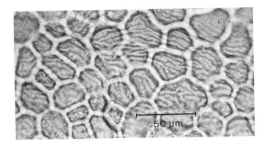

Fig. 3: Epidermis with sinuate cuticular striations

Herbal preparations: Maté is available on its own from several firms, and also in tea bags (mostly containing up to ca. 1.8 g), e.g. Mate-Gold® and roasted Mate-Gold®. It is a component of several herbal mixtures for preparing refreshing and stimulating drinks, some of which are also available in tea bags and in food shops, as well as in Blasen- und Nierentee (bladder and kidney tea) NRF.
Maté extracts are present in instant teas such as Nieroxin®-Tee.
Dried maté is a component of Lanes Lustys Herbalene, a multi-ingredient herbal laxative.

Phytomedicines: Some prepared Bladder, Kidney, Laxative, and "Blood-purifying" Teas also contain maté, e.g. Protitis®-Tee, Ramend®-Tee, Species urologicae nach Dr. May, Vital-Kopfschmerztee (headache tea). Maté extracts are also present in Phytoren®-Tropfen (drops).

Regulatory status (UK): General Sales List – Schedule 1, Table A.

Authentication: Macro- (see: Description) and microscopically. See also [4]. The leaf epidermis is covered with a thick striated cuticle (Fig. 3). There are fairly numerous calcium oxalate cluster crystals and occasional prisms in the spongy mesophyll.
On microsublimation, the caffeine can be detected as characteristic needles. The identification can also be carried out by TLC.

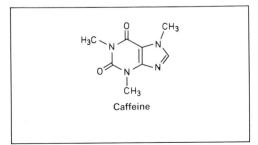

Caffeine

Extract from the German Commission E monograph (BAnz no. 85, dated 05.05.1988)

Uses
Mental and physical fatigue.

Contraindications
None known.

Side effects
None known.

Interactions with other remedies
None known.

Dosage
Unless otherwise prescribed: average daily dose, 3 g drug; preparations correspondingly.

Mode of administration
Chopped drug for infusions. Drug powder for other galenical preparations for internal use.

Effects
Analeptic, diuretic, positively inotropic, positively chronotropic, glycogenolytic, lipolytic.

Test solution: 2 g powdered drug refluxed with 10 ml of an ethanol + chloroform + water (40 + 20 + 10) mixture for 5 min. and, after cooling, filtered into a 20 ml volumetric flask, followed by rinsing the flask and the filter and making up to the mark.

Reference solutions: A, 50 mg caffeine dissolved in 10 ml of the foregoing solvent mixture; B, 50 mg theobromine dissolved in the same mixture.

Loadings: 5 μl each of the test solution and the two reference solutions A and B, as 2-cm bands.

Solvent system: ethyl acetate + methanol + water (100 + 16.5 + 13.5), 6 cm run.

Detection: chromatogram dried in a current of warm air. Observed in UV 254 nm light. Then sprayed with iodine solution, followed by ethanol + 25% hydrochloric acid (1 + 1).

Evaluation: in UV 254 nm light. Reference solutions: caffeine quenching zone in the upper third; slightly below it, the weaker theobromine quenching zone. Test solution: comparable zones, and further quenching zones in the centre and lower third (Fig. 4). Sprayed. Test and Reference solutions: dis-

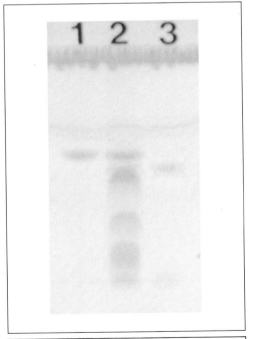

Fig. 4: TLC on 4 × 8 cm foil

1: Caffeine
2: Maté
3: Theobromine

For details, see the text

tinct brown caffeine zones, but only very faint theobromine zones; in the test solution chromatogram, possible additional brown zones.

Other TLC methods are to be found in [5].

Quantitative standards: Erg. B. 6: *No chopped fragments of twigs*, especially in the finely cut drug. *Ash*, not more than 6%.
BHP 1983: *Water-soluble extractive*, not less than 20%. *Foreign organic matter*, not more than 1%. *Moisture content*, not more than 10%. *Total ash*, not more than 8%. *Acid-insoluble ash*, not more than 2%.

Adulteration: In Brazil, there are many other *Ilex* species, some of which are also used for the preparation of maté. The imported drug comes almost entirely from cultivated plants. There is no information about possible adulterants.

Storage: Protected from light and moisture.

Literature:
[1] R. Hegnauer, Chemotaxonomie der Pflanzen, Birkhäuser, Basel – Stuttgart, 1964, vol. **3**, pp. 165 et seq.
[2] G. Gosmann, E.P. Schenkel, and O. Seligmann, J. Nat. Prod. **52**, 1367 (1989).
[3] N. Ohem, Dtsch. Apoth. Ztg. **130**, 2737 (1990).
[4] B.P. Jackson and D.W. Snowdon, Atlas of microscopy of medicinal plants, culinary herbs and spices, Belhaven Press, London, 1990, p. 160.
[5] H. Wagner, S. Bladt, and E.M. Zgainski, Plant drug analysis, Springer-Verlag, Berlin, Heidelberg, New York, Tokyo, 1984, p. 86.

Matricariae flos (DAB 10, Ph. Eur. 2), Matricaria flowers (*BAN*; BP 1988), Matricaria flower (BHP 1/1990)

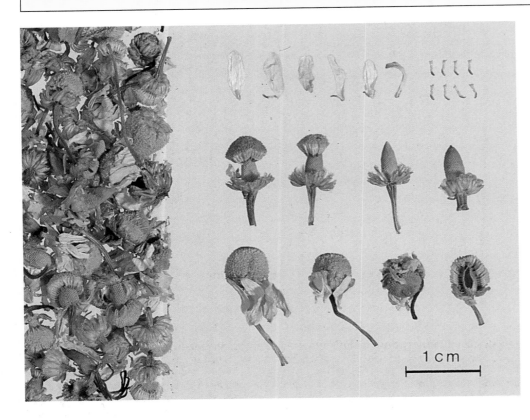

Fig. 1: Matricaria flowers

<u>Description:</u> The flower-heads have yellow tubular florets surrounded by a ring of white ligulate florets; the latter are often found on their own. The sharply conical receptacle of the inflorescence is hollow and it has no scales.

<u>Odour:</u> Characteristic, strongly aromatic.

<u>Taste:</u> Somewhat bitter.

Fig. 2: *Matricaria recutita* L.

A plant up to ca. 0.5 m in height widely distributed in waste places, having 2–3 times pinnately subdivided leaves and numerous flower-heads. In the foreground of the picture, the inflorescence of *Thlaspi arvense* L., field penny-cress (Brassicaceae = Cruciferae).

Fig. 3: *Matricaria recutita* L.

The ca. 15 white ligulate florets of the flower-head at first spread laterally and later hang downwards. The yellow tubular florets, densely packed on a hollow conical receptacle, open in succession from the bottom to the top.

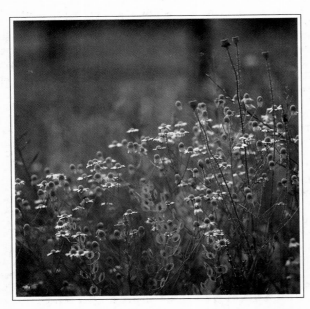

Fig. 2

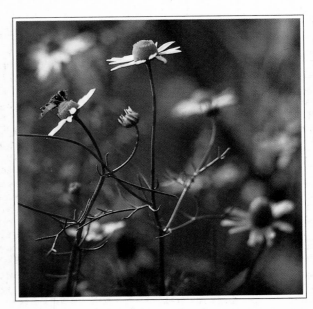

Fig. 3

DAB 10: Kamillenblüten
ÖAB: Flos Chamomillae vulgaris
Ph. Helv. VII: Matricariae flos
St. Zul. 7999.99.99

Plant source: *Matricaria recutita* L., scented mayweed or wild chamomile (Asteraceae). *Chamomilla recutita* (L.) RAUSCHERT and *Matricaria chamomilla* L. pro parte are considered to be synonyms.

Synonyms: Flos chamomillae vulgaris (Lat.), Matricaria, German or Hungarian chamomile, Pin heads (Engl.), Kamillenblüten, Kleine Kamille, Feldkamille (Ger.), Fleur de camomile (Fr.).

Origin: Originally native in southern and eastern Europe and western Asia. Nowadays, throughout Europe, North America, and also in Australia. The commercial product is derived mainly from cultivated plants and comes especially from Argentina, Egypt (not always of pharmacopoeial quality, often for the food industry), Bulgaria, Hungary, and to a small extent from Spain, former Czechoslovakia, and Germany.

Constituents: 0.3–1.5% essential oil, containing (–)-α-bisabolol (INN: levomenol), the bisabolol oxides A, B, and C, bisabolone oxide, chamazulene (from matricin through saponification, loss of water, and decarboxylation), the crimson-red, pleasantly-smelling chamaviolin, spathulenol and the *cis*- and *trans*-enyne dicyclo ethers (spiroether, polyacetylenes) as principal components. Flavonoids: including many identified methoxylated flavones and flavonols [1], apigenin (arising by hydrolysis of the 7-*O*-glucoside during drying [37]), luteolin, quercitrin, 7-mono- and 7-diglycosides and 7-monoglycosides acetylated in the sugar moiety (among them, luteolin and apigenin 7-*O*-glucosides, apigenin 7-*O*-rutinoside and 7-*O*-neohesperidoside). Sesquiterpene lactones: matricin, matricarin, desacetylmatricarin. Coumarins: umbelliferone and herniarin. Mucilage. Regarding further constituents, see [1–5].

Indications: As an antiphlogistic, spasmolytic, carminative, and stomachic. The antiphlogistic, spasmolytic, ulcer-protecting, bactericidal, and fungicidal activity has been repeatedly demonstrated in many pharmacological models, animal experiments, and in clinical tests [1, 6–10]. The main uses internally are for gastrointestinal complaints (gastritis, enteritis, colitis, flatulence, cramp-like symptoms in the digestive tract) and menstrual problems. Externally, chamomile is used for conditions affecting the skin and

mucous membranes, thus in inflammation and catarrh of the nose and throat and of the bronchi (inhalation of the vapour), mouth (washes), and erythema of the skin (poultices, baths, ointments).

The activity results from the interplay of structurally different compounds which are responsible for the therapeutic value of the drug. The antiphlogistic action of (–)-α-bisabolol [11, 14], chamazulene and matricin [14], as well as of the spiro-ethers [15], has been substantiated. Apigenin and to a lesser extent other flavonoids of the drug [1, 16], and also α-bisabolol [16] and the spiro-ethers [1, 4, 15, 17], have musculotropic spasmolytic activity. α-Bisabolol has been shown to have an antiseptic and ulcer-protecting action [18, 19]. The spiro-ethers and α-bisabolol are among the antibacterial and fungicidal components [4, 15, 20]. The detoxification of bacterial toxins [21, 22] and an effect on the metabolism of the skin [23] have also been demonstrated.

The chamomile flavones have a local anti-inflammatory effect on topical application. In an experimental model (croton oil-induced dermatitis in mice), apigenin and luteolin had a potency similar to that of indomethacin; quercetin, apigenin 7-glucoside, and rutin were less active [24–26].

Allergic skin reactions to matricaria flowers have been described in a few rare cases. The suspected allergen, the sesquiterpene lactone

anthecotulide from *Anthemis cotula* L., generally does not occur in genuine chamomile. It is found in imported drug of the bisabolol B-type from Argentina only in traces which are not enough to cause sensitization [27, 28]. The coumarin herniarin has also been mentioned as a possible allergen of matricaria flowers [29]. Information on adverse reactions to *Matricaria recutita* is summarized in [38].

The warning in the Standard Licence that infusions of chamomile should not be used near the eyes is to avoid any possible effect by irritants or particles of the drug on these sensitive organs.

Making the tea: Boiling water is poured over 1–2 g of matricaria flowers, covered, and allowed to stand for 10 min.; it is then passed through a tea strainer. (Note: up to 70% of the essential oil remains in the marc. The use of aqueous alcoholic, standardized extracts is certainly more effective.).

1 Teaspoon = ca. 1 g, 1 tablespoon = ca. 2.5 g.

Herbal teas: Tea bags (0.9–1.3 g) made by various manufacturers are available. Care should be taken to make sure that the contents consist only of flowers; sometimes, finely chopped herb is used (it is permitted as a foodstuff), which has an essential-oil content far below the pharmacopoeial requirement. Therefore, it must be ensured that tea bags contain pharmacopoeial quality material. The drug for infusion should have a homogeneous particle size not greater than 2 mm and be packed in a suitable tea bag which will hold back the small amount of fines [39]. Instant teas are also available.

Matricaria flowers are a popular component of herbal teas on the UK market [40].

Phytomedicines: In Germany, matricaria extracts alone or in combination are a component of more than 90 licenced prepared remedies [30]. The annual consumption of matricaria flowers in Germany is almost 4000 tonnes. Most preparations are antiphlogistics, e.g. Kamillosan®, Perkamillon®, Eukamillat®, Kamille Spitzner®, Matmille®, and many more, gastrointestinal remedies, skin remedies, etc.

Extract from the German Commission E monograph (BAnz no. 228, dated 05.12.1984)

Uses

Externally: Inflammation of the skin and mucous membranes and bacterial skin conditions, including those of the mouth and gums.
Inflammation and irritation of the respiratory tract (inhalations).
Complaints in the anal and genital regions (baths and washes).
Internally: Gastrointestinal spasms and inflammatory conditions of the gastrointestinal tract.

Contraindications

None known.

Side effects

None known.

Interactions

None known.

Dosage

Boiling water (ca. 150 ml) is poured over a heaped tablespoon of matricaria flowers (= ca. 3 g), covered, and after 5–10 min. passed through a tea strainer.
Unless otherwise prescribed, for gastrointestinal complaints a cup of the freshly prepared tea is drunk three or four times a day between meals. For inflammation of the mucous membranes of the mouth and throat, the freshly prepared tea is used as a wash or gargle.
External use: for poultices and rinses, 3–10% infusions; as a bath additive, 50 g to 10 l water.
Semi-solid formulations with preparations corresponding to 3–10% drug.

Mode of administration

Liquid and solid formulations for external and internal use.

Effects

Antiphlogistic, musculotropic spasmolytic, promotes wound healing, deodorant, antibacterial and inhibits bacterial toxins. Stimulates skin metabolism.

Fig. 4: A tubular floret of *Matricaria chamomilla*

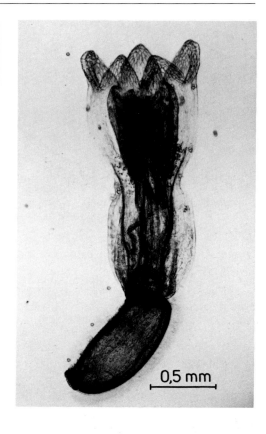

0,5 mm

About the conditions required to stabilize matricin (the main antiphlogistic constituent) in solid dosage forms (flowers, extracts), see [41].

Regulatory status (UK): General Sales List – Schedule 1, Table A.

Authentication: Macro- and microscopically, following the Ph. Eur. 2, BP 1988, etc. The presence of the hollow receptacle is an important characteristic. The tubular florets (Fig. 4) afford microscopical diagnostic features: a ring of stone cells at the base of the ovary, the peltate glandular trichomes (Fig. 5), the lengthwise-oriented mucilaginous epidermal cells of the ovary [42], and the pollen (Fig. 6). See [43] for the detailed, illustrated microscopy of the powdered drug.

Identification tests according to Ph. Eur. 2, etc., also include the detection of proazulene, determination of the volatile-oil content, and TLC separation of a concentrated dichloromethane percolate as a purity test; assignment of the zones is discussed in the Commentary [31]. In the literature, there are other TLC methods for testing the purity [e.g. 32–36]. For the detection and (semi-) quantitation of chamazulene by sublimation, see: Millefolii herba. There is an unresolved difference of opinion about whether determination of the matricin or chamazulene content of the drug and its preparations is more appropriate [44].

Wording of the package insert, from the German Standard Licence:

6.1   Uses

Gastrointestinal complaints, irritation of the mucous membranes of the mouth and throat and of the upper respiratory tract.

6.2   Mode of administration and Dosage

Hot water (ca. 150 ml) is poured over a tablespoonful of **Matricaria flowers** and after 5–10 min. passed through a tea strainer. To prepare a vapour bath, hot water is poured over 1–2 tablespoonfuls of matricaria flowers.

Unless otherwise prescribed, for gastrointestinal complaints a cup of the freshly prepared infusion is drunk three or four times a day between meals. For inflammation of the mouth and throat, the freshly prepared infusion is used as a rinse or gargle several times a day. For inflammation of the upper respiratory tract, the vapour from the freshly prepared infusion is inhaled.

Warning: The infusion should not be used near the eyes.

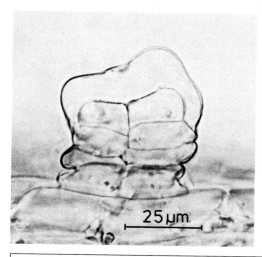

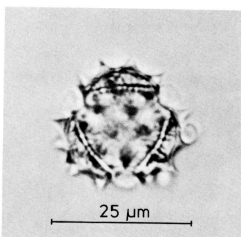

Fig. 5: Asteraceous, peltate glandular trichome

Fig. 6: Pollen grain, with short spines on the exine and three pores

Quantitative standards: Ph. Eur. 2, etc.: *Volatile oil*, not less than 0.4% of a blue-coloured product. *Appearance*, not more than 25% fragments not passing a 710 sieve. *Sulphated ash*, not more than 13.0%.

BHP 1/1990: Matricaria flower must comply with the requirements of the Ph. Eur. 2 for Matricariae flos and the BP 1988 for Matricaria flowers.

Note: Matricariae flos is the subject of an ESCOP proposed European harmonized monograph.

Adulteration: Rare, since the drug comes from cultivated plants. Almost always, it is evident from the macroscopic or microscopic examination (pith-like receptacle, 4-lobed corolla, etc.); see also [31]. Adulteration with other plant materials containing $(-)$-α-bisabolol or with non-chamomile and cheaper $(-)$-α-bisabolol can be directly detected without prior isolation through determination of the $^{13}C : ^{12}C$ ratio by combined GLC and IRMS (isotope-ratio mass spectrometry) [45]; the $^{2}H : ^{1}H$ ratio as determined by 2D-NMR spectroscopy can also be utilized [46].

Literature:
[1] H. Becker and J. Reichling, Dtsch. Apoth. Ztg. **121**, 1285 (1981).
[2] E. Flaskamp, G. Nonnenmacher, and O. Isaac, Z. Naturforsch. **36b**, 114 (1981).
[3] H. Schilcher, Die Kamille, Wissenschaftliche Verlagsgesellschaft, Stuttgart, 1987.
[4] R. Carle and O. Isaac, Dtsch. Apoth. Ztg. **125**(Suppl. I), 3 (1985).
[5] E. Luppold, Pharmazie in unserer Zeit **13**, 65 (1984).
[6] O. Isaac, Dtsch. Apoth. Ztg. **120**, 567 (1980).
[7] A. Detter, Pharm. Ztg. **126**, 1140 (1981).
[8] Th. Nasemann, Z. Allgemein. Med. **51**, 1105 (1975).
[9] H.B. Foster, H. Niklas, and S. Lutz, Planta Med. **40**, 309 (1980).
[10] R. Carle and O. Isaac, Z. Phytotherap. **8**, 67 (1987).
[11] V. Jakovlev and A.v. Schlichtegroll, Arzneim.-Forsch. **19**, 615 (1969).
[12] O. Isaac, Planta Med. **35**, 118 (1979).
[13] V. Jakovlev, O. Isaac, K. Thiemer, and R. Kunde, Planta Med. **35**, 125 (1979).
[14] V. Jakovlev, O. Isaac, and E. Flaskamp, Planta Med. **49**, 67 (1983).
[15] J. Breinlich and K. Scharmagel, Arzneim.-Forsch. **18**, 429 (1968).
[16] U. Achterrath-Tuckermann et al., Planta Med. **39**, 38 (1980).
[17] J. Breinlich, Dtsch. Apoth. Ztg. **106**, 698 (1966).
[18] O. Isaac and K. Thiemer, Arzneim.-Forsch. **25**, 1352 (1975).
[19] J. Szelenyi, O. Isaac, and K. Thiemer, Planta Med. **35**, 218 (1979).
[20] D. Slalontay, G. Verza-Petri, E. Florian, and G. Gimpel, Dtsch. Apoth. Ztg. **115**, 913 (1975).
[21] M. Kienholz, Dtsch. Apoth. Ztg. **102**, 1076 (1962).
[22] M. Kienholz, Arzneim.-Forsch. **13**, 980 (1963).
[23] K. Thiemer, R. Stadler, and O. Isaac, Arzneim.-Forsch. **23**, 756 (1973).
[24] R. Della Loggia et al., Progr. Clin. Biol. Res. **213**, 481 (1986).
[25] R. Della Loggia, Dtsch. Apoth. Ztg. **125** (Suppl. I), 9 (1985).
[26] A. Tubaro, C. Zilli, C. Redaelli, and R. Della Loggia, Planta Med. **51**, 359 (1985).
[27] B. M. Hausen, E. Busher, and R. Carle, Planta Med. **50**, 229 (1984).
[28] B. M. Hausen, Dtsch. Apoth. Ztg. **125** (Suppl. I), 24 (1985).
[29] E. Hegyi, M. Sarsunova, and K. Traubnerova, Farm. Obz. **55**, 29 (1986); C.A. **104**, 146939 (1986).
[30] Pharmazeutische Stoffliste, 4th ed., with supplements, Arzneibüro der ABDA (ed.), Frankfurt am Main, 1963–1982.
[31] Kommentar DAB 10.
[32] O. Isaac, H. Schneider, and H. Eggenschwiller, Dtsch. Apoth. Ztg. **108**, 293 (1968).
[33] J. Hölzl and G. Demuth, Dtsch. Apoth. Ztg. **113**, 671 (1973).
[34] J. Hölzl and G. Demuth, Planta Med. **27**, 37 (1975).
[35] J. Reichling and H. Becker, Dtsch. Apoth. Ztg. **117**, 275 (1977).
[36] P. Rohdewald, G. Rücker, and K.-W. Glombitza, Apothekengerechte Prüfvorschriften, Deutscher Apotheker Verlag, Stuttgart, 1986, 813.
[37] R. Bauer, and H. Wagner, Sci. Pharm. **59**, 3 (1991).
[38] B. M. Hausen, in: P.A.G.M. de Smet et al., Adverse Effects of Herbal Drugs, vol. 1, Springer-Verlag, Berlin, Heidelberg, New York, p. 243, 263.
[39] U.H. Hagenström, A. Spitzkowski, and U. Winkler, Pharmazie **45**, 211 (1990).
[40] C.A. Baldwin, L.A. Anderson, and J.D. Phillipson, Pharm. J. **239**, R10 (1987).
[41] B. Soyke, Eur. J. Pharm. Biopharm. **38**, 97 (1992).
[42] R. Länger and J. Saukel, Sci Pharm. **56**, 31 (1988).
[43] B.P. Jackson and D.W. Snowdon, Atlas of microscopy of medicinal plants, culinary herbs and spices, Belhaven Press, London, 1990, p. 162.
[44] Dtsch. Apoth. Ztg. **131**, 175, 279, 331, 505, 506 (1991).
[45] R. Carle, I. Fleischhauer, J. Beyer, and E. Reinhard, Planta Med. **56**, 456 (1990).
[46] R. Carle, C. Beyer, A. Cheminat, and E. Krempp, Phytochemistry **31**, 171 (1992).

Meliloti herba   Melilot

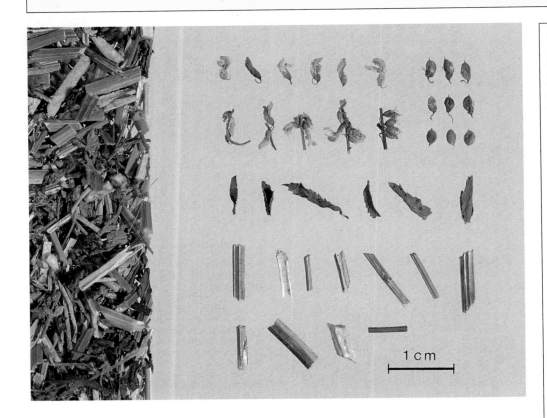

Fig. 1: Melilot

<u>Description</u>: The drug consists of broken fragments of leaf with a blunt to sharp serrate-dentate margin and glabrous or pubescent only on the lower surface along the nerves. The pieces of stem are hollow and longitudinally grooved. The bluish yellow papilionaceous flowers (first and second rows) which are arranged in one-sided racemes (second row) are characteristic. The small, straw-yellow to brown, usually glabrous pods remain closed and normally contain only one seed (top right); they should only occasionally be present in the drug.

<u>Odour</u>: Sweetish, of coumarin.

<u>Taste</u>: Bitter, somewhat pungent and salty.

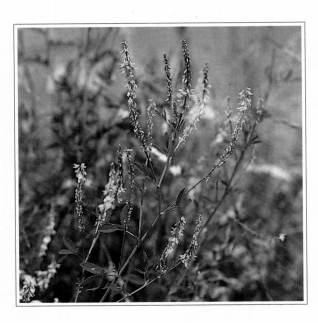

Fig. 2: *Melilotus officinalis* (L.) PALLAS

An 80 cm tall, biennial composite, frequently encountered along roadsides, with 3-foliolate leaves having an irregularly dentate margin and yellow flowers in racemes. In contrast to the very similar *Melilotus altissima*, keel of the flowers shorter than the wings and pods glabrous.

Coumarin   Melilotin   Melilotoside

Plant sources: *Melilotus officinalis* (L.) PALL., ribbed or common melilot, and/or *M. altissima* THUILL., tall melilot (Fabaceae).

Synonyms: Yellow, Sweet, or Field melilot, King's or Yellow sweet clover (Engl.), Steinkleekraut, Honigklee, Mottenklee, Bärenklee, Mallotenkraut (Ger.), Petit trèfle jaune, Trèfle des mouches, Herbe aux mouches, Herbe aux puces, Couronne royale (Fr.).

Origin: Widely distributed in Europe and Asia along roadsides (ribbed melilot) or scattered in damp localities (tall melilot). The drug is imported from eastern European countries.

Constituents: Coumarin derivatives and coumarin, partly in the form of glycosides, e.g. melilotoside, melilotin, etc.; flavonoids, especially kaempferol and quercetin derivatives; sapogenins [1] of the oleanolic-acid type and presumably also the corresponding saponins.

Indications: In the form of a tea mainly as an antiphlebitis remedy, but in *folk medicine* also as a diuretic. The German Commission E monograph [2] also listed the following indications: Disorders accompanying chronic venous insufficiency, such as pains and a feeling of heaviness in the legs, night cramps, itching, and swellings. In supportive treatment of haemorrhoids and lymphatic congestion. External uses: contusions, sprains, and superficial effusions of blood.

Animal experiments have demonstrated an acceleration of wound healing.

Side effects: In rare cases, headache.

Making the tea: Boiling water (ca. 150 ml) is poured over 1–2 teaspoonfuls of the finely chopped drug and after 5–10 min. passed through a tea strainer. As an antiphlebitis remedy, two or three cups a day are drunk. For sores and haemorrhoids, and as a poultice: the drug is thoroughly soaked with the same amount of hot water, wrapped in linen, and placed on the affected part.
↑ Teaspoon = ca. 1.6 g.

Phytomedicines: Melilot is a component of some prepared herbal remedies (teas), mostly to enhance the taste, but also as an active drug.
Melilot extracts are components of several antiphlebitis remedies, most of which have a standardized coumarin content, e.g. Venalot® (capsules, ampoules, liniment), Phlebodril-Creme, Pascovenol® (dragees, drops), etc.

Authentication: Macro- (see: Description) and microscopically. The leaves have anomocytic stomata on both surfaces. There are occasional trichomes, which are more frequent on young leaves, consisting of three cells; the basal and middle cells are thin-walled and short, and the terminal cell is long and thick-walled with a warty cuticle (Fig. 3). The septate fibres, which contain

crystals and which are associated with the vascular bundles, are another important feature. On the calyx and ovary there are glandular trichomes with a two- or three-celled stalk and a multicellular oval head (Fig. 4). The following TLC procedure [3] examines the coumarins:

Test solution: 1 g powdered drug extracted for 30 min. with 10 ml methanol on the water-bath, filtered, and the filtrate concentrated to ca. 1 ml.

Reference solution: 1% solutions of coumarin, scopoletin, and umbelliferone in methanol.

Loadings: 20 µl test solution and 5 or 10 µl reference solution, as bands on silica gel F_{254}.

Solvent system: freshly prepared, toluene + diethyl ether (1+1) saturated with 10% acetic acid.

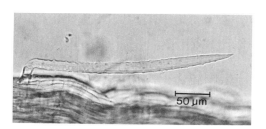

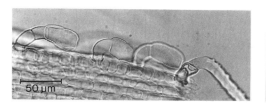

Fig. 3: Trichome with warty cuticle (see text)

Fig. 4: Glandular trichome from the calyx and ovary (the head is thickly covered with mucilage and therefore difficult to recognize as being multicellular)

Extract from the German Commission E monograph (BAnz no. 50, dated 13. 03. 1986)

Uses

Internal use: Disorders arising from chronic venous insufficiency, such as pains and heaviness in the legs, night cramps, itching, and swellings. In supportive treatment of thrombophlebitis, the post-thrombotic syndrome, haemorrhoids, and lymphatic congestion.
External use: Contusions, sprains, and superficial effusion of blood.

Contraindications

None known.

Side effects

None known.

Interactions with other remedies

None known.

Dosage

Unless otherwise prescribed:
Internal use: average daily dose, the amount of drug or preparation corresponding to 3–30 mg coumarin.
Parenteral use: the amount corresponding to 1.0–7.5 mg coumarin.
The effective dosage of Melilot preparations in fixed combinations for external use must be determined for each product.

Mode of administration

Chopped drug for making infusions and other galenical preparations for internal use.
Liquid preparations for parenteral use. Ointments, liniments, poultices, and medicated pads for external, and ointments and suppositories for rectal, use.

Effects

Anti-oedematous in inflammatory and congestive oedema, as a result of an increase in venous return and improvement in lymph kinetics.
Animal experiments have demonstrated an acceleration of wound healing.

Detection: in UV 365 nm light before and after spraying with 5% or 10% ethanolic potassium hydroxide.

Evaluation: in UV 365 nm light. Reference solution: coumarin zone not seen; scopoletin and umbelliferone as bluish white fluorescent zones at Rf ca. 0.25 and 0.4. Test solution: a series of red fluorescent zones (chlorophyll derivatives); weakly fluorescent zones corresponding to scopoletin and umbelliferone; a blue fluorescent zone at Rf ca. 0.5.

After spraying, again in UV 365 nm light. Reference solution: coumarin seen as an intense greenish yellow fluorescent zone at Rf ca. 0.65. Test solution: intense fluorescent coumarin zone now visible, along with the zones already mentioned.

Adulteration: In practice, rarely occurs. The *Melilotus* species mentioned in the older literature, *M. alba* MEDIKUS, white melilot, and *M. dentata* (WALDST. et KIT.) PERS., have no scent and are morphologically different from the genuine drug; they can also be recognized by their deviating microscopical features.

Storage: Protected from light, in well-closed containers (to prevent loss of coumarin).

Literature:
[1] S.S. Kang and W.S. Woo, J. Nat. Prod. **51**, 335 (1988).
[2] Announcement by the Federal Ministry of Health (BGA) dated 18.02.1986; BAnz dated 13.03.1986, p. 3077; Dtsch. Apoth. Ztg. **126**, 619 (1986); Pharm. Ztg. **131**, 777 (1986).
[3] H. Wagner, S. Bladt, and E.M. Zgainski, Plant drug analysis, Springer-Verlag, Berlin, Heidelberg, New York, Tokyo, 1984, p. 156.

Melissae folium   (DAB 10), Balm

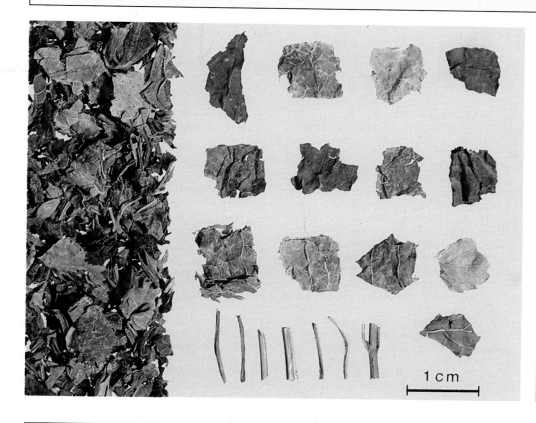

Fig. 1: Balm

Description: The more or less long-petiolate leaves are ca. 8 cm long and up to 3 cm wide, broadly ovate, and rounded or almost cordate at the base. The thin and somewhat crumpled lamina has a dark green upper surface which is slightly pubescent and a lighter green lower surface which is almost glabrous or only slightly pubescent along the veins and finely punctate (Fig. 3). The margin is irregularly crenate or serrate and the venation is thin and prominent on the lower surface.

Odour: Spicy and aromatic, reminiscent of lemon; often, only noticeable after rubbing the leaves; with material that has been stored for some time, the odour may be very faint.

Taste: Pleasantly spicy.

Fig. 2: *Melissa officinalis* L.

A herb, up to 70 cm in height, smelling strongly of lemon, with distinctly petiolate, broadly ovate, opposite and decussate leaves on 4-angled stems. Leaf venation very prominent on the lower surface and margin crenate and serrate. Pale-coloured ca. 1 cm long flowers, with a 2-lobed calyx, grouped in the axils of the leaves.

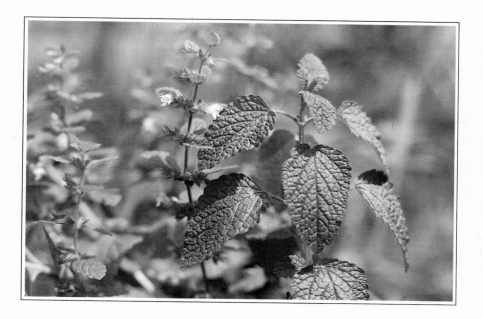

DAB 10: Melissenblätter
ÖAB: Folium Melissae
Ph. Helv. VII: Melissae folium
St. Zul. 1149.99.99

Plant source: *Melissa officinalis* L., balm (Lamiaceae).

Synonyms: Folia citronellae, Folia melissae citratae (Lat.), Melissa, Balm, Lemon or Sweet balm, Cure-all (Engl.), Melissenblätter, Zitronenkraut, Zitronenmelisse (Ger.), Feuilles de mélisse (Fr.).

Origin: Originally, native in the eastern Mediterranean region and in western Asia; cultivated in western (especially Spain), central (southern and eastern Germany), and eastern Europe. Imports of the drug come from Bulgaria and Romania. For a review of the literature, including the history of its cultivation and current research, see [1].

Constituents: 0.02–0.3% essential oil, comprising more than 70 components – >60% monoterpenes and >35% sesquiterpenes; the oxygen-containing fraction is very large-

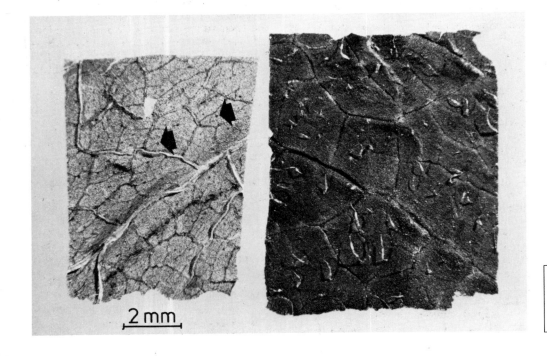

Citral b (= Neral)   Citronellal   Geraniol   Germacrene D   β-Caryophyllene

ly (ca. 90%) monoterpenoid, while the hydrocarbon fraction is mostly (ca. 90%) sesquiterpenoid. Among the principal monoterpenoid components are citronellal (ca. 30–40%) and citral a and b (geranial and neral) in the ratio 3:4–5 (ca. 10–30%); small amounts of methyl citronellate, (+)-ocimene, citronellol, geraniol and nerol, etc. are also present. The predominant sesquiterpenes include ca. 10% each of β-caryophyllene and germacrene D, along with some germacra-1(10)E,5E-dien-4-ol [13, 14]. Monoterpene glycosides, and other glycosides with a volatile aglycone, e.g. eugenyl glucoside, are also present in balm leaves [15]. The composition of the essential oil depends on various factors, including origin and climate, and whether it is obtained from leaf material of the first or second cut also plays a decisive role [4, cf. 13, 14]. When cultivated under special conditions and in a particular climate, e.g. as in Spain, the essential-oil content of some materials (chemical races?) may rise to 0.8% [5]. The drug contains ca. 4% rosmarinic acid (so-called labiate tannin), glycosidically bound chlorogenic and caffeic acids, triterpenes, and flavonoids [2, 3].

Indications: Preparations of balm have sedative, spasmolytic, and antibacterial actions. They are therefore employed for gastrointestinal disorders of nervous origin, in psychosomatic cardiac disorders, against migraine, and as a "nervine" [7, 8]. In mice, aqueous alcoholic extracts of the drug have been shown to have sedative and peripheral analgesic activity; they also induce and potentiate sleep after administering subhypnotic and hypnotic doses of pentobarbital [16]. Possibly, the polyphenolics present are responsible for the long known [6] choleretic action of balm leaf [7, 8]. Whether this is also the case for the demonstrated virostatic action [9], more especially of the herpes viruses [10], or whether this is due to the whole complex of substances is still under discussion. Very probably, the effect results from a reaction between the polyphenolics and the viral and cell-membrane proteins, the phenolic substances occupying viral receptors and thereby preventing adsorption of the virus on to the cell wall. The diminution of the thyrotrophin level in animals brought about by balm extracts is worth noting [11]. In *folk medicine,* preparations of balm are also recommended against colds (as a diaphoretic, "calming", or "strengthening" remedy), in functional disorders of the circulation ("nervous palpitations of the heart", "migraines", "hysteria", and "melancholia").

Making the tea: Boiling water is poured over 1.5–2 g of the finely chopped drug, covered, and allowed to stand for 5–10 min. before being passed through a tea strainer. 1 Teaspoon = ca. 1.0 g.

Herbal preparations: The drug is also available in tea bags (1.0–1.5 g); care has to be taken to ensure that it is of pharmacopoeial quality. In instant teas, the drug extract is usually combined with other drug extracts.

Phytomedicines: A series of preparations, grouped as plant hypnotics and sedatives contain, among other things, aqueous or more often alcoholic extracts of balm leaf. However, because of the cost, the proportion of genuine balm is usually very small. Alcoholic distillates, such as Melissa or Carmelite water, are prepared not only from balm leaf, but also make use of other drugs

Fig. 3: *Melissa officinalis*: **Paler lower surface of the leaf, showing the glandular punctation (arrows), and darker upper surface with whitish bristles**

2 mm

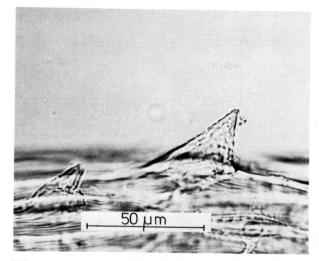

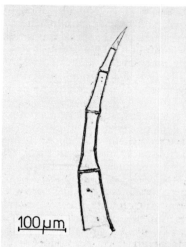

Fig. 4: Tooth-like conical trichome on the nervature of the leaf

Fig. 5: Multicellular covering trichome

containing essential oils, e.g. coriander, cardamom, nutmeg, cloves, cinnamon, angelica root, ginger, galangal root, elecampane root. In the DAB 6 formulation of Carmelite water (Spiritus Melissae compositus) the balm oil is replaced by citronella oil. Balm bath oils usually do not contain genuine balm oil but rather "Indian Melissa oil" (= citronella oil DAB 6), a relatively cheap essential oil obtained from citronella and lemon grass (*Cymbopogon* species; Poaceae). To some extent, lemon oil, or lemon oil which has been distilled over balm herb (Melissae Citratum oleum), is used as a substitute for expensive balm oil.

Regulatory status (UK): General Sales List – Schedule 1, Table A.

Authentication: Macro- (see: Description) and microscopically. Particular noteworthy are the conical or tooth-like trichomes (Fig. 4); there are other, similar trichomes which are more slender and sometimes two-celled. The three- to five-celled covering trichomes with a warty or striated cuticle (Fig. 5) are a prominent feature. The essential oil accumulates in typical 8-celled lamiaceous peltate glandular trichomes which are mostly situated in depressions on the lower leaf surface. In addition, there are various types of capitate trichomes with one- or two-celled heads and one- to three-celled

stalks. The diacytic stomata, found only on the lower leaf surface, are raised like a dome above the surface.
The DAB 10 test of identity is as follows:

Test solution: 0.30 g freshly powdered drug shaken for 2–3 min. with 5 ml dichloromethane, then filtered over ca. 2 g anhydrous sodium sulphate, followed by rinsing with a further 2 ml solvent; combined filtrates carefully taken to dryness and the residue dissolved in 0.2 ml ethyl acetate.

Reference solution: 5 µl citral and 4.0 mg guaiazulene dissolved in 10 ml toluene.

Loadings: 20 µl test solution and 10 µl reference solution, as 2-cm bands on silica gel G.

Solvent system: ethyl acetate + hexane (10 + 90), 2 × 10 cm run.

Detection: before spraying, in daylight and in UV 365 nm light; after spraying with anisaldehyde reagent and heating to 100–105 °C for 5–10 min., in daylight.

Evaluation: before spraying. Test solution: just above the starting line, two greyish green zones fluorescing intense red in UV 365 nm light (chlorophyll); a little below the solvent front a yellow zone.
After spraying. Reference solution: about the middle, the faint greyish violet citral zone; in the upper third, the orange-brown guaiazulene zone. Test solution: about the middle, the faint greyish violet citral zone, with slightly above it the pinkish red caryophyllene epoxide zone (possibly ab-

sent); in the upper third, slightly below the level of the reference guaiazulene zone, the faint greyish violet citronellal zone; near the solvent front and slightly above the level of the reference guaiazulene zone, the violet main zone (caryophyllene and other hydrocarbons); in the lower half of the chromatogram, other, mostly faint, greyish violet or reddish zones (including citronellol, geraniol).
An excellent paper by Schultze et al. [14], which describes extraction of the TLC zones and their subsequent GC/MS examination, indicates that evaluation of the chromatogram (after spraying) requires modification. The following is a suitably modified text [with comments]:
Test solution: about the middle, two close but distinct zones (the upper one one citral,

the lower one geranial) [If no reference is used, and bearing in mind the variation in colour due to the spray reagent, there could be confusion with a greenish grey zone having a somewhat higher Rf; there can be a little as 1–2% geranial/-neral in the oil, but even so it should be detectable.], with slightly above it the pinkish red caryophyllene epoxide zone (possibly overlapped by two greenish zones and therefore not visible) [Caryophyllene epoxide always appears to-be present.]; in the upper third, below the Rf of the reference guaiazulene zone, a greyish violet zone; near the top of the middle third, the distinct greyish violet citronellal zone [In fact, the proportion of citronellal can vary from undetectable to the dominant terpene present.]; near the solvent front and slightly above the Rf of the reference guaiazulene zone, the violet to greyish blue main zone (caryophyllene and other hydrocarbons) [Other apolar lipophilic constituents may affect the colour produced.]; in the lower half of the chromatogram, other, mostly faint, greyish violet or reddish zones [There is no citronellol/-geraniol band detectable in the extract, but one at a slightly lower Rf.].

A TLC separation of the leaf extract into 13 bands, better than that using the DAB 10 (9) procedure, is obtained on double development using the solvent systems: (a) hexane + ethyl acetate (90 + 10), 10 cm run, and (b) hexane + ethyl acetate (95 + 5), 14 cm run; for the detection of the fainter bands, the phosphomolybdic acid spray is rather more sensitive than the anisaldehyde reagent.

It is evident, on comparing the chromatograms of the steam-distilled oil and the extract from the leaves, that the latter contains a series of interfering constituents. Identification of Melissae folium would be better carried out by TLC of the volatile oil [14], though it has to be said that the DAB 10 does not require the oil content to be determined.

Quantitative standards: <u>DAB 10</u>: *Foreign matter*, not more than 3%. *Loss on drying*, not more than 12.0%. *Ash*, not more than 12.0%.
<u>ÖAB</u>: *Volatile oil*, not less than 0.05%. *Foreign matter*, not more than 3%. *Ash*, not more than 12.0%. *Acid-insoluble ash*, not more than 1.0%.
<u>Ph. Helv. VII</u>: *Foreign matter*, not more than 3%; stem fragments, not more than 7%; leaves of *Stachys* and *Ballota* species (see: Adulteration), absent. *Sulphated ash*, not more than 17%.
<u>BHP 1983</u>: *Total ash*, not more than 14%. *Acid-insoluble ash*, not more than 2%.

Adulteration: Happens occasionally. Leaves of *Nepeta cataria* L. var. *citriodora* (BECKER) BALBIS, cat-mint, are softly pubescent on the upper surface and velvety on the lower greyish green surface; they smell more strongly of lemon than do the leaves of balm. The covering trichomes are like those of balm; the glandular trichomes mostly have bicellular heads, though some with a one-celled stalk and four-celled head also occur. The tooth-like conical trichomes characteristic of balm are absent. Leaves of *Stachys* and *Ballota* species have needles of calcium oxalate in the mesophyll and the epidermal cells have a striated cuticle.

Storage: Protected from light and moisture in well-closed (but not plastic) containers. Under normal conditions of storage (room temperature, absence of light), the essential-oil content of the chopped drug can decrease to 30% of the initial amount within three months [12].

Literature:
[1] I. Koch-Heitzmann and W. Schultze, Dtsch. Apoth. Ztg. **124**, 2137 (1984); idem., Z. Phytotherap. **9**, 77 (1988).
[2] Kommentar DAB 10.
[3] Literature reviewing the constituents of balm:
F.W. Hefendehl, Arch. Pharm. (Weinheim) **303**, 345 (1970).
J. Morelli, Boll. Chim. Farm. **116**, 334 (1977).
G. Tittel, H. Wagner, and R. Bos, Planta Med. **46**, 91 (1982).
I. Nykänen, in: J. Adda (ed.) Progress in Flavour Research, Elsevier, Amsterdam, **1984**, p. 329.
A. Mulkens, E. Stephanon, and I. Kapetanidis, Pharm. Acta Helv. **62**, 19 (1987).
[4] W. Schultze, P. Klosa, and A. Zänglein, unpublished data.
[5] Dr. Wolf (Fa. Klosterfrau, Cologne), personal communication.
[6] E. Chabrol et al., Compt. Rend. Soc. Biol. **103**, 3 (1930).
[7] H. Braun and D. Frohne, Heilpflanzenlexikon für Ärzte und Apotheker, G. Fischer, Stuttgart – New York, 1987.
[8] R. Hänsel and H. Haas, Therapie mit Phytopharmaka, Springer, Berlin, 1984.
[9] R.A. Cohen, L.S. Kucera, and E.C. Herrmann, Proc. Soc. Exptl. Biol. Med. **117**, 431, 869 (1967).
R. R. Paris and M. Moyse, Précis de Matière Médicale, Masson, Paris, 1971, vol. **3**.
L.I. Litvinenko, T.P. Popova, A.V. Simonjan, I. G. Zoz, and V. S. Solokov, Planta Med. **27**, 372 (1975).
G. May and G. Willuhn, Arzneimittel.Forsch. **28**, 1 (1978).
[10] S. Aschoff, Z. angew. Phytotherap. **2**, 219 (1981).
[11] H. Sourgens, H. Winterhoff, H.G. Gumbinger, and F.H. Kemper, Planta Med. **45**, 78 (1982).
[12] F.-C. Czygan, unpublished observations (1980).
[13] A. Mulkens and I. Kapetanidis, Pharm. Acta Helv. **63**, 266 (1988).
[14] W. Schultze, A. Zänglein, R. Klosa, and K.-H. Kubeczka, Dtsch. Apoth. Ztg. **129**, 155 (1989).
[15] A. Mulkens and I. Kapetanidis, J. Nat. Prod. **51**, 496 (1988).
[16] R. Soulimani et al., Planta Med. **57**, 105 (1991).

Menthae crispae folium

Spearmint leaf, Spearmint (*USAN*)

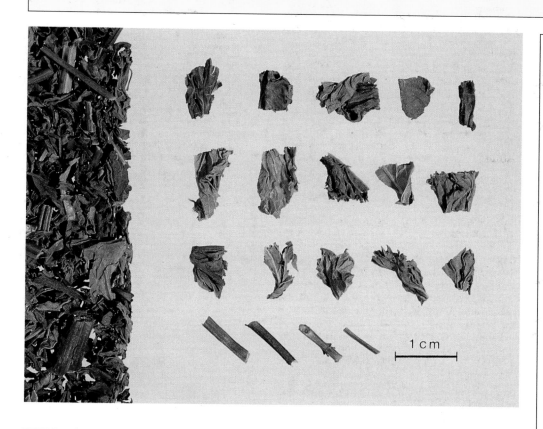

Fig. 1: Spearmint leaf

Description: The material comprises much crumpled, very brittle leaf fragments in which the irregularly and coarsely serrate margin is not always easily recognized (Fig. 3). The upper surface of the leaf is dark green and raised between the nerves, while the lower surface is light greyish green and punctate with scattered glands (hand lens); the pinnate nervature is more prominent on the lower surface. There are occasional pieces of four-angled stem.

Odour: Very spicy and characteristic.

Taste: Spicy, characteristic, not cooling (difference with peppermint).

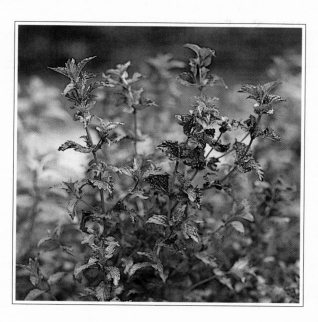

Fig. 2: *Mentha spicata* L. var. *crispa*

A perennial up to 1 m in height, bearing opposite and decussate leaves with a characteristic coarsely serrate and lacerate margin. Whorls of small, pale violet flowers arranged in long spikes.

Erg. B. 6: Folia Menthae crispae

Plant source: *Mentha spicata* L. var. *crispa*, spearmint (Lamiaceae).

Synonyms: Garden, Mackerel, or Green mint (Engl.), Krauseminzblätter (Ger.), Feuilles de menthe crépue (Fr.).

Origin: Almost entirely from cultivation, since in Europe the occurrence of plant is scattered to rare. The drug is imported from Egypt, former Yugoslavia, and Hungary.

Constituents: 0.8–2.5% essential oil containing ca. 50% carvone, as well as dihydrocarveol acetate and other monoterpenes; menthol is absent. The composition of the essential varies considerably according to its origin [1]. Older sources record the occurrence of flavonoids, tannins, and bitter substances, but confirmatory studies are required.

Indications: Spearmint leaf is used, like peppermint leaf, as a stomachic and carminative, but it cannot replace peppermint in combined bile and liver or nerve herbal teas. The essential oil of the drug is recommended for catarrhal complaints, mainly for inhalation. Large amounts of the essential oil are incorporated into mouth washes and toothpastes, as well as into chewing gum.

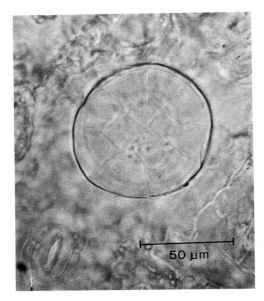

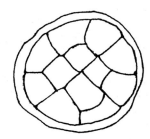

Fig. 4: Head of a peltate glandular trichome from spearmint leaf, with 12 secretory cells (cf. the above drawing)

Making the tea: Boiling water is poured over 1–1.5 g of the drug and left in a covered vessel for about 10 min. before being strained. As a carminative in mild digestive complaints, a cupful of the tea is drunk several times a day.
1 Teaspoon = ca. 0.7%.

Phytomedicines: Spearmint leaf is a component of herbal teas used in *folk medicine* for the most varied conditions; in these mixtures, it functions rather as an aromatic.

Authentication: Macro- (see: Description) and microscopically. The peltate glandular trichomes mostly have 12 secretory cells (Fig. 4) and the thin-walled covering trichomes are one- to six-celled.
For the TLC detection of carvone and menthol, see: Adulteration.

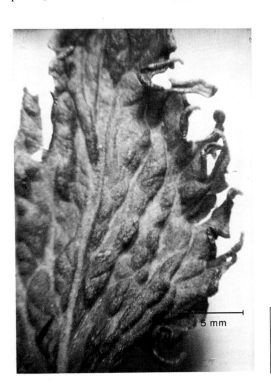

Fig. 3: Leaf fragment, showing the uneven and coarsely serrate margin (hand lens)

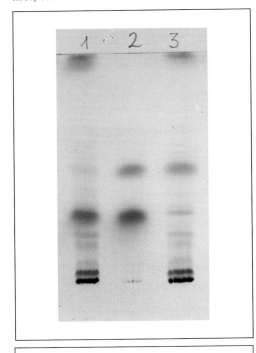

Fig. 5: TLC on 4 × 8 cm silica-gel foil

1: Peppermint leaf
2: Reference solution
3: Spearmint leaf

For details, see the text

Quantitative standard: <u>Erg. B. 6</u>: *Volatile oil,* not less than 1.0%.

Adulteration: Rare. Admixture with peppermint leaf can be determined quite simply by the difference in smell. On TLC examination, a strong menthol spot will be found; the method is as follows:

Test solution: 1 g powdered drug refluxed with 10 ml dichloromethane at 60 °C for 15 min., cooled, and filtered.

Reference solution: 5 mg carvone and 5 mg menthol dissolved in 2 ml toluene.

Loadings: 4 µl test solution and 1 µl reference solution, as bands on silica gel.

Solvent system: toluene + ethyl acetate (97 + 3), 6 cm run.

Detection: after evaporation of the solvent, sprayed with anisaldehyde reagent and heated for ca. 3 min. at 100–105 °C.

Evaluation: in daylight (in UV 366 nm light). <u>Reference solution</u>: menthol at Rf ca. 0.27 as a violet zone (sealing-wax red fluorescence) and carvone at Rf ca. 0.48 as an orange-red zone (dark violet fluorescence). <u>Test solution</u>: spearmint leaf – detection of carvone positive and of menthol negative; peppermint leaf – detection of carvone negative and of menthol positive, and a pinkish red zone at the same Rf as carvone due to limonene.

Storage: Cool, dry, and protected from light, but not in plastic containers.

Literature:
[1] J. Jaskonis and N. Ziviniene, Liet. TSR Mokslu Akad. Darb. Ser. C **1985**, 56; C.A. **103**, 3685 (1985).

Menthae piperitae folium

(DAB 10, Ph. Eur. 2, etc.), Peppermint leaf (*BAN*; BHP 1/1990), Peppermint (*USAN*; USP XXII)

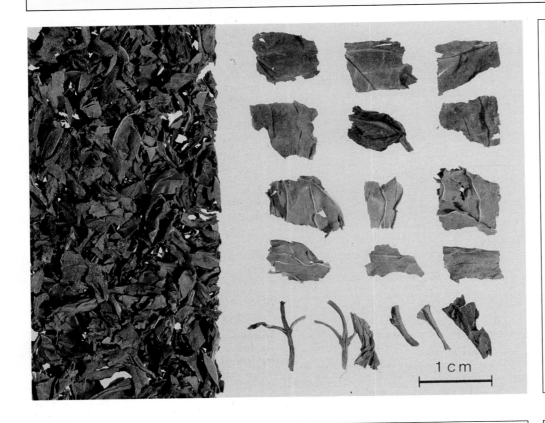

Fig. 1: Peppermint leaf

Description: The drug consists of thin, brittle, ovate to lanceolate leaves, 3–9 cm long, with pinnate, often violet tinged venation (Mitcham variety – the best quality) and a sharply serrate margin. On examination with a hand lens, the glandular trichomes can be seen as yellow dots (Fig. 3).

Odour: Characteristic, very strong.

Taste: Spicy and aromatic, and cooling.

Fig. 2: *Mentha × piperita* L.

A triple hybrid, *Mentha longifolia* × *M. rotundifolia* (= *M. spicata*) × *M. aquatica*, of English origin. A plant, with a distinctly 4-angled stem and decussate leaves, growing to a height of about 60 cm. Pale red flowers in spicate whorls.

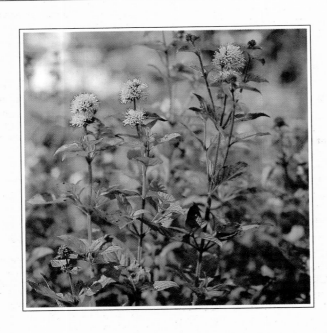

DAB 10: Pfefferminzblätter
ÖAB: Folium Menthae piperitae
Ph. Helv. VII: Menthae piperitae folium
St. Zul. 1499.99.99

Plant source: *Mentha × piperita* L., peppermint (Lamiaceae).

Synonyms: Pfefferminzblätter, Katzenkraut (Ger.), Menthe poivrée, Feuilles de menthe (Fr.).

Origin: Entirely from cultivation (for genetic reasons, only through vegetative multiplication by means of runners (stolons)). Nowadays, exports come mainly from: Bulgaria, Greece, Spain, and a few other Balkan countries; a small amount of the drug is produced in southern Germany. Northern Europe and the USA also export the leaf.

Constituents: 0.5–4% essential oil (menthol and menthol esters [especially the acetate and isovalerianate], menthone, menthofuran, and other monoterpenes, and small amounts of sesquiterpenes). The yield of oil depends on the age of the plants and on the

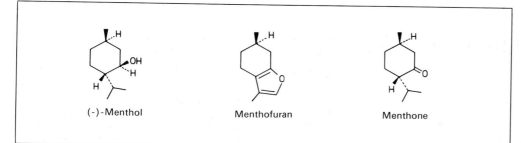

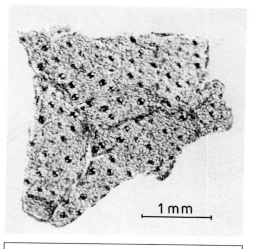

cut – the first cut in the second year tending to give the best yield, which decreases thereafter; the composition of the oil is less affected [5]. Moderate osmotic stress leads to an increase in oil yield with a decrease in biomass; the proportion of menthol/menthone is not affected, but with greater stress the proportion of sesquiterpenes increases somewhat [6]. On the other hand, exposure of plants to a continuing short photoperiod induces in young leaves the oxidative pathway from pulegone to menthofuran rather than the reductive pathway leading to menthone/menthol [7].

Flavonoids, among them a range of free lipophilic aglycones, with *O*-methylation patterns that vary with age and that point to sequential 4′- and 6′-*O*-methylation [8]. Also, 6–12% tannins; triterpenes; bitter substances (?).

Indications: As a spasmolytic, carminative, and cholagogue; mixed with other herbal drugs, also as a sedative. The action is mainly, but not entirely, due to the content of essential oil, the direct action of which on organs with smooth-muscle tissue causes a stronger spasmolysis than some of its individual components [1]. Peppermint tea brings about a considerable increase in the production of bile [2]; the effect is due to the essential oil, but presumably the flavonoids also play a part [3].

Peppermint tea is indicated in acute and chronic gastritis and enteritis, in colicky disorders of the gastrointestinal tract, and in flatulence; and also in chronic cholecystopathies. It is free from of injurious side effects on prolonged use, *provided it is not used to excess* [1, 4]. Reported side effects relate chiefly to peppermint oil and/or its constituents menthol and menthone or to products in which they are significant components of the formulation, e.g. confectionery, menthol cigarettes, peppermint-oil capsules. Peppermint teas usually contain only ca. 25% (ca. 5 mg or less) of the oil present in the drug and thus only small amounts of menthol and menthone [9, 10].

Making the tea: Boiling water is poured over 1.5 g drug, covered, and stood for

5–10 min. before being passed through a tea strainer.
1 Teaspoon = ca. 0.6 g, 1 tablespoon = ca. 1.5 g.

Herbal preparations: The drug is also available as an instant tea (usually a spray-dried extract) and in tea bags (1.3–1.5 g). Note: The contents of peppermint-tea bags when indicated to be of "herbal-tea quality" do not always conform to pharmacopoeial requirements (higher proportion of stem and lower essential-oil content).

Phytomedicines: Peppermint leaf or extracts prepared from it are included in many (ca. 50) prepared cholagogues and bile-duct remedies, e.g. Cholagogum Nattermann® (capsules, drops), etc., gastrointestinal Remedies (ca. 50), e.g. Gastricholan®, Iberogast®, Ventrodigest®, etc.), liver remedies (more than 10), hypnotics/sedatives (more than 10), e.g. Nerventee Stada®, Esberi-Nervin® drops, etc., and laxatives.

Regulatory status (UK): General Sales List – Schedule 1, Table A.

Authentication: Macro- and microscopically, following the Ph. Eur. 2, etc. The characteristic glandular trichomes have 8 secretory cells, with a ballooned cuticle (Fig. 4); the cuticle of the long covering trichomes is striated or warty (Fig. 5); crystals are absent. Leaves attacked by the mint rust, *Puccinia menthae*, must be discarded. The microscopy of the the powdered drug is described and illustrated in [11].

Quantitative standards: Ph. Eur. 2, etc.: *Volatile oil*, not less than 1.2%. *Foreign matter*, not more than 5% stem fragments greater than 1 mm in diameter; not more than 2% other foreign matter; and not more than 10% leaves with brown spots caused by *Puccinia menthae. Water*, not more than 11.0%. *Acid-insoluble ash*, not more than 1.5%.

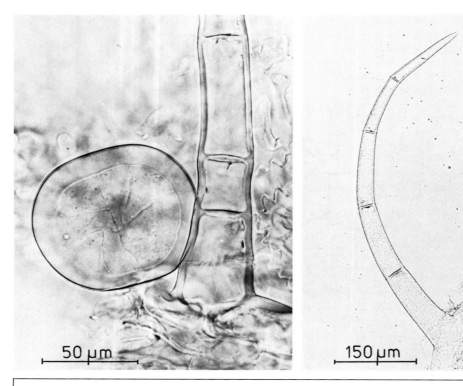

Fig. 4: Lamiaceous (peltate) glandular trichome with 8 secretory cells and the base of a covering trichome

Fig. 5: Large covering trichome with striated cuticle

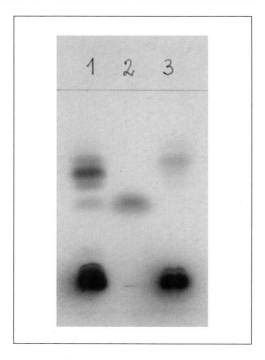

Fig. 6: TLC on 4 × 8 silica-gel foil

1: Peppermint leaf
2: Menthofuran
3: Mentha arvensis var. piperascens

For details, see the text

<u>USP XXII</u>: *Stems and other foreign organic matter*, not more than 2% stems more than 3 mm in diameter and other foreign matter.

Adulteration: Relatively rare, since the drug is derived from cultivated plants; it is necessary to ensure that inadmissable amounts of stem are not present.

In recent times, because of the increasing demand for menthol, leaf material of *Mentha arvensis* L. var. *piperascens* (L.) HOLMES, so-called Japanese mint, has come on to the market. Small amounts of it cannot be detected in Peppermint leaf because of the very similar morphological and anatomical characters. However, the TLC detection of menthofuran, which is present in *M. piperita*, whatever its origin, and which is absent or present only in traces in *M. arvensis*, offers a suitable means of differentiation:

Test solution: oil (+ xylene) carefully collected after the pharmacopoeial determination of the essential-oil content.

Reference solution: 10 mg menthofuran dissolved in 2 ml *n*-hexane.

Loadings: 1 μm test solution and 1 μm reference solution.

Solvent system: *n*-hexane, 5 cm run.

Detection: after evaporation of the solvent, sprayed with anisaldehyde reagent and then heated for ca. 1–2 min. at 100–105 °C.

Evaluation: in daylight. <u>Reference solution</u>: menthofuran as an orange-yellow zone at Rf ca. 0.5. <u>Test solution</u>: besides several violet zones, a more or less comparable orange-yellow zone at about the same Rf as the reference substance – with leaves of *M. arvensis* var. *piperascens*, this zone is absent (Fig. 6).

The Ph. Eur. 2, etc., TLC test of purity examines a dichloromethane extract run in the solvent system: ethyl acetate + toluene (5 + 95), with menthol, cineole, thymol, and menthyl acetate as reference compounds; the chromatogram is evaluated in UV 254 nm light and after being sprayed with anisaldehyde reagent and heated at 100–105 °C for 5–10 min.

Enantioselective capillary GLC of mint oils (and presumably also of oils obtained from the drug) can detect adulteration with racemic menthol and menthyl acetate, which is not otherwise possible with present official methods of analysis [12].

Storage: Cool, dry, and protected from light, but not in plastic containers.

Literature:
[1] K. Dinckler, Pharm. Zentralhalle **77**, 281 (1936).
[2] K. Steinmetzer, Wiener Klin. Wochenschr. **39**, 1418, 1455 (1926).
[3] I.K. Pasechnik, Farmakol. Toksikol. **29**, 735 (1966); C.A. **66**, 54111, cf. 36450 (1967).
[4] W.D. Erdmann, Dtsch. Apoth. Ztg. **83**, 2140 (1958).
[5] D.A. Adamovic et al., Plantes Méd. Phytothérap. **23**, 6 (1989).
[6] D.J. Charles, R.J. Joly, and J.E. Simon, Phytochemistry **29**, 2837 (1990).
[7] B. Voirin, N. Brun, and C. Bayet, Phytochemistry **29**, 749 (1990).
[8] B. Voirin and C. Bayet, Phytochemistry **31**, 2299 (1992).
[9] H. Miething and W. Holz, Pharm. Ztg. **133**, 16 (1988).
[10] I.H. Bowen and I.J. Cubbin, in P.A.G. M. de Smet, K. Keller, R. Hänsel, and R.F. Chandler (eds.) Adverse effects of herbal drugs, Springer, Berlin, Heidelberg, New York, 1992, vol. **1**, p. 171.
[11] B.P. Jackson and D.W. Snowdon, Atlas of microscopy of medicinal plants, culinary herbs and spices, Belhaven Press, London, 1990, p. 178.
[12] C. Askari et al., Arch. Pharm. (Weinheim) **325**, 35 (1992).

Menyanthidis folium   Bogbean (BHP 1/1990)

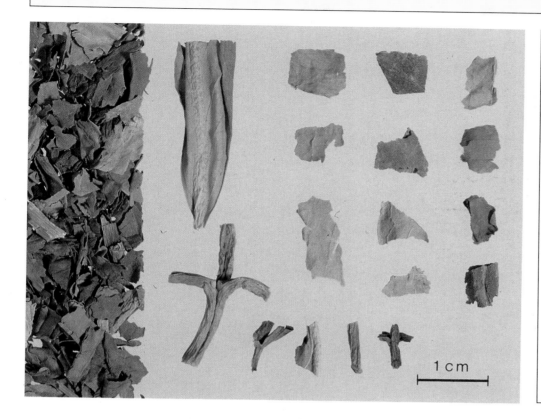

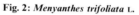
1 cm

Fig. 1: Bogbean

<u>Description</u>: The leaves are ternate ("trefoil"), with a ca. 10 cm long petiole, and the individual leaflets are 5–10 cm long, elliptic, glabrous, and with an entire margin. The leaf fragments of the cut drug are greyish green, partly with the shrivelled, brownish nerves; because on drying the aerenchyma shrivels more, the fragments of the thicker petiole are wrinkled and longitudinally grooved. Very occasionally, petiole fragments with the three points where the leaflets were attached are recognizable.

<u>Taste</u>: Very bitter.

Fig. 2: *Menyanthes trifoliata* L.

A perennial marsh plant, up to 30 cm in height, with ternate leaves. Flowers white, petals bearded on the inside.

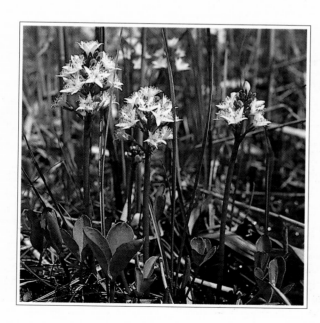

DAC 1986: Bitterkleeblätter
ÖAB: Folium Menyanthis

Plant source: *Menyanthes trifoliata* L., bogbean (Menyanthaceae).

Synonyms: Trifolii Fibrini folium, Folia Trifolii aquatici (Lat.), Bogbean or Buckbean or Marsh trefoil leaf (Engl.), Fieberkleeblätter (Ger.), Feuilles de menyanthe, Feuilles des trèfle des marais (Fr.).

Origin: Damp localities in the northern temperate zone. The drug is imported from the former USSR, Poland, former Yugoslavia, and Hungary.

Constituents: The bitter substances stated to be present are the secoiridoid glycosides dihydrofoliamenthin, menthiafolin, and loganin [1]; according to more recent studies (1988), however, foliamenthin is absent from the leaves, though present in the rhizomes [literature in 1]. The monoterpenoid alkaloids gentianine and gentianidine are possibly artefacts arising during the isolation procedure. Also present are: small amounts

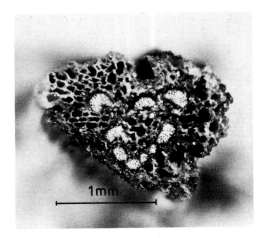

Fig. 3: Transverse surface of the leaf petiole, showing the whitish vascular bundles and spongy aerenchyma

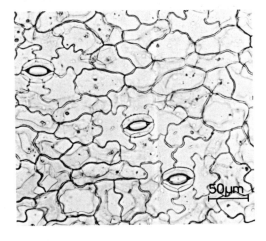

Fig. 4: Stomata on the lower surface of *Menyanthes trifoliata* leaf

cholagogic effects and scopoletin also has a spasmolytic action on the alimentary system [7].

Making the tea: Boiling water is poured over 0.5–1 g of the finely chopped drug or cold water is added to the drug and boiled for a short period; after 5–10 min., the liquid it is passed through a tea strainer. Soaking the drug in water at room temperature for several hours has also been recommended. An unsweetened cupful is taken $^{1}/_{2}$ hour before meals.
1 Teaspoon = ca. 0.9 g.

Herbal preparations: Bogbean is a component of some prepared herbal mixtures for a range of different indications.

Phytomedicines: The drug is present in several cholagogues, e.g. Gallexier®, etc., as well as geriatric remedies, e.g. Vitasana®-Lebenstropfen, etc.
In the UK, bogbean is present in over 30 anti-inflammatory (antirheumatic) preparations [8], e.g. Potter's Rheumatic Pain Tablets, etc.

of tannins; flavonoids [2]; triterpenes, including the betulinic acid derivative menyanthoside, the main saponin of the rhizomes [6]; coumarins – those isolated from the aerial parts include scoparone, braylin, and scopoletin [3, 7]; loliolide, a degradation product of xanthophyll [7]; phenol-carboxylic acids [4]; as well as ubiquitous substances.

Indications: Like Gentianae radix (gentian root) or Centaurii herba (centaury herb), the drug is used as a bitter to stimulate the appetite and the secretion of gastric juice.
Former indications for the use of this and other bitter drugs against fevers are obsolete, since there is no antipyretic activity. Scoparone and scopoletin have been shown to have antihepatotoxic, choleretic, and

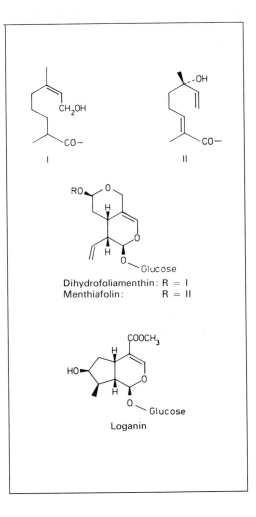

Dihydrofoliamenthin: R = I
Menthiafolin: R = II

Loganin

Extract from the German Commission E monograph
(*BAnz no. 22a, dated 01.02.90*)

Uses
Lack of appetite. Dyspeptic complaints.

Contraindications
None known.

Side effects
None known.

Interactions with other remedies
None known.

Dosage
Unless otherwise prescribed: daily dose, 1.5–3 g drug; preparations with an equivalent bitterness value.

Mode of administration
Chopped drug for infusions and other bitter-tasting preparations for internal use.

Effects
Stimulates the secretion of gastric juice and saliva.

Regulatory status (UK): General Sales List – Schedule 1, Table A.

Authentication: Macro- (see: Description) and microscopically. Apart from fine cuticular striations and the characteristic aerenchyma (in both the lamina and petiole of the leaf), there are few conspicuous features (Figs. 3 and 4). See also the BHP 1/1990.

The TLC identification and test for purity can be carried out as follows [5]:

Test solution: 1 g powdered drug extracted with 10 ml methanol at 60 °C for 10 min., filtered, and the filtrate concentrated to 2 ml.

Reference solution: 1% methanolic neohesperidin.

Loadings: 40 µl test solution and 20 µl reference solution, as bands on silica gel 60F$_{254}$.

Solvent system: ethyl acetate + methanol + water (77 + 15 + 8), 15 cm run.

Detection: sprayed with 5% ethanolic sulphuric acid, followed immediately by 1% ethanolic vanillin, then heated at 110 °C for 5–10 min. while under observation.

Evaluation: in daylight. Reference solution: a reddish orange zone at Rf ca. 0.5. Test solution: a dark blue zone at Rf ca. 0.6 and two dark blue zones in the Rf range 0.8–0.85, these latter corresponding to menthiafolin and dihydrofoliamenthin; also, dark blue zones below the solvent front (essential oils and aromatic acids) and black or brown zones above the starting line (partly due to sugars). The BHP 1/1990 TLC procedure yields a fingerprint chromatogram: ethyl acetate + anhydrous formic acid + glacial acetic acid + water (100 + 11 + 11 + 27) and then spraying with 1% methanolic diphenylboryloxyethylamine and 5% ethanolic polyethylene glycol 400.

Evaluation: in UV 366 nm light. Test solution: relative to rutin, fluorescent bands at Rx 1.5 (pale blue), 1.3 (orange), 1.2 (yellowish white), 1.0 (orange), 0.85 (pale blue).

Quantitative standards: DAC 1986: *Bitterness value*, not less than 3000. *Extractive*, not less than 35.0%. *Foreign (vegetable and mineral) matter*, not more than 2%. *Loss on drying*, not more than 10.0%. *Ash*, not more than 10.0%.

ÖAB: *Bitterness value*, not less than 4000. *Foreign matter*, not more than 2%. *Ash*, not more than 10.0%.

BHP 1/1990: *Water-soluble extractive*, not less than 23%. *Foreign matter*, not more than 2%. *Total ash*, not more than 10%. *HCl-insoluble ash*, not more than 2%.

Adulteration: Rare.

Literature:

[1] P. Junior, Planta Med. **55**, 83 (1989).

[2] P. Lebreton and M.P. Dangy-Caye, Plantes Méd. Phytothérap. **7**, 87 (1973).

[3] G. Ciaceri, Fitoterapia **43**, 134 (1972).

[4] L. Swiatek, C. Adamczyk, and R. Zadernowski, Planta Med. **52**, 530 (1986).

[5] H. Wagner, S. Bladt, and E.M. Zgainski, Plant drug analysis, Springer-Verlag, Berlin, Heidelberg, New York, Tokyo, 1984, p. 132.

[6] Z. Janeczko, J. Sendra, K. Kmiec, and C.H. Brieskorn, Phytochemistry **29**, 3885 (1990).

[7] U. Adamczyk, S.A. Brown, E.G. Lewars, and L. Swiatek, Pl. Méd. Phytothérap. **24**, 73 (1990).

[8] J.D. Phillipson and L.A. Anderson, Pharm. J. **232**, 80, 111 (1984).

Millefolii herba   (DAB 10), Yarrow (BHP 1/1990)

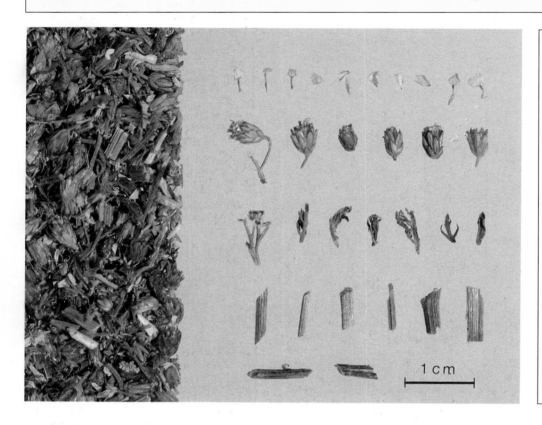

Fig. 1: Yarrow

<u>Description</u>: The elliptical flower-heads (in the Ph. Helv. VII, a separate drug) are ca. 3 mm broad and 5 mm long; and on the outside they have imbricately arranged and scarious-margined involucral bracts; they have 4–5 white or reddish ray (ligulate) florets, 3–20 disk (tubular) florets, and many narrow scarious bracts on the domed receptacle. The leaves are several times pinnately divided, so that the lamina consists mainly of thread-like or thin segments. The longitudinally ridged stem has a pith and is more or less covered with matted hairs.

<u>Odour</u>: Aromatic, but not very strong.

<u>Taste</u>: Somewhat bitter and faintly aromatic.

Fig. 2: *Achillea millefolium* L.

A widely distributed herbaceous plant, up to 70 cm in height, with characteristic narrow, oblong, several times pinnately divided leaves; small flower-heads comprising ca. five white or pink ligulate florets and a few yellow tubular florets, arranged in umbel-like panicles.

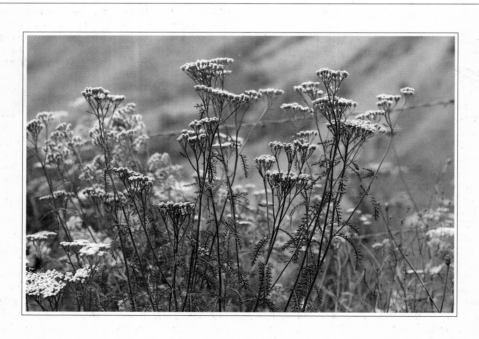

DAB 10: Schafgarbenkraut
ÖAB: Herba Millefolii
Ph. Helv. VII: Millefolii flos
St. Zul. 1249.99.99

Plant source: *Achillea millefolium* L., s.l., yarrow (Asteraceae).

Synonyms: Achillea, Millefolium, Milfoil, Nosebleed (Engl.), Schafgarbenkraut, Achilleskraut, Bauchwehkraut, Katzenkraut, Jungfraukraut (Ger.), Herbe de millefeuille, Herbe au charpentier (Fr.).

Origin: A cytogenetic and chemically polymorphic aggregate species native in Europe, northern Asia, and North America. Depending on the monographer, various species, subspecies, or even microspecies are recognized and named [1–3]; besides *Achillea millefolium* L. s.s., among those in Europe worth mentioning are: *A. setacea* WALDST. et KIT., *A. distans* WALDST. et KIT., and *A. collina* BECKER, *A. pannonica* SCHEELE, and *A. aspleniifolia* VENT. The main suppliers are south-eastern and eastern European countries. It is also obtained from the UK.

Achillicin

Leukodin

Millefin

Pontica epoxide

$H_3C-(C\equiv C)_3-CH=CH-CH-CH-CH=CH_2$

$H_3C-(C\equiv C)_3-CH=CH-C-O-CH_3$

Matricaria ester

Constituents: 0.2 to more than 1% essential oil, which, depending on the origin, may contain no or up to 50% chamazulene; the leaves are less rich than the flower-heads [11].

There is a correlation between the presence of prochamazulene and the chromosome number. As a rule, only tetraploid plants contain prochamazulene, while most other karyotypes are azulene-free [3]. The oil distilled from an octaploid had ca. 80% oxygen-containing monoterpenes, principally linalool; that from a hexaploid comprised ca. 50% mono- and sesquiterpene hydrocarbons, ca. 40% oxidized mono- and sesquiterpenes, and **no** chamazulene; and the oil from the tetraploid consisted of almost 90% mono- and especially sesquiterpene hydrocarbons and had the highest chamazulene content [12]. As many as 82 components of the essential oils have been identified [12]. In azulene-free oil, 24 identified components make up ca. 95% of the oil, the main ones being camphor (18%), sabinene (12%), 1,8-cineole (10%), α-pinene (9%), and isoartemisiaketone (9%) [4]. In azulene-containing oil, along with chamazulene (25%), β-pinene (23%), caryophyllene (10%), and α-pinene (5%), there are the other main components [5]. Achillicin (= 8-acetoxyartabsin) has been identified as one of the pro-azulenes. The sesquiterpene lactone matricin, often cited in the literature (see: Matricariae flos – Matricaria flower), has not been found. Those present include: the guaianolides 2,3-dehydrodesacetoxy- and desacetylmatricin and leukodin, the 3-oxaguaianolides 8-acetyl- and 8-angeloylegelolide [13], the germacranolides

millefin, balchanolide acetate, dihydroparthenolide [14], etc.; see also: Side effects. Polyynes: pontica epoxide, as well as *cis*- and *trans*-matricaria ester. Flavonoids: apigenin and luteolin and their 7-*O*-glucosides, and also glycosylflavones [6, 14], especially swertisin, vicenin-2 and -3, schaftoside, and isoschaftoside, etc. Phenolic acids. Triterpenes and sterols [14]; *N*-containing compounds: a range of alkamides in the subterranean parts [15], achillein (= betonicin), stachydrine, choline, glycine betaine, and the cyanogenic glycoside prunasin. Ca. 0.35% coumarins. Ca. 3–4% tannins.

Indications: Internal and external use of this drug is very similar to that of Matricariae flos (q.v.): frequent use as an antiphlogistic, spasmolytic, stomachic, carminative, and cholagogue. The main applications are in gastrointestinal complaints (inflammation, diarrhoea, flatulence, cramps). In addition, it is also employed as a bitter aromatic (for loss of appetite) and to stimulate the secretion of bile; the choleretic acitvity has been confirmed in animal experiments [7]. As with Matricariae flos, the activity may result from the interaction of compounds of different structural types, being similar and in part identical in the two drugs, e.g. chamazulene, flavonoids.

Externally, in the form of poultices, lotions, and baths, but mostly in the form of preparations with alcohol (percolates, fluid extracts), for inflammation of the skin and mucous membranes, as well as for healing wounds. Aqueous and ether extracts have antimicrobial activity against a range of bacteria [8]. A protein-carbohydrate com-

plex has been isolated from the aqueous extract, which, in animal experiments had systemic (40 mg/kg) and topical antiphlogistic activity not involving counter-irritation [9]. The sesquiterpene lactones may also take part in the antiseptic and antiphlogistic action (see: Arnicae flos and Matricariae flos). In *folk medicine*, the drug is often employed as a haemostyptic, e.g. in bleeding from haemorrhoids, and in problems of menstruation and to remove perspiration (baths).

Side effects: With allergies to Asteraceae, itching and inflammatory changes in the skin with the formation of vesicles (yarrow dermatitis) may occur, in which case the treatment must be stopped immediately. One of two recently isolated guaianolide peroxides, α-peroxy-achifolide, is believed to be responsible for the allergic contact dermatitis [16]. Like some of the other sesquiterpene lactones present, this substance contains an α-methylene-γ-lactone group, which is also essential for the antiphlogistic activity of these compounds.

Making the tea: Boiling water is poured over 2.0 g of the finely chopped drug, covered, allowed to stand for 10 min., and then passed through a tea strainer.
1 Teaspoon = ca. 1.5 g.

Herbal preparations: The drug is also available in tea bags (1.25 g or 2.0 g). Among such UK products is Potter's Wellwoman Herbs.

Phytomedicines: The drug or extracts prepared from it are a component of numerous prepared remedies, mainly cholagogues and biliary remedies, as well as powdered tea extract and tea paste, gastrointestinal remedies, etc. The drug is also an adjuvant in preparations for many other indications, such as antitussives and expectorants, antiphlebitis and varicose-vein remedies, etc., and in wound-healing ointments.
Among the products available in the UK containing the herb and/or extracts of it are: Seven Seas Rheumatic Pain Tablets, Seven Seas Catarrh Tablets, Potter's Rheumatic Pain Tablets, Potter's Tabritis Tablets, and Potter's Wellwoman Tablets. See also [17].

Regulatory status (UK): General Sales List – Schedule 1, Table A.

Authentication: Macro- (see: Description) and microscopically, following the DAC 1986; see also the BHP 1/1990, which includes the detailed microscopy of the powdered drug. The covering trichomes of the leaves (Fig. 3) are particularly diagnostic; they consist of a uniseriate, 4–6-celled stalk and a long, thick-walled, often somewhat tortuous terminal cell (Fig. 4).

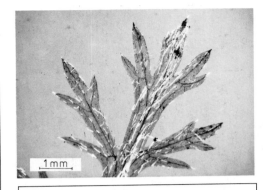

Fig. 3: Part of a pinnately divided *Achillea millefolium* leaf, showing the matted pubescence (in polarized light)

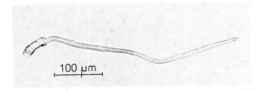

Fig. 4: Trichome with 4(-6) short basal cells and a very long, thick-walled, terminal cell

BHP 1/1990: *Water-soluble extractive*, not less than 15%. *Foreign matter*, not more than 2%. *Total ash*, not more than 10%. *HCl-insoluble ash*, not more than 2.5%.

Adulteration: In practice does not occur.

Storage: Protected from light and moisture, but not in plastic containers.

The DAC 1986 test for pro-azulenes is as follows: 1 g powdered drug is shaken for 2 min. with 10 ml chloroform; the filtrate is concentrated on the water-bath to 1 ml and, after addition of 5 ml 4-dimethyl-aminobenaldehyde reagent (0.25 g dissolved in a mixture of 50 g glacial acetic acid, 5 g phosphoric acid, and 45 g water), heated on the water-bath for 5 min.; after cooling, the solution is shaken out with 10 ml light petroleum: the lower phase should be distinctly blue in colour.

A qualitative estimate of the chamazulene content in as little as 100 mg of the flowers can be obtained by moistening them with a few drops of 1% sulphuric acid, followed by sublimation at 150 °C *in vacuo*; material poor in azulene furnishes a reddish rather than intense blue to blue-green sublimate; capillary GC of the sublimate allows quantitation [18].

The DAC 1986 TLC method of identification is as follows:

Test solution: the oil/xylene from the determination of the volatile oil content.

Reference solutions: 10 mg caryophyllene and 4 mg guaiazulene, each in 10 ml methanol.

Loadings: 30 µl of each, as bands.

Solvent system: toluene + ethyl acetate (95 + 5), 15 cm run.

Detection: sprayed with anisaldehyde reagent, followed by heating at 100–105 °C.

Evaluation: Reference and Test solutions: each two zones with the same Rf and colour; in the upper one-third, each a zone with the same Rf. Test solution: further coloured zones, the number and colour varying according to the source of the drug. An illustration of the chromatogram is to be found in [10].

Quantitative standards: DAB 10: *Volatile oil*, not less than 0.2%. with not less than 0.02% azulene. *Bitterness value*, not less than 5000. *Foreign matter*, not more than 5% stems and not more than 2% other foreign matter. *Loss on drying*, not more than 10%. *Total Ash*, not more than 10%. *HCl-insoluble ash*, not more than 1.0%.
ÖAB: *Volatile oil*, not less than 0.3%. *Foreign matter*, not more than 2%. *Ash*, not more than 8.0%.
Ph. Helv. VII: *Volatile oil*, not less than 0.20%. *Foreign matter*, not more than 3% and peduncles of inflorescences not more than 10%. *Sulphated ash*, not more than 10%.

Literature:
[1] F. Ehrendorfer, Österr. Bot. Z. **122**, 133 (1973); idem., Ber. Dtsch. Bot. Ges. **75**, 137 (1962).
[2] K.M. Valant-Vetschera, Thesis, University of Vienna, 1981.
[3] U. Kastner et al., Sci. Pharm. **60**, 87 (1992); **61**, 47 (1993).
[4] A.J. Falk, L. Bauer, and C.L. Bell, Lloydia **37**, 598 (1974).
[5] M.Y. Haggag, A.S. Shal'aby, and G. Verzar-Petri, Planta Med. **27**, 361 (1975).
[6] K.M. Valant-Vetschera, Sci. Pharm. **52**, 307 (1984); idem., Biochem. Syst. Ecol. **13**, 15, 119 (1985).
[7] E. Chabrod et al., C. R. Soc. Biol. **108**, 1100 (1931).
[8] G. Orzechowski, Pharmazie in unserer Zeit **1**, 43 (1972).
[9] A.S. Goldberg et al., J. Pharm. Sci. **58**, 938 (1972).
[10] P. Pachaly, Dünnschichtchromatographie in der Apotheke, 2nd ed., Wissenschaftliche Verlagsgesellschaft, Stuttgart, 1983.
[11] A.P. Carnat and J.L. Lamaison, Plantes Méd. Phytothérap. **24**, 238 (1990).
[12] L. Hoffmann et al., Phytochemistry **31**, 537 (1992).
[13] G. Ochir et al., Phytochemistry **30**, 4163 (1991).
[14] A. Ulubelen, S. Söksüz, and A. Schuster, Phytochemistry **29**, 3948 (1990).
[15] H. Greger and O. Hofer, Phytochemistry **28**, 2363 (1989).
[16] G. Rücker, D. Manns and J. Breuer, Arch. Pharm. (Weinheim) **324**, 979 (1991).
[17] J.D. Phillipson and L.A. Anderson, Pharm. J. **233**, 80, 111 (1984).
[18] E. Saberi, Sci. Pharm. **58**, 317 (1990).

Myrrha   (DAB 10), Myrrh (BHP 1/1990; BHC)

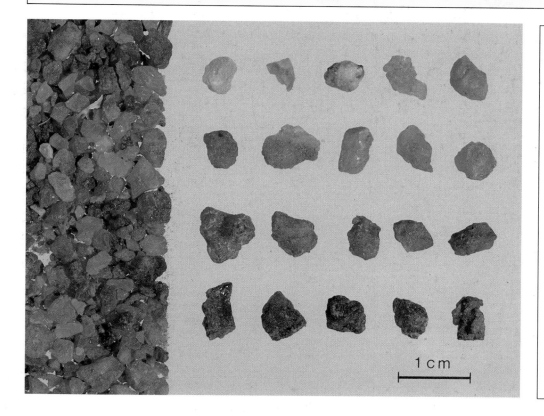

Fig. 1: Myrrh

Description: Myrrh is the air-dried oleo-gum resin that exudes from the bark of *Commiphora* species. The material comprises irregular, rounded grains or lumps of varying sizes with holes and ranging in colour from dark brown and almost black to light or dark orange-brown; some parts may be yellow or colourless to pale yellow. The surface is mostly covered with a grey to yellowish grey powder; the fracture is conchoidal and yields thin, translucent fragments.

Odour: Harsh and aromatic.

Taste: Bitter and aromatic, acrid; sticks to the teeth on chewing.

Fig. 2: *Commiphora erythraea* (EHRENB.) ENGL.

The myrrh-producing *Commiphora* species are shrubs or small trees with large, sharply pointed thorns on the stem. The unequal ternate leaves are alternate and the small flowers are arranged in terminal panicles. When damaged, the schizogenous resin ducts yield the drug myrrh.

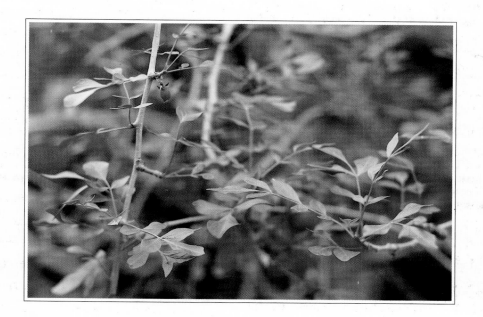

DAB 10: Myrrhe
ÖAB, Ph. Helv. VII: Myrrha

Plant sources: *C. molmol* ENGL. and other *Commiphora* species, insofar as the chemical composition of their gum-resin is comparable with that of Myrrha DAB 10 (Burseraceae).

There is considerable confusion in the literature regarding the sources of myrrh and the identity (synonymy) of the *Commiphora* species involved. The following remarks are based on the reviews by Tucker [6] and Martinetz et al. [7]. Common (or hirabol) myrrh appears to derive from *C. myrrha* (NEES) ENGL. Somalian myrrh is said to come from *C. molmol* ENGL. ex TSCHIRCH. However, the systematic (taxonomic) relationship between *C. myrrha* and *C. molmol* is not clear. The source of Abyssinian myrrh is *C. madagascariensis* JACQ. (syn. *C. abyssinica* (BERG) ENGL.).

Opopanax (= bisabol myrrh = perfumed bdellium) is stated to originate from either *C. erythraea* (EHRENB.) ENGL. or *Opopanax*

Curzerenone
(Furanoeudesmane type)

4,5-Dihydrofuranodien-6-one   2-Methoxyfuranodiene
(Furanoelemene type)

Lindestrene
(Furanogermacrane type)

Elemol

chironium KOCH. Products from many other *Commiphora* species are probably occasionally passed off as myrrh or bdellium.

Synonyms: Gummi myrrha, Myrrha vera (Lat.), Gum myrrh, Commiphora resin, Guggal gum or resin, Heerabol myrrh. (Engl.), Myrrhe, Männliche Myrrhe (Weibliche Myrrhe = Opopanax) (Ger.), Myrrhe (Fr.).

Origin: Native in Erythrea, Abyssinia, Somalia, Yemen, Sudan; and imported from these countries; various commercial varieties are distinguished, among them Somali, Yemen, and Hirabol myrrh [1, 6, 7].

Constituents: The composition is very complex and only partially known. 40–60% is soluble in ethanol and comprises a very inadequately known resin and an essential oil which has been studied in some detail [2] and found to consist (almost) entirely of sesquiterpenes. The main components are furanosesquiterpenes of the germacrane, elemane, eudesmane, and guaiane types. In addition, there are sesquiterpene hydrocarbons, e.g. β- and δ-elemene, β-bourbonene, β-caryophyllene, humulene, and sesquiterpene alcohols, e.g. elemol. Presumably, some of the furanosesquiterpenes are characteristic of pharmaceutical myrrh. 50–60% is insoluble in ethanol (= crude gum or crude mucilage) and includes 20% proteins and 65% carbohydrates which are made up of galactose, 4-O-methylglucuronic acid, and arabinose [1, 3].

Indications: Myrrh, mostly as tincture of myrrh (DAB 10, but see also the Standard Licence), is employed because of its disinfecting, deodorizing, and granulation-promoting actions in inflammatory conditions of the mouth and throat, as a paint, gargle, and rinse (especially in dentistry). Myrrh,

however, is not astringent [4]. There is no local precipitation of protein and hence no formation of a more or less surface layer of coagulated cells which provide a protective layer against chemical, bacterial, or mechanical action. The action of myrrh is not traceable to a local stimulant effect of particular constituents in the essential oil of myrrh, since tincture of myrrh is more likely to have an anti-inflammatory effect [cited from 4].

In *folk medicine*, the drug is sometimes also used internally as a carminative and expec-

torant. Alcoholic extracts are employed as fixatives in the perfumery industry.

Making the tea: Not applicable. The drug is almost always used in the form of the tincture (St. Zul. 6699.99.99 – Tincture of Myrrh) which is prepared by macerating 1 part myrrh with 5 parts 90% ethanol (DAB 10, ÖAB, Ph. Helv. VII).
Myrrh is also a component of the so-called "Swedish bitters" (see note under: Aloe capensis).

Phytomedicines: A series of preparations which include either tincture of myrrh DAB 10 or combinations with essential oil-containing drugs, e.g. Salviae folium (Salvia leaf), or tannins, e.g. Tormentillae rhizoma (Tormentil root), in the form of dental remedies and mouth washes, ointments, paints, and dragees.

Regulatory status (UK): General Sale List – Schedule 1, Table A.

Authentication: Macro- (see: Description) and microscopically. The brownish yellow powder is characterized by yellowish splinters or spherical grains of various sizes, along with fine granular material which swells in water. In chloral-hydrate mounts, there are only a few fragments of tissue from the plant source: reddish brown fragments of cork, individual and groups of polyhedral to oblong stone cells, partly with greatly thickened, pitted, and lignified walls and brownish contents; fragments of thin-walled parenchyma and sclerenchymatous fibres, and 10–25 μm irregular prismatic to polyhedral crystals of calcium oxalate.
The DAB 10 TLC proof of identity is as follows:

Test solution: 0.1 g powdered drug warmed on the water-bath for 2–3 min. with 1.0 ml 96% ethanol.

Reference solution: 5 mg each of Dimethyl Yellow, Indophenol Blue, and Sudan Red G dissolved in 10 ml dichloromethane.

Loadings: 10 μl of each solution, as 2-cm bands on silica gel G or H.

Solvent system: dichloromethane, 10 cm run.

Detection: sprayed with anisaldehyde reagent, followed by heating at 100–105 °C for 10 min.

Evaluation: Test solution: uppermost zone (furanoeudesma-1,3-diene) reddish violet, larger and more intense than zones lower down; directly below it, possibly a fainter and similarly coloured zone; at about the same Rf as the Sudan Red G reference zone,

---

Extract from the German Commission E monograph
(BAnz no. 193, dated 15.10.1987)

Uses
Topical treatment of mild inflammatory conditions of the mucous membranes of the mouth and throat.

Contraindications
None known.

Side effects
None known.

Interactions with other remedies
None known.

Dosage
Unless otherwise prescribed, tincture of myrrh: dab the affected area two to three times a day with the undiluted tincture or rinse or gargle with 5–10 drops in a glass of water.
In tooth powders, corresponding to 10% powdered drug.

Mode of administration
Powdered drug, tincture of myrrh, and other galenical preparations for topical use.

Effect
Astringent.

two further intense reddish violet zones, the upper one belonging to curzerenone and the lower one to 2-methoxyfuranodiene; usually, above the uppermost zone, a smaller bluish coloured zone; in the lower (Indophenol Blue) and upper (Dimethyl Yellow) parts, further less distinct zones; in the lower part, no intense blue zones may be present. The BHP 1/1990 also has a TLC identification procedure.

The ÖAB (cf. the BHP 1/1990) has the following test for sesquiterpenes: 0.5 g powdered myrrh is vigorously shaken with 10 ml ether for 10 min. and then filtered. After evaporation of the solvent, bromine vapour blown over the residue should only colour it deep violet to reddish violet; failure of this reaction indicates old or non-pharmacopoeial quality myrrh. Another identification test given in the ÖAB is the following: if 1 ml 6N sulphuric acid is poured over ca. 0.1 g powdered myrrh and a crystal of vanillin is then added, the liquid should turn red; the colour remains even after dilution with water. The furanosesquiterpenes characteristic of pharmacopoeial myrrh can also be detected with the following colour reaction [5]: treatment with a 1% solution of *p*-dimethylaminobenzaldehyde in 1N hydrochloric acid affords a reddish violet colour.

Quantitative standards: <u>DAB 10</u>: *Foreign (vegetable and/or mineral) matter*, not more than 2%. 96% *Ethanol-insoluble matter*, not more than 65%. *Loss on drying*, not more than 15%. *Ash*, not more than 7.0%.
<u>ÖAB</u>: *Acid value*, 19.5–22.0. *Alcohol-insoluble matter*, not more than 65% and the residue must be almost completely soluble in water giving a cloudy mucilage. *Ash*, not more than 8.0%.
<u>Ph. Helv. VII</u>: *Alcohol-insoluble matter*, not more than 70%. *Sulphated ash*, not more than 15%.

<u>BHP 1/1990</u>: 90% *Ethanol-insoluble residue*, not more than 70%. *Volatile oil*, not less than 6%. *Foreign matter*, not more than 4%. *Total ash*, not more than 9%. *HCl-insoluble ash*, not more than 5%.

Adulteration: DAB 10 quality is difficult to find commercially. Usually, large amounts of insoluble material, e.g. gum arabic, are present.
False myrrh (= bdellium resin) from *Commiphora mukul* (HOOK.) ENGL., must be considered an adulterant. It can, however, be distinguished by TLC (q.v.) from genuine myrrh [3].

Storage: Protected from light and moisture in well-closed containers; best with a desiccant, since the carbohydrate part of the drug readily absorbs water; not to be stored in powdered form.

Literature:
[1] K. Lohs and D. Martinetz, Naturwiss. Rundschau **38**, 503 (1985).
[2] C.H. Brieskorn and P. Noble, Phytochemistry **22**, 187, 1207; idem., Planta Med. **44**, 87 (1982); idem., Tetrahedron Lett. 1511 (1980).
[3] Kommentar DAB 10.
[4] R. Hänsel, Pharmazeutische Biologie (Spezieller Teil), Springer, Berlin, 190.
[5] A.R. Pinder, in: L. Zechmeister, Fortschr. Chem. Org. Naturstoffe **34**, 81 (1977).
[6] A.O. Tucker, Econ. bot. **40**, 425 (1986).
[7] D. Martinetz, K. Lohs, and J. Janzen, Weihrauch und Myrrhe, Wissenschaftliche Verlagsgesellschaft, Stuttgart, 1988.

Myrtilli folium   Bilberry leaf

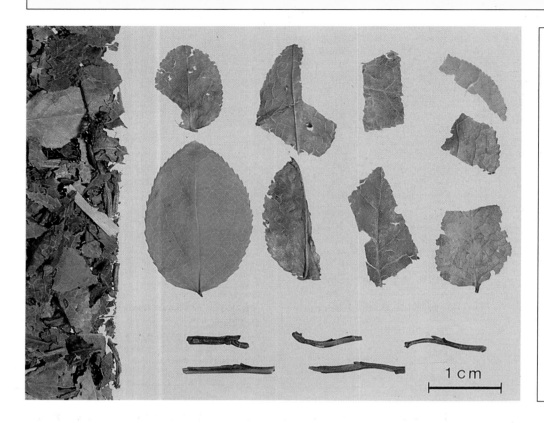

Fig. 1: Bilberry leaf

<u>Description:</u> The drug consists of small, 2–3 cm long, ovate, short-petioled small leaves which are thin to rough and stiff, depending on their age. The margin is crenate-serrate and at the end of each serration there is a stalked gland (Fig. 3); the venation is inconspicuous. The drug is odourless.

<u>Taste:</u> Faintly bitter and astringent.

Fig. 2: *Vaccinium myrtillus* L.

A deciduous dwarf shrub, 20–50 cm in height, with ovate, short-petioled leaves and pale red to greenish, axillary flowers.

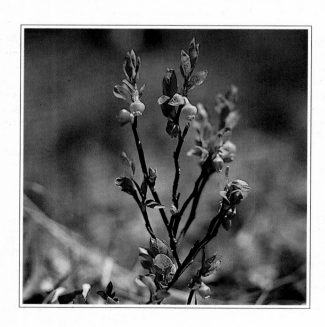

Erg. B. 6: Folia Myrtilli

Plant source: *Vaccinium myrtillus* L., bilberry (Ericaceae).

Synonyms: Myrtillus (Lat.), Blueberry, Whortleberry, Huckleberry or Hurtleberry leaf (Engl.), Heidelbeerblätter, Blaubeerblätter (Ger.), Feuilles de myrtille (Fr.).

Origin: Northern and Central Europe; imports of the drug also come from south-eastern Europe (the former USSR, Albania, former Yugoslavia).

Constituents: Catechol tannins, according to recent data 0.8–6.7% [1], leucoanthocyans [2], flavonoids (mostly glycosides of quercetin), phenol-carboxylic acids, and iridoids [3]. Arbutin and hydroquinone, mentioned in the older literature as constituents, are present only in traces or are absent altogether [3, 4]; see further: Adulteration. There are no new studies on the "glucokinin" neomyrtillin, said to be a methoxylated glucoside of gallic acid [5]. The manganese content of the drug is said to be high

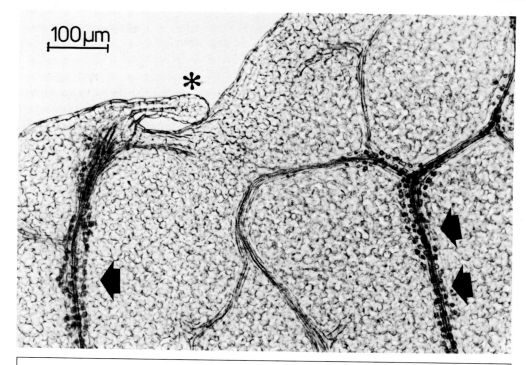

Fig. 3: *Vaccinium myrtillus*, multicellular glandular trichome (*) and files of cells containing a calcium oxalate prism running alongside the veins of the leaf (◆)

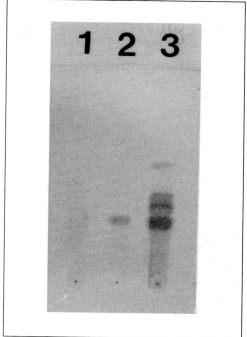

Fig. 4: TLC on 4 × 8 cm silica-gel foil
1: Bilberry leaf
2: Arbutin (reference substance)
3: Cowberry leaf

For details, see the text

[6, 7], and the chromium content – 9.0 ppm – is also remarkably high [8]. Small amounts of quinolizidine alkaloids, myrtine and epimyrtine, have been found in the aerial parts of the plant, including presumably the leaves [9].

Indications: To a modest extent, externally as an astringent in rinses and washes. In *folk medicine,* bilberry leaf is still considered to be a "blood sugar-reducing" drug and is therefore a frequent component of so-called "antidiabetic" teas [7]; about drugs with an antidiabetic action, see the critical review by Kraus and Reher [7]. Based on the observation that rats fed on a chromium-free diet showed symptoms of diabetes mellitus type II, drugs with an antidiabetic action have recently been examined for their chromium content, and bilberry leaves, as already indicated, contain a particularly large amount – 9.0 ppm. Chromium is a component of the so-called glucose tolerance factor, which is suitable for treating the diabetes mellitus type II developed in animal experiments [8]. But whether it is the chromium content of the drug that determines the possible antidiabetic action requires further research [8].

Likewise, it also has to be seen whether the flavonoids present in the drug can be used for the treatment of diabetic circulatory disorders.

Side effects: In the experimental work concerned, the effects reported were interpreted as being corresponding largely with the picture of hydroquinone poisoning; it was assumed that the leaves contained a relatively high concentration of hydroquinone. The work has never been repeated, and since it is now known that arbutin is absent or present

only in traces, the findings – if indeed reproducible – must be due to other constituents of the plant. In view of the unsubstantiated therapeutic activity and the possible risk of side effects on long-term use, medicinal utilization of bilberry leaf cannot be recommended [10].

Making the tea: Boiling water is poured over 1 g of the finely chopped drug and after 5–10 min. strained. The tea should not to be taken for a prolonged period.
1 Teaspoon = ca. 0.6 g.

Extract from the German Commission E monograph (BAnz no. 76, dated 23.04.1987)

Uses

Bilberry leaf is used for diabetes mellitus, and for both prevention and treatment of disorders and complaints of the gastrointestinal tract, the kidneys and urinary tract, and the respiratory tract, for rheumatism, arthritis, skin complaints, haemorrhoids, circulatory disorders, functional heart conditions, as well as for stimulating the metabolism and for "purifying" the blood.
Activity in the conditions indicated has not been substantiated.

Risks

With higher doses or on prolonged use, chronic intoxication may arise, the symptoms of which in animal experiments were initially cachexia, anaemia, icterus, acute excitatory states, and disturbances of tonus, and which could finally, after chronic administration of 1.5 g/kg/day, end in death.

Evaluation

Since the activity has not been substantiated, therapeutic use of bilberry leaf cannot be recommended in view of the risks involved.

Phytomedicines: A monovalent preparation, Diabetonit® 125 (dragees); the drug is a frequent component of so-called antidiabetic teas, e.g. Bad Neuenahrer Zuckertee, Diabetiker Tee Dr. Greither; the drug is also included in diuretics, e.g. Nieren-Blasen-Tee Dr. Greither, Uro-Tee, etc. Extracts are included in prepared remedies, such as Diabetylin® (tablets), Tumulca® (mixture), etc.

Authentication: Diagnostic features of the drug are: macroscopic – the serrate leaf margin with (sometimes broken) stalked glandular trichomes at the tip of the serrations; microscopic – paracytic stomata, files of cells with calcium oxalate crystals associated with the midrib, warty thick-walled glandular trichomes on the upper surface of the larger nerves, and glandular trichomes (Fig. 3).

Quantitative standard: Erg. B. 6: *Ash*, not more than 4%.

Adulteration: The leaves of the cowberry (red whortleberry), *Vaccinium vitis-idaea* (see: Uvae ursi folium – Bearberry leaf, Fig. 3) are a possible adulterant; however, they contain arbutin. This glucoside can al-

so be detected when leaves of a hybrid between *V. myrtillus* and *V. vitis idaea*, *V. × intermedium*, which are almost indistinguishable from those of genuine bearberry, are present in the drug [9].

The presence of arbutin can be established by the following TLC method:

Test solution: 4 g powdered drug refluxed with 50 ml 50% methanol for 15 min., filtered hot, and after cooling made up to 100 ml with 50% methanol; 2 ml 10% basic lead acetate solution then added and the whole mixed and filtered.

Reference solution: 5 mg arbutin dissolved in 2 ml methanol.

Loadings: 5 µl each of the test and reference solutions.

Solvent system: (a) ethyl acetate + methanol + water (77 + 13 + 10), 2 cm run; then (b) chloroform + methanol (95 + 5), 5 cm run.

Detection: after evaporation of the solvent, sprayed with 0.1% methanolic dichloroquinonechlorimide and carefully exposed to ammonia fumes (too long exposure darkens the background).

Evaluation: in daylight. Reference solution: arbutin at Rf ca. 0.3, as a bright blue spot, changing after some time towards reddish violet. Test solution: with bilberry leaves, no zone corresponding to arbutin, but only a faint, somewhat lower, greyish blue spot; with the adulterant cowberry leaves, on the other hand, a distinct arbutin zone.

Storage: Kept dry and protected from light.

Literature:

[1] N. Krstic-Pavlovic and M. Milutinovic, Jugoslav. Vocarstvo **16**, 27 (1982); C.A. **100**, 65041 (1984).
[2] J. Schönert and H. Friedrich, Pharmazie **25**, 775 (1970).
[3] H. Friedrich and J. Schönert, Planta Med. **24**, 90 (1973).
[4] Lj. Kraus and D. Dupáková, Pharmazie **19**, 41 (1964).
[5] N.K. Edgars, J. Am. Pharm. Assoc **25**, 288 (1936).
[6] Hager, vol. **6**, p. 369 (1979).
[7] Lj. Kraus and G. Reher, Dtsch. Apoth. Ztg. **122**, 2357 (1982).
[8] A. Müller, E. Diemann, and P. Sassenberg, Naturwissenschaften **75**, 155 (1988).
[9] P. Slosse and C. Hootelé, Tetrahedron **37**, 4287 (1988).
[10] D. Frohne, Z. Phytotherap. **11**, 209 (1990).

Myrtilli fructus   Bilberry fruit

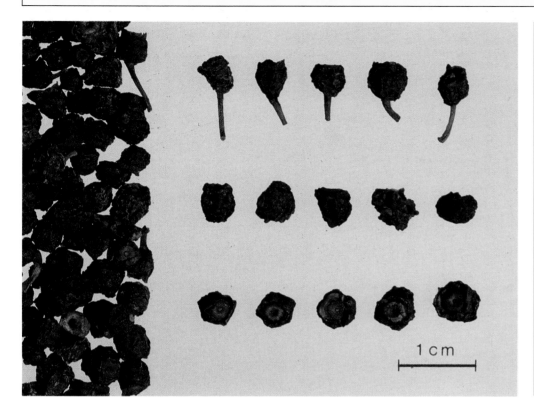

1 cm

Fig. 1: Bilberry fruit

Description: The globular, coarsely wrinkled, black berries are up to 6 mm in diameter and occasionally bear the remains of the stalk at the base and the remains of the disc and calyx at the top. In the fleshy mesocarp, there are many small, shiny, brownish red seeds.

Taste: Somewhat acidulous and sweet, weakly astringent.

An aqueous extract has a distinct reddish violet colour.

Fig. 2: *Vaccinium myrtillus* L.

Description as in Fig. 2, p. 348. Blue, mostly slightly pruinous, berries.

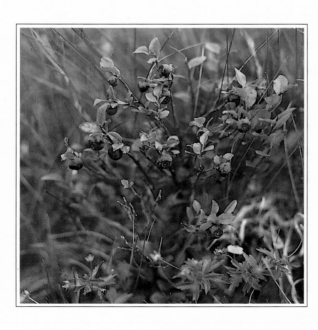

DAC 1986: Heidelbeeren
ÖAB: Fructus Myrtilli
Ph. Helv. VII: Myrtilli fructus
St. Zul. 1009.99.99

Plant source: *Vaccinium myrtillus* L., bilberry (Ericaceae).

Synonyms: Baccae Myrtilli (Lat.), (Red) Whortleberries (Engl.), Heidelbeeren, Blaubeeren, Bickbeeren, Schwarzbeeren (Ger.), Baies de myrtille (Fr.).

Origin: Northern and Central Europe; also imported from south-eastern Europe (the former USSR, Poland, Albania, former Yugoslavia).

Constituents: According to older data [1] up to 10% tannins, mostly catechol tannins; more recent analyses, using the combined phosphotungstic acid/hide powder method of the Ph. Helv. VII, suggest the presence of only about 1.5% [2]. Further, there are anthocyans, flavonoids, plant acids, invert sugar, and pectins.

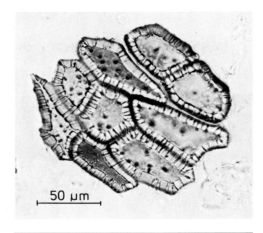

50 µm

Fig. 3: Group of stone cells from the inner fruit wall

Indications: Because of the tannin content, the drug is used as an antidiarrhoeic, especially in mild cases of enteritis. The fresh drug seems not to be suitable for the purpose – perhaps because the tannins first arise by condensation of the monomeric tannin precursors during the drying process [2].

Making the tea: Cold water is added to 5–10 g of the crushed drug, brought to the boil for 10 min., and then strained while hot.
1 Teaspoon = ca. 4 g, 1 tablespoon = ca. 10 g.

Phytomedicines: Only a few preparations, e.g. Stopftee Fides. Preparations such as Augenschutzkapseln Salus, Difrarel®, Dynef® (anthocyan pigments to improve vision?), etc., are proposed for a range of eye conditions. Cf. [2].

Authentication: Since bilberries are normally used as the whole drug, the macroscopic verification of the description is the essential requirement. It is important to make sure that the drug has not been attacked by insects and that it is not mouldy; the berries should be as soft as possible (drug that has been stored too long is hard and brittle).
Microscopically, besides occasional calcium-oxalate clusters, the stone cells of the meso- and endocarp (cf. Fig. 3) afford an important diagnostic feature.
The DAC 1986 TLC examination is based on the detection of anthocyan pigments, but it is not very specific and is therefore not described in detail here. It is recommended to use the solvent system given in the DAB 10 for Hibisci flos: *n*-butanol + 25% hydrochloric acid + anhydrous formic acid + water (70 + 12 + 12 + 6), on silica-gel foil (4 × 8 cm). The TLC examination of the aglycones set out in the DAC 1986 – required for the Standard Licence – does not afford any additional essential information.

Quantitative standards: <u>DAC 1986</u>: *Foreign matter*, not more than 2%. *Loss on drying*, not more than 12%. *Ash*, not more than 3.0%.
<u>ÖAB</u>: *Water-soluble extractive*, not less than 50%. *Ash*, not more than 2.0%.
<u>Ph. Helv. VII</u>: *Tannins*, not less than 1.5%. *Foreign matter*, not more than 1% (peduncles, leaves, and other foreign fruit – *Vaccinium uliginosum* L.). *Loss on drying*, not more than 14.0%. *Sulphated ash*, not more than 4.5%.

Adulteration: Rare. The fruit of *Vaccinium uliginosum*, bog bilberry or whortleberry, are similar to bilberries; however, they give only a faint brownish colour to an aqueous extract. For their microscopical recognition, see: Authentication.

Literature:
[1] Ch. Kröger, Pharmazie **6**, 211, 355, 603 (1952).
[2] D. Frohne, Z. Phytotherap. **11**, 209 (1990).

Nasturtii herba   Water-cress herb

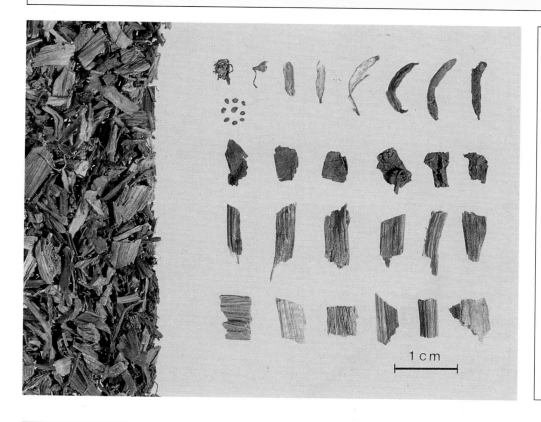

Fig. 1: Water-cress herb

<u>Description:</u> The drug consists of much shrivelled and mostly curled up light to dark green glabrous pieces of leaf with a fine venation. Also present are light brownish, compressed, broad fragments of stem, small yellowish white flowers with yellow anthers, and somewhat curved siliquae containing small brown seeds.

<u>Odour:</u> Very faintly spicy.

<u>Taste:</u> Slightly bitter and pungent.

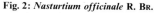
1 cm

Fig. 2: *Nasturtium officinale* R. Br.

A 30–40 cm tall perennial herb with imparipinnate leaves. Stem hollow. Flowers white, with yellow anthers.

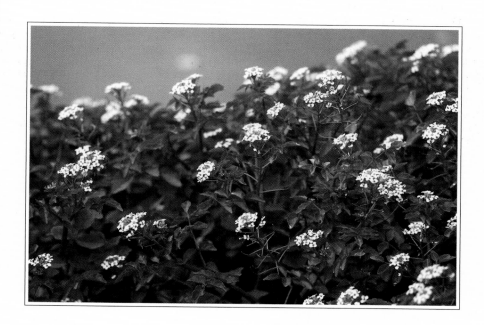

Erg. B. 6: Herba Nasturtii

Plant source: *Nasturtium officinale* R. Br., green or summer water-cress (Brassicaceae).

Synonyms: Herba Nasturtii aquatici (Lat.), Brunnenkressenkraut, Wasserkresse (Ger.), Cresson de Fontaine, Herbe aux chantes (Fr.).

Origin: Occurs scattered, along streams and in wet places; it is also cultivated on a small scale. Drug imports come from eastern and south-eastern European countries.

Constituents: The drug contains small amounts of glucosinolates (mustard-oil glycosides), e.g. gluconasturtiin, 2-phenylethyl isothiocyanate, and nitriles such as 3-phenylpropionitrile, 8-methylthiooctanone nitrile, etc. [1–3].

Indications: The drug is employed in the form of extracts for the preparation of cholagogues (see: Phytomedicines).
In <u>folk medicine</u> the drug is little used, e.g. as a stomachic, for coughs, and, rarely, for

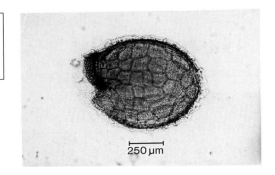

Fig. 3: Seed, showing the coarsely tesselated epidermis

250 µm

gingivitis and periodontitis. On the other hand, the fresh herb is much valued in naturotherapy as a "spring cure" or "blood purifier", mixed with fresh nettle and dandelion herbs, in the form of a salad.

Side effects: Because of the content of mustard-oil glycosides, water-cress herb should not be taken either in large amounts or for a long period of time, otherwise irritation of the gastric mucosa may develop.

Making the tea: Not common. Boiling water is poured over 2 g of the drug and after 10 min. passed through a tea strainer.
1 Teaspoon = ca. 1.7 g.

Phytomedicines: Water-cress extracts are present in several prepared cholagogues, e.g. in Cholongal Saft (juice), etc.

Authentication: Macro- (see: Description) and microscopically. The leaf epidermis comprises wavy-walled cells with anomocytic stomata. The palisade layer has broad cells and the spongy parenchyma is made up of relatively large, flat cells. The seeds have a *coarsely* tesselated epidermis (Fig. 3).

Quantitative standard: Erg. B. 6. *Ash*, not more than 12%.

Adulteration: Very rare. Contamination with *Cardamine amara* L., large bitter-cress, can be recognized by the dark violet anthers and stem with pith. The adulteration with *Berula* species mentioned in the literature is easily recognized, since these Apiaceae have flowers with five petals.

Storage: Protected from light and moisture.

Literature:
[1] E.A. Spinks, K. Sones, and G.R. Fenwick, Fette Seifen Anstrichmittel **86**, 228 (1984).
[2] A.J. MacLeod and R. Islam, J. Sci. Food Agric. **26**, 1545 (1975).
[3] D. Doernemann, W. Löffelhardt, and H. Kindl, Ca. J. Biochem. **52**, 916 (1974).

Ononidis radix   Restharrow root

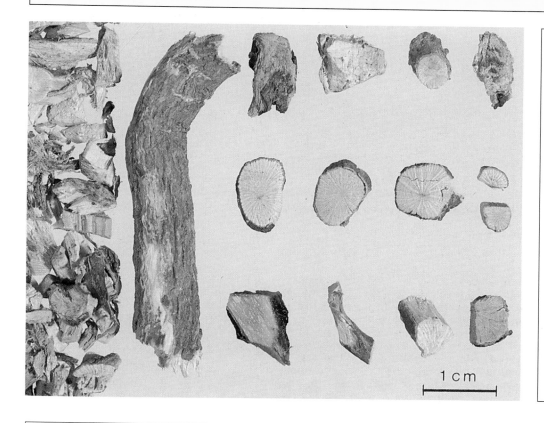

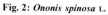

1 cm

Fig. 1: Restharrow root

<u>Description</u>: The root, which is usually flattened and twisted and bent, is greyish brown to dark brown on the outside and has deep longitudinal grooves. Characteristic of the transverse section is the clearly observable radiate structure of the xylem, brought about by the unequal width of the medullary rays (Fig. 3).

<u>Taste</u>: Somewhat harsh, sweetish, and distinctly irritating.

Fig. 2: *Ononis spinosa* L.

An up to 80 cm tall subshrub with thorns; lower leaves ternate, upper ones simple. Pinkish white papilionaceous flowers.

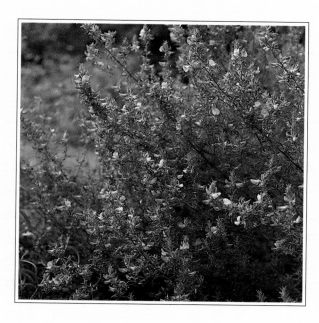

DAC 1986: Hauhechelwurzel
ÖAB: Radix Ononidis
St. Zul.: 9899.99.99

Plant source: *Ononis spinosa* L., spiny restharrow (Fabaceae).

Synonyms: Cammock root (Engl.), Hauhechelwurzel, Haudornwurzel, Ochsenbrechwurzel, Harnkrautwurzel (Ger.), Racine de bugrane (Fr.).

Origin: Native in Europe, western Asia, and North Africa. The drug is collected from the wild in south-eastern Europe (Bulgaria, Albania, former Yugoslavia, Hungary).

Constituents: 0.02–0.1% essential oil, with as main components *trans*-anethole, as well as carvone and menthol; isoflavones, especially ononin (formononetin 7-glucoside) and its 6″-malonate, and also biochanin A 7-glucoside and its 6″-malonate [1]; ordinary flavonoids occur only in the aerial parts [2]; triterpenes, especially α-onocerin (= onocol); sterols, particularly sitosterol.

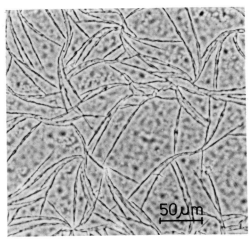

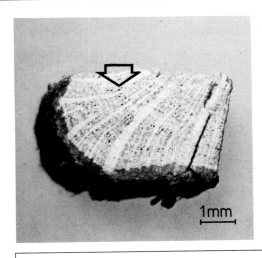

Glucose–O

Ononin

α-Onocerin (= Onocol)

Fig. 3: Transverse surface *Ononis spinosa* root, showing the whitish medullary rays and large vessels (arrow)

Fig. 4: Fine, sinuate needles of the micro-sublimate (onocol)

Indications: As a mild diuretic. The action of the drug has been repeatedly confirmed in animal experiments [3], but it has not yet proved possible to isolate any active constituents nor have constituents of known structure been tested pharmacologically.
In *folk medicine*, restharrow root is also used for gout and rheumatic complaints.

Making the tea: Boiling water is poured over 2–2.5 g of the finely chopped or coarsely powdered drug and after 20–30 min. strained.
1 Teaspoon = ca. 3 g.

Phytomedicines: Many herbal mixtures and a few prepared diuretics, e.g. Pulvhydrops® (dragees).

Authentication: Macro- (see: Description) and microscopically. With the hand lens, a darkish scaly cortex can be seen on the outside and towards the inside a thin periderm; in the xylem, there are medullary rays of greatly varying widths and often vessels with a rather large lumen (Fig. 3). The microscopical picture is characterized by the presence of numerous groups of xylem fibres accompanied by a crystal sheath; small roundish starch grains are also present.
Microsublimation (at ca. 220 °C) of the powdered drug yields fine, often slightly bent or stellately branched needles, of onocol (Fig. 4). When 1 drop conc. sulphuric acid and 1 drop ethanolic vanillin solution (1 g/100 ml) is added to this sublimate, after

a few minutes the needles are coloured bluish violet.
The following method provides a fingerprint TLC:

Test solution: 1 g powdered drug refluxed for 30 min. with 15 ml methanol and, after cooling, filtered.

Reference solution: authentic drug treated in the same way, or 10 mg each of vanillin and resorcinol dissolved in 10 ml methanol.

Loadings: 5 µl each of the test and reference solutions, as bands on silica gel.

Solvent system: toluene + chloroform + ethanol (4 + 4 + 1), 6 cm run.

Detection: in UV 365 nm light, followed by spraying with or dipping in anisaldehyde reagent and heating at 105 °C for 5–10 min.

Evaluation: Test solution: in UV 365 nm light, several blue to bluish violet fluorescent zones, with the most intense ones at Rf values in the middle; in daylight, the intense reddish violet onocol zone in the middle, just below the level of the reference vanillin zone.
The DAC 1986 TLC examination is similar; the solvent system is: toluene + ethanol + dichloromethane (45 + 10 + 45), and resorcinol and vanillin are the reference compounds; evaluation is in UV 254 and 365 nm light, and after spraying with anisaldehyde reagent and heating.

Quantitative standards: DAC 1986: *Water-soluble extractive*, not less than 15.0%. *For-*

---

*Extract from the German Commission E monograph
(BAnz no. 76, dated 23. 04. 1987)*

Uses
For irrigating the urinary tract in inflammatory conditions. Also for the prevention and treatment of kidney gravel.

Contraindications: None known.

Warning: no irrigation therapy in cases of oedema arising from cardiac or renal insufficiency.

Side effects
None known.

Interactions with other remedies
None known.

Dosage
Unless otherwise prescribed: daily dose, 6–12 g drug; preparations correspondingly.

Mode of administration
Chopped drug for infusions and other galenical preparations for internal use.

Warning: an abundant fluid intake should be ensured.

Effects
Diuretic.

Wording of the package insert, from the German Standard Licence

6.1   Uses

For increasing the amount of urine in catarrh of the bladder and of the pelvis of the kidney, for urinary gravel and the prevention of urinary calculi.

6.2   Contraindications

Accumulation of water (oedema) as a result of impaired heart and kidney function.

6.3   Dosage and Mode of administration

Boiling water (ca. 150 ml) is poured over ca. 2 teaspoonfuls (3–4 g) of **Restharrow root**, kept warm, and after about 30 mins. passed through a tea strainer.

Unless otherwise prescribed, a cup of the tea is drunk two or three times a day between meals.

6.4   Duration of use

Restharrow-root tea should only be used for a few days, since the effect gradually diminishes. After waiting for a few days, the treatment can be resumed.

6.5   Note

Store protected from light and moisture.

eign matter, not more than 2%. *Loss on drying*, not more than 10%. *Ash*, not more than 7.0%.

ÖAB: *Foreign matter*, not more than 5% (stem fragments). *Ash*, not more than 6.0%

Adulteration: Very rare. The roots of *Medicago sativa* L., lucerne or alfalfa, have a round transverse section and a distinct pith.

Literature:

[1] J. Köster, D. Strack, and W. Barz, Planta Med. **48**, 131 (1983).

[2] Th. Kartnig et al., Pharm. Acta Helv. **60**, 253 (1985).

[3] M. Rebuelta, et al., Plantes Méd. Phytothérap. **15**, 99 (1981).

Orthosiphonis folium   (DAB 10), Orthosiphon

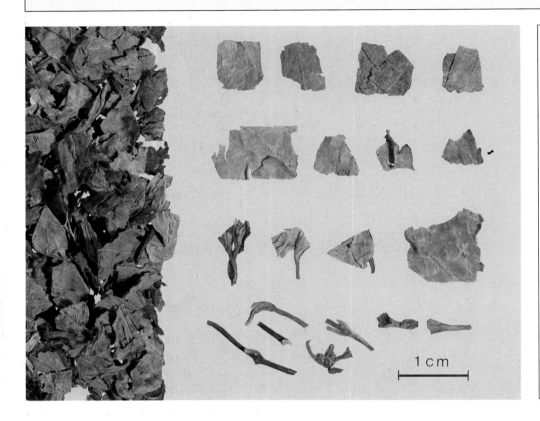

Fig. 1: Orthosiphon leaf

<u>Description:</u> The drug consists of the dried leaves and tips of the stems gathered shortly before the flowering period. The short-petioled, lanceolate-ovate, 2–7 cm long leaves are cuneate at the base and have a long acumen at the tip; the venation is pinnate and the margin is coarsely serrate. The upper surface is deep green or yellowish green and the lower surface pale greyish green; the venation on the lower surface sometimes has a violet tinge. The petioles are more or less 4-angled and, like the venation, brownish violet.

<u>Odour:</u> Very faintly aromatic.

<u>Taste:</u> Somewhat salty, slightly bitter, and astringent.

Fig. 2: *Orthosiphon aristatus* (BLUME) MIQ.

A perennial, growing to a height of 60 cm, with 4-angled stems and decussate, short-petiolate, acuminate leaves with a coarsely serrate margin. Characteristic light violet lobate flowers, arranged in whorls, with four very long and projecting blue-violet stamens and a style of similar length; it is to these that the plant owes its vernacular name: kumis kucing = cat's whiskers.

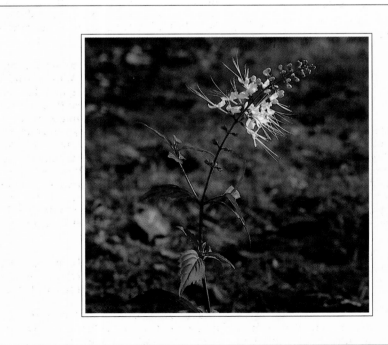

DAB 10: Orthosiphonblätter
Ph. Helv. VII: Orthosiphonis folium
St. Zul. 1159.99.99

Plant source: *Orthosiphon aristatus* (BLUME) MIQ. (syn. *O. spicatus* BACKER, BAKH.f., et STEENIS, non BENTH. and *O. stamineus* BENTH.), kumis kucing (Lamiaceae).

Synonyms: Orthosiphon leaf, Java tea (Engl.), Orthosiphonblätter, Javatee, Indischer Nierentee (Ger.), Feuilles de barbiflore, Thé de Java (Fr.), Kumis kucing (Koemis koetjing) (Indonesian, Malay).

Origin: Native in tropical Asia; it is cultivated on Java, from where it is exported.

Constituents: 0.02–0.06% essential oil (distillation with acidified or basified water affords much larger quantities), of great complexity [1]; among the ca. 60 components so far isolated sesquiterpenes. A range of phenolic constituents is present [2, 3, 9], including lipophilic flavones (higher methoxylated compounds such as sinensetin, eupatorin, scutellarein tetramethyl ether, salvigenin,

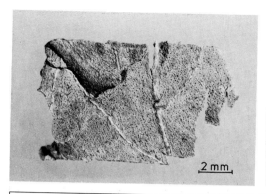

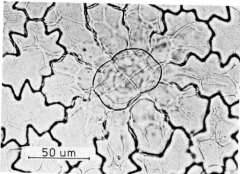

Fig. 3: Lower surface of the leaf, showing the glandular dots

Fig. 4: Peltate glandular trichomes with only four secretory cells

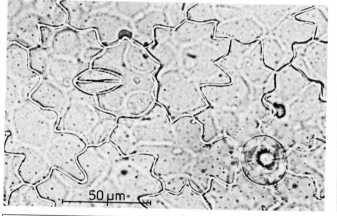

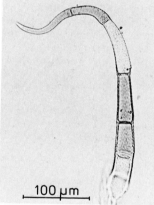

Fig. 5: Leaf epidermis, showing a diacytic stoma and a capitate glandular trichome

Fig. 6: Multicellular covering trichome with partly reddish cell sap

mixed teas as diuretic and urological remedies, e.g. Salus® Nieren-Blasentee (kidney-bladder tea), Blasen-Nieren-Tee Stada®, Hevert® Blasen und Nierentee, Nephronorm Med®, Nephrubin®, etc. It is included in the form of an extract in instant preparations of the same kind, e.g. Solubitrat®, Solvefort®, NB-tee Siegfried®, Harntee 400, etc.

Authentication: Macro- and microscopically, following the DAB 10. With a hand lens, it is possible to see the fine glandular dots on the lower surface of the leaf (Fig. 3); in contrast with many other Lamiaceae, the glandular trichomes have only 4 secretory cells (Fig. 4). The diacytic stomata (Fig. 5) are present on both leaf surfaces, but are particularly numerous on the lower surface. The multicellular covering trichomes are up to 450 µm long and often lie obliquely; they are sometimes filled with a reddish cell sap (Fig. 6) and the basal cell is more or less ventricose.

Adulteration: Occasionally noted; usually with the leaves of other *Orthosiphon* species, which are practically without smell and they can be detected by TLC.
The following TLC test of identity is based on the DAB 10 procedure and is concerned with the lipophilic flavones:

rhamnazin, etc.), flavonol glycosides, and caffeic acid derivatives (mainly rosmarinic and 2,3-dicaffeoyltartaric acids). The isolation of methylripariochromene A, reportedly in 4% yield [10], has not been confirmed [9]. Saponins may also be present, and ca. 3% potassium salts.

Indications: As a diuretic in chronic or recurrent inflammation of the renal pelvis, in bladder catarrh, kidney catarrh, irritable bladder, bacteriuria without clear symptoms. It is not simply a question of water diuresis, but there is also an increase in the excretion of sodium chloride [4–7, 12]. So far, it has not been possible to associate the diuretic action with any specific con-

stituents; presumably, it is due to the combined action of potassium salts, saponins (?), and flavonoids [8]. In a hot water extract, similar to a herbal tea, caffeic acid derivatives represent as much as 95% of the phenolic substances present [9]. The drug may have some effect in widening the ureters, thereby allowing small renal calculi to be eliminated [11].

Making the tea: Boiling water is poured over 2–3 g of the finely chopped drug, kept for 5–20 min. in a covered vessel, and then strained.
1 Teaspoon = ca. 1 g.

Phytomedicines: The drug is used as such or in combination with other herbal drugs in

Wording of the package insert, from the German Standard Licence:

5.1 Uses
For increasing urine formation, e.g. in kidney and bladder catarrh and in kidney gravel.

5.2 Contraindications
Accumulation of water (oedema) resulting from impaired cardiac and renal function.

5.3 Dosage and Mode of administration
Hot water (ca. 150 ml) is poured over ca. one teaspoonful (2–3 g) **Orthosiphon** and after ca. 15 min. passed through a tea strainer.

The tea can also be prepared with cold water and allowing it to draw for several hours.
Unless otherwise prescribed, a cup of the tea is drunk two or three times a day between meals.

5.4 Note
Store away from light and moisture.

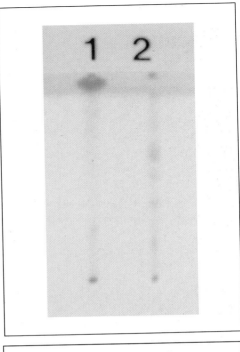

Test solution: 1 g powdered drug extracted by shaking for 15 min. with 10 ml dichloromethane, followed by filtration.

Reference solution: authentic drug treated in the same way or 1 mg scopoletin dissolved in 20 ml methanol.

Loadings: 5 µl test solution and 5 µl (authentic drug) or 3 µl (scopoletin) reference solution, as bands on silica gel.

Solvent system: chloroform + ethyl acetate (60 + 40), 5 cm run.

Detection: after complete evaporation of the solvent, examination in UV 366 and 254 nm light.

Evaluation: in UV 366 nm light. Reference solution: the intense blue fluorescent scopoletin zone at Rf 0.4–0.5. Test solution: four fluorescent zones in the region Rf 0.2–0.6, the most intense one being just below the scopoletin zone; adulterants have only weakly fluorescent zones in this region. In UV 254 nm light. Orthosiphon leaf: several quenching zones in the region Rf 0.6–0.9 and an intense blue fluorescent zone at Rf ca. 0.5 (Fig. 7); adulterants have only one

quenching zone, just below the solvent front (Fig. 7).
Illustrations of chromatograms run in the solvent system indicated are to be found in [13].

Quantitative standards: <u>DAB 10</u>: *Foreign matter*, not more than 2% and not more than 5% stems with a diameter greater than 1 mm. *Loss on drying*, not more than 11.0%. *Ash*, not more than 12.5%.
<u>Ph. Helv. VII</u>: *Foreign matter*, not more than 5% (including stems with a diameter greater than 1 mm). *Sulphated ash*, not more than 16.0%.

Fig. 7: TLC on 4 × 8 cm silica-gel foil

1: Adulterant
2: Orthosiphon leaf

For details, see the text

Literature:
[1] G.A. Schut and J.H. Zwaving, Plant Med. **52**, 240 (1986).
[2] G. Schneider and H.S.G. Tan, Dtsch. Apoth. Ztg. **113**, 201 (1973).
[3] E. Wollenweber and K. Mann, Planta Med. **51**, 459 (1985).
[4] R. Schuhmann, Über die diuretische Wirkung von Koemis Koetjing, Thesis, Marburg (1927).
[5] J. Westing, Weitere Untersuchungen über die Wirkung der Herba Orthosiphonis auf den menschlichen Harn, Thesis, Marburg (1928).
[6] F. Mercier and L.J. Mercier, Bull. Méd. **1936**, 523.
[7] S.Y. Chow, J. Formosan Med. Assoc. **78**, 11 (1979).
[8] N. Tiktinskij et al., Urol. i Nefrol. **1983**, 47; Zentralbl. Pharm. **124**, 58 (1985).
[9] W. Sumarjono et al., Planta Med. **57**, 176 (1991).
[10] J.-C. Guerin, H.-P. Reveillière, P. Ducrey, and L. Toupet, J. Nat. Prod. **52**, 171 (1989).
[11] A. Grevenstuk and F.W. Mreyen, Geneesk. Tijdschr. Nederl.-Indië **81**, 154 (1941).
[12] J. Casadebaig-Lafon et al., Pharm. Acta Helv. **64**, 220 (1989).
[13] H. Wagner, S. Bladt, and E.M. Zgainski, Plant drug analysis, Springer-Verlag, Berlin, Heidelberg, New York, Tokyo, 1984, p. 188.

Paeoniae flos   Peony flower

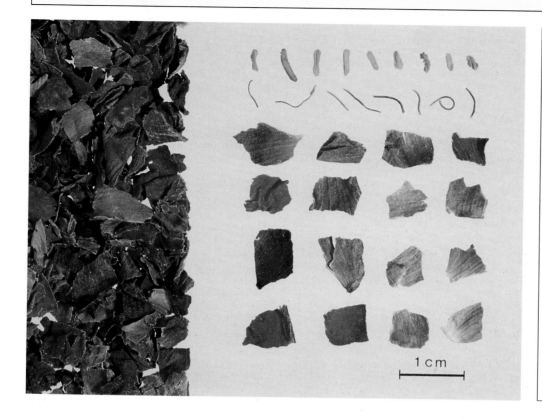

Fig. 1: Peony flower

Description: The rapidly dried, deep purple-red, somewhat wrinkled, thickish and stiff petals of the double garden form are 4–5 cm long and 3–4 cm broad. The petals are obovate, with numerous radiating veins, and a paler spot at the base; towards the upper margin, they are irregularly incised to crenate. The chopped drug consists of dark red, shrivelled, brittle fragments of the petals.

Odour: Honey-like and sweet.

Taste: Harsh and astringent.

Fig. 2: *Paeonia officinalis* L. emend. WILLD.

The wild form, a robust shrub, up to 80 cm in height, with a bulbous rhizome and large, shiny green leaves divided into numerous segments; bright red, shell-shaped flowers, reaching a diameter of ca. 10 cm, and with 5–8 petals and numerous yellow stamens. In the double garden form, from which the drug comes, the stamens are partly transformed into petals.

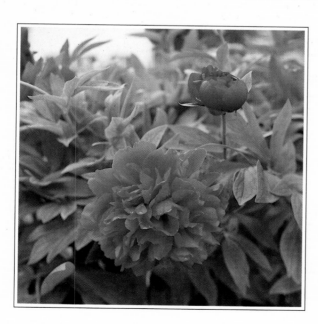

Erg. B. 6: Flores Paeoniae

Plant source: Double, red-flowered garden forms of different subspecies and varieties of *Paeonia officinalis* L. emend. WILLD., peony (Paeoniaceae).

Synonyms: Flores Rosae benedictae (Lat.), Pfingstrosenblüten, Bauernrosenblüten, Päonienblüten (Ger.), Fleurs de pivoine, Fleurs de péone (Fr.).

Origin: In open woods in southern Europe and Asia Minor; cultivated since ancient times as a decorative garden plant and as a medicinal plant; imports come from eastern European countries – Bulgaria and Turkey.

Constituents: While the roots of *Paeonia officinalis* are relative well studied, this is not the case with the flowers; most of the old data regarding the constituents need to be looked at again. The drug contains anthocyanin pigments, especially paeonin (= paeonidin 3,5-diglucoside) [1]; flavonoids, particularly derivatives of kaempferol [2]; tannins, presumably gallotannins, the presence of which has been demonstrated in the leaves and roots [3].

Indications: Only in *folk medicine*, formerly against "epilepsy", arthritis, and bowel complaints (as also the seeds and roots of the paeony) and as a cough remedy. In homoeopathy, the drug is also applied against fissures, haemorrhoids, varicose veins, etc. Nowadays, the drug is obsolete; occasionally, however, it is included in herbal teas to enhance their appearance.

Side effects: Overdoses of the flowers (and also of the seeds and roots) cause gastroenteritis with vomiting, colic, and diarrhoea [3].

Making the tea: Not very usual. Boiling water is poured over 1 teaspoon of the drug and after 5–10 min. passed through a tea strainer.
1 Teaspoon = ca. 1 g.

Phytomedicines: As a component for enhancing the appearance of herbal teas; as a homoeopathic mother tincture in antiphlebitis remedies, e.g. Aescosulf®.
Note: Peony seeds (Semen Paeoniae) were also included in the Erg. B. 6; like Radix Paeoniae, this drug was formerly used in *folk medicine* as an emetic and emmenagogue.

Authentication: Macro- (see: Description) and microscopically, following the Erg. B. 6. Among the diagnostic features are: the dark red petal fragments with large, elongated

epidermal cells showing beaded side walls and distinct, finely sinuate, cuticular striations (Fig. 3), as well as fragile spirally thickened vessels.
TLC methods for examining the anthocyanins of peony flowers are given in [4], which also illustrates the chromatograms obtained.

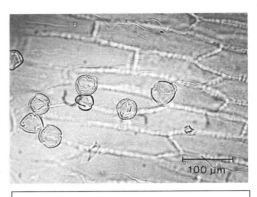

Fig. 3: Epidermis, showing the beaded cell walls and the very fine cuticular striations; triporate pollen grains are lying on top

Quantitative standards: Erg. B. 6: *Ash*, not more than 3%. *Bleached or discoloured flowers should not be present.*

Adulteration: Almost never occurs.

Storage: Protected from light and moisture; not to be stored for longer than one year, since the petals start to fade fairly rapidly and become unsightly.

Literature:
[1] R. Willstätter and Th.J. Nolan, Liebigs Ann. Chem. **408**, 136 (1915).
[2] K. Egger, Z. Naturforsch. **16b**, 430 (1961).
[3] Hager, vol. **6**, p. 384 (1977).
[4] H. Wagner, S. Bladt, and E.M. Zgainski, Plant drug analysis, Springer-Verlag, Berlin, Heidelberg, New York, Tokyo, 1984, p. 274.

Passiflorae herba   (DAB 10), Passiflora (BHP 1/1990)

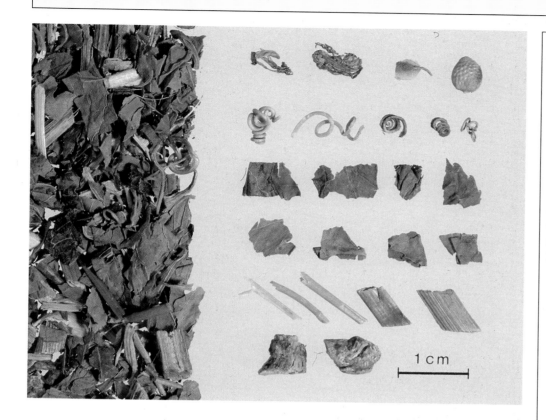

Fig. 1: Passiflora

<u>Description</u>: The thin and roundish pieces of stem are hollow. The petiolate, 6–15 cm long leaves are deeply 3-lobed and have a finely pubescent lower surface, with a finely serrate margin and reticulate venation (Fig. 3). Also present are round, glabrous, axillary tendrils which are curled up like a corkscrew; fragments of them are a conspicuous feature of the chopped drug. The long-pedicellate flowers, up to 9 cm in diameter, have 3 bracts, a calyx with 5 sepals, and a corolla comprising 5 white petals, as well as many white and purplish red filamentous appendages (coronal threads) and 5 large and prominent stamens. The greyish green, pubescent ovary is superior and the style has 3 long branches ending in capitate stigmas. The flat, greenish or brownish fruits contain many depressed punctate, brownish yellow seeds.

<u>Odour</u>: Slightly aromatic.

<u>Taste</u>: Not distinctive, bland.

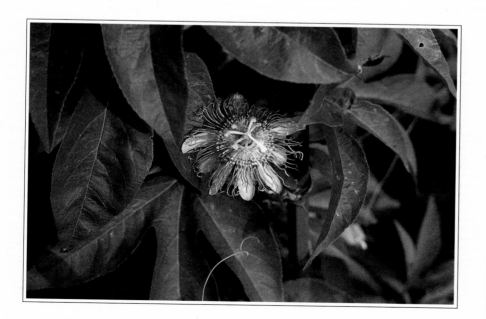

Fig. 2: *Passiflora incarnata* L.

Passion flowers are herbaceous climbers, reaching a height of several metres, with deeply lobed leaves. It is the unusual construction of the whitish violet flowers (see the description of the drug) that gave rise to the name of the plant: the coronal threads were seen as a symbol for the Crown of Thorns, the five stamens for the Wounds, and the three stigmas for the Nails on the Cross.

DAB 10: Passionsblumenkraut
Ph. Helv. VII: Passiflorae herba
St. Zul. 1619.99.99

Plant source: *Passiflora incarnata* L., passion flower (Passifloraceae).

Synonyms: Passion-flower herb, Maypop (Engl.), Passionsblumenkraut, Fleischfarbige Passionsblume (Ger.), Herbe de passiflore (Fr.).

Origin: Native to North, Central, and South America; cultivated to some extent in tropical and subtropical regions. The drug is imported from the USA and India, and it is also obtained from the West Indies.

Constituents: Up to 2.5% flavonoids, principally glucosyl derivatives such as vitexin, saponarin, orientin, homo-orientin, schaftoside, isoschaftoside, vicenin etc. [1, 2, 9, 12, 13]; ca. 0.05% maltol (3-hydroxy-2-methyl-γ-pyrone); small amounts of cyanogenic glycosides, particularly gynocardin [3]; traces of an essential oil of still unknown composition; the occurrence of harman alkaloids is not certain – but is certainly largely dependent on the stage of development of the plants [4].

Indications: As a sedative in neurasthenia, neurovegetative dystonia, difficulties in sleeping, anxiety states, restlessness, nervous disorders, especially in children.
In the countries of origin, passion-flower herb is used as a spasmolytic and as a sedative. Animal experiments have shown that extracts of the drug have a spasmolytic ac-

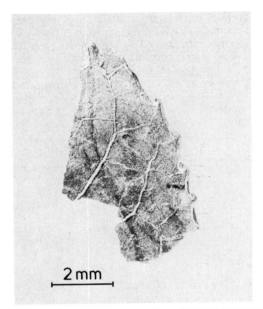
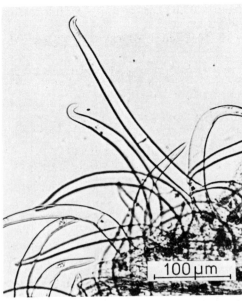

2 mm

100 µm

Fig. 3: Thin fragment of leaf showing the serrate margin

Fig. 4: Few-celled covering trichomes, some of which have a hooked tip

tivity comparable with that of papaverine [4, 5]; at the same time, there is a central depressant effect. About the neuropharmacological activity of Passiflora extracts, see [10].

Making the tea: Boiling water is poured over 2 g of the finely chopped drug and after 5–10 min. passed through a tea strainer. Two or three cups are drunk throughout the day or one or two cups are taken before going to bed.
1 Teaspoon = ca. 2 g.

Phytomedicines: The drug or extracts of it are a component especially of prepared sedatives, e.g. Plantival®, Sanadormin®, Sedinfant®, Kräuter-Dragees, Passiflora-Curarina-Tropfen, Aranidorm®, Bunetten®, etc., and also cardiotonic remedies.
In the UK, Passiflora and/or extracts of it are a component of about 40 sedative prepa-

rations [11], including Gerard 99 Tablets, Gerard House Passiflora Tablets, Gerard House Motherwort Compound Tablets, Lanes Quiet Life Tablets, Lanes Naturest, Seven Seas Restful Night Tablets, Potter's Anased Pain Relief Tablets, Potter's Passiflora, etc., etc.

Regulatory status (UK): General Sales List – Schedule 1, Table A.

Authentication: Macro- (see: Description) and microscopically, following the DAB 10. See also the BHP 1/1990. The thin-walled covering trichomes, often ending in a rounded hooked tip, which occur on stem and leaf fragments (Fig. 4), are particularly diagnostic. In the mesophyll of the leaf there are numerous small clusters of calcium oxalate (ca. 15 µm in diameter). The epidermal cells of the corolla, especially those of the inner surface, are beaded. The pollen, with diameter ca. 70 µm, has reticulate ornamentation on the exine.

The DAB 10 prescribes the following TLC identification test:

Test solution: 0.6 powdered drug shaken for 5 min. with 5 ml methanol on the water-bath at 60 °C, then filtered.

Reference solution: 2.0 mg each of hyperoside and rutin dissolved in 10 ml methanol.

Loadings: 20 µl test solution and 10 µl reference solution, as 2-cm bands on silica gel G.

Solvent system: water + anhydrous formic acid + ethyl methyl ketone + ethyl acetate (10 + 10 + 30 + 50), 12 cm run.

Detection: after 5 min. drying at 105 °C, the still warm plate sprayed with 1% methanolic diphenylboryloxyethylamine followed by 5% methanolic Macrogol 400.

Evaluation: in UV 365 nm light. Reference solution: two yellowish brown fluorescent zones, the rutin zone in the lower third and the hyperoside zone about the middle. Test solution: somewhat below the level of the reference rutin zone, an intense green fluorescent zone (saponarin) and directly below it a strong greenish yellow fluorescent zone; somewhat below the level of the reference hyperoside zone, an intense yellow fluorescent zone (iso-orientin) and immediately above this a less intense zone fluorescing pale green and after some time fluorescing greenish grey (isovitexin); directly above the level of the reference hyperoside zone, a moderately strong brownish yellow fluorescent zone (orientin); a little further up, a usually faint pale green fluorescent zone, gradually becoming fainter and dirty grey (vitexin); near the solvent front, one or two relatively strong red fluorescent chlorophyll zones; a few more faint, brownish or bluish fluorescent zones possibly also present.

For the unequivocal TLC identification of *Passiflora incarnata extracts* (including their presence in mixed preparations), three different separation procedures are required [6]: (a) butan-1-ol + glacial acetic acid + water (40 + 10 + 50; upper phase), with cellulose; (b) ethyl acetate + methyl ethyl ketone + formic acid + water (50 + 30 + 10 + 10), with silica gel 60; (c) methanol + water + formic acid (28 + 12 + 5), with HPTLC RP 18. The characteristic flavonoids, coumarins, and plant acids are detected with diphenylboryloxyethylamine. See also the BHP 1/1990 and [7, 8].

Quantitative standards: DAB 10: *Flavonoids*, not less than 0.4% calculated as hyperoside (M_r 464.4). *Foreign matter*, not more than 2%; pith-containing stem fragments greater than 3 mm in diameter should be absent (*Passiflora edulis* SIMS., *P. coerulea* L., and other *Passiflora* species); on triturating the drug with water, there should be no odour of hydrocyanic acid (*P. coerulea* L. and other *Passiflora* species); in the TLC identification test (above), the chromatogram of the test solution in the region between the saponarin and iso-orientin zones there should be at most very weak yellow or orange-yellow fluorescent zones. *Loss on drying*, not more than 10%. *Ash*, not more than 13%.

Ph. Helv. VII: *Flavonoids*, not less than 0.3%. calculated as hyperoside (M_r 464.4).

Foreign matter, not more than 3%; root fragments should not be present; *P. coerulea*, which liberates hydrocyanic acid on trituration with water, should not be present. *Sulphated ash*, not more than 17.0%.

BHP 1/1990: *Water-soluble extractive*, not less than 15%. *Foreign matter*, not more than 3%. *Total ash*, not more than 11%. *HCl-insoluble ash*, not more than 3%.

Note: Passiflorae herba forms the subject of an ESCOP proposal for a European harmonized monograph.

Adulteration: In the trade, drug material derived from other *Passiflora* species is quite often encountered. See: Authentication (above).

Literature:
[1] C. Congora, A. Proliac, and J. Raynaud, Helv. Chim. Acta **69**, 251 (1986).
[2] A. Proliac and J. Raynaud, Pharmazie **41**, 673 (1986).
[3] K.C. Spencer and D.S. Siegler, Planta Med. **50**, 356 (1984).
[4] J. Lutomski, E. Segiet, K. Szpunar, and K. Grisse, Pharmazie in unserer Zeit **10**, 45 (1981).
[5] R. Paris, Ann. Pharm. Franç. **21**, 389 (1963).
[6] Th. Kartnig, G. Kummer-Fustinioni, and B. Heydel, Sci. Pharm. **51**, 269 (1983).
[7] H. Schilcher, Dtsch. Apoth. Ztg. **107**, 849 (1967).
[8] P. Pachaly, Dtsch. Apoth. Ztg. **125**, 1223 (1985).
[9] A. Proliac and J. Raynaud, Pharm. Acta Helv. **63**, 171 (1988).
[10] E. Speroni and A. Minghetti, Planta Med. **54**, 488 (1988).
[11] J.D. Phillipson and L.A. Anderson, Pharm. J. **233**, 80, 111 (1984).
[12] H. Geiger and K.R. Markham, Z. Naturforsch. **41 c**, 949 (1986).
[13] Li Qimin et al., J. Chromatogr. **562**, 435 (1991).

Petasitidis folium   Butterbur leaf

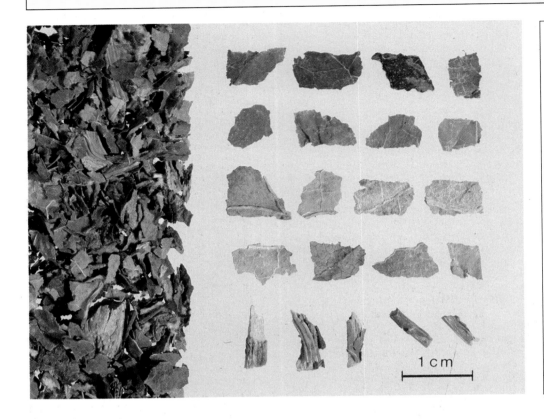

Fig. 1: Butterbur leaf

Description: The more or less firm leaf fragments are often folded together; they have a dull green, sparse to scattered pubescent upper surface and a mostly woolly to velvety tomentum on the lower surface. The reticulate venation on the lower surface is fairly prominent (Fig. 4).

Odour: Faint and characteristic.

Taste: Mucilaginous and somewhat bitter.

Figs. 2 and 3: *Petasites hybridus* (L.) P. GAERTN., B. MEYER, et SCHERB.

A shrub, growing along the damp banks of streams and rivers, with very large, long-petiolate leaves having a grey tomentous lower surface and first appearing after the flowers. Pale pink to lilac (sometimes also yellowish) flower-heads (entirely male or entirely female) comprising only tubular florets and crowded together on the bracteate stem.

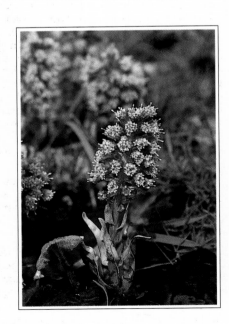

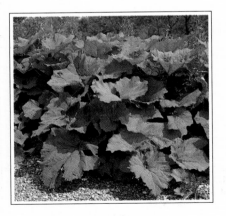

Plant source: *Petasites hydridus* (L.) P. GAERTN., B. MEYER, et SCHERB. (syn. *P. officinalis* MOENCH), butterbur (Asteraceae).

Synonyms: Folia petasites (Lat.), Pestwurzblätter, Großblättriger or Falscher Huflattich (Ger.), Feuilles de pétasite (Fr.).

Origin: Native throughout Europe, northern and western Asia, and introduced into North America. The drug comes entirely from the wild and plays little or no part in the drug *wholesale* trade.

Constituents: Esters of the eremophilane-type sesquiterpene alcohols petasol, neopetasol, and isopetasol, with petasin (0.36%), isopetasin (0.15%), and angelicoyl-neopetasol as principal components; fukinone, as well as the β-methylene-γ-lactone bakkenolide (= fukinanolide), etc.; ca. 0.1% essential oil, with dodecanal as the odoriferous substance of the drug; flavonoids: isoquercitrin, astragalin, quercetin; mucilage; tannins; traces of triterpenoid saponins and pyrrolizidine alkaloids (senecionine, integerrimine, senkirkine) [1]. Besides the pharmaceutically used petasin race, there is

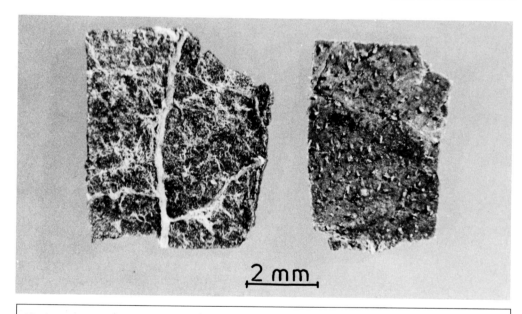

Petasol: R = H
Petasin: R = Angelicoyl

Neopetasol R = H
R = Angelicoyl
R = 3-Methylcrotonoyl
R = Methacryloyl
R = Isobutyroyl

Isopetasol R = H
R = Angelicoyl (=Isopetasin)
R = 3-Methylcrotonoyl
R = Metnacryloyl
R = Isobutyroyl

Furanopetasin

Fukinone

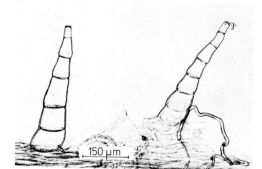

Fig. 4: Tomentous lower surface of the leaf (left) and darker upper surface with a few covering trichomes

Fig. 5: Large, multicellular trichomes with broad basal and cylindrical cells. Woolly trichome from the lower surface (right)

a petasin-free so-called furan race, containing furanoeremophilanes, which must be considered as an adulterant.

Indications: The drug is used as a spasmolytic with analgesic effects, as a kind of "phytotranquillizer", in neurodystonic functional disturbances of the gastrointestinal tract, and also for intestinal spasms, bronchial asthma, and dysmenorrhoea of different origins [2]. Petasin, isopetasin, and possibly other sesquiterpenoid compounds of similar structure [3], may be the active components; petasin has been shown to have analgesic and soporific effects after i.m. and i.v. administration in rats [4]. In *folk medicine*, butterbur leaf was formerly used as a sudorific and diuretic and also for its phlegm-dissolving properties in respiratory complaints (coughs and hoarseness). The fresh leaves were used externally for treating wounds and skin conditions. For the mutagenic and cancerogenic action of the pyrrolizidine alkaloids, see [9] and Senecionis herba.

Making the tea: Boiling water is poured over 1.2–2 g of the chopped drug and, after 5–10 min., strained. A cup of the infusion is drunk two or three times a day.
1 Teaspoon = ca. 0.6 g.

Phytomedicines: None. However, extracts from the rhizomes of other *Petasites* species are components of prepared cholagogues, sedatives, bronchospasmolytics, and spasmolytics.

Authentication: Macro- and microscopically, in accordance with the data in the DAB

10 monograph on Farfarae folium, where *Petasites* species are described as an adulterant. Fig. 5 shows the typical covering trichomes of the drug.

The TLC method given in the DAB 10 under Farfarae folium (Coltsfoot, q.v.) for verifying the absence of petasin-containing and petasin-free *Petasites* leaves is also a suitable identification test for Petasitidis folium and means of establishing the absence of the petasin-free furan race; see, in addition, [5].

Coloured illustrations of chromatograms of Petasitidis folium and details for differentiating it from *P. albus* (L.) GAERTN. and *P.*

paradoxus (RETZ.) BAUMG. are given in [6, 8].

Adulteration: Since the drug originates mostly from collections in the wild and often reaches commerce without being authenticated, adulteration with other *Petasites* species is possible. These can be recognized by macroscopic and microscopic examination, but more satisfactorily by means of TLC (see above).

Literature:

[1] J. Lüthy et al., Pharm. Acta Helv. **58**, 97 (1983).
[2] A. Crema, C. Milani, and L. Rovati, Il Farmaco (sci. ed.) **12**, 726 (1957).
[3] H. Aebi, T. Waaler, and J. Büchi, Pharm. Weekbl. **93**, 397 (1958).
[4] G. Hampel, Fr. M. 8,351 (Cl. A 61k. C 07 g); C.A. **79**, 61795 (1973).
[5] P. Pachaly, Dünnschichtchromatographie in der Apotheke, 2nd ed., Wissenschaftliche Verlagsgesellschaft m.b.H., Stuttgart, 1983.
[6] H. Wagner, S. Bladt, and E.M. Zgainski, Plant drug analysis, Springer-Verlag, Berlin, Heidelberg, New York, Tokyo, 1984, p. 192.
[7] Kommentar DAB 10 (Huflattichblätter).
[8] P. Rohdewald, G. Rücker, and K.-W. Glombitza, Apothekengerechte Prüfvorschriften, Deutscher Apothekerverlag, Stuttgart, 1986, p. 779.
[9] J. Westendorf, in P.A.G.M. de Smet, K. Keller, R. Hänsel, and R.F. Chandler (eds.) Adverse effects of herbal drugs, Springer, Berlin, Heidelberg, New York (1992), vol. 1, pp. 212–214, 225.

Petroselini fructus   Parsley seed

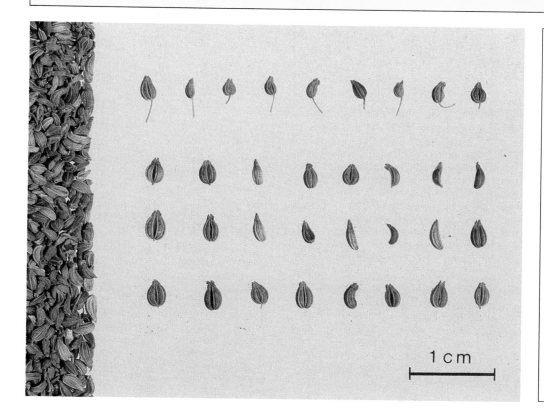

Fig. 1: Parsley seed

<u>Description:</u> The roundish, ovoid to pear-shaped, strongly laterally compressed , greenish grey to greyish brown double achenes readily split along the commisural surface to give the somewhat sickle-shaped mericarps which are up to 2 mm long and 1–2 mm broad.

Each mericarp has five, not very prominent, glabrous, straight, straw-yellow ribs; between them, there are four broad greenish grey, finely striose furrows with prominent vittae. At the base, the double achenes usually have a short, thread-like petiole and at the distal end they are tipped with the remains of the style together with the two outward curving stigmas.

<u>Odour:</u> Characteristically spicy.

<u>Taste:</u> Characteristically spicy.

Fig. 2: *Petroselinum crispum* (MILL.) A.W. HILL

A biennial umbelliferous plant, ca. 60–100 cm in height, with several times pinnately divided leaves; various cultivated forms have crispate leaves. Small greenish yellow or reddish flowers arranged in double umbels with distinct bracts and only a few foliaceous bracteoles.

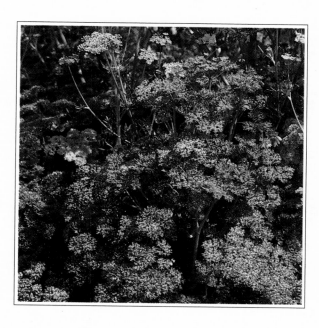

Erg. B. 6: Fructus Petroselini

Plant source: *Petroselinum crispum* (MILL.) A.W. HILL subsp. *crispum* (syn. *P. hortense* auct. non HOFFM., *P. sativum* HOFFM.), garden parsley (Apiaceae).

Synonyms: Semen Petroselini, Fructus Apii hortensis (Lat.), Parsley fruit (Engl.), Petersilienfrüchte (Ger.), Fruits de persil (Fr.).

Origin: Presumably native in the Mediterranean region; nowadays, cultivated in different races and varieties in Eurasia, North and South America, South Africa, India, Japan, and Australia. The drug comes from domestic cultivation.

Constituents: Depending on the origin and variety, 2–6% essential oil with as main components apiol, myristicin, and occasionally 1-allyl-2,3,4,5-tetramethoxybenzene. In particular chemical races, each of these compounds may represent more than 50% of the total oil [1]. Besides these phenylpropanes, there are terpenes (in some oils up

Uses

Parsley seed is used for complaints of the gastrointestinal tract and of the kidneys and urinary tract, and also to stimulate the metabolism.
The activity in the conditions indicated has not been fully substantiated.

Risks

Large doses of parsley-seed essential oil and of the phenylpropane derivative it contains, apiol, bring about vascular congestion and increased contractility of the smooth muscle of the bladder, intestines, and especially the uterus.
Parsley seed and oil are therefore often used to bring about abortion.
After taking parsley-seed preparations, the renal epithelium is irritated or damaged; cardiac arrhythmias have also been described.
Largish doses of apiol can lead to fatty liver, emaciation, extensive mucosal bleeding, and inflammatory haemorrhagic infiltration of the gastrointestinal tract, haemoglobinuria, methaemoglobinuria, and anuria.
In animal experiments, myristicin, which is present in the essential oil, has been shown to be bound to mouse-liver DNA. No hepatocancerogenic effects have been observed with either myristicin or apiol.
The toxicological risk of aqueous extracts from parsley seeds is less, because of the smaller essential-oil content.

Evaluation

Since the activity of parsley seed and its preparations has not been substantiated, in view of the risks their therapeutic use cannot be endorsed.

Apiol   Myristicin   Allyltetramethoxybenzene

to 50% α- and β-pinene, among other mono- and sesquiterpenes) [2]. Further, ca. 20% fixed oil, flavonoids (including apiin) and traces of furanocoumarins (e.g. bergapten) [3].

Indications: The drug is used as a powerful diuretic, the action being traced to the irritant (stimulant) action of the essential oil and flavonoids on the renal parenchyma [4, 5].
The apiol and myristicin content of parsley seed causes them to act as a spasmolytic and oxytocic, so that the drug is also used in *folk medicine* to treat dysmenorrhoea and menstrual problems; it is employed additionally in *folk medicine* as an emmenagogue, galactagogue, and stomachic, and externally against head lice [3]. The essential oil finds use in the food industry as an aroma component in meat, sauces, and liqueurs.

Side effects: In higher doses, pure apiol acts as an abortifacient through pelvic congestion [4, 5]. Ingestion of larger amounts of the essential oil gives rise initially to central stimulation then perhaps to a narcotic state (effect of the hallucinogenic myristicin?). In

addition, the essential oil in large doses irritates the gastrointestinal tract and the kidneys. Indications of damage to the hepatic parenchyma and cardiac arrhythmias due to overdoses of apiol is given in [3]. However that may be, with normal use of the drug, intoxication will not arise. The occasional severe polyneuritis with symmetrical paresis of the hands, feet, and ankles that used to arise from apiol abuse were traced to contamination with tricresyl phosphate [4, 5].

Making the tea: Not very usual, since the drug is rarely used on its own, but mostly in combination with other diuretic drugs.
Immediately before use, 1 g of the drug is crushed; boiling water poured over it and after 5–10 min. passed through a tea strainer. A cupful is drunk two or three times a day.
1 Teaspoon = ca. 1.4 g.

Phytomedicines: The drug is a component of diuretic teas, as well as laxative and "slimming" teas; in the form of an extract, it is included in prepared diuretic remedies.

Authentication: Macro- (see: Description) and microscopically. See also [6]. The exocarp and mesocarp have large calcium-oxalate clusters (up to 10 μm in diameter); the mesocarp has thin-walled, tangentially elongated parenchyma cells; the endocarp consists of elongated brown cells. The vittae, up to 200 μm wide, are overlayed with transverse cells which are ca. 120 μm long and up to 10 μm broad. The endosperm cells contain fixed oil and aleurone grains in which well-formed calcium-oxalate rosettes, 2–6 μm in diameter, are present.
The TLC identification, which is based on the detection of the phenylpropanes, is as follows [7]:

Test solution: steam distillate (volatile oil) diluted 1:10 with toluene.

Reference solution: eugenol and apiol, 3% in toluene.

Loadings: 5 μl test solution and 3 μl reference solution, as bands on silica gel 60F$_{254}$;

smaller amounts of the reference compounds give decreased Rf values.

Solvent system: toluene + ethyl acetate (93 + 7), 15 cm run.

Detection: sprayed with 5% ethanolic sulphuric acid, followed immediately by 1% ethanolic vanillin, and observed while being heated at 110 °C for 10 min.

Evaluation: in daylight. Reference solution: violet-brown zone at Rf ca. 0.5 (eugenol) and brown-violet zone at Rf ca. 0.75 (apiol). Test solution: two main brown-violet zones at Rf ca. 0.75 and 0.8 (apiol and myristicin), together with weaker violet-brown zones in the intermediate Rf region (eugenol or eugenol methyl ether and allyltetramethoxybenzene).
In most oils, myristicin and apiol are present in roughly equal amounts; but in other oils, one or other may be predominant and, occasionally, allyltetramethoxybenzene is the main constituent. Sometimes, a zone due to safrole can be detected above the myristicin zone [7].

Adulteration: Scarcely ever occurs in practice, as the drug originates from cultivated material.

Storage: Protected from light and moisture in well-closed containers. The drug should not be stored in powdered form.

Literature:
[1] E. Stahl and H. Jork, Arch. Pharm. (Weinheim) **297**, 273 (1964).
[2] V. Formácek and K.-H. Kubeczka, Essential oil analysis by capillary gas chromatography and carbon-13 NMR spectroscopy, Wiley, Chichester, 1982.
[3] Hager, vol. **6**, p. 542 (1977).
[4] H. Braun and D. Frohne, Heilpflanzenlexikon für Ärtze und Apotheker, Gustav Fischer Verlag, Stuttgart – New York, 1987.
[5] R.F. Weiß, Herbal Medicine, Arcanum, Gothenburg, and Beaconsfield Publishers, Beaconsfield, 1988.
[6] B.P. Jackson and D.W. Snowdon, Atlas of microscopy of medicinal plants, culinary herbs and spices, Belhaven Press, London, 1990, p. 174.
[7] H. Wagner, S. Bladt, and E.M. Zgainski, Plant drug analysis, Springer-Verlag, Berlin, Heidelberg, New York, Tokyo, 1984, p. 28.

Petroselini radix   Parsley root, Petroselinum (BHP 1983)

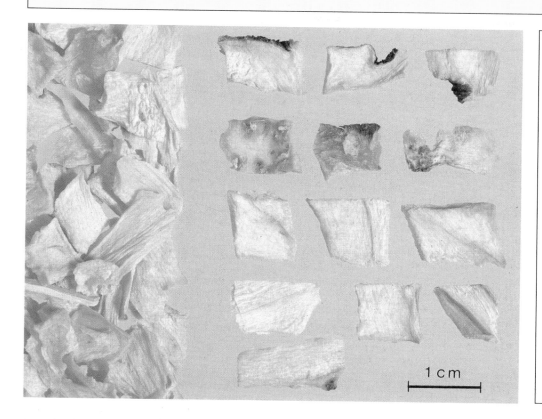

Figs. 1 and 2: Parsley root

<u>Description</u>: The whole drug consists of mostly longitudinally sliced, usually 15 cm long and ca. 2 cm thick, roots. They are somewhat twisted, yellowish white to reddish yellow, coarsely wrinkled and in the upper part transversely ringed. The fracture is sharp and rather uneven. The cut drug is characterized by yellowish white to reddish yellow pieces of root with a coarsely wrinkled surface and in places fine, brownish transverse rings. On the transverse surface of the broken surface, the broad dirty white cortex and the dark brown line of the cambium are clearly set off against the outer lemon-yellow and inner white xylem. In the bark, dark brown, shiny oil ducts are visible and the xylem especially is radially striate with brown medullary rays.

<u>Odour</u>: Characteristically aromatic.

<u>Taste</u>: Sweetish and somewhat pungent.

For illustrations of the plant source, see under: Petroselini fructus (Parsley seed)

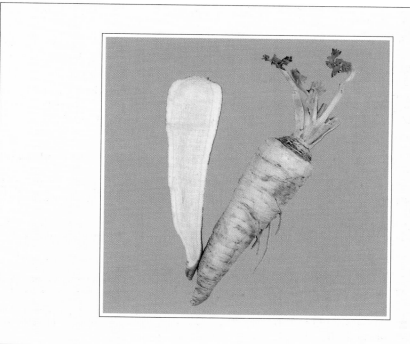

Erg. B. 6: Radix Petroselini

Plant source: *Petroselinum crispum* (MILL.) A.W. HILL subsp. *tuberosum* (BERNH. ex RCHB.) Soó, garden parsley (Apiaceae).

Synonyms: Radix Apii hortensis (Lat.), Petersilienwurzel, Wurzelpetersilie (Ger.), Racine de persil (Fr.).

Origin: Exclusively from plants cultivated as a vegetable and spice. The drug is produced in Germany and is also imported from Hungary and former Czechoslovakia.

Constituents: Up to 0.5% essential oil, with apiol and myristicin as the main components; in addition, flavonoids, e.g. apiin, polyynes, including falcarinol, furanocoumarins, among them bergapten, isoimperatorin [1, 2], and oxypeucedanin [3].

Indications: Like parlsey seeds, as a diuretic, but somewhat milder in action.

Bergapten R = —OCH₃

Isoimperatorin R =

Oxypeucedanin R =

Apiol R = —OCH₃
Myristicin R = —H

$H_2C=CH-CH_2-(C\equiv C)_2-CH_2-CH=CH-(CH_2)_6-CH_3$

Falcarinol

Extract from the German Commission E monograph (BAnz no. 43, dated 02.03.89)

Uses

For irrigation in disorders of the urinary tract. Irrigation therapy for the prevention and treatment of kidney gravel.

Contraindications

Pregnancy, inflammatory disorders of the kidneys.
Warning: No irrigation therapy in cases of impaired cardiac or renal activity.

Side effects

In rare cases, allergic reactions of the skin and mucous membranes may occur.
People with a light skin, especially, may suffer phototoxic reactions.

Interactions with other remedies

None known.

Dosage

Unless otherwise prescribed: daily dose, 6 g drug; preparations correspondingly.

Mode of administration

Comminuted drug for infusions and other galenical preparations with a comparably small essential-oil content for internal use.

Warning: Because of its toxicity, the pure essential oil should not be used.
In irrigation therapy, an adequate fluid intake must be ensured.

In *folk medicine,* it is used in the same way as parsley seeds (q.v.).

Making the tea: Boiling water is poured over 2 g of the finely chopped drug, covered, and allowed to stand for 10–15 min. before being strained. As a mild diuretic, two or three cups of the infusion are drunk in the course of the day.
1 Teaspoon = ca. 2 g.

Phytomedicines: Parsley root is an infrequent component of bladder and kidney teas.

Authentication: Macro- (see: Description) and microscopically. The periderm consists of only a few layers of suberinized cells. The broad cortex contains secretory canals with a narrow lumen, which are more frequent in the inner part of the cortex. Vessels are present in radial rows and fibres are absent. The parenchyma contains very small starch grains. See also the BHP 1983.

Quantitative standards: Erg. B. 6: *Ash,* not more than 6%.

BHP 1983: *Total ash,* not more than 8%. *Acid-insoluble ash,* not more than 1%.
Note: The BHP 1990 monograph deals with Petroselini herba (Parlsey herb).

Adulteration: In the drug trade, adulteration with the roots of *Pastinaca sativa* L., wild parsnip, is not infrequently observed. Wild turnip root has a very homogeneous and broad xylem which takes up more than half the diameter of the root; simple or paired starch grains are absent.
Parsley-root bark is stained red with iron(II) sulphate solution; that of the wild turnip is not affected.
Notes: A TLC system that will differentiate parsley root from wild-turnip root, and that will enable wild-turnip root admixtures in batches of parsley root to be recognized, has not yet been developed. This is due partly to the fact that at present morphologically very different races and types of parsley root are on the market and partly to the fact that in the two drugs there are varying amounts of myristicin. Finally, it should be noted that the essential-oil content in the parsley with large roots that is cultivated nowadays is very low – often below 0.1% [4]. (The former AB-DDR specified an essential-oil content of not less than 0.3%.)

Storage: Protected from light and moisture, in well-closed containers (not made of plastic).

Literature:
[1] Kommentar DAB 7-DDR.
[2] Hager, vol. **6**, p. 543 (1977).
[3] S.K. Chaudhury et al., Planta Med. **52**, 462 (1986).
[4] D. Warncke, personal communication (1987).

Phaseoli pericarpium   Kidney-bean pods (without seeds)

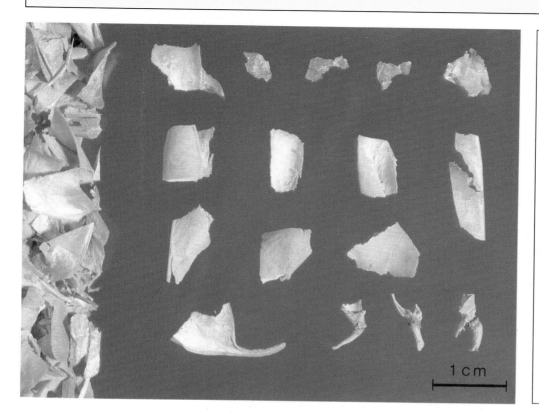

1 cm

Fig. 1: Kidney-bean pods

<u>Description</u>: The drug consists of the fruit walls freed from the seeds. The material is in the form of yellowish white, somewhat curled, thin pieces of the up to 15 cm long fruit wall. The outside surface is pale yellow and slightly wrinkled, while the inside is covered with a whitish, shiny membrane (endocarp + inner mesocarp layers). Occasionally, yellow fragments of the stalks are present.

<u>Taste</u>: Somewhat mucilaginous.

Fig. 2: *Phaseolus vulgaris* L.

A twining (up to 4 m in height) or low bushy annual, with ternate leaves and white, pale pink, or violet flowers. The illustration shows leaves, flowers, and unripe fruit.

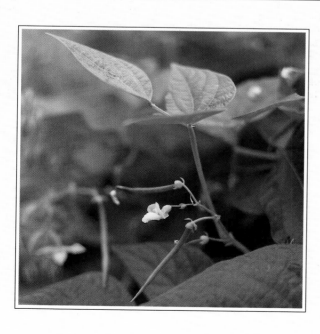

DAC 1986: Bohnenhülsen
St. Zul.: 8499.99.99 (Samenfreie Gartenbohnenhülsen)

Plant origin: *Phaseolus vulgaris* L., kidney, French, or haricot bean (Fabaceae).

Synonyms: Fructus phaseoli sine semine (Lat.), Bohnenhülsen, Schminkbohne (Ger.), Gousses d'haricot (Fr.).

Origin: An ancient cultivated plant. The drug comes entirely from cultivated plants grown in various European countries: Bulgaria, Hungary, the former USSR, former Yugoslavia.

Constituents: Numerous substances of ubiquitous occurrence are mentioned in the literature, of which up to now arginine and silicic acid have been thought perhaps to be responsible for the antidiabetic action.
Recently, the content of chromium salts has been seen as possibly significant in regard to the antidiabetic activity [2].

Indications: Used *only in folk medicine* as a diuretic and weak antidiabetic. Older indi-

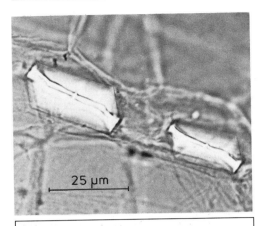

Fig. 3: Calcium-oxalate prisms with characteristic diagonal structure, from the innermost mesocarp layer of *Phaseolus*

cations of glucokinin-like constituents have so far not been confirmed. The discovery that the trace element chromium is present in the glucose tolerance factor has led to the testing of medicinal plants recommended for the treatment of diabetes mellitus type II, and it has been found that bean pods also contain a notable amount – ca. 1 ppm [2].
It is known that insulin is not effective in rats fed on a chromium-poor diet. Whether the chromium content of the bean pods is essential for the (weak) antidiabetic action requires further investigation [2].
Hence, from the point of view of current medicinal-plant research, the inclusion of the drug in the numerous herbal mixtures and phytomedicines still remains problematical. This applies to the use both as a so-called antidiabetic and as a diuretic.

Making the tea: Boiling water is poured over 2.5 g of the drug, covered, and after 10–15 min., strained.
1 Teaspoon = ca. 1.5 g, 1 tablespoon = ca. 2.5 g.

Herbal preparations: The drug is also put up in tea bags (mostly 2 g); it is a component of the bladder and kidney tea NRF 9.1.

Phytomedicines: Bean pods are present in many bladder and kidney teas, but also in prepared remedies with the same indications; in addition, also in "antidiabetics".

Among the products available in the UK is Arkocaps Phytoskin (capsules).

Authentication: Macro- (see: Description) and microscopically. The exocarp has a strongly wrinkled cuticle, roundish stomata, and cicatrices. In the outer layers, the mesocarp consists of short, spindle-shaped, thickened cells. The crystals located in the inner layers of the mesocarp are a conspicuous feature (Fig. 3).

Quantitative standards: DAC 1986: *Water-soluble extractive*, not less than 12.0%. *Foreign matter*, not more than 4% seed fragments and not more than 2% other foreign matter. *Ash*, not more than 8.0%.

Adulteration: Rarely occurs.

Literature:
[1] Lj. Kraus and G. Reher, Dtsch. Apoth. Ztg. **122**, 2357 (1982).
[2] A. Müller, E. Diemann, and P. Sassenberg, Naturwissenschaften **75**, 155 (1988).

Pimpinellae radix Burnet-saxifrage root

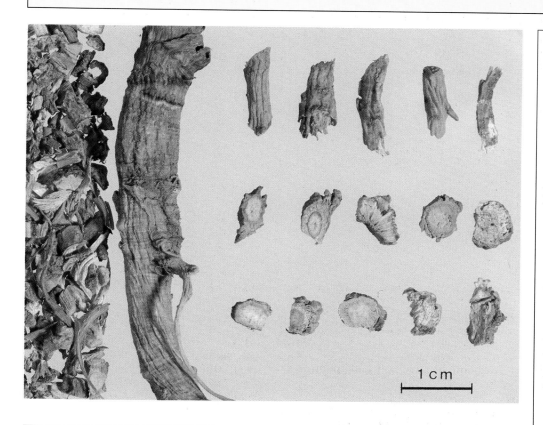

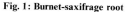

Fig. 1: Burnet-saxifrage root

<u>Description:</u> The yellowish brown to greyish yellow pieces of root are finely wrinkled longitudinally but ringed horizontally. The transverse surface shows a light yellow periderm and a broad, brownish white bark which is somewhat spongy and fissured towards the outside and which also has numerous very small, brownish yellow secretory canals (recognizable with a hand lens, Fig. 3). The relatively narrow xylem tissue inside the dark brown cambial zone is yellow and radially striate (hand lens). Rhizome fragments also have pith. The fracture may be slightly fibrous.

<u>Odour:</u> Aromatic and spicy.

<u>Taste:</u> At first spicy, then pungent, but not bitter.

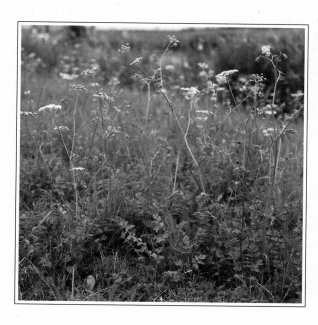

Fig. 2: *Pimpinella major* (L.) HUDS.

An up to 1 m tall shrub, with an angular stem and simple pinnate leaves. Double umbels mostly without bracts or bracteoles. Fruit glabrous.

Plant sources: *Pimpinella major* (L.) HUDS., greater burnet-saxifrage, and *P. saxifraga* L., burnet-saxifrage (Apiaceae).
Warning: Not to be confused with *Sanguisorba minor* SCOP., greater burnet (Rosaceae), which is used as a spice in salads!

Synonyms: Radix Pimpernellae albae, hircinae, saxifragae, majoris or minoris (Lat.), Bibernellwurzel, Pimpernellwurzel, Pfefferwurzel, Bockwurzel (Ger.), Racine de boucage (Fr.).

Origin: Throughout almost the whole of Europe and western Asia; introduced into North America and naturalized. The drug comes principally from the wild and is therefore very often confused or adulterated (see: Adulteration); the drug is mainly imported from former Yugoslavia.

Constituents: Ca. 0.4–0.6% essential oil, containing, among other things, geijerene, pregeijerene, β-bisabolene, 1,4-dimethylazulene, and as principal components the tiglic or 2-methylbutyric acid esters of epoxypseudoisoeugenol (not epoxyisoeugenol ester; revision of the structure in [1, 2]). According to [1], the isobutyric ester reported in [2] does not occur, but is a constituent of the oil of *Pimpinella peregrina* L. (see: Adulteration); polyacetylenes; coumarins and furanocoumarins: umbelliferone, bergapten, xanthotoxin (structures, see: Angelicae radix), scopoletin, sphondin, isobergapten, pimpinellin, and isopimpinellin (especially the furanocoumarins only in traces). Further, sitosterol and caffeic, quinic, and chlorogenic acids. Ca. 1% saponins (?), tannins.

Indications: Burnet-saxifrage root is used as an antitussive and mild expectorant in bronchitis (secretomotor and -lytic actions) as well as for infections of the upper respiratory tract (hoarseness, pharyngitis, tracheitis, angina), The action is ascribed to the essential oil and to the so far unconfirmed presence of saponins; investigations with these constituents of the drug have not yet been carried out. Infusions or tinctures of the drug are employed as a gargle for inflammation of the mouth and throat.
The epoxypseudoisoeugenol esters have insecticidal and acaricidal activity and they also inhibit plant growth [8].
In *folk medicine,* the drug is also sometimes taken as a stomachic and diuretic. It is used in preparing spirits. Alcoholic extracts are a component of some mouthwashes.

Epoxypseuodoisoeugenol ester
R = Tigloyl or 2-methylbutyryl

Isobergapten: R^1 = OCH$_3$, R^2 = H
Pimpinellin: R^1 = H,   R^2 = OCH$_3$
Isopimpinellin: R^1 = OCH$_3$, R^2 = OCH$_3$

Pregeijerene

Geijerene

Sphondin

Making the tea: Boiling water is poured over 3–10 g of the very finely cut drug; adding cold water and briefly boiling is also customary. As a cough remedy, a cup is taken three or four times a day, sweetened with honey.
1 Teaspoon = ca. 2.5 g.

Phytomedicines: Burnet-saxifrage root or extracts made from it are components of bronchial remedies, e.g. Melrosum®, etc., arthritis remedies, and remedies for the circulation, e.g. Befelka®-Tinktur.

Authentication: Macroscopically, including odour and taste, and microscopically. The round starch grains are ca. 4–8 µm in diameter and the secretory canals are less than 120 µm wide. Disclosure of adulteration, which according to [1] is nevertheless problematical for *P. peregrina*, is possible through TLC of the coumarins [3]; the method is carried out as indicated in the monograph on Angelicae radix:

Evaluation: in UV 366 nm light. Burnet-saxifrage root extract: an intense blue fluorescent base-line zone and five to maximally eight fainter blue or blue-green fluorescent zones between Rf 0.1 and 0.65 (Angelicae radix: Fig. 3); more strongly fluorescent zones in the upper part of the chromatogram point to adulteration with the root of *Heracleum sphondylium*.
TLC of the coumarins from the roots of Apiaceae is dealt with in [4, 5].

Quantitative standard: *Ash*, not more than 6.5%.

Adulteration: Extremely frequent; sometimes, the genuine drug is unobtainable. Most often, it is adulterated with hogweed or cow parsnip root (from *Heracleum sphondylium* L.), which is known in commerce as Radix Pimpinellae franconiae, with wild parsnip root (from *Pastinaca sativa* L.), and with the roots of other *Pimpinella* species. In

---

Extract from the German Commission E monograph
(BAnz no. 101, dated 01. 06. 90)

Uses
Catarrh of the upper respiratory tract.

Contraindications
None known.

Side effects
None known.

Interactions with other remedies
None known.

Dosage
Unless otherwise prescribed: daily dose, 6–12 g drug; 6–15 ml burnet-saxifrage tincture (1 : 5).

Mode of administration
Comminuted drug for infusions and other galenical preparations for internal use.

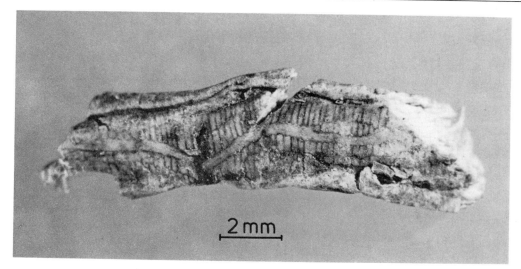

Fig. 3: Fragment of *Pimpinella major* root, showing the transparent, yellowish brown, secretory canals

recent years, *Pimpinella peregrina* L., which originates from southern Europe, Asia Minor, and Egypt, is being increasingly cultivated in southern Germany and is being offered as Radix Pimpinellae DAB 6. The composition of the essential oil and coumarins of *P. peregrina* and *P. saxifraga*, as well as *P. major*, is extremely similar, so that according to [1] admission of the cultivated *P. peregrina* as an additional source of the drug is worth considering. A decision as to which species is present can only be made with certainty through GC of the essential oil.

The roots of *P. peregrina* have a whitish to light brown bark (*P. saxifraga*, a dark brown bark), and the upper part of fully developed roots has a diameter greater than 2 cm (*P. saxifraga* and *P. major*, not more than 1.5 cm). Proof of adulteration can be established macro- and microscopically [7] and also by means of TLC (see: Authentication). See further, the monograph of Angelicae radix (Fig. 3).

Storage: Protected from light, in well-closed containers (not made of plastic). The drug is readily attacked by insects.

Literature
[1] K.-H. Kubeczka and I. Bohn, Dtsch. Apoth. Ztg. **125**, 399 (1985).
[2] R. Martin, J. Reichling, and H. Becker, Planta Med. **51**, 198 (1985).
[3] H. Wagner, S. Bladt, and E.M. Zgainski, Plant drug analysis, Springer-Verlag, Berlin, Heidelberg, New York, Tokyo, 1984, p. 152.
[4] L. Hörhammer, H. Wagner, and D. Kraemer-Heydweiller, Dtsch. Apoth. Ztg. **106**, 267 (1966).
[5] O.-B. Genius, Dtsch. Apoth. Ztg. **121**, 386 (1981).
[6] K.-H. Kubeczka, I. Bohn, and V. Formácek, in: Essential oil research, E.-J. Brunke (ed.), de Gruyter, Berlin – New York, p. 279 (1986).
[7] Berger, vol. **5**, p. 332 (1960).
[8] J. Reichling, B. Merkel, and P. Hofmeister, J. Nat. Prod. **54**, 1416 (1991).

Plantaginis lanceolatae folium
Plantain leaf

Plantaginis lanceolatae herba
(DAB 10), Plantain herb

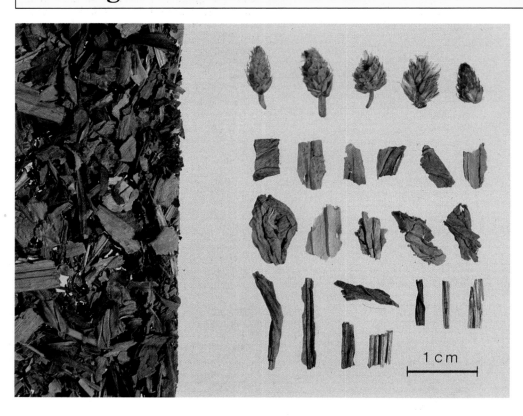

Fig. 1: Plantain herb

<u>Description:</u> The light to greyish green, glabrous or sparsely pubescent, pieces of leaf have almost parallel (Fig. 3) whitish green nerves that are prominent on the lower surface. Longitudinally grooved, green to brownish black fragments of petiole and fragments of the brown, cylindrical flowering spike with its crowded, membranaceous bracts are also present (top row, Fig. 1)

<u>Taste:</u> Mucilaginous, somewhat bitter and salty.

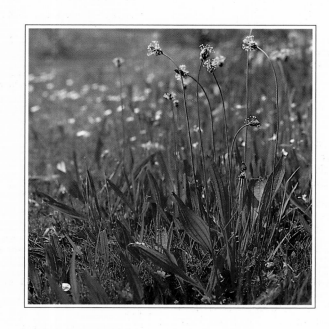

Fig. 2: *Plantago lanceolata* L.

A widely distributed perennial with a basal rosette of leaves 20 cm long and linear-lanceolate and with parallel venation. Insignificant brownish flowers appearing in cylindrical spikes on long, ridged, stalks overtopping the leaves. Conspicuous projecting, yellowish white stamens.

DAB 10: Spitzwegerichkraut
ÖAB: Folium Plantaginis
Ph. Helv. VII: Plantaginis folium
St. Zul. 1289.99.99

Plant source: *Plantago lanceolata* L., ribwort plantain (Plantaginaceae).

Synonyms: Ribwort (Engl.), Spitzwegerich-blätter or -kraut, Heil- or Wundwegerich (Ger.), Feuilles (Herbe) de plantain, Psyllium blond d'Allemagne (Fr.).

Origin: Distributed throughout Europe and northern and central Asia. The drug is derived mainly from cultivated plants and only partly from the wild. Imports come from Bulgaria, the former USSR, former Yugoslavia, Romania, Hungary, Poland, and the Netherlands. It is also grown in the eastern part of Germany.

Constituents: Iridoid glycosides, including 0.3–2.5% aucubin (= rhinanthin) and 0.3–1.1% catalpol and asperuloside [1]. The au-cubin content as determined by HPLC is almost half as much as that determined pho-tometrically, e.g. in six samples 1.16–1.21% as against 2.03–2.21% [2]. (After hydrolysis, aucubin is converted into dark brown poly-mers, which are responsible for the dark colour of drug material that has been care-lessly dried.) Ca. 6.5% mucilage, comprising at least four polysaccharides: probably a rhamnogalacturonan, an arabinogalactan, and a glucomannan [3]. Tannins, phenolic carboxylic acids: *p*-hydroxybenzoic, proto-catechuic, and gentisic acids, etc.; chloro-genic and neochlorogenic acids. The cou-marin aesculetin. Flavonoids, among them apigenin, luteolin, and scutellarein. Over 1% silicic acid. Inorganic substances with a high proportion of zinc and potassium. The oc-

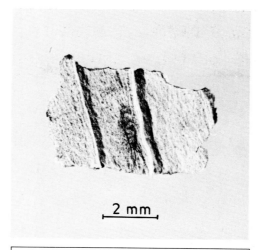

Fig. 3: Leaf fragment, showing the quasi-parallel ve-nation

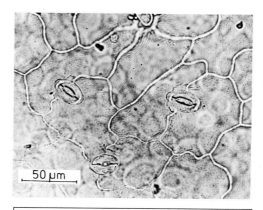

Fig. 4: Diacytic stomata (centre), immediately next to an anomocytic one (below)

currence of saponins is controversial. Ac-cording to newer studies, a haemolytically and antimicrobially active saponin is present in the leaves [4].

Indications: Plantain herb is used to allevi-ate irritation in catarrh of the upper respira-tory tract (effect of the mucilage and also of the tannin).
Macerates, fluid extracts, syrups, press juice from the fresh plant, and pastilles are all used for treating inflammation of the mouth and throat.
Aqueous extracts prepared in the cold, fluid extracts, and the press juice have been shown to have *in-vitro* bacteriostatic and

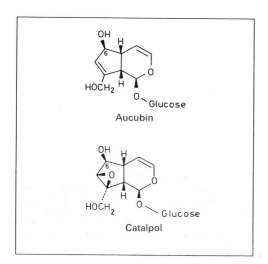

Aucubin

Catalpol

bactericidal activity, while aqueous infu-sions and decoctions are inactive [5, 6]. The antibacterial action is due to the aglycone, aucubigenin, which is liberated from aucu-bin by the β-glucosidase present in the plant, or to a degradation product derived from it; the polymerizates are inactive. In boiling the drug with water, the β-glucosidase is dena-tured by the heating, and the hydrolysis of aucubin thereby prevented. 1 ml of a 2% aqueous solution of aucubin together with β-glucosidase has the same activity against *Staphylococcus aureus* as 600 I.U. penicillin. When making the tea, the major part of the aucubin goes into the aqueous extract and a cupful (1.5 g drug, 150 ml water) contains ca. 14 mg aucubin [2].
Decocts of plantain leaves after i.v. adminis-tration in mice induced interferon formation [7].
Aucubin has very low toxicity and is said to have hepatoprotective activity (chloroform, α-amanitin) [8].
In *folk medicine*, the press juice of the fresh herb is applied externally as a wound-heal-ing and inflammation-inhibiting remedy (antibacterial activity, tannins). An ointment prepared from the dried leaves (10% leaf powder) is used in the same way [9]. The drug is also considered to be a haemostyptic [10].
Note: The BHP 1983 has a monograph enti-tled Plantago major, which deals with the leaves of the plant, said to have diuretic and antihaemorrhagic actions.

Extract from the German Commission E monograph
(BAnz no. 223, dated 30. 11. 1985)

Uses
Internally: catarrh of the respiratory passages; in-flammation of the mucous membranes of the mouth and throat.
Externally: inflamed skin.

Contraindications
None known.

Side effects
None known.

Interactions with other remedies
None known.

Dosage
Unless otherwise prescribed: average daily dose, 3–6 g drug; preparations correspondingly.

Mode of administration
Chopped drug and other galenical preparations for internal and external use.

Effects
Soothing, astringent, antibacterial.

Side effects: None, when used as prescribed. Pure aucubin when administered internally is said to cause gastroenteritis and symptoms of central paralysis.

Making the tea: Boiling water is poured over 2–4 g of the chopped drug (or cold water can be used and brought to the boil for a short while) and after 10 min. passed through a tea strainer.
1 Teaspoon = ca. 0.7 g.

Herbal preparations: The drug is also available in tea bags (0.9 g). Extracts of the drug are a component of instant antitussive teas, e.g. Bronchostad®.

Phytomedicines: The drug or extracts prepared from it are a component of many prepared antitussives and expectorants (ca. 25) and bronchospasmolytics (2).

Authentication: Macro- (see: Description) and microscopically. In surface view, both epidermises have sinuous polygonal cells with stomata surrounded by two to four subsidiary cells, the majority having two subsidiary cells oriented at right angles to the opening (diacytic, Fig. 4). The cuticle is often coarsely striated. The "jointed" trichomes are characteristic (Fig. 5) and occur particularly on the nerves and at the margin of the leaves. "Jointed" trichomes with a second (or more) cell(s) overlapping the previous one like a joint or claw are less numerous. Often, these trichomes are broken off at the "joint" (Fig. 5). There are, in addition, 35–40 µm long trichomes with a unicellular stalk and a head consisting of several rows of small cells (Fig. 6), as well as very long, thin-walled, frequently twisted, covering trichomes which often have partially collapsed cells.
An assured differentiation from *P. major* L., greater or rat-tail plantain, and *P. media* L., hoary plantain, is only possible on the basis of the morphological and anatomical fea-

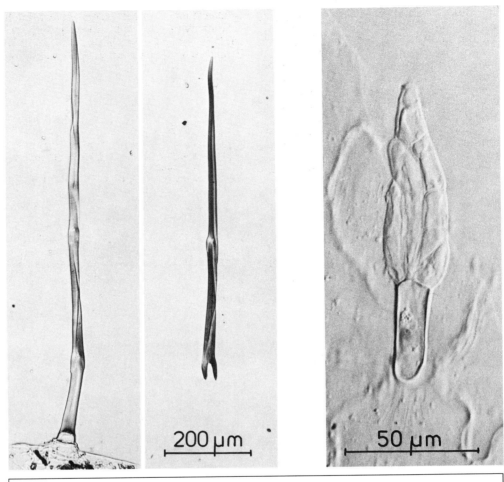

Fig. 5: Trichome, the individual cells of which are "jointed" (right, the lower cells separated)

Fig. 6: A pointed multicellular glandular trichome

tures [see 13], since the species all contain aucubin.
Nevertheless, the DAB 10 includes the following TLC identification test:

Test solution: 0.5 g powdered drug shaken for 5 min. with 5 ml methanol on the water-bath at 65 °C and, after cooling, filtered.

Reference solution: 5 mg Naphthol Yellow dissolved in 1.0 ml methanol.

Loadings: 20 µl test solution and 10 µl reference solution, as 2-cm bands on silica gel H.

Solvent system: water + 98% acetic acid + ethyl acetate (20 + 20 + 60), 10 cm run.

Detection: Sprayed with freshly prepared dimethylaminobenzaldehyde solution (0.2 g dissolved without warming in a mixture of 4.5 ml water and 5.5 ml 36% hydrochloric acid) and heated at 100–105 °C for 10 min. while under observation.

Evaluation: In daylight. Test solution: in the lower half, at about the same level as the yellow reference zone, the strong aucubin zone slowly changing through brownish grey to bluish grey; a few, mostly similarly coloured zones also present; at the solvent front, a narrow, dark chlorophyll zone.
In [11, cf. 12], the solvent system is: *n*-propanol + toluene + glacial acetic acid + water (25 + 20 + 10 + 10), with aucubin as reference substance and benzidine as the detecting agent. The chromatogram is illustrated in [11]; aucubin appears as a brown zone at Rf ca. 0.35.

Quantitative standards: Herba − <u>DAB 10</u>: *Swelling index*, not less than 6. *Foreign matter*, not more than 5% dark to very dark brown fragments; not more than 2% other foreign matter. *Loss on drying*, not more than 10.0%. *Ash*, not more than 15.0%.
Folium − <u>ÖAB</u>: *Foreign matter*, not more than 3%. *Ash*, not more than 12.0%. *Acid-insoluble ash*, not more than 1.5%.
<u>Ph. Helv. VII</u>: *Water-soluble extractive*, not less than 30%. *Foreign matter*, not more than 3%; discoloured and brown leaves, not more than 10%. *Sulphated ash*, not more than 16.0%.

Adulteration: Very rare. Occasionally, adulteration with the similar looking leaves of *Digitalis lanata* used to happen, but is readily detected by microscopical examination (cf. the Ph. Helv. VII).

Literature:
[1] A. Bianco et al., J. Nat. Prod. **47**, 901 (1984).
[2] H. Miething, W. Holz and R. Hänsel, Pharm. Ztg. **131**, 746 (1986).
[3] M. Bräutigam and G. Franz, Planta Med. **51**, 293 (1985); Dtsch. Apoth. Ztg. **125**, 58 (1985).
[4] D. Tarle, J. Petričič and M. Kupinič, Farm. Glas. **37**, 351 (1981); C.A. **96**, 40797 (1982).
[5] J. Ehlich, Dtsch. Apoth. Ztg. **106**, 428 (1960).
[6] M. Felklowá, Pharm. Zentralhalle **97**, 61 (1958).
[7] J. Plachcinska et al., Fitoterapia **55**, 346 (1984).
[8] I.M. Chang, H.S. Yun and K.H. Yan, Yakhak Hoechi **28**, 35 (1984); C.A. **101**, 163663 (1984).
[9] R.K. Aliew, J. Amer. pharm. Assoc., Sci. Ed. **39**, 24 (1950).
[10] E. Keeser, Dtsch. med. Wschr. **65**, 375 (1939).
[11] H. Wagner, S. Bladt, and E.M. Zgainski, Plant drug analysis, Springer-Verlag, Berlin, Heidelberg, New York, Tokyo, 1984, p. 136.
[12] P. Rohdewald, G. Rücker and K.W. Glombitza, Apothekengerechte Prüfvorschriften. Deutscher Apotheker-Verlag Stuttgart 1986, S. 993.
[13] W. Schier, Dtsch. Apoth. Ztg. **130**, 1457 (1990).

Plantaginis ovatae semen

(DAB 10), Plantago seed (USP XXII, partly),
Plantago ovata (BHP 1983)

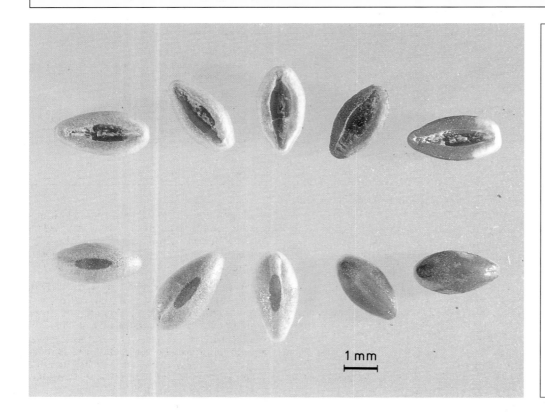

Description: The oval, boat-shaped, 1.5–3.5 mm long seeds vary considerably in colour – from pale pink to greyish brown and even reddish yellow. On the convex surface, there is a reddish brown oval fleck (lower row), while the concave surface is grooved and has a distinct scar (hilum; upper row). When placed in water, the seeds swell rapidly and become surrounded by a colourless, transparent layer of mucilage.

Taste: Bland and mucilaginous.

Fig. 2: *Plantago ovata* Forssk.

A low annual herb with a very soft and short pubescence. Leaves linear and flowers grouped in very short spikes.

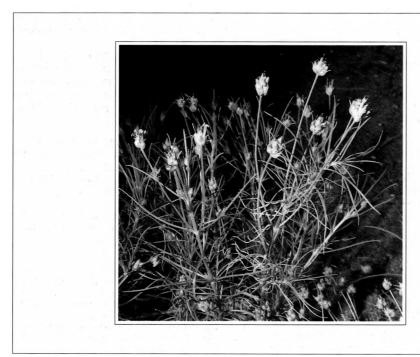

DAB 10: Flohsamen, Indische
St. Zul. 1549.99.99

Plant source: *Plantago ovata* Forssk. (syn. *P. ispaghula* Roxb.) (Plantaginaceae).

Synonyms: Semen ispaghulae (Lat.), Ispaghula seed, Spogel seeds, Isfagul, Pale psyllium seeds, Blond or Indian psyllium, Indian Plantago seed (Engl.), Indische Flohsamen, Indisches Psyllium (Ger.), Ispagul (Fr.).

Origin: Native in Iran and India; cultivated there and in neighbouring countries. The drug is imported from India, Pakistan, and Iran.

Constituents: 20–30% mucilage which is located only in the epidermis of the testa. It consists of up to 85% weakly acidic arabinoxylans with a small proportion of rhamnose and galacturonic acid [1]. The seeds contain fixed oil, protein, and very small amounts of iridoids, such as aucubin.

Indications: The seeds are taken, together with abundant fluid, as a laxative, because

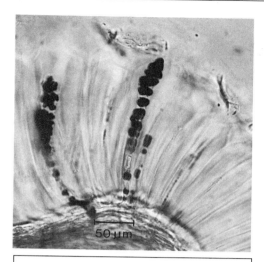

Fig. 3: Mucilaginous epidermis in transverse section, showing embedded starch grains (stained dark with iodine)

of their considerable swelling power. The dilation stimulus caused by the ensuing increased volume of the intestinal contents leads to defaecation; the mucilage facilitates the smooth passage of the intestinal contents.

The drug is contraindicated in cases of intestinal obstruction.

The repeatedly mentioned lipid-lowering effect of ispaghula seed is very slight. After an intake of 15 g drug per day over a period of two weeks, the decrease in the serum cholesterol level was less than 5% [2].

Making the tea: Not applicable. As a laxative, ca. 10 g drug is pre-swollen with ca. 100 ml water and, after being taken, is followed by drinking at least 200 ml water; it is taken morning and evening.
1 Teaspoon = ca. 4.7 g.

Herbal preparations: Among the multi-ingredient products available in the UK are: Potter's Cleansing Herb and Gerard House Priory Cleansing Herbs.

Phytomedicines: Some prepared laxatives contain only ispaghula seed or the testa, e.g. Metamucil®, Agiocur®-Granulat, Bio-Bekunis®-Granulat, etc.; some preparations contain in addition standardized senna-fruit extracts, e.g. Agiolax®-Granulat, Laxiplant®-Granulat, etc.

Throughout the English-speaking world, there is a large number of proprietary preparations containing ispaghula seed or testa; among those on the UK market are: Colven®, Fybogel® (granules in sachets), Isogel® (granules), Manevac® (granules), Metamucil® (oral powder; also in the USA), Regulan® (oral powder in sachets), etc.

Regulatory status (UK): General Sales List – Schedule 1, Table A.

Authentication: Macro- and microscopically, following the DAB 10. The most important criterion of quality is the swelling number, which must be at least 9. In practice, with good quality drugs higher values are observed, mostly between 11 and 14. Unlike plantain seed, ispaghula seed contain a scattering of starch grains in the epidermis (Fig. 3). See also [3].

Note: The BP 1988 (and BHP 1/1990) monograph is on Ispaghula husk (*BAN*; the epidermis and collapsed adjacent layers removed from the ripe seeds of *P. ovata*; Plantaginis ovatae testa).

Note: The USP XXII includes the seeds of *Plantago ovata*, *P. psyllium* L. (Psyllii semen, q.v.), and *P. indica* auct. (syn. *P. arenaria*

WALDST. et KIT.) (Psyllii semen, q.v.) all under the monograph entitled "Plantago seed". **Note:** Plantaginis ovatae semen is the subject of an ESCOP proposal for a European harmonized monograph.

Quantitative standards: DAB 10: *Swelling index*, not less than 9. *Foreign matter*, not more than 3%. *Loss on drying*, not more than 10.0%. *Ash*, not more than 4.0%.
USP XXII: *Water absorption*, equivalent to a swelling index of not less than ca. 10. *Foreign organic matter*, not more than 0.50%. *Total ash*, not more than 4.0%. *Acid-insoluble ash*, not more than 1.0%.
BHP 1983: *Absorbency*, equivalent to a swelling index of not less than ca. 12. *Foreign organic matter*, not more than 3%. *Total ash*, not more than 6%. *Acid-insoluble ash*, not more than 3%.
Ispaghula husk – BP 1988 (and BHP 1/1990): *Swelling power*, 1 g in 90 ml water for 24 hours, made up to 100 ml and stood for 5 hours, volume of mucilage not less than 40 ml. *Loss on drying*, not more than 12.0%. *Ash*, not more than 4.5%.

Adulteration: Occasionally, the seeds of other *Plantago* species, e.g. *P. major* L., greater or rat-tail plantain, and *P. media* L., hoary plantain, are seen; their colour is different and the seeds swell very little in water.

Storage: Protected from light. The comminuted drug should not be kept longer than 24 hours.

Literature:
[1] J.F. Kennedy, J. Singh, and D.A.T. Southgate, Carbohydrate Res. **75**, 265 (1979); C.A. **91**, 135932 (1979).
[2] A.N. Howard and J. Marks, Arterioscler. Brain Dis. **1983**, 203; C.A. **100**, 67113 (1984).
[3] B.P. Jackson and D.W. Snowdon, Atlas of microscopy of medicinal plants, culinary herbs and spices, Belhaven Press, London, 1990, p. 136.

Polygalae radix   Senega root (Ph. Eur. 2, BP 1988), Senega (BHP 1990)

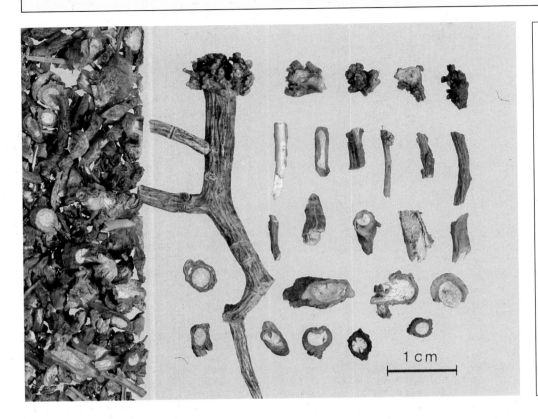

Fig. 1: Senega root

Description: The spindle-shaped, curved, or somewhat spirally twisted root is yellowish brown to dark brown; at the top, it has a broad crown on which the numerous remains of buds and broken-off bases of stems can be seen. On the inside of the curve, there is a keeled swelling (which is no longer recognizable in the soaked drug) and, on the outside, transverse folds. The transverse section shows a white phloem and a yellow xylem which, opposite the keeled side, is flattened or appears as if wedges have been cut out of it (broad wedge-shaped medullary rays) (Fig. 3). The fracture is cartilaginous and uneven.

Odour: Characteristic, mostly somewhat "rancid" or reminiscent of methyl salicylate.

Taste: Slightly harsh and somewhat pungent.

DAB 10: Senegawurzel
ÖAB: Radix Senegae
Ph. Helv. VII: Polygalae radix

Plant sources: *Polygala senega* L. (Polygalaceae). The Ph. Eur. 2 monograph allows certain other (unnamed) related *Polygala* species or a mixture of species. According to the Kommentar DAB 10 [4], the species concerned is primarily *P. tenuifolia* WILLD., Japanese Senega, which comes from temperate Asia (India and Japan). See also below, under: Adulteration.

Synonyms: Radix Polygalae senegae (Lat.), (Seneca) Snake root (Engl.), Senegawurzel, Klapperschlangenwurzel, Virginische Schlangenwurzel (Ger.), Racine de sénéga, Racine de Polygala (Fr.).

Origin: Native in the forests of North America; the drug is imported from India, Japan, Canada, and the USA.

Constituents: 6–12% saponins, a mixture of triterpene glycosides (senegasaponins A-D) with presenegenin as the main sapogenin

(the haemolytic index of the drug is ca. 3000–5000); ca. 5% lipids; various mono- and oligosaccharides, including 1,5-anhydro-D-glucitol and its derivatives; methyl salicylate and its glucoside; traces of essential oil.

Indications: Because of its saponin content, as an expectorant in bronchitis with the production of thick or little sputum, in catarrh of the respiratory tract and emphysema.

On i.p. administration in rats, the saponins isolated from the plant cause an increase in the ACTH, corticosterone, and glucose blood levels [1].

Side effects: Only on overdosage: nausea, diarrhoea, stomach upsets, dizziness.

Making the tea: 0.5 g of the finely chopped or coarsely powdered drug is placed in cold water, slowly brought to the boil, and after 10 min. poured through a tea strainer. As a

---

Extract from the German Commission E monograph (BAnz no. 50, dated 13. 03. 1986)

Uses
Catarrh of the upper respiratory tract.

Contraindications
None known.

Side effects
Gastrointestinal irritation on prolonged use.

Interactions with other remedies
None known.

Dosage
Unless otherwise prescribed: daily dose, 1.5–3.0 g drug, 1.5–3 g fluid extract (as in the Erg. B. 6), 2.5–7.5 g tincture (as in the Erg. B. 6); preparations correspondingly.

Mode of administration
Chopped drug for decoctions and other galenical preparations for internal use.

Effects
Secretolytic, expectorant.

secretolytic, a cup is drunk two or three times a day – in serious cases every 2 hours, but then the possible occurrence of side effects should be borne in mind.
1 Teaspoon = ca. 2.5 g.

Phytomedicines: As the fluid extract or dry extract, a component of some prepared antitussives.
An extract of the drug is a component of the UK multi-ingredient liquid preparation Potter's Chest Mixture, for example.

Regulatory status (UK): General Sales List – Schedule 1, Table A.

Authentication: Macro- (see: Description) and microscopically. See also [5]. The drug does not contain starch or calcium-oxalate crystals; stone cells and phloem fibres are also absent, but in the parenchyma of the cortex there are oil droplets. In the xylem, there are numerous thin-walled tracheids with slit-shaped pits, lignified vessels up to 60 μm in diameter, and some lignified parenchyma cells.
After pouring boiling water on to 0.1 g powdered drug and cooling, the solution on shaking gives a stable foam.
The Ph. Eur. 2 TLC examination for purity is as follows:

Test solution: 1.0 g powdered drug refluxed for 15 min. with 10 ml 70% ethanol, then filtered and cooled.

Reference solution: 10 mg aescin dissolved in 10 ml 70% ethanol.

Loadings: 10 μl test solution and 10 and 40 μl reference solution, as 2-cm bands on silica gel G.

Solvent system: upper phase of: 98% acetic acid + water + butan-1-ol (10+40+50), 12 cm run.

Detection and Evaluation: dried at 100–105 °C and sprayed with anisaldehyde reagent and again heated at 100–105 °C till the red saponin bands are visible. Test solu-

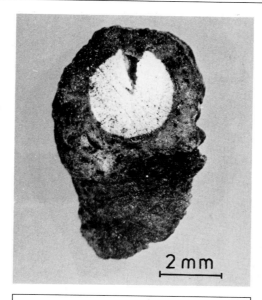

2 mm

Fig. 3: **Transverse surface of the root, showing the keel-like ridge (bottom) and on the opposite side a wedge-shaped sector cut out of the xylem (top)**

tion: in the lower and middle Rf range, 3–5 red zones at about the same level as the greyish violet bands of the aescin reference solution.
Sprayed with 20% phosphomolybdic acid in anhydrous ethanol and heated at 100–105 °C till the saponin zones turn blue. Intensity and size of the test-solution zones must be in between those of the aescin zones of the two reference solutions.
See also [2–4]. Another useful method [4] uses the solvent system: chloroform + methanol + water (64+50+10), and detection with Komarowsky reagent (1 ml 50% ethanolic sulphuric acid and 10 ml 2% methanolic 4-hydroxybenzaldehyde, mixed shortly before use; after spraying, the plate is heated at 100 °C for 5–10 min. while under observation).

Quantitative standards: Ph. Eur. 2, etc., Ph. Helv. VII: *Foreign matter*, not more than 2%. *Acid-insoluble ash*, not more than 3.0%. *Sulphated ash*, not more than 8.0%.
ÖAB: *Haemolytic index*, not less than 2500. *Foreign matter*, in the powdered drug no starch grains or calcium oxalate crystals may be present. *Ash*, not more than 5.0%.
BHP 1990: Senega complies with the Ph. Eur. 2 monograph on Polygalae radix and the BP 1988 monographs on Senega Root or Powdered Senega Root.

Adulteration: Happens occasionally, mainly with the roots of other *Polygala* species; often, they can be recognized macroscopically, but with more certainty on microscopical examination (starch, crystals, stone cells, etc.). However, cf. above under: Plant sources.
The smaller roots of Southern or White Senega, which comes from the southern USA, are derived from *P. alba* NUTT. and *P. boykini* NUTT. Pakistan Senega is stated to come from *Andrachne aspera* SPRENG. (Euphorbiaceae) [6]. Syrian Senega, from *Pergularia marginata* (DC.) KITTEL (Caryophyllaceae) and Indian Senega, from *Glinus oppositifolius* (L.) A.DC. (Molluginaceae or Aizoaceae) can be recognized by their deviating chromatograms in the TLC test of identity [4].

Literature
[1] H. Yokojama. S. Hiai, H. Oura, and T. Hayashi, Yakugaku Zasshi **102**, 555 (1982); C.A. **97**, 156258 (1982).
[2] E. Stahl, Arch. Pharm. (Weinheim) **306**, 693 (1973).
[3] H. Wagner, S. Bladt, and E.M. Zgainski, Plant drug analysis, Springer-Verlag, Berlin, Heidelberg, New York, Tokyo, 1984, pp. 234, 244.
[4] Kommentar DAB 10.
[5] B. P. Jackson and D.W. Snowdon, Atlas of microscopy of medicinal plants, culinary herbs and spices, Belhaven Press, London, 1990, p. 212.
[6] W.C. Evans, Trease and Evans' Pharmacognosy, 13th ed., Baillière Tindall, London – Philadelphia – Toronto – Sydney – Tokyo, 1989, p. 498.

Polygoni avicularis herba   Knotgrass herb

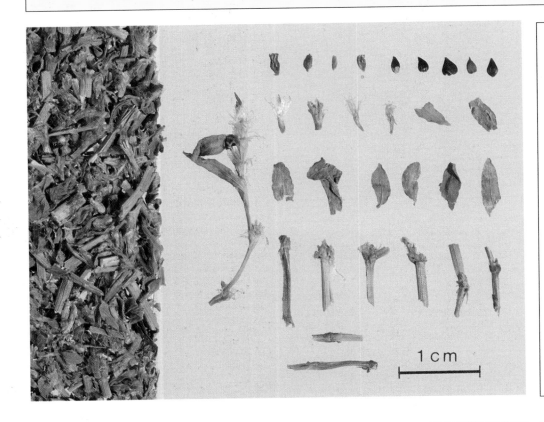

Fig. 1: Knotgrass herb

Description: The 0.5–2 mm thick, cylindrical or slightly angular, longitudinally striated stem bears sessile or short-petiolate, glabrous, entire leaves, which differ widely in shape and size according to the locality. The sheath-like stipules (ocrea), which are particularly characteristic of the drug, have the form of a lacerated membrane which is white and brown at the base. The small axillary flowers have five greenish white perianth segments, the tips of which are often coloured red. The fruits are small, brown and triangular nuts. The roots, which are always present, are thin, brownish, with occasional hair-thin lateral roots (see also Fig. 3).

Fig. 2: *Polygonum aviculare* L.

A highly polymorphous annual, widespread in fields, waste places, and along paths and roads, with prostrate, branched shoots and elliptic to narrow, ca. 3 cm long leaves with transparent ocrea. Small, greenish to reddish, axillary flowers appearing in groups of 1–5.

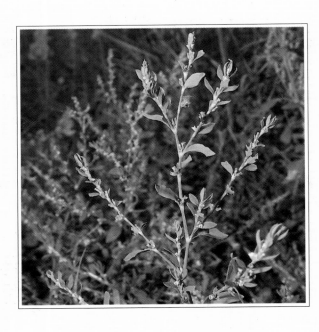

ÖAB: Herba Polygoni
Erg. B. 6: Herba Polygoni avicularis

Plant source: *Polygonum aviculare* L. s.l., knotgrass (Polygonaceae).

Synonyms: Herba Sanguinalis, Herba Centumnodii (Lat.), Vogelknöterichkraut, Blutkraut, Weidemannscher Tee, Russischer Knöterichtee (Ger.), Herbe de renouée des oiseaux (Fr.).

Origin: Cosmopolitan in the temperate zones. The drug is imported from eastern European countries: the former USSR, Hungary, Albania, Bulgaria, Poland, and former Yugoslavia.

Constituents: 0.2–1% flavonoids: derivatives of kaempferol, quercetin, and myrcetin, especially avicularin (= quercetin 3-arabinoside); mucilage, which on hydrolysis affords galacturonic acid, glucose, galactose, arabinose, and rhamnose [1]; some tannin; ca. 1% silicic acid, a small part of which is present as water-soluble silicates; phenolcarboxylic acids, coumarin derivatives (such as umbelliferone and scopoletin), as well as a number of ubiquitous plant substances.

Indications: The drug is used almost exclusively in *folk medicine* as an expectorant and secretolytic for coughs and bronchial catarrh, and further as an adjuvant in pulmonary disorders (like other silicic acid-containing drugs). as well as against night sweats in patients with tuberculosis. In *folk medicine*, the drug is also employed as a diuretic, a haemostyptic in certain kinds of bleeding, and for skin conditions.

In pharmacological experiments, knotgrass extracts have been shown to be active ACE (angiotensin converting enzyme) inhibitors, which very probably involves the tannins

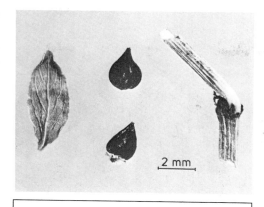

Fig. 3: Oblong-lanceolate leaflet (left), triangular brown-black nutlets (middle), and a longitudinally striated fragment of stem with a node (right)

Extract from the German Commission E monograph (BAnz no. 76, dated 23. 04. 1987)

Uses

Mild catarrh of the respiratory tract; inflammation of the mucous membranes of the mouth and throat.

Contraindications

None known.

Side effects

None known.

Interactions with other remedies

None known.

Dosage

Unless otherwise prescribed: daily dose, 4–6 g drug; preparations correspondingly.

Mode of administration

Chopped drug for infusions and other galenical preparations for internal and topical use.

Effects

Astringent, *in-vitro* ACE inhibition.

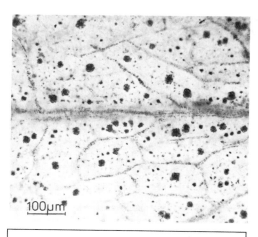

Fig. 4: Abundant occurrence of calcium-oxalate clusters (some very large) in the leaf

present [2]; conclusions regarding a possible antihypertonic effect cannot be drawn from these *in-vitro* experiments. The flavonoid fraction of the drug inhibits thrombocyte aggregation, presumably through an effect on cyclo-oxygenase [3].

Making the tea: 1.5 g of the chopped drug is put into cold water, heated to boiling, and after 10 min. strained. As an adjuvant for coughs and bronchial catarrh, a cup of the tea is drunk three to five times a day.
1 Teaspoon = ca. 1.4 g.

Phytomedicines: The drug is included in several cough teas and bronchial teas; extracts of it are a component of a few prepared antitussives, e.g. Tussiflorin® Hustensaft (juice), diuretics, etc.

Authentication: Macro- (see: Description) and microscopically. In the mesophyll of the leaves, and in the stems, there are numerous, partly very large, clusters crystals of calcium oxalate (Fig. 4). On warming with conc. potassium hydroxide solution, the epidermis of the leaves and a few cells of the mesophyll stain red to reddish violet. Leaf fragments are stained almost black with iron(III) chloride solution.

Quantitative standards: Erg. B. 6: *Ash*, not more than 10%.
ÖAB: *Foreign matter*, not more than 1%. *Ash*, not more than 8.0%.

Adulteration: In practice, does not occur.

Literature:
[1] A.I. Yakovlev, G.I. Churilov and A.I. Ginak, Khim Prir. Soedin **1985**, 619; C.A. **104**, 85430 (1986).
[2] J. Inokuchi et al., Chem. Pharm. Bull. **33**, 264 (1985); C.A. **102**, 197701 (1985).
[3] A.G. Panosyan a.a. Khim.-Farm. Zh. **20**, 190 (1986); C.A. **104**, 199798 (1986).

Primulae flos   Primula (BHP 1983)

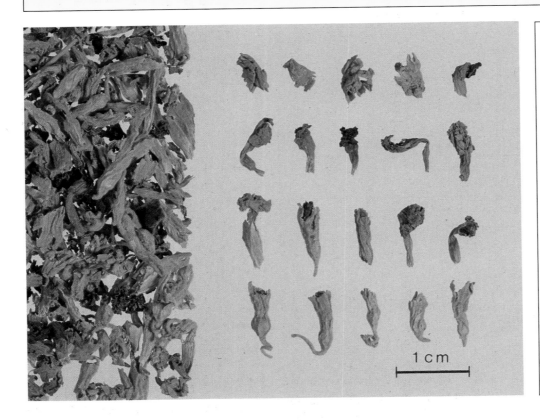

1 cm

Fig. 1: Primula flower

Description: The drug consists of either the entire flowers or only of the petals, stamens, and ovaries (Flores primulae sine calycibus); this latter drug is little used and must be declared ("without the calyx"). The ca. 15 mm long corolla tube is light yellow to brownish yellow with a lemon-yellow margin; it terminates in five obcordate lobes (the shape can only be seen after soaking in water), which have an orange-yellow spot at the base that fades on drying. The margin and lobes of the corolla may be partly green in colour (see: Authentication). The calyx is greenish brown with five prominent ribs and short pointed teeth.

Odour: Faint, characteristic, reminiscent of honey.

Taste: Faintly sweetish.

Fig. 2: *Primula veris* L.

A ca. 20 cm tall pubescent herb, with coarsely wrinkled leaf blades of the sessile basal rosette narrowing abruptly into the petioles. Golden-yellow gamopetalous, scented flowers, with an orange-red fleck in the centre, appearing in groups of up to 30 arranged in a nodding one-sided umbel.

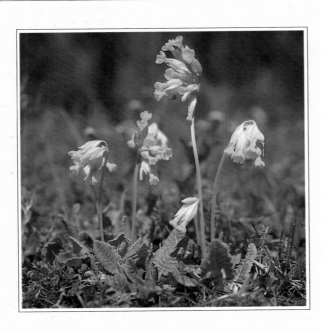

Erg. B. 6: Flores Primulae cum Calycibus
Erg. B. 6: Flores Primulae sine Calycibus
St. Zul. 1659.99.99 (Schlüsselblumenblüten)

Plant source: *Primula veris* L. (syn. *P. officinalis* (L.) HILL), cowslip; the St.Zul. also permits the flowers of *P. elatior* (L.) HILL, oxlip (Primulaceae).

Synonyms: Flores Paralyseos (Lat.), Paigle(s), Peagle (Engl.), Primelblüten, Schlüsselblumen, Aurikeln (Ger.), Fleurs de primevère officinale (Fr.).

Origin: Found throughout central and western Asia and Europe in sunny meadows and light undergrowth; in certain parts, locally absent. Drug imports come from Bulgaria, Albania, former Yugoslavia, Romania, and the former USSR.

Constituents: Small amounts of saponins, especially primula acid, mainly in the sepals (up to 2%). In the other parts of the flowers, there is almost no saponin, but instead flavonoids [1], the chief components being gossypetin, kaempferol dirhamnoside and 3-

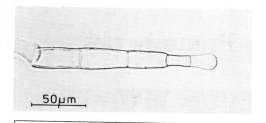

Gossypetin

Fig. 3: Covering trichome, showing the pear-shaped terminal cell

gentiotrioside, quercetin, etc.; carotenoids; traces of essential oil; enzymes (primverase).

Indications: As a mild secretolytic and expectorant for coughs, bronchitis, and colds. In *folk medicine* as a nervine for headaches, neuralgia, shaking of the limbs, as a hydrotic (sudorific, hydragogue), also as a "heart tonic" in vertigo and cardiac weakness; all these indications are empirical and without a proper foundation.

Side effects: Allergy to primulas may give rise to skin reactions. Serious overdosage may cause stomach upsets and vertigo.

Making the tea: Boiling water is poured over 2–4 g of the drug and after 10 min. passed through a tea strainer. As a bronchial tea, a cupful sweetened with honey is drunk several times a day.
1 Teaspoon = ca 1.3 g.

Phytomedicines: Primula flower is a component of some prepared antitussives, e.g. Salus® Bronchial-Tee, etc., and of so-called "blood-cleansing" and "arterial and circulation" teas.

Authentication: Macro- (see: Description) and microscopically. Among the diagnostic features are: the thickened epidermal cells of the corolla, which are finely beaded and have cuticular striations, and on the sepals covering trichomes with their pear-shaped

Extract from the German Commission E monograph (BAnz no. 122, dated 06.07.1988)

Uses
Catarrh of the respiratory tract.

Contraindications
Known allergy to primulas.

Side effects
Stomach upsets and vertigo may occasionally occur.

Interactions with other remedies
None known.

Dosage
Unless otherwise prescribed: daily dose 2–4 g drug; 2.5–7.5 g tincture (as in Erg. B. 6); preparations correspondingly.

Mode of administration
Chopped drug for infusions and other galenical preparations for internal use.

Effects
Secretolytic, expectorant.

terminal cells (Fig. 3); similar trichomes are to be found on the petals. See also the BHP 1983.
The StZul. has the following TLC test of identity:

Test solution: 1.0 g powdered drug refluxed for 15 min. with 10 ml methanol and filtered.

Reference solution: 10 mg hyperoside and 10 mg rutin dissolved in 10 ml methanol.

Loadings: 40 µl test solution and 10 µl reference solution, as 1-cm bands on silica gel HF_{254}.

Solvent system: upper phase of: ethyl acetate + glacial acetic acid + water (80 + 20 + 50), 15 cm run.

Detection: after removal of the solvent, sprayed with vanillin + antimony(III) chloride in chloroform (1 + 2 in 47).

Visualization: in UV 365 nm light. Test solution: at about the Rf of the reference hyperoside zone, two fluorescent zones; at about the level of the reference rutin zone and in the lower Rf range, further yellow coloured zones. In daylight. Test solution: in the upper Rf region below the solvent front, sometimes one or two reddish violet zones.
The flavonoids can be examined by TLC on silica gel in the solvent system: ethyl acetate + formic acid + glacial acetic acid + water (100 + 11 + 11 + 27), using diphenylboryloxyethylamine as the detecting agent. The orange fluorescent bands appearing in the lower part of the chromatogram are due to quercetin and gossypetin glycosides and the green fluorescent bands to kaempferol diglycosides and flavonol triglycosides [2].

Quantitative standards: St.Zul. 1659.99.99: *Green flowers*, not more than 30%. *Foreign matter*, not more than 2%. *Loss on drying*, not more than 12.0%. *Ash*, not more than 8.0%.
Erg. B. 6: *Green flowers*, not more than 30%. *Ash*, not more than 8% (Flores Primulae cum Calycibus) or 6% (Flores Primulae sine Calycibus).

Adulteration: As already indicated, in the Erg. B. 6 the flowers of *P. elatior* are considered an adulterant. They are sulphur yellow and do not have orange-yellow spots in the corolla tube; the calyx is not swollen as in *P. veris*; and the teeth of the sepals have long tips. The St.Zul., on the other hand, expressly permits the flowers of *P. elatior*.

Wording of the package insert, from the German Standard Licence:

6.1 Uses
As supportive treatment in promoting the secretion of phlegm and alleviation of irritation in catarrh of the upper respiratory tract.

6.2 Side effects
If used as prescribed, none known.
Warning: After contact between the skin and the flowers, in rare cases there may be hypersensitivity (allergy) in the form of reddening of the skin and the formation of small vesicles.

6.3 Dosage and Mode of administration
Boiling water (ca. 150 ml) is poured over ca. 1–2 teaspoonfuls (2–4 g) of **Primula flower** and after 10 min. passed through a tea strainer.
Unless otherwise prescribed, a cup of the infusion is drunk as hot as possible several times a day, especially in the morning after waking and at night before going to bed.

6.4 Note
Store protected from light and moisture.

Literature:
[1] J. B. Harborne, Phytochemistry **7**, 1215 (1968).
[2] H. Wagner, S. Bladt, and E.M. Zgainski, Plant drug analysis, Springer-Verlag, Berlin, Heidelberg, New York, Tokyo, 1984, p. 176.

Primulae radix   (DAB 10), Primula root

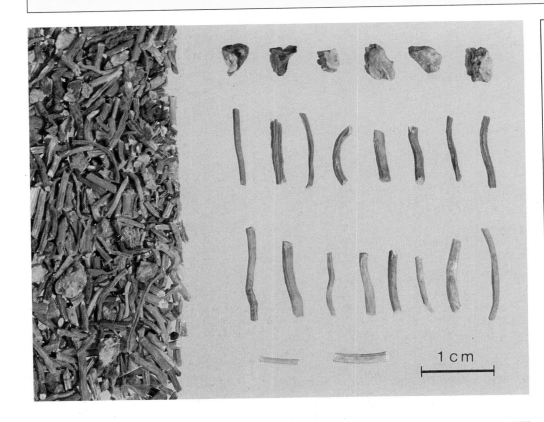

Fig. 1: Primula root

Description: The drug consists of rhizomes and roots. The 2–5 mm thick and 1–5 cm long rhizomes which are densely covered with roots, are greyish brown, tortuous, verrucose and tuberculate. The roots, which are only ca. 1 mm thick and several cm in length, are whitish yellow (*Primula veris*) or pale brown to reddish brown (*Primula elatior*), brittle, with inconspicuous longitudinal grooves.

Odour: Faint, characteristic, reminiscent of methyl salicylate (*Primula elatior*) or anise (*Primula veris*).

Taste: Obnoxiously irritating.

Care needs to be taken when powdering the drug, as the dust is highly sternutatory.

Figs. 2 and 3: *Primula elatior* (L.) HILL

The oxlip is somewhat larger than the cowslip (see: Primulae flos, Fig. 2), has almost no scent, and the inflorescences have fewer (1–20) flowers, which are pale yellow with a somewhat darker centre.

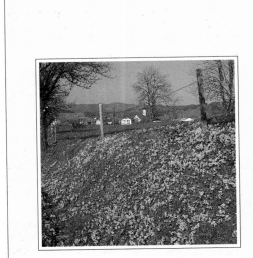

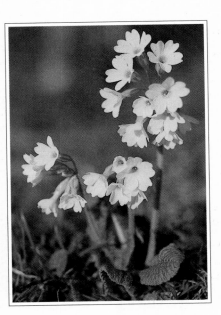

**DAB 10: Primelwurzel
ÖAB: Radix Primulae**

Plant sources: *Primula veris* L. (syn. *P. officinalis* (L.) HILL), cowslip, and *P. elatior* (L.) HILL, oxlip (Primulaceae).

Synonyms: Rhizoma Primulae, Radix Paralyseos (Lat.), Primelwurzel, Schlüsselblumenwurzel (Ger.), Racine de primevère officinale (Fr.).

Origin: Distributed in central and western Asia and Europe, but absent in certain localities. The roots of this perennial are best harvested in the third year. The drug is imported from former Yugoslavia, Turkey, and Bulgaria.

Constituents: 5–10% triterpenoid saponins (in *P. veris* derived from several, closely related aglycones, such as priverogenin A, B, etc., in *P. elatior* from protoprimulagenin A [1]); phenolic glycosides, especially primulaverin (= primulaveroside), which on enzymic degradation during drying yield the characteristic aroma substances of the plant,

Principal saponin from Primula elatior

Priverogenin A : R = -CHO
Priverogenin B : R = -CH₂OH

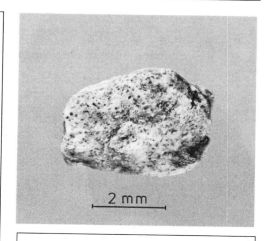

Fig. 4: Light-coloured fragment of rhizome, showing the tannin-containing idioblasts (inclusions; dark spots)

e.g. methyl 5-methoxysalicylate; rare sugars and sugar alcohols; small amounts of tannin (only in *P. veris*).

Indications: On the basis of its saponin content, as a secretomotor and secretolytic expectorant in bronchitis, catarrh of the respiratory tract, coughs, colds, and phlegm in the broncho- pulmonary system.
In *folk medicine,* primula root is also employed in whooping cough, asthma, gout, and neuralgic complaints.

Side effects: Only on overdosage: the symptoms are nausea and diarrhoea.

Making the tea: 0.2–0.5 g of the finely chopped or coarsely powdered drug is placed in cold water, heated to boiling, and after standing for 5 min. strained. As an expectorant, a cupful, sweetened with honey, is drunk every two or three hours.
1 Teaspoon = ca. 3.5 g.

Herbal preparations: Dry extracts of primula root are a component of instant expectorant teas, e.g. Solubifix® (bronchial tea), etc.

Phytomedicines: The drug is a component of some mixed herbal teas, but it is much more often used in the form of extracts (tincture, fluid extract, dry extract, syrup), combined with other drug extracts, in prepared antitussives and expectorants, e.g. Primotussan® (drops), Perdiphen®, (juice), and many more.

Authentication: Macro- and microscopically, following the DAB 10. The light-coloured pieces of rhizome when examined with a hand lens show the tannin idioblasts quite distinctly (Fig. 4). The rhizome of *Primula elatior* has yellowish green, heavily pitted stone cells in the pith. The starch grains are simple or compound, the individual grains being sack-, club-, or rod-shaped and 5–15 μm long.
The DAB 10 TLC proof of identity allows the two *Primula* species to be differentiated through the detection of their characteristic saponins [1, 2]:

Test solution: 1.0 g powdered drug refluxed for 15 min. with 10 ml 70% ethanol and filtered.

Reference solutions: a. 10 mg saponin dissolved in 1.0 ml 70% ethanol. b. 2.0 mg aescin dissolved in 0.2 ml 70% ethanol.

Loadings: 20 μl of each solution, as 2-cm bands on silica gel GF₂₅₄.

Solvent system: upper phase of: 98% acetic acid + water + butan-1-ol (10+40+50), 12 cm run.

Detection: after drying at 100–105 °C, examined in UV 254 and 365 nm light and the quenching and fluorescent zones outlined; then sprayed with anisaldehyde reagent and heated at 100–105 °C for 5–10 min. while under observation.

Evaluation: in UV 254 nm light. Reference solutions a and b: quenching zones visible. Test solution: quenching zones just below the solvent front and at about the level of the reference aescin zone and just above it.

Extract from the German Commission E monograph
(BAnz no. 122, dated 06. 07. 1988)

Uses
Catarrh of the respiratory tract.

Contraindications
None known.

Side effects
Stomach upsets and nausea may sometimes occur.

Interactions with other remedies
None known.

Dosage
Unless otherwise prescribed: daily dose, 0.5–1.5 g drug, 1.5–3 g tincture (as in ÖAB 9); preparations correspondingly.

Mode of administration
Powdered drug for infusions, cold macerates and other galenical preparations for internal use.

Effects
Secretolytic, expectorant.

In UV 365 nm light. Test solution: near the saponin zone, no pale blue to greenish fluorescent zones (admixture of *Cynanchum vincetoxicum* roots). Sprayed chromatogram. Reference solutions: a. saponin as 3 brown to brownish zones; b. aescin as a bluish violet zone. Test solution: at about the level of the reference aescin zone, a clear and prominent dark violet zone, with below it at about the level of the saponin quenching zone another similarly coloured zone; weak violet, yellowish, and brownish green zones may also be present.

Another procedure, using the solvent system: chloroform + methanol + water (64 + 50 + 10) and vanillin/sulphuric acid or antimony(III) chloride as detecting agent is described in [4].

Quantitative standards: DAB 10: *Foreign (vegetable and/or mineral) matter*, not more than 2%. *Loss on drying*, not more than 10.0%. *Ash*, not more than 11.0%.
ÖAB: *Haemolytic index*, not less than 3000. *Foreign matter*, remains of flower peduncles and leaf bases may not be present. *Ash*, not more than 8.0%.

Adulteration: The very similar looking roots and rhizomes of *Vincetoxicum hirundinaria* MEDIKUS (syn. *V. officinale* MOENCH) (Asclepiadaceae) have been encountered both in the drug trade and in practice. The roots of this (poisonous) adulterant can be recognized microscopically by the very broad xylem with diarch vascular bundles and by the abundant occurrence of numerous calcium-oxalate clusters in the parenchyma of the cortex.

In addition, *Vincetoxicum* can be detected by means of a colour reaction [3]: 0.5 g powdered drug is refluxed with 10 ml toluene for 15 min.; 0.25 ml of the filtrate is evaporated to dryness and 0.25 ml of a mixture of 5 ml conc. sulphuric acid and 0.4 ml 10.5% iron(III) chloride solution added to the residue. If *Vincetoxicum* roots are present, the solution turns weak violet and becomes bluish green in the course of the following 30 min.; the coloration is due to the presence of (toxic) steroid glycosides in *Vincetoxicum*. In the DAB 10 TLC examination (above), these steroids can be seen as light blue to greenish fluorescent zones at Rf ca. 0.1–0.35.

Literature:
[1] Kommentar, DAB 10.
[2] E. Stahl, Arch. Pharm. (Weinheim), **306**, 693 (1973).
[3] L. Langhammer, Dtsch. Apoth. Ztg. **104**, 1183 (1964).
[4] H. Wagner, S. Bladt, and E.M. Zgainski, Plant drug analysis, Springer-Verlag, Berlin, Heidelberg, New York, Tokyo, 1984, pp. 234, 236.

Pruni spinosae flos   Blackthorn flower

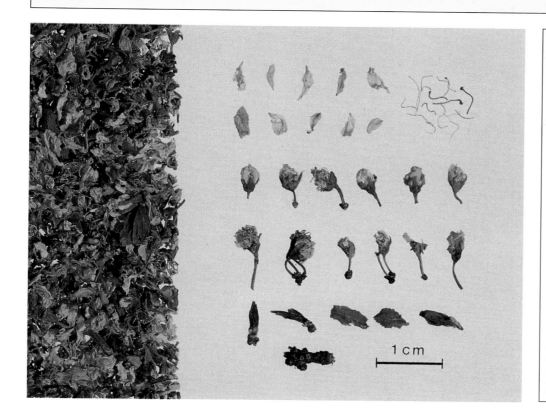

Fig. 1: Blackthorn flower

<u>Description:</u> The whole drug consists of the very small, shortly pedicellate, whitish yellow to brownish flowers; these have a small, brown hypanthium, on the upper margin of which there are five, usually 2 mm long, broadly lanceolate and entire sepals; five yellowish white, 4–6 mm long, ovate petals with a short spur; and numerous stamens with long filaments and ovoid anthers. At the base of the hypanthium, there is a unilocular ovary which has a long style and a capitate stigma.

The cut drug consists of the whole, 6–8 mm flowers, and occasional fallen, yellowish white, oval petals. Only a few cartilaginous pieces of twigs (bottom row) should be present.

<u>Taste:</u> Slightly bitter.

Fig. 2: *Prunus spinosa* L.

A much branched, thorny shrub, with a very dark coloured bark, up to 4 m in height. 5-part white flowers, ca. 10–15 mm in diameter, appearing before the 3–4 cm long, ovate, serrulate-margined, dull green leaves. Sourish and astringent, blue-black spherical fruits – one-seeded drupes.

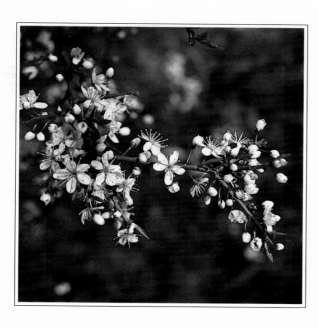

Erg. B. 6: Flores Pruni spinosae.

Plant source: *Prunus spinosa* L., blackthorn (Rosaceae).

Synonyms: Flores Acaciae germanicae or nostratis (Lat.), Schlehenblüten, Schwarzdornblüten (Ger.), Fleurs de prunellier, Fleurs d'épine noire (Fr.).

Origin: In light thickets and hedges and on sunny slopes in Europe and western Asia (absent in the north), the Caucasus and North Africa. Naturalized in North America. The drug is collected in the wild and imported from eastern and south-eastern Europe: Albania, Bulgaria, former Yugoslavia, and Hungary.

Constituents: Quercetin and kaempferol glycosides, including quercitrin, rutin, and hyperoside. Cyanogenic glycosides (amygdalin), if indeed present, are only in the fresh flowers [1]. The coumarins mentioned in many books on medicinal plants as a constituent of the plant are not recorded in the scientific literature.

Indications: Only in *folk medicine,* as a mild laxative, diuretic, diaphoretic, and expectorant. In homoeopathy, for "cardiac weakness" and "nerve pains in the head".

Note: Blackthorn fruit and leaf are also occasionally employed in *folk medicine,* e.g. the fruit juice as a gargle for inflammation of the mouth, gums, and back of the throat; blackthorn syrup and wine as a purgative and diuretic; a jam made from the fruit for a weak stomach; and the leaf, like the flower and fruit, as an astringent and diuretic.

Side effects: In normal doses, not to be expected.

Making the tea: Boiling water is poured over 1–2 heaped teaspoonfuls, allowed to stand for 5–10 min. with occasional stirring, and then strained. One or two cups during the day, or two cups in the evening, are drunk according to need.
1 Teaspoon = ca. 1.0 g.

Phytomedicines: Blackthorn flower is a component of some laxative and so-called "blood-purifying" teas, e.g. Kneipp-Abführtee; extracts of blackthorn flower are present in some expectorants, laxatives, and a few other prepared remedies.

Authentication: Macro- (see: Description) and microscopically. The epidermis of the hypanthium has a distinctly striated and crinkled cuticle (Fig. 3) and it also has unicellular, ca. 150 µm long, pointed trichomes (Fig. 4). The endothecium has solid, thickened ridges (Fig. 5). The pollen grains are spherical with a thin exine and three pores.

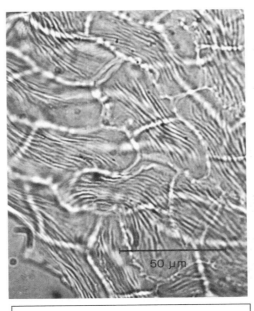

Fig. 3: Epidermis of the hypanthium, showing the sinuate, striated cuticle

Unicellular, short, conical trichomes are present on the pedicels of the flowers.
The flavonoids can be examined by TLC in the solvent system: ethyl acetate + formic acid + glacial acetic acid + water (100 + 11 + 11 + 27) and detected after spraying with diphenylboryloxyethylamine and polyethylene glycol 400; there are at least eight strong yellowish orange fluorescent zones in the Rf range 0.4–0.9 and two bluish fluorescent bands at Rf 0.5–0.6 [2].

Quantitative standard: Erg. B. 6: *Ash,* not more than 8%.

Adulteration: The drug should not be contaminated with pieces of stem, thorns, and leaf remains. Adulteration with the flowers of the bird cherry, *Prunus padus* L. (syn. *Padus avium* MILL.), as described in [1], is rare; these flowers are larger, have reflexed sepals, and on the inner epidermis of the floral axis they have many thin-walled, tubular trichomes; the teeth of the sepals have large glandular shaggy trichomes.

Storage: Protected from light and moisture; if possible, the drug should not be stored longer than a year, since it becomes dark brown and unsightly.

Literature:
[1] Hager, vol. **6**, p. 952 (1977).
[2] H. Wagner, S. Bladt, and E.M. Zgainski, Plant drug analysis, Springer-Verlag, Berlin, Heidelberg, New York, Tokyo, 1984, p. 180.

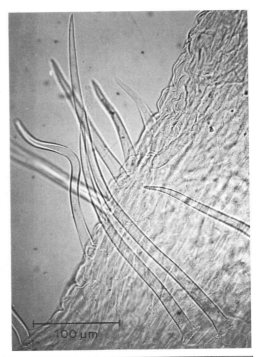

Fig. 4: Unicellular, pointed trichomes from the hypanthium

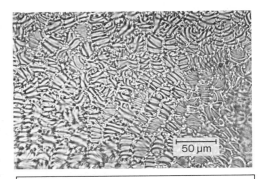

Fig. 5: Endothecium with clasp-like bands of thickening

Psyllii semen   (DAB 10), Plantago seed (USP XXII, partly), Psyllium

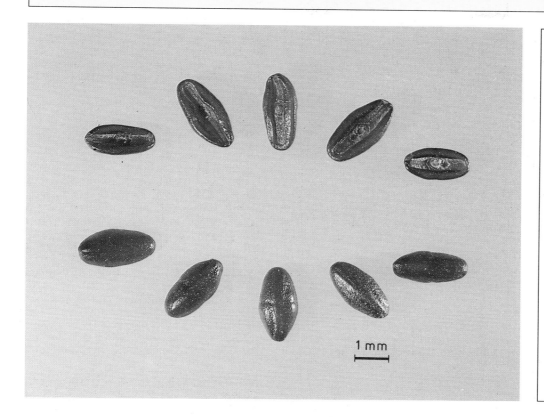

1 mm

Fig. 1: Psyllium

<u>Description:</u> The dark reddish brown, shiny, oblong-ovoid seeds are 2–3 mm long. On the convex side, there is a continuous groove, which in the middle has a paler, round scar. The seeds swell greatly in water and are soon surrounded by a colourless, transparent layer of mucilage.

<u>Taste:</u> Bland and mucilaginous.

Fig. 2: *Plantago psyllium* L.

A low, annual herb with lanceolate to narrowly linear leaves. Flowers grouped in a short spike.

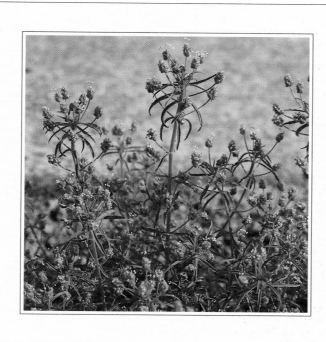

DAB 10: Flohsamen
Ph. Helv. VII: Psyllii semen
St. Zul. 1509.99.99

Plant sources: *Plantago afra* L. (syn. *P. psyllium* L. 1762 non 1753) and *P. indica* L. (syn. *P. arenaria* WALDST. et KIT.) (Plantaginaceae).

Synonyms: Semen Pulicariae (Lat.), Flea-wort seed (Engl.), Flohsamen, Heusamen (Ger.), Semences (graines) de puces (Fr.).

Origin: Native to the Mediterranean region, where it is also cultivated (especially in France). The drug is imported from France and elsewhere. in commerce, the drug is known variously as Dark, Spanish, French, Brown, or Black psyllium.

Constituents: 10–12% mucilage, which is located exclusively in the epidermis of the testa (as in the case of linseed); it is built up mainly from xylose and galacturonic acid, as well as arabinose and rhamnose. The seeds contain fixed oil, hemicellulose, protein, small amounts of iridoid glycosides, e.g. aucubin, and traces of alkaloids, e.g. plantagonine and indicaine.

Indications: As a drug capable of a considerable degree of swelling, it is taken <u>together with abundant fluid</u>, as a laxative for treating constipation. By increasing the volume of the bowel contents it brings about a dilation stimulus which leads to defaecation; at the same time, the swollen mass of mucilage facilitates the smooth passage of the bowel contents.

Psyllium is contraindicated in cases of intestinal occlusion.

Making the tea: Not applicable. As a laxative, morning and evening, ca. 10 g of the drug is pre- swollen with some water (ca. 100 ml) and this mixture is taken, and this is then followed by drinking at least 200 ml fluid.

1 Teaspoon = ca. 4.7 g.

Phytomedicines: Rarely used in Germany; more often, ispaghula seed (Plantaginis ovatae semen, q.v.) is taken. There are several prepared remedies in France and the USA containing psyllium.

Authentication: Macro- and microscopically, following the DAB 10. See also the BHP 1983.

Quantitative standards: <u>DAB 10:</u> *Swelling index*, not less than 10 (good quality drugs, mostly between 14 and 19). *Foreign vegetable and/or mineral matter*, not more than 2%. *Loss on drying*, not more than 10.0%. *Ash*, not more than 4.0%.
<u>Ph. Helv. VII:</u> *Swelling index*. not less than 10. *Foreign matter*, not more than 1% immature and green seeds and other foreign matter; neither seeds with a darkish central spot on the ridge and the cells of the external epidermis of the tegument of which swell in a 0.15% methylene blue solution only to a height of 20–45 μm (*P. lanceolata* and *P. major*) nor seeds with a light brown or greyish brown surface (*P. ovata* and *P. sempervirens*) should be present. *Loss on drying*, not more than 14.0%. *Sulphated ash*, not more than 6.0%.
<u>USP XXII:</u> *Water absorption – P. psyllium* not less than 14 and *P. indica* not less than 10. See further: Plantaginis ovatae semen.
<u>BHP 1983:</u> *Absorbency*, equivalent to a swelling index of ca. 14. *Foreign organic matter*, not more than 3%. *Total ash*, not more than 5%. *Acid-insoluble ash*, not more than 1%.

Adulteration: Very rare. Seeds of other *Plantago* species are very dark brown and light reddish brown and swell only slightly in water.

Pulmonariae herba

(DAB 10), Pulmonaria (BHP 1983), Lungwort

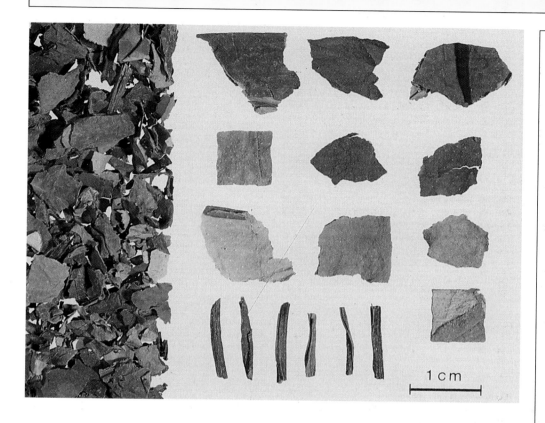

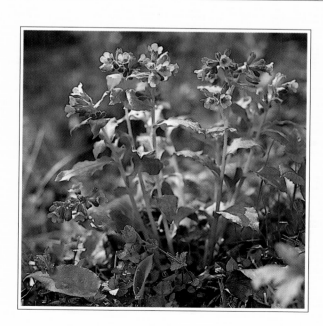

Fig. 1: Lungwort

<u>Description</u>: The chopped drug consists of mostly square cut, bristly (Fig. 3) and occasionally flecked leaf fragments which are partly loose and partly rolled up together; the lower surface is pale green and the upper surface dark green. Stem fragments with brownish black shrivelled leaf petioles and entire, brown, bristly calices, or fragments of them, may also be present.

<u>Odour</u>: Not characteristic.

<u>Taste</u>: Somewhat mucilaginous.

Fig. 2: *Pulmonaria officinalis* L.

A 20 cm tall perennial growing preferentially in deciduous woods on chalky soil. Cordate and petiolate basal leaves, often flecked with white, appearing after the end of flowering. Flower colour changing with age from light red to blue-violet.

DAB 10: Lungenkraut

Plant source: *Pulmonaria officinalis* L. (syn. *P. maculosa* (LIEBL.) GAMS), lungwort (Boraginaceae).

Synonyms: Jerusalem sage or cowslip (Engl.), Lungenkraut, Hirschmangold, Unserer-Lieben-Frauen-Milchkraut (Ger.), Pulmonaire, Herbe de pulmonaire officinale, Herbe aux poumons (Fr.).

Origin: Native in Europe. The drug is collected in the wild in south-eastern and eastern Europe, especially former Yugoslavia and Bulgaria.

Constituents: Mucilage and other carbohydrates (among them, fructans); up to 15% inorganic matter, with up to ca. 3% total silicic acid (soluble and insoluble); flavonoids, e.g. kaempferol, quercetin; allantoin (characteristic of Boraginaceae); saponins are absent [1]. The occurrence of pyrrolizidine alkaloids, some of which are hepatotoxic, is suspected [2], but detailed gas-chromatographic investigations of material from different sources has not enabled any alkaloids to be detected [3].

Indications: Although formerly much valued, nowadays the drug has scarcely any medicinal significance [4].
The drug is thus now only used in *folk medicine* for its mild soothing and expectorant properties in alleviating throat irritation; sometimes, it is also employed as a demulcent and antidiarrhoeic [1]. In an older work, the drug is described as causing an increase in diuresis [5].
As with other silicic acid-containing plants, lungwort herb was formerly used as a remedy against lung diseases (hence the name), e.g. tuberculosis. This entirely obsolete use was no doubt connected with the doctrine of signatures, since the broadly lanceolate, flecked leaves are reminiscent of human lung tissue.

Making the tea: 1.5 g of the finely chopped drug is placed in cold water and briefly boiled or boiling water is poured over it and after 10 min. passed through a tea strainer. As a bronchial tea (in folk medicine), a cupful sweetened with honey is swallowed, a mouthful at a time, several times a day.
1 Teaspoon = ca. 0.7 g.

Herbal preparations: Instant cough teas, e.g. Bronchostad®, Bronchiflux®, etc.

Extract from the German Commission E monograph
(BAnz no. 193, dated 15. 10. 1987)

Uses
Lungwort preparations are employed in complaints and disorders of the respiratory and gastrointestinal tracts, as well as the kidneys and lower urinary tract, and also as an astringent and for treating wounds. The activity of the drug in treating the conditions indicated has not been adequately demonstrated.

Hazards
None known.

Evaluation
Since the activity of lungwort preparations in the claimed applications has not been adequately substantiated, therapeutic use of the drug cannot be justified.

Phytomedicines: The drug and extracts prepared from it are components especially of cough teas or liquid antitussives.
Among the UK preparations containing an extract of lungwort is Potter's Balm of Gilead.

Authentication: Macro- (see: Description) and microscopically, following the DAB 10; see also the BHP 1983. The diagnostic features include: up to 2 mm long, unicellular bristles, more or less retort-shaped at the base and 150–170 µm broad, thick-walled, and narrowing towards the tip (Fig. 4); unicellular, less thickened, sharply conical bristles which are ca. 50 µm broad at the base and 100–200 µm long; and glandular trichomes with a 3–4-celled stalk and a club-shaped or spherical head. Almost all the leaf, flower, and stem fragments have these trichomes. Leaf fragments also have thick-walled, partly pitted epidermal cells – those on the upper surface have somewhat sinuous walls and those on the lower surface are more strongly sinuous in outline. The pollen grains are ca. 35 µm in diameter, shortly cylindrical, smooth, and have five pores arranged longitudinally. The cells of the endothecium exhibit spiral or stellate thickening.

Quantitative standards: DAB 10: *Foreign (vegetable and mineral) matter*, not more than 2%. *Loss on drying*, not more than 10%. *Ash*, not more than 20%.
BHP 1983: *Total ash*, not more than 15%.

Adulteration: The drug is sometimes adulterated with other *Pulmonaria* species, particularly *P. mollis* WULFEN ex HORNEM. A leaf of this plant, soaked in water, has a velvety feel, while a leaf of *P. officinalis* feels

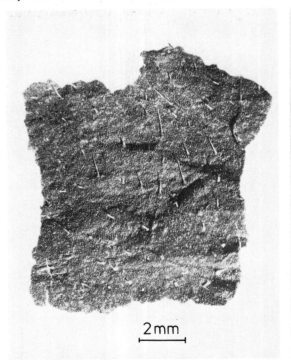

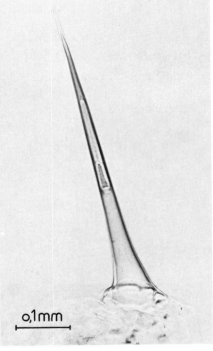

2mm

0,1mm

Fig. 3: Upper surface of *Pulmonaria officinalis* leaves, showing the bristly hairs

Fig. 4: Multicellular bristle with spherical swelling at the base

rough. The unicellular pointed bristles which are typical of the genuine drug are absent from *P. mollis* and instead there are, particularly on the rosette leaves, many 3- or 4-celled glandular trichomes with spherical or club-shaped terminal cells.
Differentiation by means of TLC is also possible:

Test solution: 2 g powdered drug refluxed for 15 min. with 10 ml methanol and, after cooling, filtered.

Reference solution: 5 mg hyperoside dissolved in 10 ml methanol.

Loadings: 4 µl test solution and 2 µl reference solution, as bands on silica gel.

Solvent system: ethyl acetate + anhydrous formic acid + water (88 + 6 + 6), 6 cm run.

Detection: after drying in a current of hot air, sprayed with 1% methanolic diphenylboryloxyethylamine, followed by 5% methanolic polyethylene glycol 400.

Evaluation: in UV 366 nm light. <u>Reference solution</u>: a yellow fluorescent zone at Rf ca. 0.4 (hyperoside). <u>Test solution</u>: at about the same Rf, a greenish rather than yellow fluorescent zone.

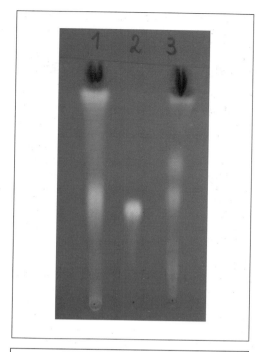

Fig. 5: TLC on 4 × 8 cm silica-gel foil

1: Lungwort
2: Hyperoside (reference compound)
3: *Pulmonaria mollis* **(adulterant)**

For details, see the text

P. mollis (an adulterant) extract: directly above the level of the hyperoside zone, a yellow to yellowish orange zone fluorescing orange in UV 366 nm light and just above that zone another, fainter, yellowish one.
The DAB 10 TLC proof of identity specifies the solvent system: ethyl acetate + anhydrous formic acid + water (84 + 8 + 8) and chlorogenic and caffeic acids as reference compounds.

Literature:
[1] Hager, vol. **6a**, p. 972 (1977).
[2] Th. Danninger, U. Hagemann, V. Schmidt, and P.S. Schönhöfer, Pharm. Ztg. **128**, 289 (1983).
[3] J. Lüthi et al., Pharm. Acta Helv. **59**, 242 (1984).
[4] R. F. Weiß, Herbal Medicine, Arcanum, Gothenburg, and Beaconsfield Publishers, Beaconsfield, 1988.
[5] R. Jaretzky, K. Breitwieser, and F. Neuwald, Arch. Pharm. (Weinheim) **276**, 552 (1938).

Quassiae lignum   Quassia (BHP 1/1990)

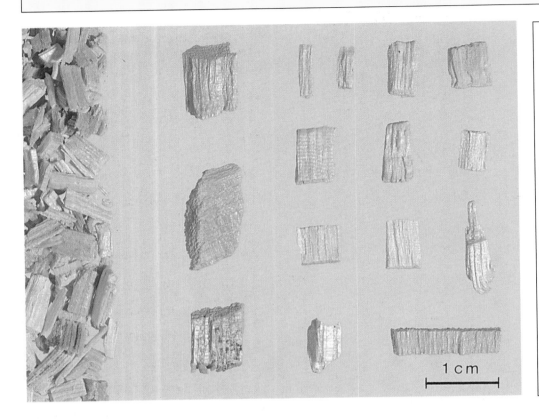

1 cm

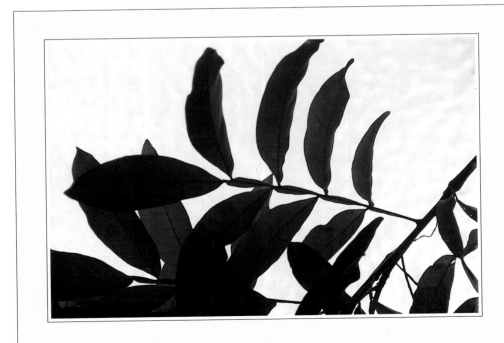

Fig. 1: Quassia

Description: The drug consists of pale yellow, fairly light, readily split pieces of wood.

Taste: Intensely bitter.

Fig. 2: *Quassia amara* L.

A 2–5 m tall bush or tree with pinnate leaves on winged rachides.

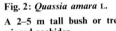

DAB 6: Lignum Quassiae

Plant sources: *Quassia amara* L., Surinam quassia, and *Picrasma excelsa* (SWEET) G. PLANCH., Jamaica quassia (Simaroubaceae).

Synonyms: Picrasma, Quassia or Bitter wood (Engl.), Bitterholz, Quassiaholz (Ger.), Bois de quassia, bois amer (Fr.).

Origin: Surinam quassia comes from Guyana, Colombia, Panama, and Argentina, while Jamaica quassia is from the Lesser Antilles, the Caribbean islands, and northern Venezuela.

Constituents: 0.05% to more than 2% bitter substances of the seco-triterpene type; the main components are quassin (bitterness value 17×10^6), neoquassin, and 18-hydroxyquassin [1, 5].
Several β-carboline alkaloids have been shown to be present [2, 5].

Indications: A now rarely used bitter, for stimulating the appetite and as a digestive. Use of the drug as an anthelmintic and insecticide is obsolete [1].

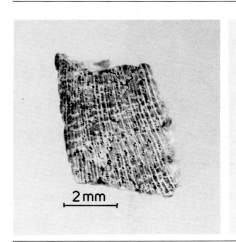

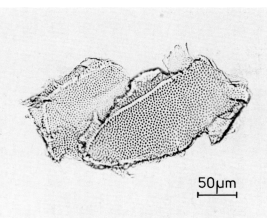

Fig. 3: Transverse section of the wood of *Quassia amara*, showing the pale narrow medullary rays and scattered large open vessels

Fig. 4: Characteristic, finely pitted fragment of a vessel wall

Side effects: Large amounts of quassia irritate the mucous membrane of the stomach and can lead to vomiting.
Administered *parenterally*, the bitter substance quassin is toxic, leading to a decrease in cardiac frequency, muscular tremors, and paralysis.

Making the tea: Boiling water is poured over 0.5 g of the finely cut or powdered quassia wood and after 10–15 min. strained; a cupful is drunk about 30 min. before meals. The drug should not be taken during pregnancy (risk of vomiting).
1 Teaspoon = ca. 2.5 g.

Phytomedicines: Quassia is a component of several prepared stomachics and cholagogues, partly as a homoeopathic mother tincture and partly as an extract, e.g. Heparcholan®; it is also present in the "alterative" Stropheupas® forte.

Authentication: Microscopically, the drug can be recognized by the presence of false annual rings (bands of parenchyma). Surinam quassia has medullary rays that are 1–2 rows of cells wide and 20–25 rows of cells high. Oxalate crystals are almost completely absent. Jamaican bitterwood has medullary rays that are 2–5 rows of cells wide, and single crystals or crystal sand is present (Figs. 3 and 4).
Note: The BHP 1/1990 monograph on Quassia deals with *Picrasma excelsa* (Jamaica quassia).
A suitable TLC procedure for examining Quassiae lignum is as follows [3]:

Test solution: 1 g powdered drug extracted for 10 min. with 10 ml methanol at 60 °C on the water-bath, filtered, and the filtrate evaporated to ca. 2 ml.

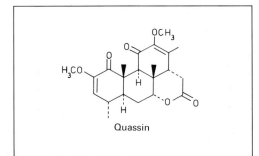

Quassin

Reference solution: 1% methanolic quassin.

Loadings: 40 µl test solution and 20 µl test solution, as bands on silica gel 60F$_{254}$.

Solvent system: chloroform + methanol (95 + 5), 15 cm run.

Detection: Liebermann-Burchard reagent (UV 365 nm light) or vanillin-sulphuric acid reagent (daylight).

Evaluation: in UV 365 nm light. Reference solution: quassin, no fluorescence. Test solution: ca. 11 weak blue and green fluorescent zones in the range Rf 0.1–1.0, belonging partly to alkaloids and coumarins. In daylight. Reference solution: quassin, a violet zone at Rf ca. 0.55. Test solution: four violet to purplish zones at Rf ca. 0.55 (quassin), 0.7, 0.95, and at the solvent front.
The BHP 1/1990 TLC procedure obtains a fingerprint chromatogram from a methanolic extract of the drug run in: chloroform + methanol (9 + 1), with quercetin as reference substance and anisaldehyde-acetic acid/-sulphuric acid as the detecting agent.

Quantitative standards: BHP 1/1990 (*Picrasma excelsa*): *Water-soluble extractive*, not less than 4%. *Foreign matter*, not more than 2%. *Total ash*, not more than 6%.
Note: The BHP 1983 required the material to comply with the BPC 1973 test for bitterness (5 g macerated with 100 ml 70% ethanol for 24 hours, filtered, and 1 ml diluted with water to 500 ml – this solution not less bitter than a 0.00002% aqueous solution of quassin).
For the quantitative determination of the bitter substances, see [4].

Adulteration: In practice does not occur.

Literature:
[1] Hager, vol. **6A**, p. 1000 (1977).
[2] P. Barbetti, G. Grandolini, G. Fardella, and I. Chiappini, Planta Med. **53**, 289 (1987).
[3] H. Wagner, S. Bladt, and E.M. Zgainski, Plant drug analysis, Springer-Verlag, Berlin, Heidelberg, New York, Tokyo, 1984, p. 134.
[4] Th. Nestler, Neue Inhaltstoffe von Lignum Quassiae und eine neue Gehaltsbestimmung der Quassia-Bitterstoffe (New constituents of Quassia wood and a new determination of the bitter substance content), Thesis, Munich (1979).

Quercus cortex Oak bark

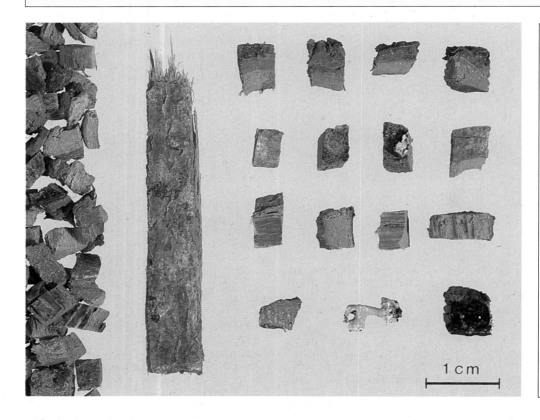

Fig. 1: Oak bark

Description: The bark is from younger branches and twigs and is up to 4 mm thick, greyish brown on the outside and often already with small areas of periderm (Fig. 4); the so-called "silver bark", which is up to 2 mm thick and has a shiny surface, is now scarcely ever found in commerce. The inner surface of oak bark is brownish red, with prominent longitudinal ridges. In the cross section, groups of stone cells can be recognized with a hand lens. The fracture is fibrous to splintery.

Odour: Tannin-like, especially after moistening.

Taste: Slightly bitter and highly astringent.

Fig. 2: *Quercus robur* L.

An up to 50 m tall tree with a huge crown, standing alone or in mixed forest. Leaves sinuate-lobate and almost sessile (difference from *Qu. petraea* (MATT.) LIEBL.). Inflorescence with a long peduncle (sessile in *Qu. petraea*).

Fig. 3: Thin branches and autumn foliage of *Quercus robur* L.

The bark of the young twigs is shiny ("silver bark").

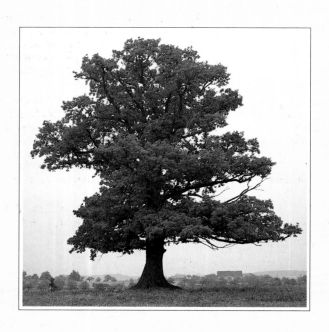

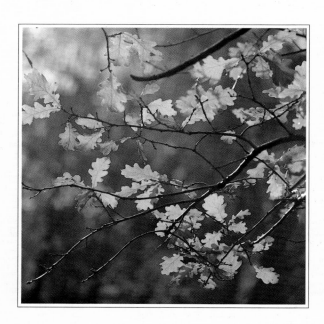

DAC 1986: Eichenrinde
ÖAB: Cortex Quercus
Ph. Helv. VII: Quercus cortex
St. Zul.: 9099.99.99

Plant sources: *Quercus robur* L. (syn. *Qu. pedunculata* EHRH.), pedunculate or common oak, and *Qu. petraea* (MATT.) LIEBL. (syn. *Qu. sessiliflora* SALISB.), sessile or durmast oak (Fagaceae).

Synonyms: Quercus, Tanner's bark (Engl.), Eichenrinde, Eichenlohe (Ger.), Écorce de chêne (Fr.).

Origin: The material comes from the eastern part of Germany and is also imported from eastern and south-eastern Europe.

Constituents: Condensed tannins: catechins, oligomeric proanthocyanidins, and to some extent ellagitannins [1]; the content is highly variable 8–20%, and depends not only on the time of harvesting and the age of the branches, but also on the method of assay employed [2, 3].

Indications: As an astringent, principally for external use (baths, poultices in chilblains, oral paints). It is sometimes employed internally in small doses as a stomachic; see: Phytomedicines.

Making the tea: 1 g of the finely cut or coarsely powdered drug is added to cold water, boiled for a short period of time, and after a few minutes passed through a tea strainer. For external use: 10% decoction.
1 Teaspoon = ca. 3 g, 1 tablespoon = ca. 6 g.

Phytomedicines: The drug is sometimes included in prepared herbal mixtures, and also

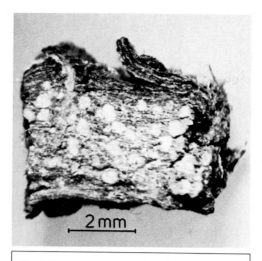

Fig. 4: Transverse broken surface of the bark of *Quercus robur*, showing the periderm and whitish groups of stone cells

in a number of prepared gastrointestinal remedies, e.g. Entero-sanol® (dragees, capsules, juice). For external use (preparation of baths), a number of firms market ready-to-use oak-bark extracts.

Authentication: Macro- (see: Description). For microscopical examination, it is convenient to scrape some material off the pieces of bark and to make a mount of the powder. The most obvious feature is the yellowish groups of fibres surrounded by a calcium-oxalate prism sheath; in addition, there are stone cells with thick, lignified walls, singly

or in groups, and often attached to the groups of fibres. Besides frequent clusters of calcium oxalate, there are also single crystals and a small quantity of small starch grains. Occasionally, scraps of periderm are encountered. The powder, as well as the cut drug, gives a dark colour with iron(III) chloride solution (tannins) and a red colour with vanillin/hydrochloric acid (catechol tannins).

Quantitative standards: DAC 1986: *Tannin*, not less than 10% precipitable with hide powder. *Foreign matter*, not more than 2%. *Ash*, not more than 6.0%.
ÖAB: *Foreign matter*, not more than 5% (fragments of cortex). *Ash*, not more than 6.0%.
Ph. Helv. VII: *Tannins*, not less than 12.0%. *Foreign matter*, not more than 1%; only a little suberized bark present and in section showing only occasional secondary formation of a suberized layer. *Sulphated ash*, not more than 8.0%.

Adulteration: Chopped thin twigs are often encountered in the drug trade [4], but because of the low tannin content of the woody tissue they are inferior. The same is true for the bark from older trunks, the drug then consisting mainly of periderm. Both can be recognized macro- and microscopically.

Storage: Protected from light and moisture. The amount of extractable tannin decreases on storage [5].

Literature:
[1] B.Z. Ahn and F. Gstirner, Arch. Pharm. (Weinheim) **304**, 666 (1971).
[2] H. Glasl, Dtsch. Apoth. Ztg. **123**, 1979 (1983).
[3] M. Luckner, O. Bessler, and P. Schröder, Pharmazie **19**, 748, 751 (1964).
[4] W. Schier, Dtsch. Apoth. Ztg. **121**, 323 (1981).
[5] C.H. Brieskorn, Pharmazie **2**, 489 (1947).

Wording of the package insert, from the German Standard Licence

6.1 Uses
Inflammation of the gums and mucous membranes of the throat, excessive sweating of the feet, supplementary treatment of chilblains and anal fissures.

6.2 Dosage and Mode of administration
For rinses and gargles, 2 tablespoonfuls of **Oak bark** in 500 ml water and for hip baths, etc., 500 g in 4–5 litres are boiled for 15–20 mins. and the liquid then poured off.
Unless otherwise prescribed, for inflammation of the mouth and throat gargle the undiluted decoction is used as a gargle several times a day. As a hip bath or foot bath, the decoction should be used at body temperature twice a day for 15–20 mins.

6.3 Note
Store away from light and moisture.

Extract from the German Commission E monograph (BAnz no. 22a, dated 01.02.90)

Uses
Externally: inflammatory skin complaints.
Internally: non-specific, acute cases of diarrhoea.
Topical treatment of mild inflammation of the mouth and throat, as well as in the genital and anal region.

Contraindications
Internally: none known.
Externally: skin damage over a large area.
Baths: independent of the particular active constituents, not to be taken in cases of
    weeping eczema and skin damage covering a large area
    febrile and infectious disorders
    cardiac insufficiency, stages III and IV (NYHA)
    hypertonia, stage IV (WHO)

Side effects
None known.

Interactions with other remedies
Externally: none known.
Internally: the absorption of alkaloids and other basic drugs may be reduced or inhibited.

Dosage
Unless otherwise prescribed:
Internally: 3 g drug; preparations correspondingly.
For lotions, poultices, and gargles: 20 g drug to 1 litre water; preparations correspondingly.
For complete or partial baths: 5 g drug to 1 litre water; preparations correspondingly.

Mode of administration
Chopped drug for decoctions and other galenical preparations for internal and topical use.

Duration of use
Should diarrhoea last for more than 3–4 days, a doctor should be consulted.
Other areas of use, not longer than 2–3 weeks.

Effects
Astringent, virostatic.

Quillajae cortex Quillaia (*BAN*; BP 1988; BHP 1990)

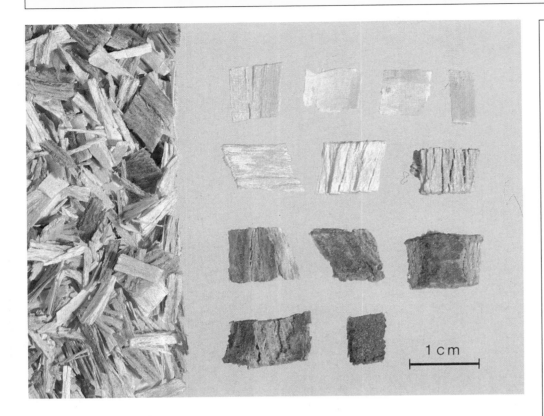

Fig. 1: Quillaja bark

<u>Description:</u> The drug consists of the stem bark freed from the cortex, in the form of flat or only slightly channelled, light pink to yellowish white, pieces; on the outside, they have coarse longitudinal striations and occasional brown patches, and the inner surface is almost entirely smooth. The fracture is fibrous and splintery, and on the surfaces of the fracture glistening crystals (prisms of calcium oxalate) can be seen with the naked eye (but better with a hand lens).

<u>Taste:</u> At first mucilaginous and sweetish, then acrid.

Warning! Inhalation of the powder causes sneezing, i.e. the powder is sternutatory.

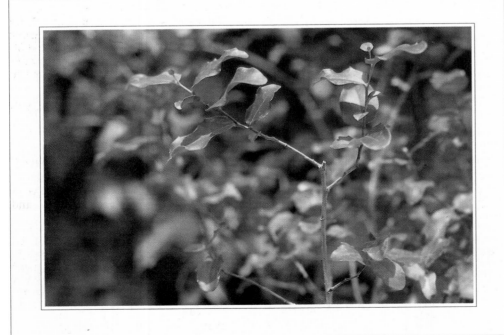

Fig. 2: *Quillaja saponaria* MOLINA

A ca. 15 m tall evergreen tree with firm, leathery leaves having an entire margin and white 5-part flowers in axillary corymbs. Five carpels partially fused at the base and forming, when the fruit is ripe, a 5-part stellate dehiscent fruit with numerous seeds.

DAC 1986: Seifenrinde
ÖAB: Cortex Quillajae
Ph. Helv. VII: Quillajae cortex

Plant source: *Quillaja saponaria* MOLINA (Rosaceae).

Synonyms: Cortex saponariae (Lat.), Quillaja, Quillaia or Soap or Quercus oak bark, Panama wood or bark (Engl.), Seifenrinde, Panama- or Waschrinde (Ger.), Écorce de quillaya, Écorce de saponaire (Fr.).

Origin: Native in Chile, Peru, and Bolivia; the drug is imported from Chile.

Constituents: ca. 10% saponins, a mixture of different triterpene glycosides with quillaic acid as the main sapogenin [8]; further, ca. 10–15% tannin; abundant calcium oxalate; starch.

Indications: Based on the saponin content, as an expectorant in respiratory complaints, but nowadays largely replaced by other drugs (Primulae radix (primrose root), Senegae radix (senega root), etc.). The drug still has a certain importance as a foaming agent in the food industry, for making hair shampoos, scalp lotions, toothpastes, and mouth washes.

In recent years, several groups have independently established that after oral administration in experimental animals the saponins of quillaja bark (like those of quillaja root) are able to reduce serum cholesterol levels [2–4]. This is ascribed to a reaction between the saponins and the bile acids, resulting in micelle formation [5] and leading to inhibition of cholesterol uptake. Quillaja saponins raise antibody production in the mouse [6], even after oral administraton; the immune response after viral infections is accelerated [7].

It remains to be seen whether in the future these findings will be of possible medical interest.

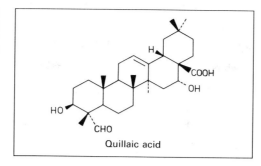

Quillaic acid

Side effects: Only to be expected with overdoses, which lead to irritation of the gastrointestinal tract with stomach pains, diarrhoea, and suchlike complaints. In animals (rats, mice) fed 0.7 g/kg/day over a period of 108 weeks, quillaja extracts were found to be non-toxic [1].

Making the tea: Nowadays not very usual. According to the ÖAB, the usual single dose is 0.2 g moderately finely chopped drug as a decoction.
1 Teaspoon = ca. 2.3 g.

Phytomedicines: Extracts of the drug are present in a very few prepared antitussive remedies.

Authentication: Macro- (see: Description) and microscopically, following the DAC 1986; see also the BP 1988 and [9]. The 2- to 5-seriate medullary rays which traverse the bark contain groups of 300–1000 µm long, strongly thickened and lignified fibres which shine in polarized light (Fig. 3). The prisms of calcium oxalate, up to more than 120 µm long, are a conspicuous feature (Fig. 4).
5 ml boiling water poured over 0.1 g drug, after cooling and shaking, gives a stable foam.
TLC proof of identity (modified from Ph. Helv. VII):

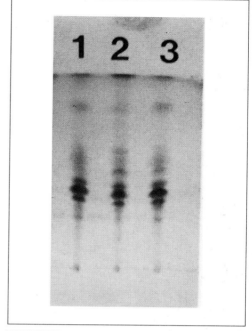

Fig. 5: TLC on 4 × 8 cm silica-gel foil
1, 2, and 3: Quillaja bark (different origins)
For details, see the text

Test solution; 1.0 g powdered drug refluxed for 30 min. with 20 ml ethanol and filtered; the filtrate concentrated, and 20 ml 7% hydrochloric acid added to the residue and refluxed for 30 min.; after cooling, the hydrolysate extracted three times with 40 ml chloroform and the combined organic phases then washed with 5 ml water and filtered over anhydrous sodium sulphate; after taking to dryness, the residue dissolved in 5 ml chloroform.

Reference solution: not applicable (according to the Ph. Helv. VII).

Loading: 5 µl test solution.

Mobile phase: chloroform + methanol (60 + 5), 5 cm run.

Detection: after evaporation of the solvent, sprayed with anisaldehyde reagent and heated to 105 °C for 3–5 min.

Evaluation: immediately in daylight. Test solution: in the middle and upper Rf range, several bluish green, bluish grey, and bluish violet zones, three in the middle range being particularly strong. The composition of individual samples may vary somewhat, depending on the provenance (Fig. 5).
The DAC 1986 TLC method makes use of the solvent system: dichloromethane +

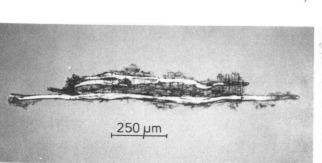

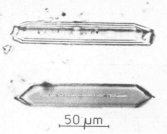

Fig. 3: Irregular, thick-walled, brightly shining fibres (polarized light)

Fig. 4: Large prisms of calcium oxalate from quillaja bark

methanol (92 + 8). TLC procedures for the analysis of the saponins rather than aglycones are to be found in [10].

Quantitative standards: <u>BP 1988</u>: 40% *ethanol-soluble extractive*, not less than 22.0%. *Acid-insoluble ash*, not more than 1.0%. *Foreign matter*, not more than 2.0%. <u>DAC 1986</u>: *Water-soluble extractive*, not less than 17.0%. *Foreign matter*, not more than 2%. *Ash*, not more than 10%. <u>ÖAB</u>: *Haemolytic index*, not less than 3000. *Foreign matter*, not more than 3%. *Ash*, not more than 10.0%

<u>Ph. Helv. VII</u>: *Haemolytic index*, at least 8 Ph. Helv. units/g. *Foreign matter*, not more than 3%. *Sulphated ash*, not more than 14.0%.

Adulteration: Rarely occurs in practice and would be easily recognized on microscopical examination.

Literature:

[1] J.P. Drake et al., Food Chem. Toxicol. **20**, 15 (1982).
[2] D.G. Oakenfull et al., Nutr. Rep. Int. **29**, 1039 (1984).
[3] G.S. Sidhu and D.G. Oakenfull, Br. J. Nutr. **55**, 643 (1986).
[4] A.V. Rao and C.W. Kendall, Food Chem. Toxicol. **24**, 441 (1986).
[5] D.G. Oakenfull, Aust. J. Chem. **39**, 1671 (1986); C.A. **105**, 221287 (1986).
[6] M.T. Scott et al., Int. Arch. Allergy Appl. Immunol. **77**, 409 (1985).
[7] I. Maharaj, K.J. Froh and J.B. Campbell, Can. J. Microbiol. **32**, 414 (1986).
[8] R. Higuchi, Y. Tokimitsu, and T. Komori, Phytochemistry **27**, 1165 (1988).
[9] B.P. Jackson and D.W. Snowdon, Atlas of microscopy of medicinal plants, culinary herbs and spices, Belhaven Press, London, 1990, p. 194.
[10] H. Wagner, S. Bladt, and E.M. Zgainski, Plant drug analysis, Springer Verlag, Berlin, Heidelberg, New York, Tokyo 1984.

Ratanhiae radix

(DAB 10, Ph. Eur. 2, etc.), Rhatany root (*BAN*; BP 1988, BHP 1/1990)

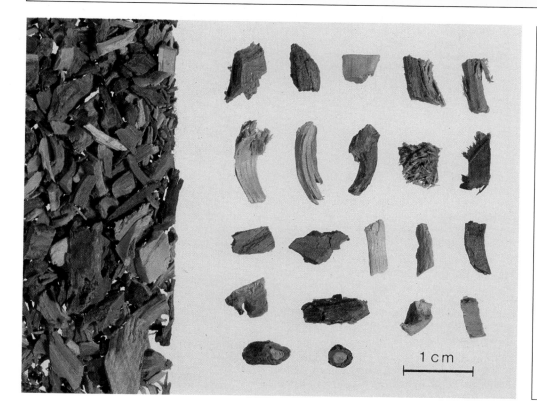

Fig. 1: Rhatany root

Description: The reddish brown, 1–3 cm thick, roots have a narrow bark which in older material is scaly and in young material smooth; it readily separates from the wood. The finely porous xylem has many narrow medullary rays, the sapwood being light brownish and the heartwood darker in colour; the fracture is fibrous on the outside and splintery on the inside.

Taste: Astringent and slightly bitter.

Fig. 2: *Krameria triandra* RUIZ et PAV.

A shrub, growing to a height of not more than 1 m, with long procumbent branches bearing closely positioned, ca. 1 cm long, oblong-ovate, silky pubescent leaves. Axillary pedicellate flowers with four pubescent sepals, grey on the outside and purple on the inside, and four purplish red petals, three stamens, and a superior ovary.

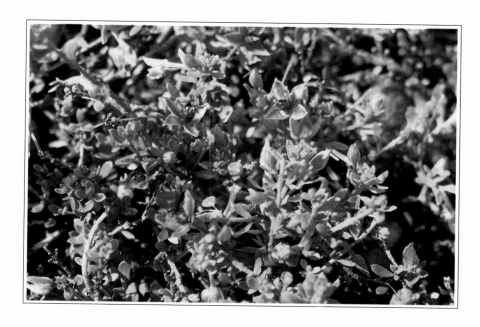

DAB 10: Ratanhiawurzel
ÖAB: Radix Ratanhiae
Ph. Helv. VII: Ratanhiae radix
St. Zul. 1179.99.99

Plant source: *Krameria triandra* RUIZ et PAV. (Krameriaceae).

Synonyms: Krameria root, Peruvian rhatany (Engl.), Rhatanhiawurzel, Rote Ratanhia, Peru- or Payta-Ratanhia (Ger.), Racine de ratanhia (Fr.).

Origin: A low undershrub native to the Bolivian and Peruvian Andes. Drug imports come from Peru and Ecuador and also from Bolivia.

Constituents [1]: Up to 15% condensed (catechol) tannins, which are localized particularly in the bark; on prolonged storage the content decreases, owing to increasing condensation of the tannins (conversion to insoluble phlobaphenes, so-called krameria red). Other constituents: lipophilic benzofuran derivatives [2], starch, sugar, *N*-methyltyrosine, etc.

Indications: On the basis of the high tannin content, as an astringent, mainly in the form of the tincture; as a gargle and especially as an oral paint, for inflammation of the gums, fissures in the tongue, stomatitis, pharyngitis, and less often also in angina. When in use, tincture of rhatany is often mixed with tincture of myrrh.

The drug has been employed internally as an antidiarrhoeic in enteritis, but is no longer so widely used; the same is true of its external application to chilblains or leg sores.

Making the tea: (if it is preferred not to use the tincture) boiling water is poured over 1.5–2 g of the coarsely powdered root, covered, and kept on the boil for 10–15 min. before being strained.
1 Teaspoon = ca. 3 g.

Phytomedicines: Rhatany tincture is present in a few prepared mouth and throat remedies, e.g. Echtrosept®, Repha-Os® Mundspray, Salviathymol®, etc.

Authentication: Macro- (see: Description) and microscopically, following the Ph. Eur. 2, etc.; see also [7]. About the quantitative spectrophotometric determination of tannin according to DAB 10, using phosphotungstic acid, see the remarks by Glasl [3] and Stahl and Jahn [4].

Quantitative standards: Ph. Eur. 2, etc.: *Tannin content*, not less than 10.0%. *Foreign matter*, not more than 2% and not more than 5% fragments of the root tuft or roots with a diameter greater than 25 mm; roots without bark should be present only in very small amounts. *Sulphated ash*, not more than 6.0%.
BHP 1/1990: specifies that rhatany root should comply with the requirements of the Ph. Eur. 2 and the BP 1988 monographs, and similarly for the powdered drug.

Adulteration: Occurs, especially with the roots of other *Krameria* species; see also [1]. According to Schier [5], "the genuine drug no longer appears to be on the market at all." In the genuine drug, almost all cells (especially those of the bark) have a brownish red content, while in the commercial drug there are usually only a few such cells. Since evidently it is difficult to obtain the genuine drug, replacing it, e.g. by Tormentillae rhizoma (tormentil root), should be considered [6].

Literature:
[1] Kommentar DAB 10.
[2] E. Stahl and I. Ittel, Planta Med. **42**, 144 (1981).
[3] H. Glasl, Dtsch. Apoth. Ztg. **123**, 1979 (1983).
[4] E. Stahl and H. Jahn, Arch. Pharm. (Weinheim) **317**, 573 (1984).
[5] W. Schier, Dtsch. Apoth. Ztg. **121**, 323 (1981); *idem*, Z. Phytotherap. **4**, 537 (1983).
[6] W.F. Daems, Dtsch. Apoth. Ztg. **121**, 46 (1981).
[7] B.P. Jackson and D.W. Snowdon, Atlas of microscopy of medicinal plants, culinary herbs and spices, Belhaven Press, London, 1990, p. 198.

Rhamni cathartici fructus (DAB 10), Buckthorn fruit

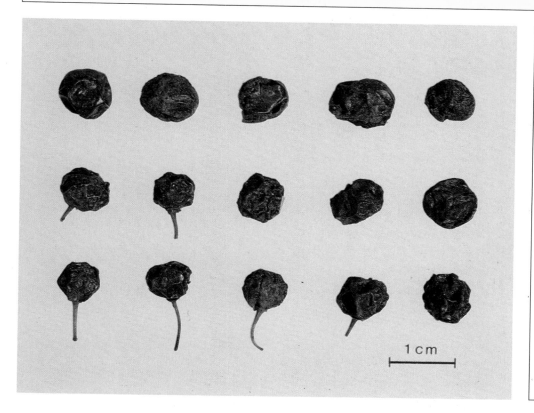

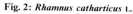

1 cm

Fig. 1: Buckthorn fruit

<u>Description</u>: The shiny, black, spherical, approximately pea-sized drupes (diameter 5–8 mm) have a wrinkled and shrunken surface. At the top, there are the remains of the 4-part pistil. The stalk, or part of it, which is often still present, is thin and somewhat curved. Inside, the four locules each contain a hard, obovoid, keeled seed.

<u>Taste</u>: At first sweetish, then bitter and somewhat sharp.

Fig. 2: *Rhamnus catharticus* L.

An up to 3 m tall bush, with opposite, finely serrate leaves, on branches often terminating in a spine. Small yellowish green, axillary flowers arranged in cymes. Fruit shiny and black when ripe.

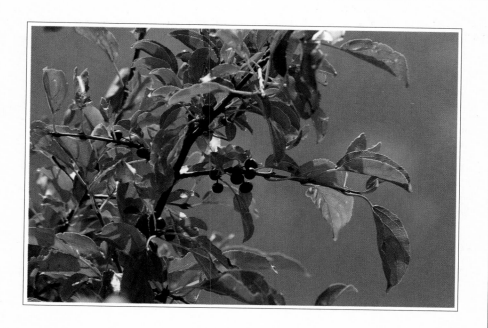

DAB 10: Kreuzdornbeeren
St. Zul.: 1089.99.99

Plant source: *Rhamnus catharticus* L., buckthorn (Rhamnaceae).

Synonyms: Baccae spinae cervinae (Lat.), Rhamnus (Engl.), Kreuzdornbeeren, Purgierbeeren, Wegdornbeeren (Ger.), Fruits de neprun purgatif (Fr.).

Origin: Distributed in Europe, North Africa, and Asia. The drug comes from the wild and is imported mainly from the former USSR.

Constituents: 2–5% anthraquinone glycosides; it is not yet clear what compounds are present, but presumably glucofrangulins and frangulins are the main components (see: Frangulae cortex (Frangula bark)).
The drug contains 3–4% tannins and ca. 1% flavonoids, pectins, mono- and oligosaccharides, as well as ascorbic acid [1].

Indications: In constipation, as a laxative acting on the large intestine, when evacua-

**Extract from the German Commission
E monograph
(BAnz no. 101, dated 01. 06. 90)**

Uses

Constipation. Disorders in which an easy evacuation
of the bowels with a soft stool is desired, e.g. with
anal fissures, haemorrhoids, and after rectal-anal operations.

Contraindications

Intestinal obstruction. During pregnancy and lactation, only after consultation with a doctor.

Side effects

With larger doses, cramp-like gastrointestinal upsets
may occur. In such cases, the dose should be reduced.

Warning: With chronic use/abuse, loss of electrolyte,
especially potassium, may take place. Pigments are
deposited in the intestinal mucosa (melanosis coli).

Interactions with other remedies

None known.

Warning: With chronic use/abuse, potassium depletion may potentiate the action of cardiac glycosides.

Dosage

Unless otherwise prescribed: daily dose, 2–5 g drug,
corresponding to 20–200 mg hydroxyanthracene
derivatives calculated as glucofrangulin.

Mode of administration

Comminuted drug for infusions and other galenical
preaprations for internal use.

Duration of use

Laxatives containing anthracene derivatives should
not be taken for a prolonged period of time.

Effect

Laxative.

**Wording of the package insert, from the
German Standard Licence:**

6.1   Uses

Constipation: all complaints in which an easy evacuation with a soft stool is desired, e.g. anal fissures,
haemorrhoids, and after rectal-anal operations.

6.2   Contraindications

Buckthorn preparations are not be used in cases of
intestinal obstruction or during pregnancy and lactation.

6.3   Side effects

When correctly used, not known.
On frequent and prolonged use or with overdoses,
there may be an increased loss of water and salts,
especially potassium salts. Moreover, there may be
deposition of pigment in the mucous membrane of
the intestine (melanosis coli).

6.4   Interactions with other remedies

Owing to an increased loss of potassium, the effects
of cardiac glycosides may be potentiated.

6.5   Dosage and Mode of administration

Boiling water (ca. 150 ml) is poured over ca. 2 teaspoonfuls (3–5 g) of **Buckthorn fruit** and after 10–
15 min. passed through a tea strainer.
Unless otherwise prescribed, a cup of the freshly prepared tea is drunk in the morning and/or in the
evening before going to sleep.

6.6   Duration of use

Buckthorn-fruit tea should be taken for only a few
days. For longer use, a doctor should be consulted.

Warning: To restore normal bowel function, a
roughage-rich diet and adequate fluid intake, and as
much exercise as possible, should be ensured.

6.7   Note

Store away from light and moisture.

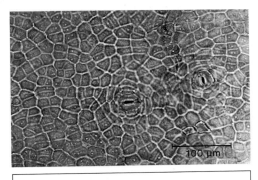

**Fig. 3: Exocarp, showing the isodiametric cells with
sunken stomata**

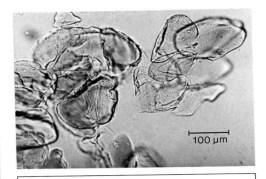

**Fig. 4: Secretory cells of the mesocarp with orange-
yellow content**

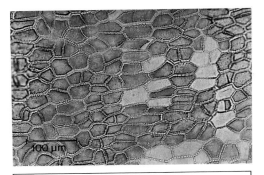

**Fig. 5: Pigment layer of the seed testa (in the light-co-
loured cells, the pigment has dropped out)**

tion with a soft stool is indicated. In *folk
medicine,* the drug is also used as a diuretic
and in so-called "blood-purifying remedies".

Side effects: Only likely on frequent or prolonged use; as with other anthracene-glycoside drugs, there is loss of water and electrolytes. The drug should not be used during
pregnancy or lactation.

Making the tea: Boiling water is poured
over ca. 4 g of the comminuted drug and
after 10–15 min. passed through a tea strainer. A cupful is drunk in the evening and, if
necessary, also in the morning and after-
noon. It has also been recommended to soak
the drug in cold water, then boil it up for
2–3 min., and strain while still warm.
1 Teaspoon = ca. 3.8 g.

Phytomedicines: The drug is a component of
some mixed teas which are mostly indicated
to be laxative, digestive, liver and bile, or
stomach and bowel teas. The dried expressed juice of the fruit, along with other

active ingredients, is present in Laxysat®-
Dragees.

Authentication: Macro- (see: Description)
and microscopically, following the DAB 10.
The diagnostic features include: the isodiametric cells of the exocarp with sunken
stomata (Fig. 3); the secretory cells of the
mesocarp with an orange-yellow content
(Fig. 4) which colours very dark brown with
iron(III) chloride solution; and the pigment
layer of the seed testa (Fig. 5).
The following method is a suitable TLC
identity test:

Test solution: 0.5 g powdered drug boiled
briefly with 5 ml 70% aqueous ethanol; after cooling, centrifuged and the supernatant
used directly for the TLC.

Reference solutions: (a) 10 mg aloin dissolved in 5 ml 70% aqueous ethanol (solution must be freshly prepared); (b) 5 mg
frangulin dissolved in 10 ml methanol.

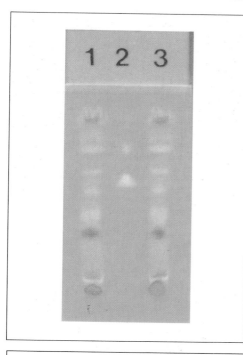

Fig. 6: TLC on 4 × 8 cm silica-gel foil

1 and 3: Buckthorn fruit (different origins)
2: Reference substances

For details, see the text

Loadings: 3 µl test solution as a band; 2 µl reference solution (a) and 5 µl reference solution (b), both as spots.

Solvent system: ethyl acetate + methanol + water (77 + 13 + 10), 6 cm run.

Detection: layer dried in a current of hot air; sprayed with 5% potassium hydroxide in 50% aqueous ethanol and observed while heating at 100–105 °C for 15 min.

Evaluation: In daylight. Reference solutions: frangulin in the upper third as a reddish spot; aloin as a yellowish brown spot slightly below it. Test solution: a reddish band at the same level as the reference frangulin spot and between the starting line and the aloin spot an intense yellowish zone; other fainter zones also present.
UV 366 nm light. Test solutions: frangulin spot, weak red; aloin spot, yellow. Test solution: a weak red fluorescent zone at the same level as the reference frangulin spot; a faint blue fluorescent zone at the same level as the reference aloin spot, and immediately below it a red fluorescent zone and a reddish fluorecent zone in the lower third; other, mostly reddish, fluorescent zones also present (Fig. 6).
The DAB 10 specifies examination in the solvent system: ethyl acetate + methanol + water (100 + 17 + 13), with aloin as reference substance, and subsequent evaluation in daylight only.

Quantitative standards: DAB 10: *Hydroxyanthracene derivatives*, not less than 4.0% calculated as glucofrangulin (M_r 578.5). *Foreign (vegetable and/or mineral) matter*, not more than 2%. *Loss on drying*, not more than 10%. *Ash*, not more than 4%.

Adulteration: Occurs mostly as a consequence of confusion during collection with the fruit of frangula, *Frangula alnus* MILL. An essential difference between the two is that frangula fruit have individual, round secretory glands with a large lumen, instead of secretory cells.

Storage: Protected from light, dry.

Literature:
[1] J. Slepetys, Liet. TSR Mokslu Akad. Darb., Ser. C **1985**, 51; C.A. **102**, 201197 (1985).

Rhamni purshiani cortex

(DAB 10, Ph. Eur. 2, etc.), Cascara (*BAN*; BP 1988), Cascara sagrada (*USAN*; USP XXII), Cascara bark (BHP 1/1990)

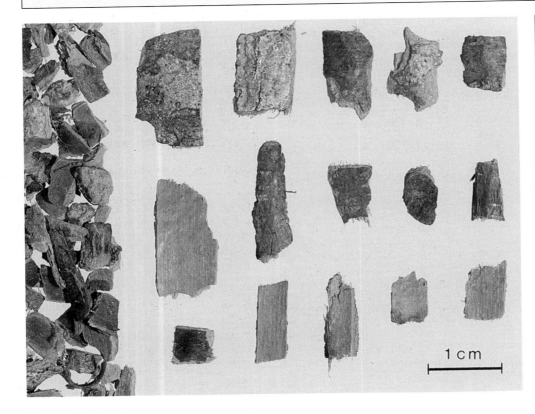

Fig. 1: Cascara bark

Description: The drug consists of quilled, channelled, or almost flat pieces, 1–5 mm thick and varying in length and width. The outer surface is grey to greyish brown, fairly smooth, mostly slightly shiny, with occasional horizontally elongated lenticels, and often covered with lichen and epiphytic moss (Fig. 2). On careful scraping, red-coloured tissue becomes visible. The inner surface is yellowish brown, cinnamon-brown to dark brown, and finely striated longitudinally. If the inner surface is spotted with 6N ammonia solution, it takes on a red colour (Bornträger reaction). In the outer part the fracture is short and granular, and in the inner part somewhat fibrous.

Odour: Characteristic, but not very pronounced.

Taste: Bitter, producing nausea.

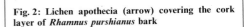

1 cm

Fig. 2: Lichen apothecia (arrow) covering the cork layer of *Rhamnus purshianus* bark

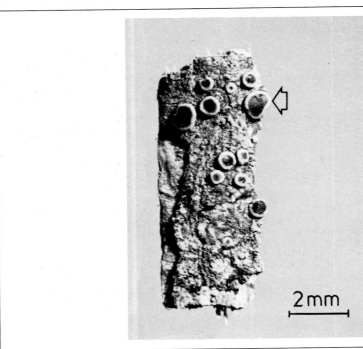

2 mm

DAB 10: Cascararinde
ÖAB: Cortex Rhamni purshianae
Ph. Helv. VII: Rhamni purshiani cortex
St. Zul. 8699.99.99

Plant source: *Rhamnus purshianus* DC.* (syn. *Frangula purshiana* (DC.) A. GRAY ex J.C. COOPER) (Rhamnaceae).

Synonyms: Cortex Cascarae sagradae (Latin), Rhamnus, Sacred bark, Bitter or Chittem bark (Engl.), Cascararinde, Amerikani-

---

* The genus name *Rhamnus* has been considered both as feminine and as masculine, thus giving rise to the alternative species epithets *purshiana* and *purshianus* found in the literature. The names of trees ending in -os were accounted feminine in Greek, and when latinized in classical times such words as *juniperus, prunus, quercus, rhamnus,* etc. (which later became generic names) usually kept the original gender. But early botanists, like Lobelin, C. Bauhin, and Linnaeus, used the word *Rhamnus* as if it were masculine (see: Hegi, *Flora von Mitteleuropa,* vol. 5/1, p. 329; W. T. Stearn, *Botanical Latin*). Since then, practice has varied – and it continues to vary; here, we follow the usage of the *Flora Europaea* and treat the word as masculine.

sche Faulbaumrinde (Ger.), Ecorce de cascara (Fr.).

Origin: Native to the Pacific coast of North America. The drug also comes from plantations in the American states of Washington and Oregon, as well as from western Canada.

Constituents: A complex mixture of various hydroxyanthracene derivatives, mainly of the C(10)-glucosylanthrone type (cf. Aloes) (70–90%), including aloins A and B and 11-desoxy-aloins A and B (= chrysaloins) (10–30%) as well as their *O*-glucosides, the cascarosides A and B (diastereoisomeric pair derived from 8-*O*-glucosylaloin) and the cascarosides C and D (diastereoisomeric pair derived from 8-*O*-glucosyl-11-desoxyaloin). As the characteristic principal constituents of the drug, they comprise ca. 60–70% of the total anthracene derivatives present. There are also 10–20% anthraquinone *O*-glucosides, e.g. aloe-emodin and frangula-emodin 8-*O*-glucosides, along with the aglycones aloe-emodin, chrysophanol, frangulaemodin, and physcion (for the structures, see: Rhei radix (rhubarb root)). Small amounts of iso- and heterodianthrones are also present. – The occurrence of bitter substances and methylhydrocotoin is disputed [1, 2]. – Storage (for at least a year), or heating in a stream of air, is supposed to decrease the content of anthrones, the primary form of the anthracene derivatives, (see: Authentication, and the data under: Frangulae cortex).

Indications: As a laxative acting on the large intestine, like Frangulae cortex (q.v.).

Making the tea: Boiling water is poured over 2 g of the finely cut drug and allowed to stand for 10 min. and then strained.
1 Teaspoon = ca. 2.5 g.

Phytomedicines: In several preparations, together with other laxatives, as a herbal tea, dry extract for infusions, as well as in solid and liquid dosage forms.
A similar range of products is available in the UK.

Authentication: Macro- (see: Description) and microscopically, following the Ph. Eur. 2, etc.; for detailed microscopy of the powdered drug, see [4]. Among the diagnostic features are: groups of stone cells and groups of fibres surrounded by a crystal sheath, medullary rays up to 5 rows of cells broad; the powder is stained red with alkali hydroxide solutions. Tests for the presence of fresh bark (which is not permitted!) and for adulteration with *Rhamnus alpinus* L. ssp. *fallax* and *R.catharticus* L., see: Frangulae cortex.

The following TLC test of identity is set out in the Ph. Eur. 2, etc.:

Test solution: 0.5 g powdered drug heated to boiling with 5 ml 70% ethanol, cooled, centrifuged, and the supernatant poured off immediately; to be used within 30 min.

Reference solution: 20 mg aloin dissolved in 10 ml 70% ethanol.

Loadings: 10 µl of each solution, as 2-cm bands on silica gel G.

Solvent system: water + methanol + ethyl acetate (13 + 17 + 100), 10 cm run.

Detection and Evaluation: after 5 min. drying in the air, on immediate spraying with fresh 0.1% nitrosodimethylaniline in pyridine: no greyish blue zones visible. Then, oversprayed with 5% ethanolic potassium hydroxide, heated at 100–105 °C for 15 min., and evaluated at once. Reference

---

Extract from the German Commission E monograph (BAnz no. 228, dated 05.12.1984)

Uses
Conditions in which easy defaecation with a soft stool is desirable, e.g. anal fissures, haemorrhoids, after rectal-anal operations, constipation.

Contraindications
Ileus of whatever origin; use during pregnancy and lactation, only after consultation with a doctor.

Side effects
None known.
With chronic use/abuse: loss of electrolytes, especially potassium. Deposition of pigment in the intestinal mucosa (melanosis coli).
In the fresh condition, the drug contains anthrones and must therefore be stored for at least a year before use or be artificially altered by heating in the presence of air.
With inappropriate use, e.g. of fresh drug, severe vomiting, possibly accompanied by spasms.

Interactions
None known.
With chronic use/abuse, the potassium deficiency may lead to potentiation of the effects of cardiotonic glycosides.

Dosage
Unless otherwise prescribed: average daily dose, 20–160 mg hydroxyanthracene derivatives.

Mode of administration
Finely cut drug, drug powder, or dry extract for infusions, decoctions, cold macerates, or elixirs. Liquid and solid dosage forms exclusively for oral use.

Duration of use
Anthraquinone-containing laxatives should not be taken for long periods of time.

Effects
The substances bring about an active secretion of electrolytes and water in the lumen of the small intestine, and they inhibit the absorption of electrolytes and water from the large intestine. The increase in volume of the bowel contents strengthens the dilatation pressure in the intestine and stimulates peristalsis.

Wording of the package insert, from the German Standard Licence:

5.1 Uses
Constipation; all disorders in which an easy evacuation of the bowel with a soft stool is desired, e.g. in cases of anal fissures, haemorrhoids, and after rectal-anal operations.

5.2 Contraindications
Preparations of cascara bark should not be used in cases of intestinal obstruction or during pregnancy and lactation.

5.3 Side effects
Used as prescribed, none known. With frequent and prolonged use, or when used to excess, an increased loss of water and salts, especially potassium salts, may take place. In addition, deposition of pigment in the intestinal mucosa (melanosis coli) may occur.

5.4 Interactions with other remedies
Because of the increased loss of potassium, the action of cardiac glycosides may be potentiated.

5.5 Dosage and Mode of administration
Boiling water (ca. 150 ml) is poured over about half a teaspoonful of **Cascara bark** and after 10–15 min. passed through a tea strainer.
Unless otherwise prescribed, a cup of the freshly prepared tea is drunk in the morning and/or at night before going to sleep.

5.6 Duration of use
Cascara-bark tea should only be taken for a few days. For longer use, a doctor should be consulted.
Warning: to restore normal functioning of the intestine, a roughage-rich diet with sufficient fluid intake, and as much exercise as possible, should be ensured.

5.7 Note
Protected from light and moisture.

	R¹	R²
Cascaroside A	β-D-Glucose	OH
Cascaroside C	β-D-Glucose	H
Aloin A	H	OH
(+)-11-Desoxyaloin	H	H

	R¹	R²
Cascaroside B	β-D-Glucose	OH
Cascaroside D	β-D-Glucose	H
Aloin B	H	OH
(−)-11-Desoxyaloin	H	H

solution: reddish brown aloin zone at Rf ca. 0.4–0.5. Test solution: several reddish brown zones of varying intensities, of the 4 faint ones 3 in the middle and 1 in the lower third; an intense zone in the upper third.
In UV 365 nm light. Reference solution: aloin zone an intense yellowish brown fluorescence. Test solution: several zones with similar fluorescence and especially below the aloin band (cascarosides). Blue fluorescent zones must be absent (other *Rhamnus* species) and so also a reddish orange fluorescent band between those of the aloin and cascarosides (*R. frangula*).
Coloured illustrations of chromatograms are to be found in [3].

Quantitative standards: Ph. Eur. 2: *Hydroxyanthracene glycosides*, not less than 8.0%, of which not less than 60% consists of the cascarosides, both calculated as cascaroside A (M_r 581). *Foreign vegetable and mineral matter*, not more than 1.0%. *Sulphated ash*, not more than 6.0%.
USP XXII: *Total hydroxyanthracene derivatives*, 7%, not less than 60% of which consists of cascarosides calculated as cascaroside A.
BHP 1/1990: Cascara bark, also in the powdered form, must comply with the appropriate monographs in the Ph. Eur. 2 and BP 1988.

Adulteration: Occasionally with bark from other *Rhamnus* species; see under: Frangulae cortex.

Storage: Protected from moisture and light. Before use, the drug must be aged (artificially or by at least 1 year's storage; see under: Authentication).

Literature:
[1] Hager, vol. **6b**, p. 83 (1979).
[2] Kommentar DAB 10.
[3] H. Wagner, S. Bladt, and E.M. Zgainski, Plant drug analysis, Springer-Verlag, Berlin, Heidelberg, New York, Tokyo, 1984, p. 104.
[4] B.P. Jackson and D.W. Snowdon, Atlas of microscopy of medicinal plants, culinary herbs and spices, Belhaven Press, London, 1990, p. 46.

Rhei radix   (DAB 10, Ph. Eur. 2, etc.), Rhubarb (*BAN*; BP 1988, BHP 1/1990)

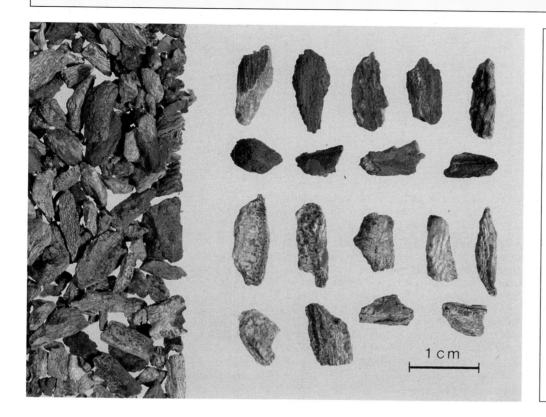

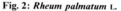

1 cm

Fig. 1: Rhubarb

<u>Description:</u> The drug consists of the peeled underground organs (turnip-shaped roots with very small rhizomes). The ochre-yellow to brownish pieces are often covered on the outside with powder and they exhibit orange striations or an orange-red mottling. The fracture is granular and crumbly (not fibrous) and reddish brown.

<u>Odour:</u> Characteristic and faintly smoky.

<u>Taste:</u> Somewhat bitter and harsh.

Fig. 2: *Rheum palmatum* L.

A 2 m tall perennial with conspicuous, palmately lobed, large leaves, the individual lobes being more or less deeply divided. Purplish red to white, 6-part flowers arranged in racemes or panicles; fruits winged.

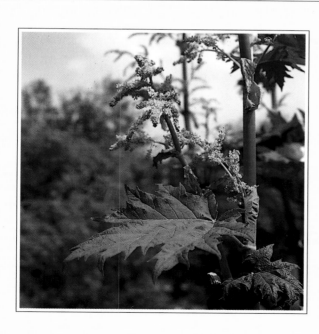

DAB 10: Rhabarbarwurzel
ÖAB: Radix Rhei
Ph. Helv. VII: Rhei radix
St. Zul. 1189.99.98

Plant sources: *Rheum palmatum* L. s.l. and/or *R. officinale* BAILLON, Chinese rhubarb (Polygonaceae), as well as hybrids of these species.

Synonyms: Rhizoma Rhei (a botanically incorrect expression), Radix Rhei sinensis, Radix Rhabarbari (Lat.), Rheum, Rhubarb rhizome or root (Engl.), Rhabarberwurzel (Ger.), Racine de rhubarbe (Fr.).

Origin: Native in north-western China and Tibet, cultivated to some extent in Europe. The drug is imported from China and India; Pakistan also supplies rhubarb, which mostly does not meet pharmacopoeial standards (see: Adulteration). About the complexities of the grading system for Chinese rhubarb, see [5, 11].

Constituents [1]: 3–12% hydroxyanthracene derivatives; the figures indicated not only

	R¹	R²
Rheum-emodin	CH₃	OH
Aloe-emodin	CH₂OH	H
Rhein	COOH	H
Chrysophanol	CH₃	H
Physcion	CH₃	OCH₃

Rhaponticin: R = β-D-Glucose
Rhapontigenin: R = H

reflect the variable content [2], but also depend greatly on the substance – aglycone, glycoside – on which they are based. Ca. 60–80% of the mixture comprises anthraquinone glycosides (of the five aglycones emodin, aloe-emodin, rhein, chrysophanol, and physcion) and ca. 10–25% dianthrone glycosides; minor cytotoxic anthraquinone glycosides – pulmatin (1,8-dihydroxy-3-methylanthraquinone 1-O-β-D-glucoside) and the congeners chrysophanein and physcionin [6]. Chromone glucosides, including aloesone [7]. Ca. 1% stilbene glucosides, 4'-O-methyl-piceid and rhaponticin (3,5-dihydroxy- and 3,5,3'-trihydroxy-4'-methoxystilbene 3-β-D-glucopyranoside, respectively) [8]. Ca. 5–10% tannins, a mixture of gallotannins and related compounds (galloyl-, hydroxycinnamoyl- (p-coumaroyl-), galloyldihydrocinnamoylglucoses, galloyl-sucroses, etc.) [9, 10]. Ca. 2–3% flavonoids (rutin, etc.).

Indications: Because of its content of anthracene derivatives and tannins, depending on the dose, as a laxative (1.0–2.0 g) or as an astringent and stomachic (0.1–0.2 g) – an example of intersecting dose-response curves; however, the drug is used mainly as a laxative, for constipation, when haemorrhoids or anal injuries are present and after rectal operations. About the mechanism of action, see: Aloe barbadensis/capensis. Use is also made of the laxative action in liver and biliary disorders, which not infrequently are accompanied by constipation; hence, the drug and drug extracts are a component of many cholagogues.
On the other hand, use as an astringent, e.g. as an antidiarrhoeal, has greatly decreased. Because of the bitter taste of the anthracene glycosides, small amounts of rhubarb are used, e.g. in the form of alcoholic extracts (Tinctura Rhei vinosa) as a stomachic.
It is known that one of the components of the tannin mixture (galloyldihydrocinnamoylglucose) has analgesic and anti-inflammatory actions which are comparable with those of phenylbutazone and acetylsalicylic acid, respectively [3]. The stilbene glucosides are moderately active α-glucosidase inhibitors [8].

Side effects: If used as prescribed, none known. Like all anthracene-glycoside drugs, rhubarb should not be used continuously over for a prolonged period, since this disturbs the water and electrolyte balance. Rhubarb should not be taken during pregnancy (reflex stimulation of the uterus) or during lactation (a proportion of the aglycones reaches the mother's milk) or in cases of intestinal obstrucion (danger of intestinal rupture).
Anthraquinones are partly conjugated with glucuronic and sulphuric acids and are excreted in the urine, which then takes on a deep yellowish brown colour and which on being made alkaline becomes red to reddish brown.

Making the tea: As a laxative, 1.0–2.0 g of the coarsely powdered drug, as a stomachic 0.1–0.2 g powdered drug, is stirred with sufficient liquid (if desired, cinnamon, ginger, or peppermint oil can be added according to taste) or boiling water is poured over it and strained after 5 min.
1 Teaspoon = ca. 2.5 g.

Phytomedicines: The drug or extracts prepared from it are frequent components of prepared laxatives, cholagogues, and gastrointestinal remedies. They are also present in "slimming cures", "spring cures", and so-called "blood-cleansing" teas. The drug is almost always a component of the so-called "Swedish (herbal) bitters" (see the note under: Aloe capensis).

Regulatory status (UK): General Sales List – Schedule 1, Table A.

Authentication: Macro- and microsopically, following the Ph. Eur. 2, etc.; see also [11] for the illustrated microscopy of the powdered drug. Examination with a hand lens shows the distinctive mottling (streaking) caused by abnormal development of the leptocentric vascular bundles in the xylem (Fig. 3). Microscopical examination reveals the large cluster crystals of calcium oxalate and the highly characteristic unlignified reticulately thickened vessels.
On microsublimation at 140–160 °C, a yellow crystalline sublimate (Fig. 5) is obtained, which, on addition of dilute potassium hy-

---

Extract from the German Commission E monograph (BAnz no. 228, 05. 12. 1984)

Uses

Constipation.
For all disorders in which defaecation with a soft stool is desired, e.g. anal fissures, haemorrhoids, after rectal-anal operations.
Small doses are indicated as an astringent in stomach and bowel catarrh.

Contraindications

Ileus of whatever origin; during pregnancy and lactation, only after consultation with a doctor.

Side effects

None known.
With chronic use/abuse: loss of electrolytes, especially of potassium; pigmentation of the intestinal mucosa (melanosis coli).

Interactions

None known.
With chronic use/abuse, the potassium deficiency may potentiate the effects of cardiotonic glycosides.

Dosage

Unless otherwise prescribed: average daily dose as laxative, 30–120 mg hydroxyanthracene derivatives, corresponding to 1.2–4.8 g drug; average daily dose as stomachic, 3–9 mg hydroxyanthracene derivatives, corresponding to 0.12–0.36 g drug.

Mode of administration

Finely chopped drug, powdered drug, or powdered dry extract for infusions, decoctions. As liquid or solid formulations exclusively for oral use.

Duration of use

Anthraquinone laxatives should not be taken for prolonged periods of time.

Effects

The anthraquinone glycosides are hydrolysed microbiologically in the large intestine to the aglycones, which are absorbed to a certain extent. They are reduced by bacteria to the actual active substances – the anthranols and anthrones. The laxative effect is due to inhibition of the uptake of water and electrolytes in the large intestine and to an effect on intestinal motility.

droxide solution, dissolves to give a red colour.

The surest test of identity is the TLC examination given in the Ph. Eur. 2; all five aglycones are detected in the hydrolysate:

Test solution: 50 mg powdered drug heated for 15 min. with a mixture of 1 ml 36% hydrochloric acid and 30 ml water, cooled, and extracted with 25 ml diethyl ether; the ether phase dried over anhydrous sodium sulphate, filtered, taken to dryness, and the residue dissolved in 0.5 ml diethyl ether.

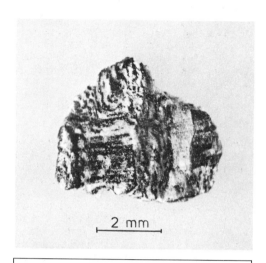

Fig. 3: Fragment of the root, showing the characteristic mottling (streaking)

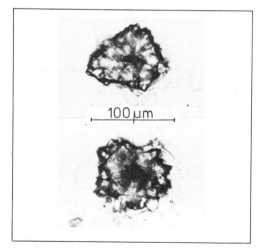

Fig. 4: Large calcium oxalate cluster crystals, from rhubarb

Wording of the package insert, from the German Standard Licence:

5.1   Uses

Constipation; all complaints in which an easy evacuation with a soft stool is desirable, e.g. anal fissures, haemorrhoids, and after rectal-anal operations.

5.2   Contraindications

Rhubarb preparations should not be used in cases of intestinal obstruction or during pregnancy and lactation.

5.3   Side effects

If used as prescribed, none known. On frequent and prolonged use, or with an overdose, an increased loss of water and salts, especially potassium salts, may occur.

5.4   Interactions with other remedies

Because of the possible loss of potassium, the effect of cardiotonic glycosides may be potentiated.

5.5   Dosage and Mode of administration

Hot water (ca. 150 ml) is poured over ca. $\frac{1}{2}$–1 flat teaspoonful of finely chopped **Rhubarb root** and after 10–15 min. passed through a tea strainer.
Unless otherwise prescribed, for constipation a cup of the freshly prepared infusion is drunk in the morning and/or at night before going to bed. For stomach and bowel catarrh, a tablespoonful of the infusion is taken several times.

5.6   Duration of use

Rhubarb tea should only be taken for a few days. For longer use, a doctor should be consulted.

Warning: To re-establish normal bowel function, a diet with sufficient roughage, an adequate fluid intake, and as much exercise as possible should be ensured.

5.7   Note

Store protected from light and moisture.

Reference solution: 5 mg emodin dissolved in 5 ml diethyl ether.

Loadings: 20 μl of each solution, as 2-cm bands on silica gel G.

Solvent system: anhydrous formic acid + ethyl acetate + light petroleum (b. range 50–70 °C) (1 + 25 + 75), 10 cm run.

Detection and **Evaluation:** in UV 365 nm light. Test solution: orange fluorescent zones at Rf ca. 0.55 (chrysophanol), ca. 0.50 (physcion), ca. 0.40 (emodin, corresponding to the zone of the reference solution), ca. 0.25 (rhein), and ca. 0.15 (aloe-emodin). On exposure to ammonia vapour, all should turn red.

The Ph. Eur. 2 TLC test for *Rheum rhaponticum* is as follows:

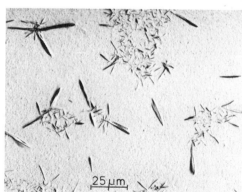

Fig. 5: Yellowish needles of the microsublimate

Test solution: 0.2 g powdered drug refluxed for 5 min. with 2 ml methanol, cooled, and filtered.

Reference solution: 10 mg rhaponticin dissolved in 10 ml methanol.

Loadings: 20 μl of each solution, as 2-cm bands on silica gel G.

Solvent system: methanol + chloroform (20 + 80), 12 cm run.

Detection: sprayed with phosphomolybdic acid solution (4 g phosphomolybdic acid dissolved in water and made up to 40 ml, then carefully added to it with cooling 60 ml 96% sulphuric acid; to be freshly prepared as required).

Evaluation: Test solution: **no** blue fluorescent zone at the starting line (rhaponticin), corresponding to the zone in the chromatogram of the reference solution.

Quantitative standards: Ph. Eur. 2, etc.: *Hydroxyanthracene derivatives*, not less than 2.5% calculated as rhein (M_r 284.2). *Foreign matter*, not more than 1%. *HCl-insoluble ash*, not more than 1.0%.
BHP 1/1990: Rhubarb, or its powder complies with the requirements of the appropriate monographs in the Ph. Eur. 2 and BP 1988.

Adulteration: Observed now and then, especially with *Rheum rhaponticum* L. (rhapontic), but also with *R. rhabarbarum* L. and other *Rheum* species; they all contain a much smaller amount of anthracene derivatives than does the pharmaceutical drug. The detection is based on the occurrence of stilbene derivatives, especially rhaponticin (= rhaponticoside): if a fragment of the drug is drawn across a piece of moistened filter paper which is then examined under UV 366 nm light, there should be no blue fluorescent streak (fluorescence due to the stilbenes). The Ph. Eur. 2 TLC examination for rhaponticin-containing *Rheum* species (above) is somewhat longer but more reliable [1].

The drug imported from Pakistan in recent years has often turned out to be an adulterant [4]; in the TLC examination for anthraquinones (Ph. Eur. 2 identification test) no rhein and aloe-emodin is found; it is not yet known from which *Rheum* species this drug comes.

Holes in pieces of the drug may be caused by insect attack or they may be bore holes (for hanging the drug up to dry).

An HPLC method is available for the simultaneous quantitative determination of the phenolic constituents (anthraquinones, anthrones, phenylbutanones, stilbenes, tannins, etc.). Commercial rhubarbs can be classified in several groups based on their chromatographic profiles [12].

Literature:
[1] Kommentar DAB 10.
[2] E.H.C. Verhaeren, M. Dreessen, and J. Lemli, Planta Med. **45**, 15 (1982).
[3] G.I. Nonaka, I. Nishioka, T. Nagasawa, and H. Oura, Chem. Pharm. Bull. **29**, 2862 (1981).
[4] E. Stahl, H. Menßen, and H. Jahn, Dtsch. Apoth. Ztg. **125**, 1478 (1985).
[5] W.C. Evans, Trease and Evans' Pharmacognosy, 13th ed., Baillière Tindall, London, p. 409.
[6] I. Kubo, I. Soediro, S. Soetarno, and S. Sastrodihardjo, Phytochemistry **31**, 1063 (1992).
[7] Y. Kashiwada, G.I. Nonaka, and I. Nishioka, Phytochemistry **29**, 1007 (1990).
[8] I. Kubo and Y. Murai, J. Nat. Prod. **54**, 1115 (1991).
[9] Y. Kashiwada, G.I. Nonaka, and I. Nishioka, Phytochemistry **27**, 1469 (1988).
[10] Y. Kashiwada, G.I. Nonaka, and I. Nishioka, Phytochemistry **27**, 1473 (1988).
[11] B.P. Jackson and D.W. Snowdon, Atlas of microscopy of medicinal plants, culinary herbs and spices, Belhaven Press, London, 1990, p. 200.
[12] Y. Kashiwada, G.I. Nonaka, and I. Nishioka, Chem. Pharm. Bull. **37**, 999 (1989).

Rhoeados flos   Red-poppy petal

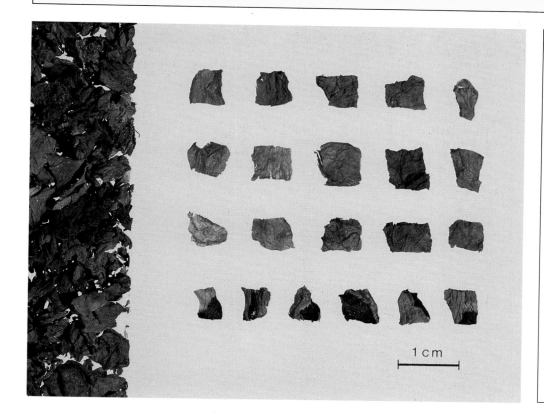

Fig. 1: Red-poppy petal

<u>Description</u>: The dark reddish violet, mostly crushed and folded petals have a velvety feel to the touch. They are broadly ovate, up to 6 cm long, with an entire margin, and narrowing at the base where there is a black spot. The vascular bundles radiating from the base of the petals anastomose in a continuous arc at the same distance from the margin. On soaking in water, the black spot at the base of the petals (bottom row) and the nerves radiating from it become distinct.

<u>Taste</u>: Slightly bitter and somewhat mucilaginous.

Fig. 2: *Papaver rhoeas* L.

An annual, up to 80 cm in height, frequently encountered at the edge of cornfields, with bristly hairs and once or twice pinnately divided leaves. Initially nodding buds becoming erect shortly before opening; petals four, often with a black spot at the base. Capsule, about 1 cm long, narrow, and with ca. 10 stigma rays.

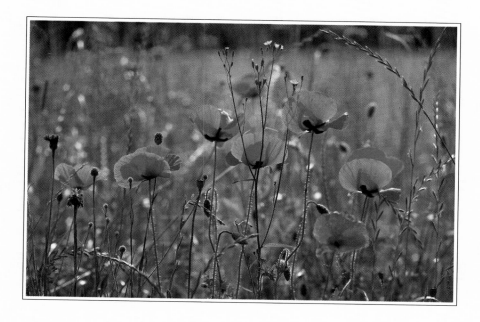

Erg. B. 6: Flores Rhoeados

Plant source: *Papaver rhoeas* L., common or field poppy (Papaveraceae).

Synonyms: Rhoeados, Red- or Corn-poppy flowers (Engl.), Klatschmohnblüten (Ger.), Fleurs de coquelicot (Fr.).

Origin: In cornfields, among weeds (mass occurrence, e.g. at the edges of newly constructed roads and motorways); almost cosmopolitan. Collected from the wild and imported mainly from eastern and south-eastern Europe (Albania, for example) and also from Morocco.

Constituents [1]: Anthocyan glycosides, especially those with cyanidin as aglycone, in particular mecocyanin (= cyanidin 3-sophoroside) [2] (for almost 50 years thought to be cyanidin 3-gentiobioside [3]), cyanin [4], and others. Up to 0.12% isoquinoline alkaloids, of which up to ca. 50% is rhoeadine. Further, mucilage and ubiquitous substances.

Indications: No medicinally well-founded uses are known; occasionally in <u>folk medicine</u> it is used to prepare a syrup for coughs and hoarseness in small children and a tea for aches, insomnia, and as a sedative. Formerly, it was also employed for colouring sweets, and nowadays it is used to enhance the appearance of herbal teas.

Side effects: Occasionally, poisoning in children has been described in books on medicinal plants. Cows are said to have become poisoned, with convulsions and coma, after taking fodder grossly contaminated with the field poppy. In rats, rhoeadine causes cramps and in rabbits stimulates respiration [cited from 1].

Making the tea: Not usual. 2 teaspoons of the drug are brewed up with boiling water, allowed to stand for 10 min., and passed through a tea strainer. To dissolve phlegm in bronchial catarrh, a cupful is drunk two or three times a day, if desired sweetened with honey.
1 Teaspoon = ca. 0.8 g.

Phytomedicines: The drug is a component of so-called "digestive teas", such as Presselin® and as an adjunct in various teas to enhance their appearance.

Extract from the German Commission E monograph
(BAnz no. 85, dated 05.05.1988)

Uses
Red-poppy petal is used for respiratory complaints, for disturbed sleep, and as a sedative and for the relief of pain.
Effectiveness in the conditions indicated has not been established.

Risks
None known.

Evaluation
Since the effectiveness of red-poppy petal in the conditions indicated has not been established, its therapeutic use cannot be recommended.
There is no objection to its incorporation as a supplement in herbal teas.

Authentication: Macro- (see: Description) and microscopically, following the Erg. B. 6: The diagnostic features of the reddish violet drug include the elongated, wavy-walled epidermal cells of the petals and occasional small, roundish stomata. Sticking to the fragments of petal are numerous roundish pollen grains, up to 30 μm in diameter, with a finely verrucose exine and three pores (Fig. 3).

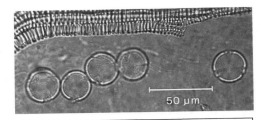

Fig. 3: Tricolpate pollen grains with finely verrucose exine

Adulteration: Rare; contamination may occur with *Papaver dubium* L., long-headed poppy, the petals of which are smaller and 2.5–3.5 cm wide.

Storage: Protected from light and moisture; it should not be kept for more than a year, since the the drug becomes unsightly and the colour fades.

Literature:
[1] Hager, vol. **6**, 444 (1977).
[2] J.B. Harborne, Phytochemistry **22**, 85 (1983).
[3] R. Willstätter and F. Weil, Liebigs Ann. Chem. **412**, 231 (1917).
[4] L. Schmid and R. Huber, Monatsh. Chem. **57**, 383 (1931).

Ribis nigri folium   Black currant leaf

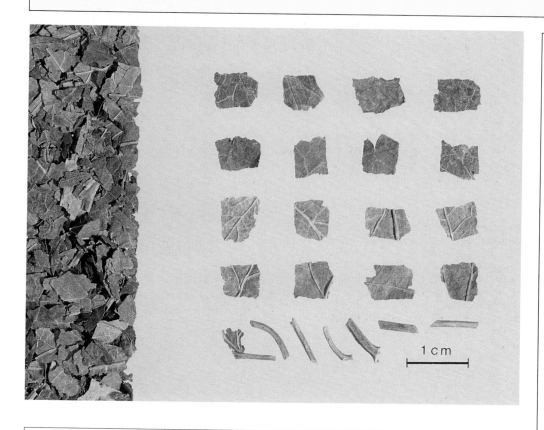

Fig. 1: Black currant leaf

<u>Description:</u> The slightly wrinkled leaf fragments have a dark green upper surface and a pale greyish green lower surface, with a widely spaced reticulate venation which is particularly distinct on the lower surface. The midrib and lateral nerves are sparsely pubescent. A scattering of dots can be seen on the lower surface, which is due to the presence of shiny yellowish glandular trichomes (hand lens). Fragments with the leaf margin show the coarsely serrate, pointed teeth (2nd row). Yellowish green, grooved leaf petioles (5th row) are frequent.

The drug has no odour or taste.

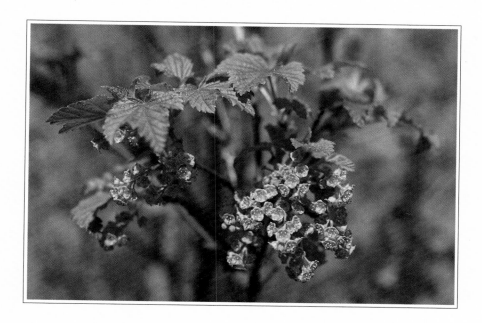

Fig. 2: *Ribes nigrum* L.

Ca. 2 m tall shrub with 3–5-lobed, doubly serrate leaves. 5-part greenish white flowers arranged in racemose inflorescences and brownish black fruits with attached calyx remains.

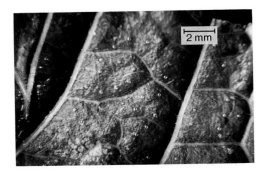

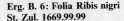

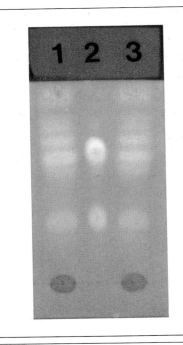

Fig. 3: Glandular trichomes on the lower surface of the leaf (hand lens)

Erg. B. 6: Folia Ribis nigri
St. Zul. 1669.99.99

Plant source: *Ribes nigrum* L., black currant (Grossulariaceae).

Synonyms: Schwarze Johannisbeerblätter, Gichtbeerblätter, Cassistee (Ger.), Feuilles de cassis (Fr.).

Origin: Grows wild in central and eastern Europe, but in temperate regions mostly cultivated. The drug is imported chiefly from Poland, Hungary, Romania, and former Yugoslavia.

Constituents: Ca. 0.5% flavonoids, especially derivatives of kaempferol and quercetin [1]; myricetin and isorhamnetin glycosides have also been detected [2]. There is little assured information about further constituents; the presence of essential oil, proanthocyanidins, oligosaccharides, diterpenes, ascorbic acid, and enzymes is reported, but without any details.

Indications: Mainly in *folk medicine* as a diuretic; and exclusively in *folk medicine* for arthritis, rheumatic complaints, diarrhoea, spasmodic cough, and, rarely, for external use in treating wounds – in all cases, the use is purely empirical.
Sakuranetin, a flavonoid present in the drug, has been shown to have fungicidal activity [3].

Making the tea: Boiling water (or add cold water and boil briefly) is poured over 2–4 g of the finely chopped drug, covered and left for 5–10 min., and then strained. A cupful is drunk several times a day.
1 Teaspoon = ca. 1.0 g.

Phytomedicines: The drug is an occasional component in diuretic tea mixtures, in "herbal teas", and in so-called "blood-purifying teas".
Note: The BP 1988 has a monograph on black currant syrup, made from the fresh ripe fruit, which is used as a dietary supplement especially for children and as a flavouring agent.

Authentication: Macro- (see: Description), microscopically, and by means of TLC (cf. St. Zul.). Among the diagnostic features are: the epidermis of the lower leaf surface, with its numerous anomocytic stomata and glandular trichomes (150–250 µm in diameter) (Figs. 3 and 4), and the curved, unicellular, pointed covering trichomes which are often present over the vascular bundles.
The TLC test of identity (fingerprint chromatogram) is as follows:

Test solution: 1 g powdered drug refluxed for 10 min. with 10 ml methanol filtered while still warm.

Reference solution: 5 mg rutin, 10 mg chlorogenic acid, and 10 mg isoquercitrin dissolved in 10 ml methanol.

Fig. 5: TLC on 4 × 8 cm silica-gel foil
1 and 3: Black currant leaf (different origins)
2: Reference substances
For details, see the text

Loadings: 5 µl test solution as a band and 1 µl reference solution as a spot.

Solvent system: ethyl acetate + anhydrous formic acid + water (80 + 8 + 12), 6 cm run.

Detection: plate dried in a current of hot air and sprayed with 1% methanolic diphenyl-

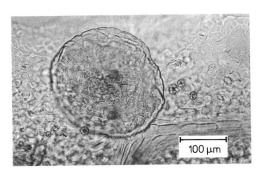

Fig. 4: Multicellular glandular trichome, embedded in the epidermis

boryloxyethylamine and then with 5% methanolic polyethylene glycol 400, followed by heating briefly at 100–105 °C.

Evaluation: in UV 366 nm light. <u>Reference solution</u>: spots at Rf ca. 0.3 (rutin, orange-yellow fluorescence), ca. 0.6 (isoquercitrin, yellowish orange fluorescence), and ca. 0.65 (chlorogenic acid, blue fluorescence). <u>Test solution</u>: a red fluorescent band just below the solvent front (chlorophyll), two orange fluorescent bands just above and below the level of the chlorogenic-acid spot, and an orange fluorescent band near the level of the rutin spot; between the level of the chlorogenic-acid spot and the solvent front, a bluish fluorescent band; additional weak fluorescent bands present (Fig. 5). An orange fluorescent zone just above the starting line indicates the presence of other *Ribes* species.

Quantitative standards: <u>St.Zul. 1669.99.99</u>: *Foreign* (*vegetable and/or mineral*) *matter*, not more than 2%. *Loss on drying*, not more than 10.0%. *Ash*, not more than 10.0%.

Adulteration: In practice seldom occurs, since the drug comes almost entirely from cultivated plants.

Storage: Dry and protected from light.

Literature:
[1] O. Calamita, J. Malinowski, and H. Strzelecka, Acta Polon. Pharm. **40**, 383 (1983); C.A. **100**, 171573 (1984).
[2] O. Rolland, A.M. Binsard, and J. Raynaud, Plantes Méd. Phytothérap. **11**, 222 (1977).
[3] B.D.L. Fitt, G.J. Smith, and D. Hornby, Plant Soil **66**, 405 (1982); C.A. **97**, 195966 (1982).

Rosae pseudofructus   (DAB 10), Rose hips (BHP 1983)

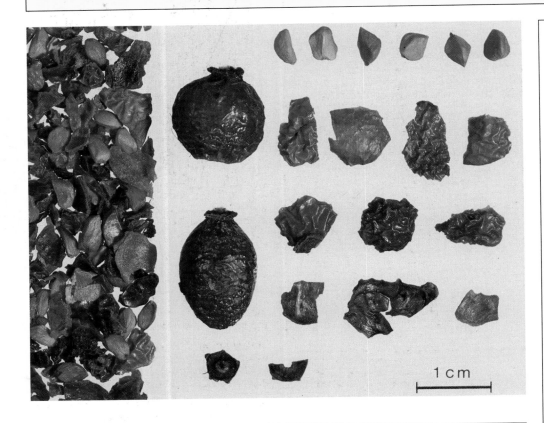

Fig. 1: Hips (upper row, "pips" (achenes), i.e. the actual fruits – not the seeds)

The drug consists of the dried hypanthia from various species of the genus *Rosa* L. with the fruit enclosed in them (wrongly called "pips" or "seeds"). The definition in DAB 10, which only admits dog-rose *hips*, reads as follows: Dog-rose hips consist of the ripe, opened, and dried hypanthia of the false fruit [the hip] largely freed of the fruit [pips] and the hairs attached to the receptacle.

__Description:__ The whole drug is about 1–2 cm long and 0.5–1.5 cm thick, roundish to ovoid, soft and fleshy, glossy and light to dark reddish brown, much shrunken and wrinkled. At the upper end, there is a stubby pentagonal disc, resulting from the shedding of most of the sepals. In the middle of the disc is a ca. 1 mm broad hole through which the remains of the styles protrude. The hollow receptacle is covered on the inside with light-coloured, stiff hairs (note the spiral ornamentation, Fig. 5) and contains ca. 5 mm long and 3 mm wide, yellowish brown, angular ovoid, three- to several-sided, fruits which are flattened on the contact face (Fig. 1).
The cut drug consists of red, fleshy, translucent, horny pieces which are curled at the edges and smooth on the outside and covered with prickly hairs on the inside (Fig. 4).

__Odour:__ Fruity.

__Taste:__ Sweetish and sour.

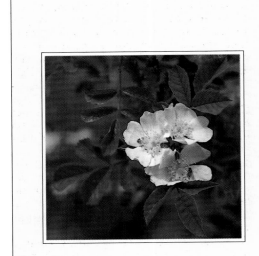

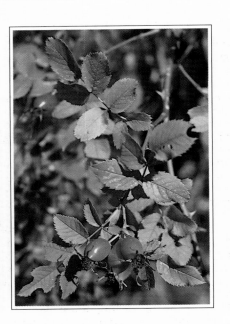

Fig. 2: *Rosa canina* L.

A shrub up to 5 m in height with pendent, thorny branches. Leaves pinnate, flowers ca. 5 cm in diameter with five pale pink to white petals.

Fig. 3: *Rosa canina* L., with hips

Note: Different drugs are official
DAB 10: Hagebuttenschalen
Ph. Helv. VII: Cynosbati fructus (Hagebutten)
Erg. B. 6: Fructus Cynosbati cum semine (Hagebutten)
Erg. B. 6: Fructus Cynosbati sine semine (Hagebuttenschalen)

Plant origin: Various *Rosa* species, especially the polymorphous *R. canina* L., dog rose; the Ph. Helv. VII also admits *R. pendulina* L. (Rosaceae).

Synonyms: Cynosbati fructus cum semine, Fructus Rosae or Cynorrhoidi (Lat.), Hip, Sweet or Wild briar fruits, Cynosbatos (Engl.), Hagebutten and many hundreds of other names within the German-speaking world [1], Cynorrhodon (Fr.).

Origin: *Rosa canina*: native in Europe, Western and Central Asia, and North Africa; naturalized in eastern North America. – *Rosa pendulina* var. *pendulina* (= *R. cinnamomea*, *R. alpina*): native in the mountains of southern and central Europe and in the Vosges. Nowadays, the drug is imported from many different countries: Chile, the former USSR, Bulgaria, Romania, China, Hungary, and former Yugoslavia.

Constituents: L-Ascorbic acid is the essential constituent, and according to [2], up to 1.7% may be present. The also drug contains pectins, tannins, sugar, and plant acids. Red and yellow pigments, especially carotenoids (mainly different isomers of rubixanthin, lycopene, and β-carotene, only the last one of which is a precursor of vitamin A); traces of flavonoids and anthocyans [3, 4].

Indications: For supportive therapy in cases of vitamin-C deficiency.
The mild laxative and diuretic action which lies at the basis of its use in *folk medicine* is supposedly due to the pectin and plant-acid content. However, this has been disputed, and it has been shown that an infusion of hips does not have a diuretic effect [5]. Nowadays, because of their acid taste, hips are much used in breakfast teas. A pleasant-tasting and vitamin-C-rich jam can be made with fresh hips from which the pips have been removed.

Making the tea: Boiling water is poured over 2–2.5 g of the crushed hips, allowed to draw for 10–15 min., and then strained.
1 Teaspoon = ca. 3.5 g.

Herbal preparations: The drug, usually mixed with Hibiscus flowers, is very often offered in tea bags or packets as a refreshing tea, without medicinal indications.

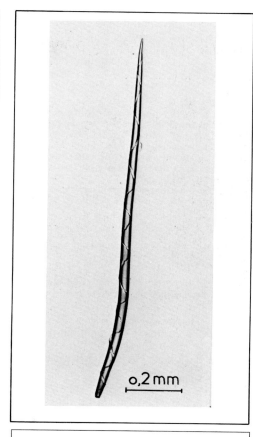

Fig. 5: **Thick-walled bristles, which narrow at both ends, from the inside "fruit wall" (hypanthium)**

Phytomedicines: In urological and diuretic preparations, and a few roborants and tonics.

Authentication: Macro- (see: Description) and microscopically; particularly noteworthy are the numerous unicellular, thick-walled, sharply pointed trichomes from the inner wall of the hip, which narrow at the base and are 2000 μm long and 30–45 μm broad (Fig. 5). The ascorbic-acid test of Merck (art. no. 10023) is suitable for the semi-quantitative estimation of vitamin C. The colour reaction depends on the reduction of the yellow phosphomolybdate complex by ascorbic acid to give molybdenum blue. The quantitative determination of vitamin C is done iodo-metrically (Ph. Helv. VII) or with 2,6-dichlorophenolindophenol (DAB 10 and [6], Tillmann reaction).
The DAB 10 TLC identity test is based on the detection of the carotenoids, but differentiation of the species of hips used as start-

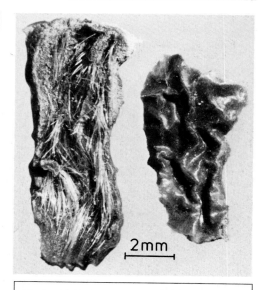

Fig. 4: **Wrinkled outer surface (right) and hairy inner surface of *Rosa canina* hips**

ing material for the drug is not possible on the basis of the carotenoid profile:

Test solution: 5 g powdered drug extracted for 5 min. on the water-bath with 20 ml methanol, then cooled and concentrated under reduced to ca. 3 ml.

Reference solution: 1 mg Sudan Red G dissolved in 2.0 ml dichloromethane.

Loadings: 20 μl test solution and 10 μl reference solution, as 2-cm bands on silica gel G.

Solvent system: ethyl acetate + hexane (50 + 50), 10 cm run.

Detection and Evaluation: after evaporation of the solvent, first examined in daylight. Reference solution: a red zone. Test solution: several yellow zones, the uppermost being the most distinct. Then sprayed with anisaldehyde reagent and heated at 100–105 °C for 5–10 min. while under observation. Test solution: uppermost part of the chromatogram, intense violet and other coloured zones visible; just below the level of the reference substance, a series of four zones, the second from the top being reddish violet and the others bluish violet to brownish – the two outer zones paler than the others; between these four zones and the intense coloured zone at the solvent front, and in the lower part of the chromatogram, only weakly coloured zones.
Only the hips from *Rosa pimpinellifolia* L. (syn. *R. spinosissima* L., p.p.), burnet rose, and the garden *R. foetida* HERRM. (syn. *R.*

Extract from the German Commission E monograph (BAnz no. 164, dated 01. 09. 90)

Uses

Preparations of rose hips are used for the prevention and treatment of colds, chills, etc., and influenza-type infections, infectious diseases, for the prevention and treatment of vitamin C deficiencies, to increase resistance, gastric-juice deficiency, bowel disorders, to aid digestion, also for gallstones, for biliary complaints and colic, complaints and disorders of the lower urinary tract, oedema, for "strengthening the kidneys", as a diuretic, for arthritis, rheumatic disorders, as an astringent, and as an eyewash.

The activity in most of the aforementioned indications has not been substantiated. The activity in treating or preventing possible vitamin-C deficiency is questionable in view of the low and rapidly decreasing vitamin C content of the drug.

Risks

None known.

Evaluation

Since the activity has not been or has not been adequately substantiated, simply on the grounds of the rapidly decreasing vitamin-C content of the drug its therapeutic application cannot be recommended.

The consumption of rose-hips preparations as a vitamin C-containing food supplement is primarily the concern of the food industry.

There are no objections to the use of the drug as a taste enhancer in herbal tea mixtures.

---

lutea MILL.) have traces of carotene, but no rubixanthin or lycopene; their dark violet colour is due to anthocyans, including cyanin [4].

Quantitative standards: Reminder – the DAB 10 drug is the dried opened hip largely freed of the pips, while the Ph. Helv. VII drug is essentially the dried whole hip.

<u>DAB 10</u>: *Ascorbic acid*, not less than 0.3% (M_r 176.1); according to our studies, in recent years ordinary commercial samples have only rarely reached this figure; the Ph. Helv. VII (below) takes this situation into account and does not specify a minimum vitamin C content. *Foreign matter*, not more than 3% fruit and not more than 1% other foreign matter; the starting zone of the chromatogram discussed above before being sprayed should only be yellow and certainly not reddish or red (Hibiscus flowers). *Loss on drying*, not more than 9.0%. *Ash*, not more than 7.0%.

<u>Ph. Helv. VII</u>: *Achenes* (fruits), not more than 55%. *Foreign matter*, not more than 1%; hypanthia of other colours, not more than 10%. *Sulphated ash*, not more than 8.0%.

Literature:

[1] W. Mitzka and L.E Schmidt (eds.), Deutscher Sprachatlas, Marburg, 1952.
[2] Hager, vol. **6B**, p. 165 (1979).
[3] Kommentar 2. AB-DDR.
[4] F.-C. Czygan and C. Wiese, unpublished results (1987). The carotinoid composition of 86 samples of ripe hips derived from 17 species was examined as part of a diploma project at the University of Würzburg.
[5] R. Jaretzky, Pharm. Zentralh. **82**, 229 (1941).
[6] R. Fischer, K. Gloris, and G. Seibt, Dtsch. Apoth. Ztg. **113**, 629 (1973).

Rosae pseudofructus "semen"   Rose hip "seeds"

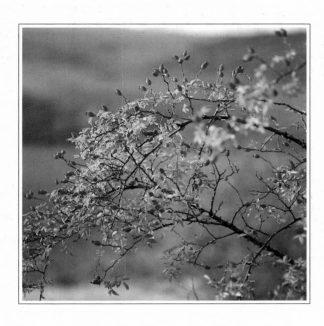

Description: The drug is the whole fruit (the "pips") and not the "seeds" of *Rosa* species. They are 3–5 mm long, ca. 2–3 mm broad, pale yellow to yellowish brown, angular ovoid, three- to several-sided and flattened on the surface of contact (see: Rosae pseudofructus, Fig. 1).

Fig. 1: *Rosa canina* L. For the Description, see: Rosae pseudofructus, Fig. 2.

Erg. B. 6: Semen Cynosbati

Plant source: As for Rosae pseudofructus (q.v.).

Synonyms: Cynosbati "semen" (Lat.), Hagebutten-Kerne, Hagebuttennüßchen (Ger.), Graine de Cynorrhodon, Graine d'eglantine (Fr.).

Origin: As for Rosae pseudofructus (Rose hips); they are obtained during the production of Fructus Cynosbati sine semine.

Constituents: Up to 10% fixed oil; up to 0.3% essential oil; traces of vitamin C (according to [1]; in our analyses, no vitamin C was detected in any of the samples investigated); inorganic substances [1].

Indications: In *folk medicine,* the drug is used as a diuretic in kidney and bladder complaints, lithiasis (possibly an indication from the doctrine of signatures); it is also employed against arthritis, rheumatism, and sciatica.

Extract from the German Commission E monograph (BAnz no. 164, dated 01. 09. 90)

Uses

Preparations of rose hip "seeds" are used in kidney and urinary tract disorders and complaints, for oedema, as a diuretic, for rheumatism and rheumatic complaints, arthritis, sciatica, for colds and chills, etc., as a laxative, for feverish complaints, as an astringent, for vitamin C deficiency and for "purifying the blood".
Efficacy in the conditions listed has not been demonstrated.

Risks

None known.

Evaluation

Since activity has not been substantiated, the therapeutic application cannot be recommended.

Making the tea: Boiling water is poured over 1–2 g of the drug which has just been coarsely powdered and after 10–15 min. passed through a tea strainer. As a diuretic, several cups of the tea are drunk throughout the day.
1 Teaspoon = ca. 3.5 g.

Phytomedicines: The drug is a component of several diuretics.

Authentication: Macro- (see: Description) and microscopically, following the Erg. B. 6 or [1]; see also the BHP 1983: Rosa.

Adulteration: Practically never.

Storage: Protected from light and moisture.

Literature:
[1] Hager, vol. **6B**, p. 167 (1979).

Rosmarini folium   Rosemary, Rosmarinus (BHP 1983)

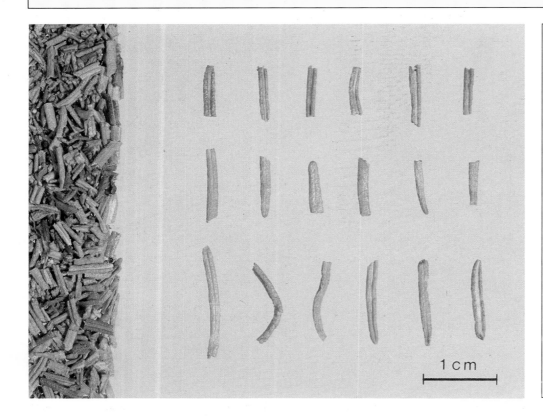

Fig. 1: Rosemary

Description: The up to 3 cm long and up to 4 mm wide leaves are narrowly lanceolate, sessile, leathery and very brittle, and with a revolute margin (upper row). Young leaves are pubescent on the upper surface, while older leaves are glabrous. They are wrinkled and grooved because of the sunken midrib which projects conspicuously from the densely woolly lower surface.

Odour: Spicy and harsh, almost camphor-like.

Taste: Spicy and harsh, bitter and aromatic, somewhat pungent.

Fig. 2: *Rosmarinus officinalis* L.

A scented, evergreen shrub (ca. 1 m in height) bearing sessile, narrowly linear, almost acicular leaves with a revolute margin and covered with a white felted tomentum. Pale bluish to light bluish violet axillary labiaceous flowers, with the two stamens projecting far beyond the corolla.

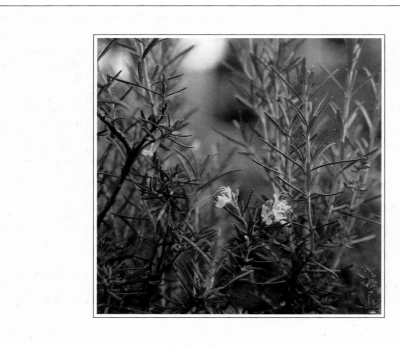

DAC 1986: Rosmarinblätter
St. Zul. 1219.99.99

Plant source: *Rosmarinus officinalis* L., rosemary (Lamiaceae).

Synonyms: Folia Anthos, Folia Roris marini (Lat.), Rosmarinblätter, Krankraut- or Kranzenkrautblätter (Ger.), Feuilles de rosmarin (Fr.).

Origin: Native in the Mediterranean region and there cultivated in many countries. The drug is imported from Spain, Morocco, former Yugoslavia, and Tunisia.

Constituents: 1.0–2.5% essential oil, with as main components 1,8-cineole (15–30%), camphor (15–25%), α-pinene (up to 25%), and other monoterpenes (among them borneol and limonene) [1]. The composition of the essential oil varies according to the stage of development and the origin of the leaves [1–3]. Also present: rosmarinic acid, diterpenoid bitter substances (carnosol (=picrosalvin), rosmanol, rosmadial, etc. [4–6]), triterpene acids (e.g. ursolic acid [4, 7,

8]), triterpene alcohols (e.g. α- and β-amyrin, betulin [9]), flavonoids (e.g. luteolin, genkwanin (7-*O*-methylapigenin), diosmetin, and corresponding glycosides [10]).

Note: The DAB 10 and Ph. Helv. VII monographs relate not to Rosmarini folium as such, but rather to rosemary oil (Rosmarini aetheroleum), the oil obtained by steam distillation from the leaves and leafy stems.

Indications: Owing to the essential-oil content, as a carminative and stomachic in digestive upsets, flatulence, feeling of distension, but also to stimulate the appetite and gastric secretion. Less often, it is also used as a (weakly active) choleretic, which is based on the content of bitter substances The rise in biliary flow is brought about by a rapidly appearing cholagogic action, followed by a slower choleretic effect [12].

Externally, in the form of an oil or ointment, the drug is applied as an analgesic liniment for rheumatism of the muscles and joints, and in the form of the drug or essential oil as an additive to baths for local stimulation of the circulation.

In *folk medicine,* rosemary is put on dressings for poorly healing wounds and for eczema; it is also utilized as an insecticide [2]. The leaves are a valued spice, especially in Italy and France.

The drug is widely employed as a preservative and antioxidant, e.g. for meat and fat; rosmanol and carnosol are particularly active in this respect [5]. In addition, the plant is an ingredient in the preparation of liqueurs, e.g. Bénédictine and Danziger Goldwasser [2].

Side effects: With the application of large amounts of rosemary oil (but hardly of the leaves), there is a danger of gastroenteritis and nephritis [11]. A 15% alcoholic extract showed no signs of toxicity in rats at doses of 2 g/kg i.p. [12]. However, rosemary preparations should not be taken during pregnancy (toxic side effects from components of the essential oil).

Making the tea: Boiling water is poured over 2 g of the finely chopped drug and after 15 min. passed through a tea strainer.

For external use, e.g. for baths, 50 g of the drug is boiled for a short while with 1 litre of water, then covered and allowed to stand for 15–30 min.; the aqueous extract separated from the drug is added to the bath. For making rosemary wine, 20 g drug of the drug is put into 1 litre of wine and left for 5 days with occasional shaking.

1 Teaspoon = ca. 2 g.

Phytomedicines: Especially rosemary oil, in combined preparations for external use as a liniment in the form of ointments, embrocations, and alcoholic extracts; in bath oils

Extract from the German Commission E monograph
(BAnz no. 223, dated 30.11.1985)

Uses
Internally: dyspeptic complaints; in supportive treatment for rheumatic disorders.
External use: circulatory disorders.

Contraindications
None known.

Side effects
None known.

Interactions with other remedies
None known.

Dosage
Internally: daily dose: 4–6 g drug, 10–20 drops essential oil; preparations correspondingly.
Externally: 50 g to a full bath; 6–10% essential oil in semi-solid and liquid preparations; other preparations correspondingly.

Mode of administration
Chopped drug for infusions; drug powder, dry extract, and other galenical preparations for internal and external use.

Effects
Experimentally: spasmolytic on the bile duct and small intestine, positively inotropic, increases coronary blood supply.
In man: skin irritant, stimulates the blood circulation (when used externally).

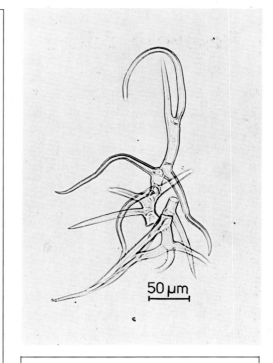

Fig. 3: Much branched covering trichome from the lower surface of the leaf of *Rosmarinus officinalis*

and bath additives; internally, as rosemary wine or as the drug extract, in gastrointestinal remedies (stomachics and carminatives).

Regulatory status (UK): General Sales List – Schedule 1, Table A.

Authentication: Macro- (see: Description) and microscopically. The multicellular, much-branched covering trichomes, which are up to 300 µm long (Fig. 3) and which mostly occur in densely tangled masses, are a particularly diagnostic feature. The cracks in the thick cuticle, which are reminiscent of "ice floes", is another important microscopical character. The hypodermis is composed of one to several layers of large irregularly rounded to ovoid cells, with thickened anticlinal walls, which are oriented towards the veins of the leaf. For the detailed microscopy of the powdered drug, see [13].

The DAB 10 TLC identity test for rosemary oil is as follows:

Test solution: 20 µl oil dissolved in 1.0 ml toluene.

Reference solution: 5 mg each of borneol and bornyl acetate and 10 µl cineole dissolved in 10 ml toluene.

Loadings: 10 µl of each solution, as 2-cm bands on silica gel G.

Solvent system: dichloromethane, 2 × 10 cm run.

Detection: sprayed with anisaldehyde reagent and heated for 5–10 min. at 100–105 °C while being observed.

Evaluation: in daylight. Reference solution: the bluish green to greyish blue zones of borneol in the lower half and of bornyl acetate just above the halfway mark, and the bluish grey cineole zone about the middle. Test solution: zones similar in position, colour, and of about the same intensity of colour; other, reddish violet zones may be present.

The following method for the TLC examination of rosemary leaf is given in [14], together with coloured illustrations of the chromatograms obtained:

Test solution: 3 g coarsely powdered leaf refluxed for 1 hour with 100 ml diethyl ether; filtrate evaporated to ca. 3 ml and the solution used for chromatography.

Reference solution: 1% methanolic carnosol (picrosalvin).

1,8-Cineole　Borneol:　　R = H　　Camphor
Bornyl acetate: R = COCH

Rosmarinic acid

Genkwanin　R^1 = H, R^2 = OH, R^3 = CH_3
Luteolin　　R^1 = R^2 = OH, R^3 = H
Diosmetin　R^1 = OH, R^2 = OCH_3, R^3 = H

Carnosol
(= Picrosalvin)

Rosmanol

Loadings: 40 µl test solution and 20 µl reference solution, on silica gel 60F$_{254}$.

Solvent system: chloroform + methanol (97 + 3), 15 cm run.

Detection: 10% aqueous iron(III) chloride reagent, or 5% ethanolic sulphuric acid and then 1% ethanolic vanillin followed by heating at 110 °C for 5–10 min. while under observation.

Evaluation: Test solution: during extraction, carnosol undergoes ring opening to carnosolic acid – a yellow brown zone at Rf ca. 0.2, becoming greenish brown with iron(III) chloride; a second, intense coloured zone at

Rf ca. 0.4; after the vanillin/sulphuric acid treatment, terpenoid compounds of the essential oil as violet zones. In UV 365 nm light, rosmarinic acid and sinensetin (a flavonoid) as blue fluorescent zones.

The essential-oil content is determined according to standard procedures.

Quantitative standards: <u>DAC 1986</u>: *Volatile oil*, not less than 1.2%. *Foreign matter*, not more than 10% brown woody stems and not more than 2% other foreign matter (the leaves of two other Lamiaceae: *Ledum palustre* L., marsh rosemary, and *Teucrium montanum* L., are mentioned). *Loss on drying*, not more than 10%. *Ash*, not more than 7.0%.

Adulteration: Rarely occurs in practice.

Storage: Protected against moisture and light in well-closed glass or metal (but not plastic) containers.

Literature:
[1] V. Formáček and K.-H. Kubeczka, Essential Oils Analysis by Capillary Gas Chromatography and Carbon-13 NMR Spectroscopy. J. Wiley u. Sons. Chichester etc. 1982.
[2] Hager, Band **6B**, 172 (1979).
[3] Kommentar DAB 10, Rosmarinöl.
[4] E. Wenkert, A. Fuchs and J.D. McChesney, J. org. Chem. **30**, 2931 (1965).
[5] R. Inatani, N. Nakatani und H. Fuwa, Agric Biol. Chem. **47**, 521 (1983).
[6] N. Nakatani and R. Inatani, Agric. Biol. Chem. **47**, 353 (1983).
[7] C.H. Brieskorn and G. Zweyrohn, Pharmazie **25**, 488 (1970).
[8] C.H. Brieskorn, Dtsch. Apoth. Ztg. **105**, 1524 (1965).
[9] C.H. Brieskorn, M. Decken, U. Degel and A. Atallah, Arch. Pharm. (Weinheim) **299**, 663 (1966).
[10] C.H. Brieskorn, H.J. Michelk and W. Biechele, Dtsch. Lebensm. Rundsch. **69**, 245 (1973).
[11] H. Braun und D. Frohne, Heilpflanzenlexikon für Ärzte und Apotheker, Gustav Fischer Verlag, Stuttgart/New York 1987.
[12] J.J. Mongold et al., Pl. Méd. phytothérap. **25**, 6 (1991).
[13] B.P. Jackson and D.W. Snowdon, Atlas of microscopy of medicinal plants, culinary herbs and spices, Belhaven Press, London, 1990, p. 202.
[14] H. Wagner, S. Bladt, and E.M. Zgainski, Plant drug analysis, Springer-Verlag, Berlin, Heidelberg, New York, Tokyo, 1984, p. 142.

Wording of the package, from the German Standard Licence:

7.1　**Uses**
Internally: flatulence, feeling of distension, and mild cramp-like gastrointestinal and biliary upsets.
Externally: in supportive treatment for rheumatism of the muscles and joints.

7.2　**Contraindications**
Preparations of rosemary should not be taken during pregnancy.

7.3　**Dosage and Mode of administration**
Internally: hot water (ca. 150 ml) is poured over 1 teaspoonful (2 g) of **Rosemary** and after 15 min. passed through a tea strainer.

Unless otherwise prescribed, a cup of the freshly prepared tea is drunk warm three or four times a day between meals.
Externally: unless otherwise prescribed, ca. 100 g of **Rosemary** are added to 20 litres of water in which to bathe the affected part(s).

7.4　**Note**
Store protected from light and moisture.

Rubi fruticosi folium   Bramble leaf

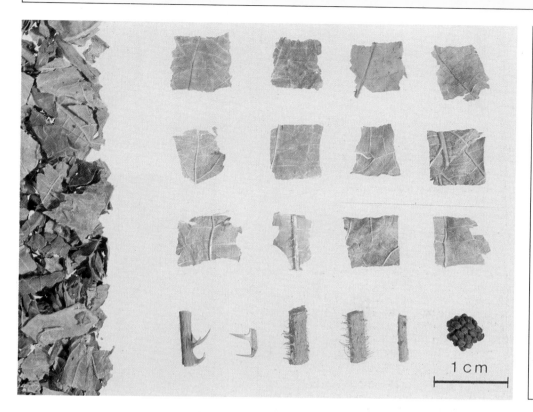

Fig. 1: Bramble leaf

<u>Description:</u> The 3–5-partite leaves, with ovate leaflets up to 7 cm long, have a serrate margin. The cut drug consists of small pieces of leaf, the midrib of which is prominent on the lower surface and bears fine whitish prickles (fig. 4). The thicker petioles or fragments of shoots (sometimes the herb is also seen in commerce), have more distinct prickles. The upper surface of the leaf is green, while its lower surface usually has only a sparse indumentum.

<u>Taste:</u> Astringent.

Fig. 2: *Rubus fruticosus* L. s.l.

A highly variable, up to 3-m tall, shrub with prickly shoots. Digitate leaves with a serrate margin. Flowers white or pink.

Fig. 3: *Rubus fruticosus* L. s.l., shoot with ripe and unripe fruits.

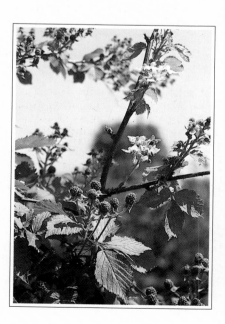

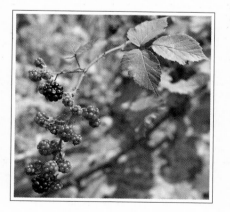

DAC 1986: Brombeerblätter
St. Zul. 1449.99.99

Plant source: *Rubus fruticosus* L. s.l., bramble or blackberry (Rosaceae).

Synonyms: Bro(h)mbeere, Kratzbeere (Ger.), Feuilles de ronce noire (Fr.).

Origin: Europe; the drug is collected from the wild and imported from the former USSR, former Yugoslavia, Bulgaria, Albania, and Hungary.

Constituents: 8(-14?) % hydrolysable tannins (gallotannins) [1]; dimeric ellagitannins [2, 3]; plant acids, including citric and isocitric acids [4]; flavonoids; pentacyclic triterpene acids [5, 6].

Indications: On the basis of the tannin content, it can be used as an astringent and antidiarrhoeic.
Bramble leaf is used (alone or in mixtures with other drugs) especially as "Deutscher Haustee" (German household tea) and "Frühstückstee" (breakfast tea). To obtain a

Fig. 4: Pubescent lower surface of *Rubus fruticosus* leaf, showing the prickles on the midrib

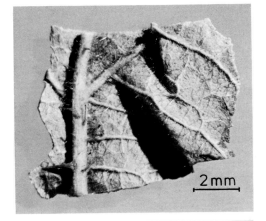

Fig. 5: TLC on 4 × 8 cm silica-gel foil
1 and 3: Bramble leaf (different origins)
2: Reference substances
For details, see the text

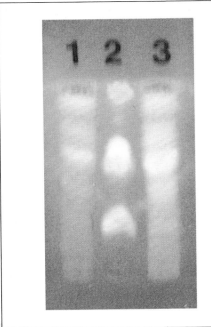

taste similar to that of ordinary tea, the leaves are likewise fermented and they then become blackish in colour. Details of the fermentation and use of the drug as a household tea can be found in [7].

Making the tea: Boiling water is poured over 1.5 g of the finely cut drug and after 10–15 min. passed through a tea strainer. 1 Teaspoon = ca. 0.6 g.

Herbal teas: Bramble leaf is present in a series of herbal teas for very different indications. Aqueous extracts of the fermented drug are, among others, constituents of instant teas.

Phytomedicines: A few preparations such as the antidiabetic Nervosana Mixtur®.

Authentication: Macro- and microscopically, following the DAC 1986. The prickles are an important diagnostic character (see: Description). In addition, there are the occasional thick-walled bristly hairs on the upper surface of the leaves, present especially over the nerves and with intersecting spiral lines (observed in numerous Rosaceae), and the stellate trichomes which are a feature of the lower surface of the leaves. Glandular trichomes with a multicellular stalk are very rare. Cluster crystals of calcium oxalate – again, frequently present in Rosaceae – occur in the mesophyll.
The following TLC method is a suitable test of identity – it provides a fingerprint chromatogram:

Test solution: 1 g powdered drug refluxed for ca. 10 min. with 10 ml methanol, filtered, the filtrate taken to dryness, and the residue dissolved in 2.0 ml methanol.

Reference solution: 10 mg rutin, 10 mg quercetin, 5 mg hyperoside, and 20 mg chlorogenic acid dissolved in 10 ml methanol.

Loadings: 3 µl test solution as a band and 1 µl reference solution, on silica gel.

Solvent system: ethyl acetate + anhydrous formic acid + water (88 + 6 + 6), 5 cm run.

Detection: after complete removal of the solvent in a current of hot air, sprayed with 1% methanolic diphenylboryloxyethylamine and then with 5% ethanolic polyethylene glycol 400.

Evaluation: in UV 366 nm light. Reference solution: reference compounds with the following approximate Rf values and fluorescence: rutin 0.25, orange-yellow; hyperoside ca. 0.53, orange-yellow; chlorogenic acid 0.60 (but not clearly separated from hyperoside) greenish blue; quercetin directly below the solvent front. Test solution: an orange fluorescent zone at about the level of the hyperoside spot; slightly below and just above this zone, two bluish fluorescent zones; near the solvent front, a red fluorescent zone (chlorophyll) and below it a bluish fluorescent zone; at the same level as the rutin spot, a (possibly very weak) orange fluorescent zone (Fig. 5).

The TLC procedure given in the St.Zul. 1449.99.99 makes use of silica gel G (15 cm run) in the solvent system: ethyl acetate + anhydrous formic acid + water (20 + 2 + 3), with chlorogenic acid and isoquercitrin as reference compounds; the detection and evaluation are essentially the same as above.

Quantitative standards: DAC 1986: *Foreign matter*, not more than 5% flowers and stems and not more than 2% other foreign matter. *Loss on drying*, not more than 10.0%. *Ash*, not more than 8.0%.

St.Zul. 1449.99.99: *Foreign matter*, not more than 4% flowers and stems more than 3 mm thick. *Loss on drying*, not more than 10%. *Ash*, not more than 8.0%.

Adulteration: Raspberry leaves, Rubi idaei folium (q.v.), are very downy on the lower surface, the tomentum in contrast to bramble leaves consisting of matted, slender trichomes.

Occasionally, batches of bramble leaf are found in commerce that derive from thornless forms ("American blackberry").

Literature:
[1] G. Marczal, Pharm. Zentralh. **100**, 181 (1961).
[2] R.K. Gupta et al., J. Chem. Soc., Perkin Trans. I, 2525 (1982).
[3] K. Lund, Thesis, Freiburg i. Br., 1986.
[4] C. Wollmann, R. Pohloudek-Fabini, and H. Wollmann, Pharmazie **19**, 456 (1964).
[5] A. Sarkar and S.N. Ganguly, Phytochemistry **17**, 1983 (1978).
[6] M. Mukherjee, K.L. Ghatak, S.N. Ganguly, and S. Antoulas, Phytochemistry **23**, 2581 (1984).
[7] K. Koch, Pharmazie **3**, 29 (1948).

Rubi idaei folium   Raspberry leaf, Rubus (BHP 1983)

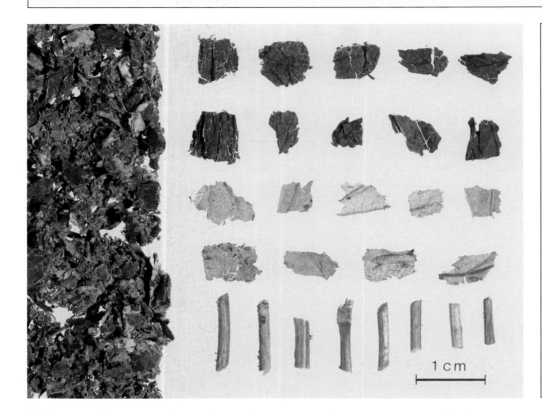

Fig. 1: Raspberry leaf

Description: The cut drug is made up of leaf fragments which are sparsely pubescent on the dark green to brownish green upper surface and which have a dense, silver-grey tomentum on the lower surface; the fragments also exhibit pinnate venation (Fig. 4); the leaf fragments clump together because of this dense tomentum. The drug is further characterized by the presence of some fragments with a sharply serrate margin and by large, green or reddish tinged, petiole fragments and a few pieces of stem. The petiole and lower part of the midrib occasionally bear very small prickles.

Taste: Somewhat harsh and bitter.

Fig. 2: *Rubus idaeus* L.

A 1–2 m tall shrub with stems bearing numerous small prickles. Leaves 3–5-partite; lower surface densely tomentose. Flowers with 5 white petals; after flowering, sepals reflexed.

Fig. 3: *Rubus idaeus* L. with ripe fruit

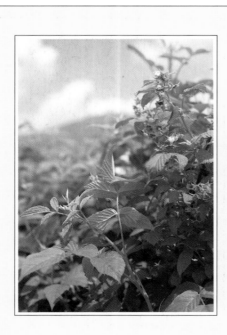

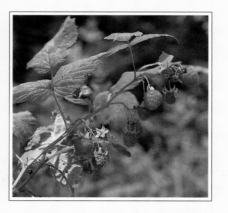

Erg. B. 6: Folia Rubi idaei

Plant source: *Rubus idaeus* L., raspberry (Rosaceae).

Synonyms: Himbeerblätter (Ger.), Feuille de framboisier (Fr.).

Origin: Native in Europe, North America, and in temperate Asia; the drug is collected from the wild in central and eastern Europe (the former USSR, former Yugoslavia, Hungary, Bulgaria).

Constituents: Gallo- and ellagitannins; flavonoids; also some vitamin C [1].

Indications: Almost exclusively in *folk medicine,* on the basis of the tannin content as an antidiarrhoeic and as an astringent gargle for inflammation of the mouth and throat, less often for chronic skin conditions. As a component of diet beverages.
It is included in many herbal mixtures to "stabilize" the mixture and prevent the components separating out.

Extract from the German Commission E monograph (BAnz no. 193, dated 15. 10. 1987)

Uses

Raspberry leaf is used for disorders of the gastrointestinal tract, the respiratory tract, the cardiovascular system, and the mouth and throat, and also for skin rashes and inflammation, influenza, fever, menstrual problems, diabetes, vitamin deficiency, as a diaphoretic, diuretic, and choleretic, and also to "purify the blood and skin".
The foregoing indications have not been substantiated.

Risks

None known.

Evaluation

Since activity in the indications cited has not been proved, therapeutic application of the drug cannot be advocated.

Making the tea: Boiling water is poured over 1.5 g finely of the chopped drug and after 5 min. passed through a tea strainer.
1 Teaspoon = ca. 0.8 g.

Phytomedicines: Together with other drugs in many laxative and "blood-purifying" teas; in household and breakfast teas. The Erg. B. 6 has a kind of German herbal tea made up of: 500 parts raspberry leaves, 450 parts strawberry leaves, and 50 parts sweet woodruff herb (*Asperula odorata* L.).
Among the available UK products containing extracts of the drug are present in Potter's Raspberry Leaf Tablets and Gerard House Helonias Compound Tablets.

Authentication: Macro- (see: Description); microscopically, the drug is characterized by leaf fragments with on the lower surface very many unicellular, slender trichomes which are often twisted and tangled together, and on the upper surface, especially over the nerves, stiff, pointed, unicellular trichomes (Fig. 5), which in the upper part are often so thickened as to obliterate the lumen and which may show spiral markings which give the effect of intersecting lines on the wall, and by glandular trichomes with a biseriate stalk and multicellular head. There are, in addition, large oxalate clusters in the mesophyll (Fig. 5). The microscopy of the powdered drug is also described and illustrated in [2].
The following fingerprint TLC procedure is a suitable test of identity:

Test solution: 1 g powdered drug refluxed for 10 min. with 10 ml methanol, filtered, the filtrate taken to dryness and the residue dissolved in 2.0 ml methanol.

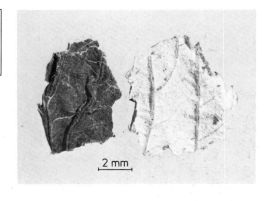

Fig. 4: Leaf fragments: sparsely pubescent, darkish upper surface (left) and lower surface with felted tomentum (right)

2 mm

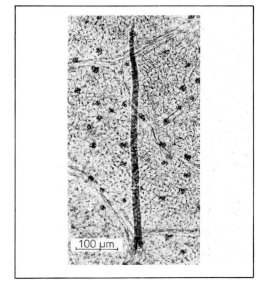

Fig. 5: Upper surface of the leaf, with a large covering trichome and numerous cluster crystals of calcium oxalate in the mesophyll

100 µm

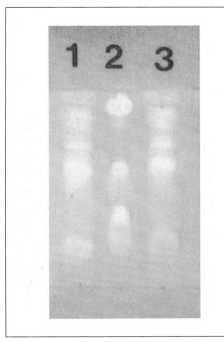

Fig. 6: TLC on 4 × 8 cm silica-gel foil

1 and 3: Raspberry leaf (different origins)
2: Reference substances

For details, see the text

Reference solution: 10 mg rutin, 5 mg hyperoside, and 10 mg quercetin dissolved in 10 ml methanol.

Loadings: 3 µl test solution as a band and 1 µl reference solution, on silica gel.

Solvent system: ethyl acetate + anhydrous formic acid + water (88 + 6 + 6), 5 cm run.

Detection: after complete evaporation of the solvent in a current of hot air, sprayed with 1% methanolic diphenylboryloxyethylamine and then with 5% ethanolic polyethylene glycol 400.

Evaluation: in UV 366 nm light. <u>Reference solution</u>: the rutin spot in the lower third, the hyperoside spot about the middle, and the quercetin spot just below the solvent front, all three spots exhibiting an orange-yellow fluorescence. <u>Test solution</u>: an orange-yellow fluorescent zone near the Rf of hyperoside, and slightly above it, and as far as the Rf of the quercetin spot, 3–4 bluish fluorescent zones; directly below the solvent front, a red fluorescent zone (chlorophylls); level with, or slightly lower than, the rutin spot, an orange fluorescent zone (Fig. 6).

Quantitative standards: <u>Erg. B. 6</u>: *Ash*, not more than 8%.
<u>BHP 1983</u>: *Water-soluble extractive*, not less than 15%. *Total ash*, not more than 8%. *Acid-insoluble ash*, not more than 1.5%.

Adulteration: Occasionally, and mostly by confusion, with bramble leaves. For the diagnostic features, see: Rubi fruticosi folium (Bramble leaf).

Literature:
[1] Hager, vol. **6B**, p. 186 (1979).
[2] B.P. Jackson and D.W. Snowdon, Atlas of microscopy of medicinal plants, culinary herbs and spices, Belhaven Press, London, 1990, p. 196.

Salicis cortex   (DAB 10), Salix (BHP 1983), Willow bark

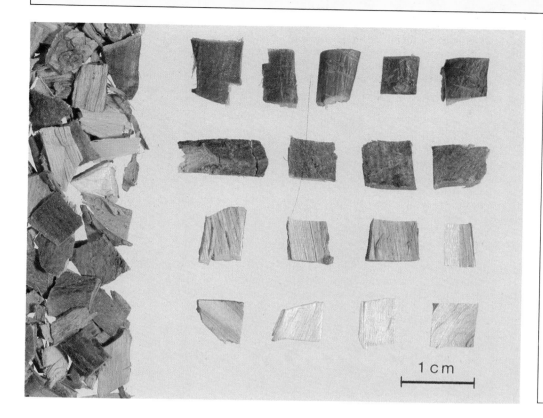

Fig. 1: Willow bark

<u>Description:</u> The 1–2 mm thick, quite often channelled pieces of bark have a glossy, greenish yellow or brownish grey outer surface, which is smooth or often shows faint longitudinal striations. Depending on the species, the almost white, pale yellow, or, usually, cinnamon brown inner surface is smooth or has fine longitudinal striations. The fracture is short and, because of the many fibres, fibrous and splintery.

<u>Taste:</u> Astringent and bitter.

Fig. 2: *Salix* sp. L.

Species supplying the drug: dioecious trees or shrubs bearing oblong to lanceolate leaves, mostly with a finely serrate margin and glabrous or pubescent, depending on the species. Bark from 2–3 year old branches.

Fig. 3: *Salix* sp. L.

Flowers of willow species in erect catkins, the male ones with protruding yellow stamens, the female ones green.

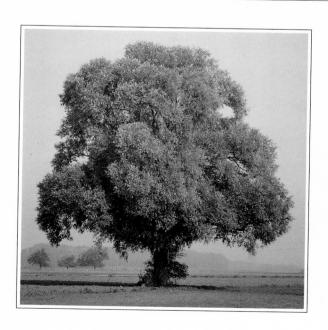

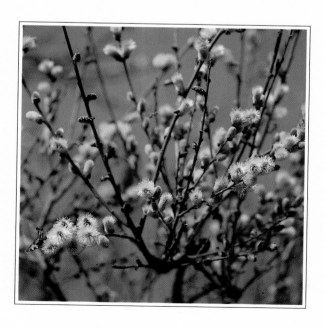

Plant sources: The plant source(s) of the drug is (are) not defined, and in practice it originates, among others, from such species as: *Salix alba* L., white willow, *S. purpurea* L., purple osier, *S. daphnoides* VILL., *S. viminalis* L., common osier, *S. caprea* L., goat willow, *S. nigricans* SM., dark-leaved willow, *S. fragilis* L., crack willow, *S. pentandra* L., bay willow, etc. (Salicaceae).
In principle, only the salicin-rich species, *S. purpurea*, *S. daphnoides*, and *S. fragilis*, should be used, since the other species usually do not have the desired or required amount of salicin (see: Constituents). The DAB 10 indicates *S. purpurea*, *S. daphnoides*, and other *Salix* species.

Synonyms: (White or European) Willow bark, Weidenrinde, Fieberweidenrinde, Maiholzrinde (Ger.), Écorce de saule (Fr.).

Origin: Native in Europe and Asia, and to some extent also in North America. Imports of the drug come from former Yugoslavia, Bulgaria, Hungary, and Romania.

Constituents: 1.5 to more than 11% phenolic glycosides, the composition varying qualitatively and quantitatively according to the plant source [1–3, 12]: the salicylates salicin, salicortin, tremulacin, populin, fragilin, as well as salireposide, triandrin, vimalin, picein, grandidentatin and 3′- and 4′-acetyl-salicortin. Aromatic aldehydes and acids: salidroside, vanillin, syringa-aldehyde, syringin; salicylic, vanillic, syringic, *p*-hydroxybenzoic, *p*-coumaric, caffeic, and ferulic acids. Salicyl alcohol (= saligenin). Flavonoids: isoquercitrin, naringin and its 7-*O*-glucoside, (+)- and (−)-naringin 5β-*O*-glucoside, the chalcone isosalipurposide, (+)-catechol. 8–20% Tannins.
The following species have a high salicin content: *S. purpurea* (6–8.5%), *S. daphnoides* (4.9–5.6%), and *S. fragilis* (3.9–10.2%); cf. *S. alba* (0.49–0.98%) [3, 4].

Indications: For mild feverish colds and infections (influenza), acute and chronic rheumatic disorders, mild headaches, and pain caused by inflammation. It is mainly salicin and the salicyl glycosides which form salicin after hydrolysis of the acyl group that represent a salicylic-acid pro-drug and that like it have antipyretic, analgesic/antirheumatic, and antiseptic actions. Salicin is split by the intestinal flora into saligenin (salicyl alcohol) and glucose. Saligenin is absorbed and oxidized in the blood and liver to salicylic acid. It is excreted in the urine mainly as salicyluric acid, but also as salicyl glucuronide, salicylic acid, gentisic acid, and unchanged saligenin.

More than 86% of salicin or saligenin is absorbed, and this affords a constant plasma salicylate level for several hours [5, 6]. Over 50% of salicortin is converted into salicin *in vitro* in synthetic gastric juice within 6 hours at 37 °C [4]. Because of the protracted formation of the active principle of the drug, use against acute headaches is inappropriate. The effective dose required daily is 60–120 mg salicin [7]. Salicin-containing plant drugs are reviewed in [13]. The enzymic decomposition of salicin and derivatives is examined in [14].
Willow bark is the phytotherapeutic precursor of acetylsalicylic acid (Aspirin®); and in times when medicines have been in short supply, notable clinical results have been achieved with it [8].

Side effects: Salicylate side effects are not to be expected with the amount of salicylate derived from the drug administered. Possible gastrointestinal troubles are due to the tannins present in the drug. With known hypersensitivity to salicylates, the possibility of the expected reactions (urticaria, rhinitis, asthma, bronchial spasms) being elicited must be borne in mind; however, the likelihood of their appearance with sodium salicylate, and hence with willow bark, is considered to be slight.
In-vitro tests show that, as with salicylic acid but not acetylsalicylic acid, salicin and sal-

Salicin → (Intestinal flora) → Saligenin + Glucose → (Oxidation) → Salicylic acid

Salicortin

Fragilin: R = 6-O-Acetylglucose
Populin: R = 6-O-Benzoylglucose

Triandrin: R = H
Vimalin: R = CH₃

icortin inhibit cyclooxygenase. Irreversible inhibition of thrombocytes is thus unlikely; there should be no increased interaction with blood coagulants and hence no danger of haemorrhage during the final months of pregnancy [13].

Making the tea: 2–3 g of the finely chopped or coarsely powdered drug is put into cold water, heated to boiling, and after 5 min. passed through a tea strainer. A cup of the tea is drunk three or four times a day.
1 Teaspoon = ca. 1.5 g.

Phytomedicines: Willow-bark extracts are a component of some prepared analgesics and antirheumatics, hypnotics and sedatives, and gastrointestinal remedies.

Regulatory status (UK): General Sales List – Schedule 1, Table A.

Authentication: Macro- (see: Description) and microscopically, following the DAB 10; see also the BHP 1983. The diagnostic features include the up to 600 μm long, very narrow, and hence very thick-walled, phloem fibres which are surrounded by a crystal sheath containing prisms of calcium oxalate. The parenchyma of the cortex is thick-walled and pitted, and often has beaded walls; it has large cluster crystals of calcium oxalate and it is stained red with 80% sulphuric acid. The medullary rays in the secondary bark are uniseriate. As a rule, stone cells are absent, but they do occur in the primary bark of *Salix alba* and *S. fragilis*. The following TLC test of identity is essentially the same as that given in the DAB 10:

Test solution: 1 g powdered drug refluxed with 50 ml methanol, filtered, and the cooled filtrate shaken for 2–3 min. with 0.5 g polyamide powder, again filtered, taken to dryness, and the residue dissolved in 3 ml methanol.

Reference solution: 2 mg salicin, 5 mg cianidanol (catechol), and 5 mg glucose dissolved in 1 ml methanol + water (1 + 1).

Loadings: 2 and 5 μl test solution and 2 μl reference solution, as bands on silica gel.

Solvent system: ethyl acetate + anhydrous formic acid + water (80 + 13 + 7), 6 cm run.

Detection: after drying at 100–105 °C for ca. 2 min., sprayed with a mixture prepared from 19 ml 0.5% ethanolic thymol and 1 ml conc. sulphuric acid, then heated at 120 °C for ca. 2–3 min. and examined at once in daylight.

Evaluation: Reference solution: glucose, in the lower third as an orangish red band, salicin about the middle as a red to reddish brown band, and catechol (cianidanol) as an orangish brown band. Test solution: three corresponding bands and, in addition, below the glucose band two pinkish red to brownish red bands (Fig. 4); further, weakly coloured bands possibly also be present.
Other TLC systems for separating and detecting the salicyl glycosides are to be found in [9, 10, cf. 15].

Quantitative standards: DAB 10: *Total salicin*, not less than 1.0% calculated as salicin (M_r 286.3); many *Salix* species do not reach this figure. *Foreign matter*, not more than 3.0%. *Loss on drying*, not more than 11%. *Ash*, not more than 10%.
BHP 1983: *Water-soluble extractive*, not less than 10%. *Total ash*, not more than 8%. *Acid-insoluble ash*, not more than 1%.

Adulteration: Hardly ever occurs. It should be remembered that besides the salicin-rich barks, there are barks on the market that contain very little salicin. The quantitative determination of the salicin is only possible after separation from ballast substances, e.g. by means of HPLC [3, 4, 11].

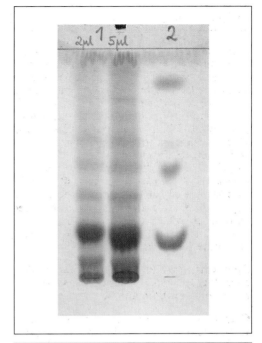

Fig. 4: TLC on 4 × 8 cm foil
1 Willow bark
2 Reference compounds
For details, see the text

Literature:
[1] H. Thieme, Planta Med. **13**, 431 (1965).
[2] H. Thieme, Pharmazie **20**, 570 (1965).
[3] B. Meier, O. Sticher, and A. Bettschart, Dtsch. Apoth. Ztg. **125**, 341 (1985).
[4] B. Meier, D. Lehmann, O. Sticher, and A. Bettschart, Pharm. Acta Helv. **60**, 269 (1985).
[5] E. Steinegger and H. Hövel, Pharm. Acta Helv. **47**, 133 (1972).
[6] E. Steinegger and H. Hövel, Pharm. Acta Helv. **47**, 222 (1972).
[7] Commission E monograph.
[8] R.A. Mayer and M. Mayer, Pharmazie **4**, 77 (1949).
[9] R.C. S. Audette, G. Blunden, J.W. Steele, and C.S.C. Wong, J. Chromatogr. **25**, 367 (1966).
[10] B. Meier, D. Lehmann, O. Sticher, and A. Bettschart, Dtsch. Apoth. Ztg. **127**, 2401 (1987).
[11] O. Sticher, C. Egloff, and A. Bettschart, Planta Med. **42**, 126 (1981).
[12] R. Julkunen-Tiitto, Phytochemistry **28**, 2115 (1989).
[13] B. Meier and M. Liebi, Z. Phytotherap. **11**, 50 (1990).
[14] R. Julkunen-Tiitto and B. Meier, J. Nat. Prod. **55**, 1204 (1992).
[15] H. Wagner, S. Bladt, and E.M. Zgainski, Plant drug analysis, Springer-Verlag, Berlin, Heidelberg, New York, Tokyo, 1984, p. 282.

Salviae folium (DAB 10), Red sage

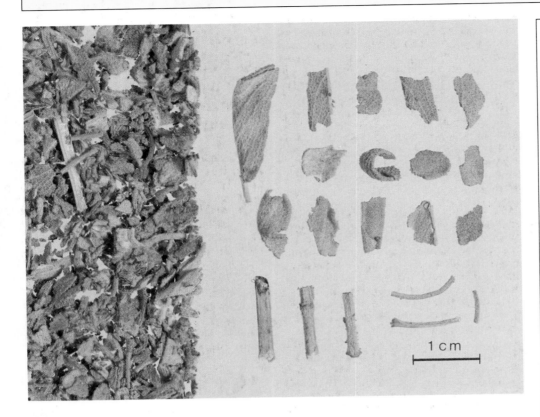

Fig. 1: Red sage

<u>Description</u>: The long-petiolate, 3–10 cm long and up to 3 cm wide, oval, oblong-ovate, to lanceolate leaves are densely pubescent on both surfaces; they have a distinctly crenulate margin and deeply depressed venation which is very prominent on the lower surface, and a lamina which is rounded and sometimes singly or doubly auriculate at the base.

The cut drug consists of small leaf fragments, which, because of the dense tomentum, cling together; the fine pubescence on both surfaces and the reticulate venation on the lower surface are easily recognized.

<u>Odour</u>: Intensely spicy and aromatic.

<u>Taste</u>: Spicy, bitter, and astringent.

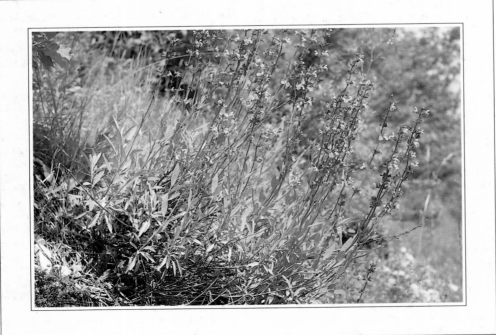

Fig. 2: *Salvia officinalis* L.

A ca. 70 cm tall subshrub, becoming woody at the base and with characteristically smelling, oblong leaves; lamina, because of the velvety tomentum, greyish green, especially on the lower surface, and often auriculate at the base. Ca. 2 cm long flowers, mostly with a bluish violet corolla, arranged in whorls forming a loose spike.

DAB 10: Salbeiblätter
ÖAB: Folium Salviae
Ph. Helv. VII: Salviae folium
St. Zul. 1229.99.99

Plant source: *Salvia officinalis* L., garden or red sage (Lamiaceae). The pharmacopoeial specification corresponds only with subsp. *minor* (GMELIN) GAMS and subsp. *major* (GARSAULT) GAMS, but not with subsp. *lavandulifolia* (VAHL) GAMS (which according to the Flora Europaea is a separate species). Recent morphological/anatomical studies support the view that the subspecies of *S. officinale* should be treated as independent species: subsp. *minor* = *S. officinale* s.s., subsp. *major* = *S. tomentosa* MILLER, and subsp. *lavandulifolia* = *S. lavandulifolia* VAHL [4].

Synonyms: Garden or Broad-leafed sage, Sawge (Engl.), Salbeiblätter, Edelsalbei, Gartensalbei (Ger.), Feuilles de sauge officinale, Feuilles de sauge commune (Fr.).

Extract from the German Commission E monograph
(BAnz no. 90, dated 15. 05. 1985)

Uses

Externally: inflammation of the mucous membranes of the mouth and throat.
Internally: dyspeptic complaints, excessive secretion of sweat.

Contraindications

The pure essential oil and alcoholic extracts should not be taken during pregnancy.

Side effects

On prolonged use of alcoholic extracts and the pure essential oil, epileptiform convulsions may occur.

Interactions

None known.

Dosage

Unless otherwise prescribed:
Internally: daily dose 4–6 g drug, 0.1–0.3 g essential oil, 2.5–7.5 g tincture (as in Erg. B. 6), 1.5–3 g fluid extract (as in Erg. B. 6).
As a gargle and rinse: 2.5 g drug as infusion or 2–3 drops of the essential oil to 100 ml water or 5 g alcoholic extract to a glass of water.
As a paint: undiluted alcoholic extract.

Mode of administration

Chopped drug for infusions, alcoholic extracts, and distillates for gargling, rinsing, and painting, and for internal use and the fresh press juice of the plant.

Effects

Antibacterial, fungistatic, virostatic, astringent, secretion-promoting, sweat-inhibiting.

Note

A separate monograph has been prepared for Salvia triloba.

Origin: Native in the Mediterranean region, especially in the Adriatic; cultivated to some extent in various European countries. Imports of the drug come from Albania and former Yugoslavia.

Constituents: 1–2.5% essential oil, consisting of thujone (up to ca. 35–60%) and other monoterpenes (particularly cineole) and small amounts of sesquiterpenes; 3–7% tannins, including rosmarinic acid; diterpenoid bitter substances, e.g. carnosol (= picrosalvin), carnosic acid 12-methyl ether γ-lactone, rosmanol and its 7-methyl ether, manool, etc.; triterpenes, e.g. oleanolic acid and derivatives [1, 5]. Extraction of an ethanol extract with supercritical carbon dioxide yields a product with greater antioxidant activity than butylated hydroxytoluene [5].

Indications: As an antiphlogistic for inflammation of the mouth and throat, for gingivitis and stomatitis, mainly in the form of a gargle, but also as a tea for digestive complaints, flatulence, inflammation of the intestinal mucosa, in diarrhoea.
As an antisudorific (antihydrotic), e.g. against night sweats in tuberculosis patients, but also against excessive sweat formation of psychosomatic origin.
Use of the drug in the two areas indicated is purely empirical. Pharmacological experiments with isolated constituents are still lacking; however, the antisudorific action has been demonstrated in animal experiments and clinically in man, e.g. pilocarpine-induced sweating is rapidly curtailed.
In *folk medicine,* because of an inhibiting effect on the secretion of milk, garden sage is also used to aid the cessation of lactation; it is also said (but not proved) to have mild hypotensive and emmenagogic effects.
Although not a cholagogue, the drug is sometimes used in this way in mixtures with other drugs (action of bitter substances?).

Side effects: Only likely with overdoses (more than 15 g sage leaves/dose) or on prolonged use. The toxic constituent of the essential oil, thujone, causes symptoms such as tachycardia, hot flushes, convulsions, and dizziness.

Making the tea: Depending on the indication; as a gargle, boiling water is poured over 3 g of the chopped drug and strained after 10 min.; against night sweats, the infusion prepared like the previous one, but the drink is allowed to cool; for gastrointestinal complaints, boiling water is poured over 1.5–2.0 g of the finely chopped drug and strained after 5 min.
1 Teaspoon = ca. 1.5 g.

Herbal preparations: The chopped drug is also available in tea bags (1.0 or 1.6 g).

Phytomedicines: The drug, extracts made from it (tincture, fluid extract), or the essential oil are components of some prepared mouth and throat remedies, e.g. Salus® Salbei-Tropfen (drops), Salviathymol®, etc., Gastrointestinal Remedies, e.g. Enterosanol® (dragees, juice, capsules), etc., and cholagogues and some other remedies. Products available in the UK include Seven Seas Catarrh Tablets, Arkopharma Phytomenopause, etc.

Regulatory status (UK): General Sales – List Schedule 1, Table A.

Authentication: Macro- (see: Description) and microscopically, following the DAB 10. See also [4, 6] and the BHP 1983. It should be noted that the covering trichomes on the upper and lower surfaces of the leaf are the same (distinction from Salviae trilobae folium – Greek sage): ca. 200–600 µm long, not more than 20 µm wide at the base, and with a short, strongly thickened basal cell (Fig. 4). The DAB 10 TLC procedure examines the composition of the essential oil:

Test solution: 0.30 g freshly powdered drug shaken for 2–3 min. with 5 ml dichloromethane and filtered over ca. 2 g anhydrous sodium sulphate.

Reference solution: 3.0 mg borneol, 5 µl bornyl acetate, and 10 µl cineole dissolved in 10 ml toluene.

Loadings: 30 µl test solution and 10 µl reference solution, as 2-cm bands on silica gel G.

Solvent system: acetone + ethyl acetate + di-chloromethane (2 + 3 + 95), 10 cm run.

Detection: sprayed with anisaldehyde reagent, followed by heating at 100–105 °C for 5–10 min. while under observation.

Evaluation: in daylight. Reference solution: the lowest zone, the brownish grey borneol zone; slightly above, the greyish violet to blue cineole zone; and above that, the brownish grey bornyl acetate zone. Test solution: these three zones, approximately equal in intensity; directly below the bornyl acetate zone, the weakly coloured reddish violet thujone zone; and somewhat below that, the weakly coloured pinkish red caryophyllene epoxide zone, followed by an intense violet zone; just below the cineole zone, another violet zone of similar intensity (viridiflorol); in the lowest part of the chromatogram, other violet or greenish yellow zones, some of them very prominent; in the upper part of the chromatogram, two intense violet to blue zones (terpene and sesquiterpene hydrocarbons).

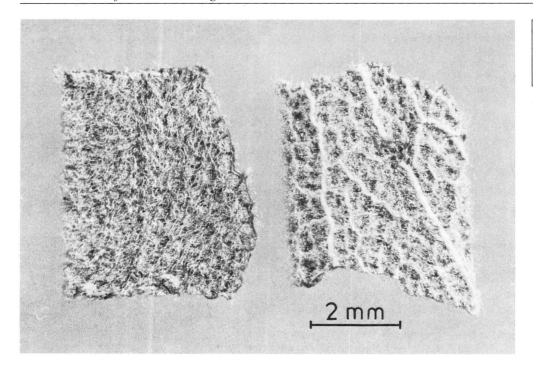

In UV 365 nm light. <u>Test solution</u>: thujone, directly below the bornyl acetate zone, as an intense sealing-wax red fluorescent zone; cineole, a bluish green fluorescent zone; borneol and bornyl acetate zones, almost no fluorescence.

TLC study of the flavonoids is also useful in aiding the identification (see: Adulteration).

Wording of the package insert, from the German Standard Licence:

6.1   Uses

Inflammation of the gums and the mucous membranes of the mouth and throat; pressure spots caused by prostheses; in supportive treatment of gastrointestinal catarrh.

6.2   Dosage and Mode of administration

For treating gastrointestinal complaints, boiling water is poured over half a teaspoonful (1–3 g), and for inflammation in the mouth, over one teaspoonful (ca. 3 g), of **Red sage** and after 10 min. passed through a tea strainer.

Unless otherwise prescribed, for gastrointestinal complaints a cup of the warm tea is drunk several times a day half-an-hour before meals.

For inflammation of the mucous membranes of the mouth and throat, the still warm infusion is used as a rinse or gargle several times a day.

6.3   Duration of use

Infusions of red sage should not be taken over a long period of time.

6.4   Note

Store protected from light and moisture.

Quantitative standards: <u>DAB 10</u>: *Thujone-rich volatile oil*, not less than 1.5%. *Foreign matter*, not more than 3% stem fragments and not more than 2% other foreign matter. *Loss on drying*, not more than 10.0%. *Ash*, not more than 10.0%.

<u>ÖAB</u>: *Volatile oil*, not less than 1.5%. *Foreign matter*, not more than 3% stem fragments. *Ash*, not more than 8.0%.

<u>Ph. Helv. VII</u>: *Volatile oil*, not less than 1.5%. *Foreign matter*, not more than 3% stems; leaves of *S. triloba* absent. *Sulphated ash*, not more than 12.0%.

BHP 1983: *Foreign organic matter*, not more than 3%. *Total ash*, not more than 8%.

Adulteration: Occasionally with the leaves of other *Salvia* species, principally those of *S. triloba* L.f., Greek sage; these have a white, velvety tomentum on both surfaces, which is denser than that of *S. officinalis* (compare Fig. 3 and Salviae trilobae folium: Fig. 3). The trichomes on the upper surface are not tortuous and whip-like, but are straight and stiff, and mostly 30–40 μm wide at the base (Salviae trilobae folium: Fig. 4).

In the DAB 10 TLC examination set out above, adulteration can be recognized by the divergent composition (a higher cineole and lower thujone content). Differentiation is also possible on the basis of the flavonoid profile; the TLC procedure is as follows:

Test solution: 1 g powdered drug refluxed for 10 min. with 10 ml methanol, filtered, the filtrate taken to dryness, and the residue dissolved in 4.0 ml methanol.

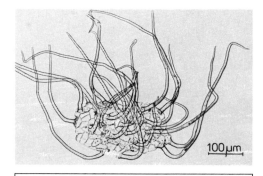

Fig. 4: Long, multicellular, tortuous covering trichomes, from the upper leaf surface

Reference solution: 10 mg rutin and 5 mg hyperoside dissolved in 10 ml methanol.

Loadings: 2 μl test solution and 2 μl reference solution, as bands on silica gel.

Mobile phase: ethyl acetate + anhydrous formic acid + water (88 + 6 + 6), 5 cm run.

Detection: after drying in a current of hot air, sprayed with 1% methanolic diphenylboryloxyethylamine, followed by 5% ethanolic polyethylene glycol 400.

Evaluation: in UV 366 nm light. <u>Reference solution</u>: orange-yellow fluorescent zones, rutin at Rf ca. 0.2 and hyperoside at Rf ca.

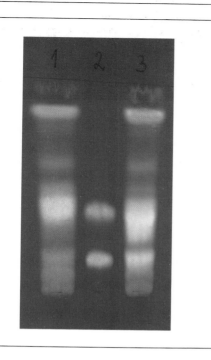

Fig. 5: TLC on 4 × 8 cm foil

1: Red sage
2: Rutin and hyperoside (reference compounds)
3: Greek sage

For details, see the text

with anisaldehyde reagent also allows red sage and Greek sage to be distinguished by: (a) the greater intensity of the violet-red double (α- and β-) thujone zone in the red sage (*S. officinalis*) chromatogram and (b) the very intense cineole zone in the Greek sage (*S. triloba*) chromatogram [7].

Storage: Protected from light, in well-closed (but not plastic) containers. Stability on storage [2, 3]: this depends on the degree of comminution (the coarsely powdered drug keeps better than the finely powdered one) and on the packaging (vacuum packs are better than double-thickness paper bags).

0.45; Test solution (*S. officinalis*): several yellowish orange and bluish fluorescent zones between Rf 0.2 and 0.9, especially just above the level of the hyperoside zone. Test solution (*S. triloba*): similar zones, but the main ones are below the level of the hyperoside zone (Fig. 5).

The solvent system: toluene + ethyl acetate (95 + 5) with silica gel F 60_{254} and detection

Literature:
[1] Kommentar DAB 10.
[2] D. Fehr, Pharm. Ztg. **127**, 111 (1982).
[3] L. Kreutzig, Pharm. Ztg. **127**, 893 (1982).
[4] R. Länger, Th. Ruckenbauer, J. Jurenitsch, and W. Kubelka, Sci. Pharm. **59**, 321 (1991).
[5] Z. Djarmati et al., Phytochemistry **31**, 1307 (1992).
[6] B.P. Jackson and D.W. Snowdon, Atlas of microscopy of medicinal plants, culinary herbs and spices, Belhaven Press, London, 1990, p. 204.
[7] P. Pachaly, Dtsch. Apoth. Ztg. **130**, 169 (1990).

Salviae trilobae folium   (DAB 10), Greek sage

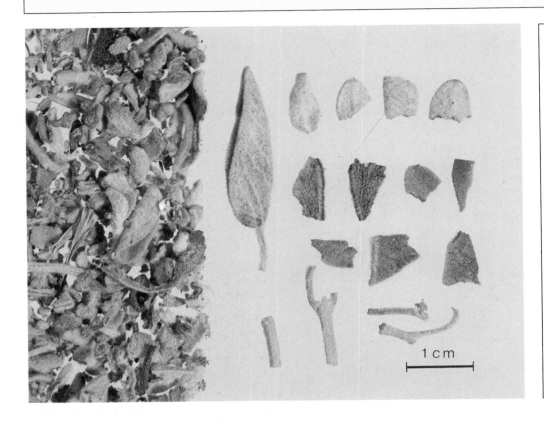

Fig. 1: Greek sage

<u>Description:</u> The oblong-ovate to more or less lance-olate, petiolate leaves often have one or two small lateral lobes at the obtuse base. The leaves are densely tomentose on both surfaces, more so on the lower surface than on the upper, making the finely reticulate venation and the undulate crenate leaf margin indistinct. The fragments of the petiole and the 4-angled stems are also covered with a dense white tomentum.

<u>Odour:</u> Spicy and, on rubbing, clearly reminiscent of eucalyptus oil (high cineole content!).

<u>Taste:</u> Aromatic and spicy, somewhat bitter, slightly astringent.

Fig. 2: *Salvia triloba* L.f.

Owing to the denser pubescence, especially on the upper surface, the leaves of Greek sage are thicker and more greyish velvety than those of *Salvia officinalis*; at the base of the lamina, there are often also two lateral lobes (hence the name). Otherwise, the habit of the plant is much the same as that of garden sage.

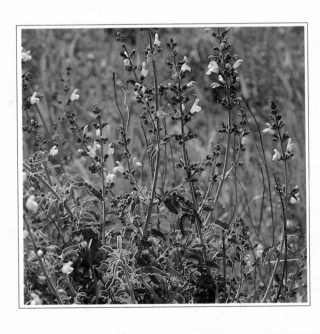

DAB 10: Salbei, dreilappiger
Ph. Helv. VII: Salviae trilobae folium

Plant source: *Salvia triloba* L.f., Greek sage (Lamiaceae).

Synonyms: Dreilappiger Salbei (Ger.), Feuilles de sauge à trois lobes (Fr.).

Origin: A subshrub occurring in Greece, parts of Italy, and on Crete and Cyprus. The drug is imported from Turkey, Greece, and the former USSR.

Constituents: 2–3% essential oil, consisting of up to more than 60% cineole and with ca. 5% thujone; the oil contains other mono- and sesquiterpenes [1]; ca. 5% tannins, including a considerable proportion of rosmarinic acid [2]; ca. 2% flavonoids, including salvigenin; diterpenes (carnosol) and triterpenes (ursolic acid, etc.) like those in garden sage.

Indications: As an antiphlogistic in the same way as garden sage (Salviae folium, q.v.), more especially for inflammation of the

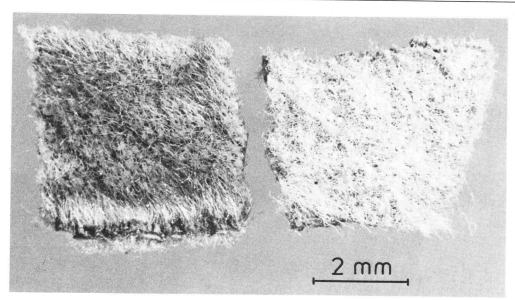

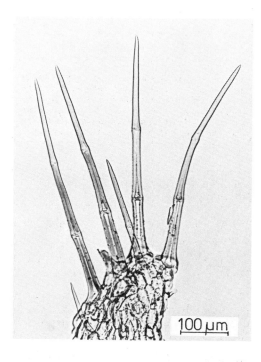

mouth and throat. Whether the drug can be used as an antisudorific (antihydrotic) has not yet been checked.

Making the tea: Boiling water is poured over 3 g of the finely chopped drug and after 10 min. passed through a tea strainer. 1 Teaspoon = ca. 1.3 g.

Phytomedicines: The drug is a very rare component of prepared remedies, used in the same way as garden sage leaves.

Fig. 4: Stiff, thick-walled trichomes, from the upper surface of the leaf

Authentication: Macro- (see: Description) and microscopically, following the DAB 10. The leaves are much more densely tomentose than those of garden sage (compare Fig. 3 and Salviae folium: Fig. 3); the trichomes on the upper leaf surface are 30–40 µm wide at the base and straight (Fig. 4). The DAB 10 proof of identity is based on TLC examination of the essential oil; for the procedure, see under Salviae folium: Authentication. **Evaluation** of the chromatogram is as follows:

Evaluation: Test solution: cineole, an intense greyish violet to blue zone; the borneol and bornyl acetate zones, less strongly coloured than the corresponding zones of the reference solution; slightly below the bornyl acetate zone, the weak pinkish red caryophyllene epoxide zone; slightly below the cineole zone, the violet viridiflorol zone; in the lowest part of the chromatogram, other violet or greenish yellow zones, some very promi-

nent; in the upper part of the chromatogram, two strong violet to blue zones (terpene and sesquiterpene hydrocarbons). In UV 365 nm light. Test solution: no intense sealing-wax red zone (thujone) present directly below the bornyl acetate zone; bluish grey fluorescent cineole zone; almost non-fluorescent borneol and bornyl acetate zones.

For the identification by TLC of the flavonoids, see under Salviae folium: Adulteration.

Quantitative standards: <u>DAB 10</u>: *Volatile oil,* not less than 1.8%. *Foreign matter,* not more than 8% stem fragments and not more than 2% other foreign matter. *Loss on drying,* not more than 10.0%. *Ash,* not more than 10.0%.

<u>Ph. Helv. VII</u>: *Volatile oil,* not less than 1.8%. *Foreign matter,* not more than 1% and not more than 10% stems; leaves of *S. officinalis* absent. *Sulphated ash,* not more than 12.0%.

Adulteration: Rare, and most likely by confusion with garden sage leaves, which, however, can be recognized by the microscopical characters and by TLC; see: Authentication.

Storage: Protected from light, in well-closed (but not plastic) containers.

Literature:
[1] E. Putievsky, U. Ravid, and N. Dudai, J. Nat. Prod. **49**, 1015 (1986).
[2] L. Gracza and P. Ruff, Arch. Pharm. (Weinheim) **317**, 339 (1984).

Sambuci flos   (DAB 10), Elder flower (BHP 1/1990)

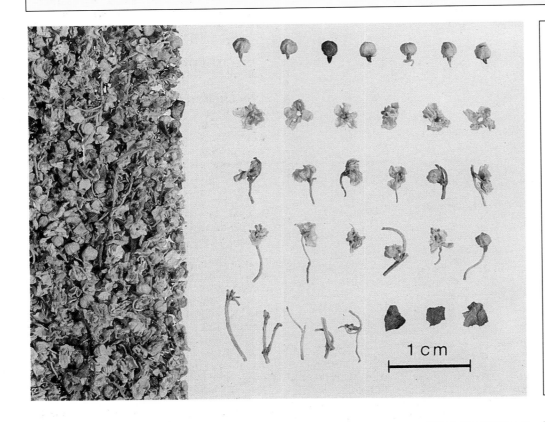

Fig. 1: Elder flower

Description: It is the individual flowers, stripped from the inflorescences (cymes, thyrses) and sieved, but also to some extent the cut up cymes, that are found in commerce. The small, 3–4 mm broad, yellowish white flowers have a fused 5-lobed corolla, 5 stamens, a 5-lobed calyx, and an inferior ovary with a short style and 3 stigmas. Usually, the corollas with attached stamens are separate and, less often, also buds. Green, longitudinally grooved pedicels are present occasionally and in products which have not been properly garbled in large amounts.

Odour: Faint and characteristic.

Taste: Mucilaginous and sweet.

1 cm

Fig. 2: *Sambucus nigra* L.

An up to 6 m tall shrub with large pinnate leaves. Flowers white, in cymes. Branches with a white porous pith. Ripe fruits black, with a dark violet juice.

Fig. 3: *Sambucus nigra*, inflorescence

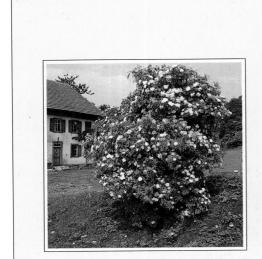

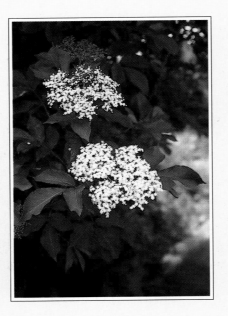

DAB 10: Holunderblüten
ÖAB: Flos Sambuci
Ph. Helv. VII: Sambuci flos
St. Zul. 1019.99.99

Plant source: *Sambucus nigra* L., elder (Caprifoliaceae).

Synonyms: Sambucus, Bourtree flowers, Black or European elder (Engl.), Holunderblüten, Aalhornblüten, Fliedertee, Schwitztee (Ger.), Fleurs de sureau (Fr.).

Origin: Native throughout Europe, West and Central Asia, North Africa. The drug is obtained from the wild, mainly in the former USSR, former Yugoslavia, Bulgaria, Hungary, and Romania, but also in the UK.

Constituents: 0.03–0.14% essential oil of a buttery consistency, owing to the high proportion of free fatty acids (66%, main component palmitic acid) and C_{14-31} *n*-alkanes (7.2%); so far, 63 components have been identified [1]. Ca. 1.8% flavonoids, almost exclusively flavonols and their glycosides, with rutin as the chief component (up to

Rutin

Chlorogenic acid

α-Amyrin : R = CH₃
Ursolic acid: R = COOH

Sambunigrin

1.92%), and also isoquercitrin, hyperoside, astragalin, and quercitrin; ca. 3% chlorogenic acid; *p*-coumaric acid, caffeic and ferulic acids and their β-glucose esters; traces of mandelonitrile β-glucoside (sambunigrin); triterpenes: ca. 1% α- and β-amyrin, occurring mainly as fatty-acid esters; triterpene acids: ca. 0.85% ursolic and oleanolic acids, 20β-hydroxyursolic acid; ca. 0.11% sterols, free, esterified, and glycosidic; mucilage, tannins [1–5].

Indications: As a diaphoretic in feverish chills, etc., in which large amounts of the infusion – often in combination with lime flowers – are drunk as hot as possible. The drug supposedly increases the response of the sweat glands to heat stimuli [6, 7]. The active principles are unknown, and it is disputed whether the effect really is based on its constituents. Wiechowski [6] observed a distinct increase in diaphoresis in healthy subjects, but other authors ascribe the effect simply to the large amounts of hot fluid taken and consider the drug to be simply a flavouring agent. It is often used for this latter purpose, e.g. in laxatives.
In *folk medicine,* the drug is also used in the preparation of gargles.

Making the tea: Boiling water is poured over 3 g of elder flower and after 5–10 min. passed through a tea strainer.
1 Teaspoon = ca. 1.5 g.

Herbal preparations: The drug is also available in tea bags (mostly 1 g).

Phytomedicines: The drug is included in many mixed teas. Drug extracts are present in a few prepared antitussives, e.g. Sinupret® (dragees, drops) for sinusitis, slimming cures, etc.

---

*Extract from the German Commission E monograph
(BAnz no. 50, dated 13. 03. 1986)*

Uses
Chills, catarrhal complaints, etc.

Contraindications
None known.

Side effects
None known.

Interactions with other remedies
None known.

Dosage
Unless otherwise prescribed: average daily dose, 10–15 g drug; preparations correspondingly.

Mode of administration
Drug as such and other galenical forms for infusions; one or two cups drunk as hot as possible several times a day.

Effects
Diaphoretic; increases the bronchial secretion.

Elder flower is included in various UK multi-ingredient preparations for rheumatic pains, e.g. Potter's Tabritis (tablets), Seven Seas Rheumatic Pain Tablets, etc., and for respiratory tract complaints, e.g. Potter's Life Drops, Potter's Elderflowers, Peppermint with Composition Essence, etc.; cf. [10].

Regulatory status (UK): General Sales List – Schedule 1, Table A.

Authentication: Macro- and microscopically, following the DAB 10 or [9]; see also the BHP 1/1990. The abundant occurrence of cells with crystal sand is diagnostic (Fig. 4); the tricolpate pollen grains have a very finely punctate exine (Fig. 5).
The TLC flavonoid profile is a useful identification test [11]:

Test solution: 1 g powdered drug extracted with 10 ml methanol for 5 min. on the water-bath at ca. 60 °C and filtered.

Reference solution: 0.05% each of rutin, chlorogenic acid, and hyperoside in methanol

Loadings: 25–30 μl test solution and 10 μl reference solution, as bands on silica gel 60 F₂₅₄.

Solvent system: ethyl acetate + formic acid + glacial acetic acid + water (100 + 11 + 11 + 27), 15 cm run.

Detection: sprayed with 1% methanolic diphenylboryloxyethylamine, followed by 5% ethanolic polyethylene glycol 400.

Evaluation: in UV 365 nm light. Reference solution: fluorescent zones at ca. Rf 0.35 (orange, rutin), ca. 0.45 (bluish, chlorogenic acid), and ca. 0.55 (orange, hyperoside). Test

---

Wording of the package insert, from the German Standard Licence:

6.1 **Uses**
A diaphoretic for the treatment of feverish, catarrhal complaints.

6.2 **Dosage and Mode of administration**
Boiling water (ca. 150 ml) is poured over about 2 teaspoonfuls (3–4 g) of **Elder flower** and after 5 min. passed through a tea strainer.
Unless otherwise prescribed, one or two cups of the freshly prepared infusion is drunk as hot as possible several times a day, especially during the latter part of the day.

6.3 **Note**
Store away from light and moisture.

Fig. 4: Cells in all parts with crystal sand

Fig. 5: Tricolpate pollen grain with finely punctate exine

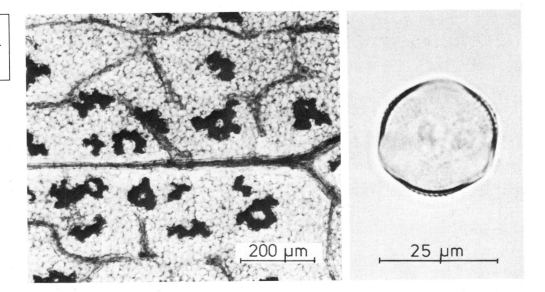

200 µm

25 µm

solution: two orange fluorescent zones, one at Rf ca. 0.35 (rutin) and the other at Rf ca. 0.6 (isoquercitrin), each with a weak, yellowish green fluorescent zone just above it; bluish fluorescent zones at Rf ca. 0.45 and 0.9, corresponding to chlorogenic and caffeic acids.

The BHP 1/1990 TLC identification test (fingerprint chromatogram) is based on the method just described. Illustrations of the TLC flavonoid profile are to be found in [8, 9, 11].

Quantitative standards: <u>DAB 10</u>: *Total flavonoids*, not less than 0.8% calculated as isoquercitrin (M_r 464.4). *Foreign matter*, not more than 10% pedicels and not more than 1% other foreign matter. *Loss on drying*, not more than 10%. *Ash*, not more than 10%.

<u>ÖAB</u>: *Foreign matter*, not more than 3% (stalks more than 1 mm thick). *Ash*, not more than 9.0%.

<u>Ph. Helv. VII</u>: *Flavonoids*, not less than 0.70% calculated as isoquercitrin (M_r 464.4). *Foreign matter*, not more than 8% fragments of the cymes and not more than 15% brown, discoloured flowers. *Sulphated ash*, not more than 12.0%.

<u>BHP 1/1990</u>: *Water-soluble extractive*, not less than 25%. *Foreign matter*, not more than 2%. *Total ash*, not more than 10%. *HCl-insoluble ash*, not more than 2%.

Adulteration: In practice, the flowers of *Sambucus ebulus* L., dwarf elder or danewort (pedicels, reddish; anthers, red; petals, pink with nerves anastomosing at the tips) are a rare adulterant.

Literature:

[1] B. Toulemonde and H.M.J. Richard, J. Agric. Food Chem. **31**, 365 (1983).
[2] W. Richter and G. Willuhn, Dtsch. Apoth. Ztg. **114**, 947 (1974).
[3] R. Hänsel and M. Kussmaul, Arch. Pharm. (Weinheim) **308**, 790 (1975).
[4] G. Willuhn and W. Richter, Planta Med. **31**, 328 (1977).
[5] W. Richter and G. Willuhn, Pharm. Ztg. **122**, 1567 (1977).
[6] W. Wiechowski, Med. Klin. **23**, 590 (1927).
[7] K.J. Schmersahl, Naturwissenschaften **51**, 361 (1964).
[8] P. Pachaly, Dünnschichtchromatographie in der Apotheke. Wiss. Verlagsgesellschaft, 2. Aufl., Stuttgart 1983.
[9] P. Rohdewald, G. Rücker and K.-W. Glombitza, Apothekengerechte Prüfvorschriften, S. 771. Deutscher Apotheker Verlag, Stuttgart 1986.
[10] Martindale, 29th ed., p. 779.
[11] H. Wagner, S. Bladt, and E.M. Zgainski, Plant drug analysis, Springer-Verlag, Berlin, Heidelberg, New York, Tokyo, 1984, p. 178.

Sambuci fructus   Elder fruit

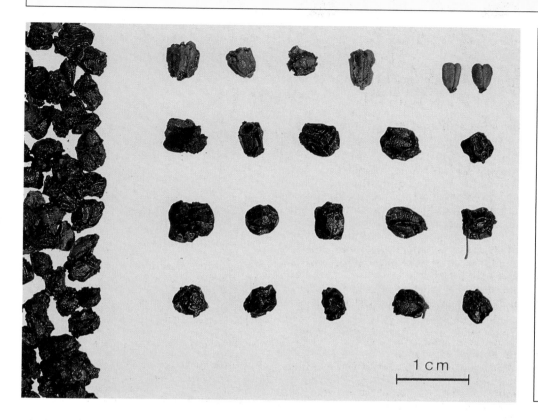

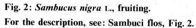
1 cm

Fig. 1: Elder fruit

<u>Description</u>: The much wrinkled, more or less spherical drupes are dark violet-black and slightly glossy. As a rule, they contain three, somewhat elongated stones (top right), each of which has a seed inside the hard endocarp. Occasionally, fruit stalks are present.

<u>Odour</u>: Characteristic.

<u>Taste</u>: Sweet and sourish, with a characteristic aroma.

Fig. 2: *Sambucus nigra* L., fruiting.
For the description, see: Sambuci flos, Fig. 2.

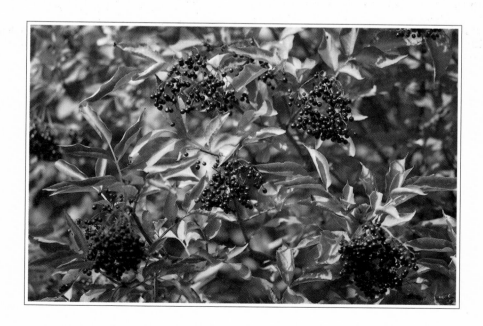

Plant source: *Sambucus nigra* L., elder (Caprifoliaceae).

Synonyms: Baccae (Drupae, Grana) Sambuci (nigrae) (Lat.), Holunderbeeren (Ger.), Baies de sureau (Fr.).

Origin: Native throughout Europe, West and Central Asia, North Africa. The drupes are collected from the wild, and the drug is imported from Russia, Poland, Hungary, Portugal, and Bulgaria.

Constituents: the flavonoid glycosides rutin, isoquercitrin, and hyperoside; 3% tannins [1]; the anthocyan glycosides (0.2–1%) sambucin, sambucyanin, and chrysanthemin (= cyanidin 3-rhamnoglucoside, 3-xyloglucoside, and 3-glucoside, respectively), and as diglycosides the 5-*O*-glucoside derivatives of sambucyanin and chrysanthemin [2–5]; ca. 0.01% essential oil with 34 identified aroma compounds [6–8]; in the seeds, the cyanogenic glycosides sambunigrin, prunasin, zierin, and holocalin [9]. 7.5% Sugar (glucose and fructose); plant acids (citric acid and malic acid); ca. 0.03% vitamin C.

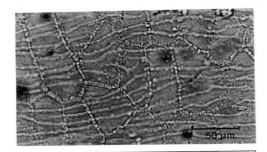

Fig. 3: Epidermis of the exocarp, showing the beaded thickening of the cell walls and the coarse cuticular striations

Sambucin: R = β-ᴅ-rhamnosylglucose
Sambucyanin: R = β-ᴅ-xylosylglucose
Chrysanthemin: R = β-ᴅ-glucose

Indications: Nowadays, the drug is only rarely used as a laxative, diuretic, and diaphoretic for catarrhal complaints. The fresh ripe fruits are used for making juice and jams. The juice (Roob Sambuci, Succus Sambuci inspissatus Ph. Helv. V) is taken in large doses as a purgative, as well as a diuretic and diaphoretic; in *folk medicine,* freshly pressed, it is also a specific against sciatica and neuralgia [1, 10]. Owing to the relatively high anthocyan content, elder fruit is also a source of natural colouring matter for the food industry.

Side effects: Taking the *raw* or insufficiently cooked fruit can lead to nausea and vomiting [11, 12].

Making the tea: Not very usual. Cold water is added to ca. 10 g drug, allowed to stand for several minutes, and then slowly brought to the boil for a short time, allowed to stand for 5–10 min., and then strained. As a mild diuretic or as supportive treatment for feverish catarrhal complaints a cup is drunk several times a day, if desired slightly sweetened and with the addition of some lemon juice. 1 Teaspoon = ca. 3.2 g.

Phytomedicines: The drug is a component of some tea preparations. A fluid extract of the fruit is present in Arthrodynat®-Tropfen.

Authentication: Macro- (see: Description) and microscopically based on the sclerenchymatous elements of the stones. Below a thin parenchyma, these have strongly thickened, short, radially elongated, strongly indented sclereids with a very irregular outline and below them two layers of thickened fibres with sharp, rounded, or irregularly forked ends. The epidermis of the fruit wall is also a diagnostic feature (Fig. 3).

Adulteration: Practically never encountered.

Literature:
[1] Hager, Band **6**, 259 (1979).
[2] R. Reichel and W. Reichwald, Pharmazie **32**, 40 (1977).
[3] K. Broenum-Hansen and S.H. Hansen, J. Chromatogr. **262**, 385 (1983).
[4] K. Broenum-Hansen, F. Jacobsen and J.M. Fink, J. Food Technol. **20**, 703 (1985).
[5] E. Pogorzelski, Przem. Spozyw **37**, 167 (1983); C.A. **100**, 21524 (1984).
[6] J. Davidek et al., Lebensm.-Wiss. und Technol. **15**, 181 (1982).
[7] K. Mikova et al., Lebensm.-Wiss. u. Technol. **17**, 311 (1984).
[8] A. Askar and H. Treptow, Ernährung/Nutrition **9**, 309 (1985).
[9] E. Pogorzelski, J. Sci. Food Agricol. **33**, 496 (1982).
[10] G. Madaus, Lehrbuch der biologischen Heilmittel, S. 2418, Georg Olms-Verlag, Hildesheim, New York 1976.
[11] R. Bergmann, Flüssiges Obst **46**, 8 (1979).
[12] F. Kuhlmann, Lebensm. Rdsch. **75**, 390 (1979).

Santali lignum rubri   Red sandalwood

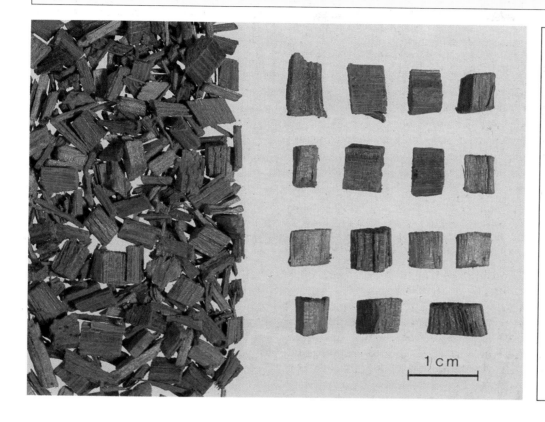

Fig. 1: Red sandalwood
Description: The drug consists of the heartwood from which the light-coloured sapwood has been removed. It is dense and heavy, but readily split; the thicker pieces, cubes or discs, are dark violet, almost black in colour. In the cut drug, the chips of wood are dark blood-red, with dots or pinholes (vessels, readily seen with the naked eye); on tangential and radial surfaces, lighter transverse striations (bands of parenchyma) and fine streaks (medullary rays) can be seen.

Odour: On rubbing, very faintly spicy.

Taste: Weakly astringent.

Erg. B. 6: Lignum Santali rubri

Plant source: *Pterocarpus santalinus* L. (Fabaceae).

Synonyms: Red sanderswood or saunderswood, Rubywood (Engl.), Sandelholz, Rotsandelholz (Ger.), Bois de santal rouge (Fr.).
Note: White sandalwood (Erg. B. 6) comes from *Santalum album* L. (Santalaceae); this drug is not a dyewood, but contains essential oil.

Origin: A tree native to India and cultivated in the Philippines. Imports of the drug come from these two countries.

Constituents [1–3]: Red pigments, derivatives of benzoxanthenone, with the two main pigments santalins A and B; a small amount of essential oil (including cedrol, pterocarpol, isopterocarpol, pterocarpotriol, eudesmol, etc.), and sesquiterpenes; triterpenes and sterols; phenol-carboxylic

Santalin A   R = H
Santalin B   R = CH₃

Pterocarpol

acids; pterocarpans and isoflavones; stilbene derivatives.

Indications: To enhance the appearance of herbal mixtures and, in powdered form, to colour tooth powders.
In *folk medicine*, use of the drug in gastrointestinal complaints or as a diuretic (and also as an antidiarrhoeic) is not founded on scientific evidence and consequently there is no justification for its use. Formerly, the drug played a significant role as a dye for wool, but nowadays it is replaced by synthetic dyes.

Making the tea: Not applicable. For the preparation of coloured solutions, e.g. for colouring eggshells, 10–20 g sandalwood is boiled with 1 litre water for ca. 15 min. and then strained.

Authentication: Macro- (see: Description) and microscopically. The bulk of the wood consists of dark red, thick-walled, long xylem fibres with a wide lumen. The up to

*Extract from the German Commission
E monograph
(BAnz no. 193, dated 15. 10. 1987)*

Uses

Red sandalwood is used for complaints and disorders of the gastrointestinal tract, as a diuretic, astringent, "blood-purifier", as well as for coughs.

Risks

None known.

Evaluation

Since evidence regarding activity is lacking, the therapeutic use of red sandalwood cannot be justified.

300 µm wide, pitted vessels are not infrequently plugged by red-coloured tyloses. Septate fibres containing crystals and uniseriate medullary rays are also present.

With potassium hydroxide solution or ammonia, the wood is stained very deep red to black.

Quantitative standard: Erg. B. 6: *Ash*, not more than 3%.

Adulteration: In practice very rare; it is readily apparent from the deviating microscopical features and the different colour obtained on treatment with potassium hydroxide solution.

Literature:

[1] T.R. Seshadri, Phytochemistry **11**, 881 (1972).
[2] N. Kumar and T.R. Seshadri, Phytochemistry **14**, 521 (1975); *ibid.*, **15**, 1417 (1976).
[3] N. Kumar, B. Ravindranath, and T.R. Seshadri, Phytochemistry **13**, 633 (1974).

Saponariae rubrae radix   Soapwort root

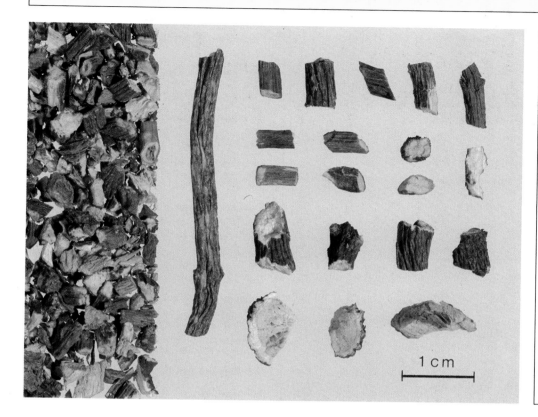

1 cm

Fig. 1: Soapwort root

<u>Description:</u> **The round, reddish brown, 1–5 mm thick pieces of root have a short, not fibrous, fracture. The transverse section (hand lens) shows a pale whitish bark and inside the cambial ring a lemon-yellow, non-radiate xylem (Fig. 3).**

<u>Taste:</u> **At first sweetish and bitter, then harsh.**

Fig. 2: *Saponaria officinalis* L.

A ca. 50 cm tall perennial with underground stolons, found in gravel along rivers. White flowers in compact panicles at the ends of mostly unbranched stems bearing long, narrow, opposite leaves.

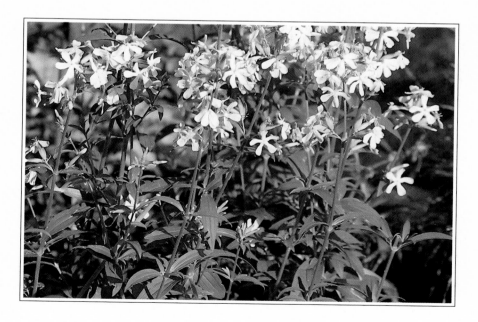

DAC 1986: Rote Seifenwurzel

Plant source: *Saponaria officinalis* L., soapwort (Caryophyllaceae).

Synonyms: Seifenwurzel, Waschwurzel (Ger.), Racine de saponaire (Fr.).

Origin: Native in Europe and western to central Asia; also often cultivated. Imports of the drug come from Turkey, China, and Iran.

Constituents: Ca. 2–5% saponins, a mixture of triterpene glycosides. According to more recent investigations, the main sapogenin is not the often-mentioned gypsogenin, but rather quillaic acid [1]. See: Quillaiae cortex (quillaja bark). Also, various sugars and carbohydrates.

Indications: On the basis of the saponin content, as an expectorant in bronchitis, but nowadays like Quillaiae cortex (quillaja bark) replaced by other drugs (Primulae radix, Senegae radix).

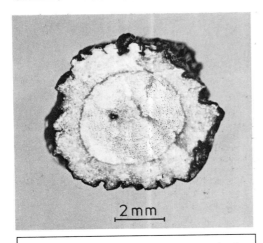

2 mm

Fig. 3: Transverse surface of soapwort root, showing the pale yellow, somewhat porous xylem and whitish phloem

Extract from the German Commission E monograph (BAnz no. 80, dated 27.04.89)

Uses
Catarrh of the upper respiratory tract.

Contraindications
None known.

Side effects
In rare cases, gastric irritation.

Interactions with other remedies
None known.

Dosage
Unless otherwise prescribed: daily dose, 1.5 g drug; preparations correspondingly.

Mode of administration
Chopped drug for infusions and other galenical preparations for internal use.

Effects
Expectorant, arising from irritation of the gastric mucosa; in higher doses, a cellular toxin.

5 ml boiling water poured over 0.1 g powdered drug, after cooling, gives a stable foam on shaking.

The DAC 1986 TLC identification test examines the saponin profile of the drug. About detection of the saponins with Nile Blue after TLC, see [4]. The following TLC method for separation of the saponins is to be found in [5]:

Test solution: 2 g powdered drug refluxed with 70% ethanol for 10 min., filtered, and the filtrate concentrated to ca. 5 ml

Reference solution: 0.1 % solution of standard saponin from *Gypsophila* sp. in methanol.

Loadings: 25–40 µl test solution and 10 µl reference solution, as bands on silica gel 60F$_{254}$.

Solvent system: chloroform + methanol + water (64 + 50 + 10), prepared exactly with *analytical* grade ethanol.

Detection: sprayed with 20% antimony(III) chloride in chloroform, followed by heating for 5–6 min. at 100 °C.

Evaluation: in daylight and in UV 365 nm light. Test solution: a large number of overlapping violet or dark violet (daylight) or greenish blue fluorescent (UV 365 nm light) zones in the Rf range 0.05–0.5.

Adulteration: In practice, does not occur.

In *folk medicine*, the drug is sometimes still used for skin complaints and in rheumatic disorders.

Its applications as a foaming agent are similar to those of Quillaiae radix (q.v.). In pharmacological studies of saponin-containing extracts of this drug, antiphlogistic effects have been demonstrated (rat-paw carrageenan-induced oedema); *in vitro*, the saponins inhibit prostaglandin synthetase [2]; at the same time, analgesic effects have been noted. The saponins of soapwort also have a spermicidal action, which has not (yet) been put to use [3].

About the ability of the saponins to lower serum cholesterol, see: Quillaiae cortex.

Making the tea: Rarely done nowadays; as for Quillaiae cortex (q.v.), but using 0.4 g of the moderately finely chopped drug.
1 Teaspoon = ca. 2.6 g.

Phytomedicines: The drug and extracts made from it are present in a few prepared antitussives.

Authentication: Macro- (see: Description) and microscopically, following the DAC 1986. In the phloem and xylem parenchyma, there are crystal clusters of calcium oxalate; the vessels are only 10–60 µm wide and are scattered irregularly throughout the xylem parenchyma. Starch is absent.

Literature:
[1] M. Henry, J.D. Brion, and J.L. Guignard, Plantes Méd. Phytothérap. **15**, 192 (1981).
[2] B. Cebo, J. Krupinska, H. Sobanski, J. Mazur, and R. Czarnecki, Herba Pol. **22**, 154 (1976); C.A. **88**, 31943 (1978).
[3] A. Abd Elbary and S.A. Nour, Pharmazie **34**, 560 (1979).
[4] H.P. Franck, Dtsch. Apoth. Ztg. **115**, 1206 (1975).
[5] H. Wagner, S. Bladt, and E.M. Zgainski, Plant drug analysis, Springer-Verlag, Berlin – Heidelberg – New York – Tokyo, 1984, p. 236.

Scoparii herba   Broom, Scoparium (BHP 1983)

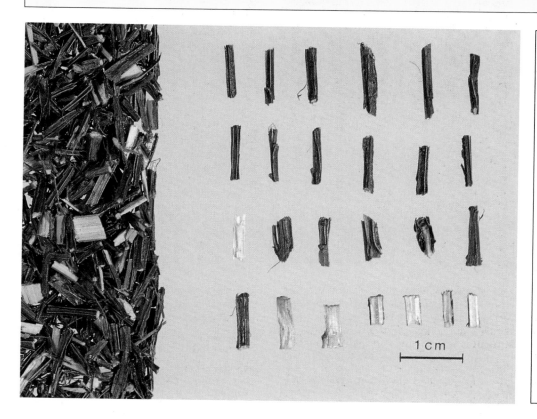

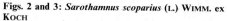

1 cm

Fig. 1: Broom

Description: The dark brown, ca. 2–3 mm thick fragments of woody twigs have five distinctly angles which are light green in colour. On some fragments, remains of the silky-haired leaflets and the yellowish brown flower buds can be recognized. However, the pieces of leaf and flower form only a small proportion compared with the fragments of twigs.

Taste: Very bitter.

Figs. 2 and 3: *Sarothamnus scoparius* (L.) WIMM. ex KOCH

Bushes, up to 2m in height, with 5-sided, green, rod-like twigs and small deciduous leaves. Yellow papilionaceous flowers up to 25 mm long with a spirally twisted style.

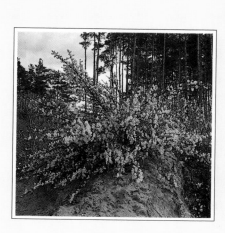

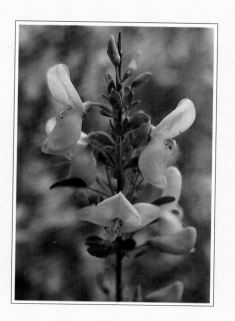

DAC 1986: Besenginsterkraut
St. Zul. 1439.99.99

Plant source: *Sarothamnus scoparius* (L.) WIMM. ex KOCH (syn.: *Cytisus scoparius* (L.) LINK), broom (Fabaceae).

Synonyms: Herba Spartii scoparii, Herba Genistae scopariae, Scoparii cacumina (Lat.), Scotch or Irish broom tops, Besom (Engl.), Besenginsterkraut, Ginsterkraut (Ger.), Herbe de genêt à balais (Fr.).

Origin: Occurs throughout central, southern, and eastern Europe. The drug comes from the eastern part of Germany and is also imported from former Yugoslavia and Bulgaria.

Constituents: 0.8–1.5% quinolizidine alkaloids, principally (−)-sparteine, together with some lupanine, 4-hydroxylupanine, 13-hydroxylupanine, ammodendrine, and traces of a further 20 or so alkaloids [1, 2]. The alkaloids are located mainly in the stem; elsewhere, they are found particularly in the epidermis and sub-epidermis [3]. 0.2–

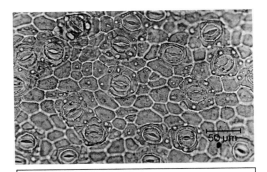

Fig. 4: Epidermis of the stem, showing numerous stomata, mostly surrounded by four small subsidiary cells

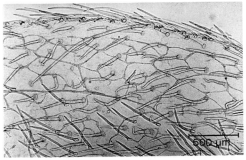

Fig. 5: Dense indumentum on the lower surface of the leaf

especially for improving cardiac circulation, and less often in diuretics.

Authentication: Macroscopically (see: description). The fragments of the twigs with their five distinct, light green, raised angles are characteristic. Microscopically, brown thick-walled polygonal cells and numerous stomata are typical of the fragments of the stem epidermis (Fig. 4). The indumentum of the leaves consists of tangled 3-celled trichomes, up to 600 µm long and with a finely warty cuticle, pointing in different directions; the two short basal cells are flattened and thick-walled (Fig. 5).
The following is a suitable TLC identification test:

Test solution: 0.5 g powdered drug refluxed with 10 ml 1N sulphuric acid for 10 min., cooled, and filtered, the flask and filter being washed with a little water. Filtrate + 5 ml dil. ammonium hydroxide solution shaken with 50 ml diethyl ether. Organic phase dried over anhydrous sodium sulphate, evaporated to dryness and the residue taken up in 5 ml diethyl ether.

Reference solution: 10 mg sparteine sulphate + 0.05 ml dil. ammonium hydroxide solution dissolved in 20 ml methanol.

Loadings: 10 µl test solution and 6 µl reference solution, as bands on silica gel.

Solvent system: chloroform + methanol + conc. ammonium hydroxide (100 + 18 + 2), 6 cm run.

Detection: plate dried in a current of warm air and sprayed with Dragendorff reagent.

Evaluation: in daylight. Reference solution: sparteine as a brown zone at about the middle or in the lower third. Test solution: a brown zone at the same Rf and immediately above it a somewhat fainter brown spot; usually also a continuous orange-brown front or double front, presumably due to a reaction product arising from the solvent system used (chloroform + NH_3 → ?) (Fig. 6).
The DAC 1986 TLC procedure employs the solvent system: heptane + diethylamine (90 + 10); the sparteine zone is found in the upper third of the chromatogram.

Quantitative standards: DAC 1986: *Total alkaloid*, not less than 0.7% calculated as sparteine (M_r 234.4). *Foreign matter*, not more than 2%. *Loss on drying*, not more than 8.0%. *Ash*, not more than 6.0%.
St.Zul. 1439.99.99: *Alkaloid*, not less than 0.8% calculated as sparteine.
BHP 1983: *Water-soluble extractive*, not less than 9%. *Foreign organic matter*, not more than 2%. *Total ash*, not more than 1.5%. *Acid-insoluble ash*, not more than 2%.

0.6% Flavonoids such as spiraeoside, isoquercitrin, genitoside, scoparoside, and other kaempferol and quercetin derivatives [4, 5]. Also isoflavones, e.g. sarothamnoside, have been detected [6]. The drug contains coumarins, caffeic-acid derivatives, and traces of an essential oil [7]. Lectins (phytohaemagglutinins) occur in the seeds.

Indications: Broom, prepared as a tea, is used to improve regulation of the circulation. The activity is determined mainly by the alkaloid content – hence the requirement for an alkaloid determination in the Standard Licence. The principal alkaloid, sparteine, is an anti-arrhythmic which inhibits the transport of sodium ions across the cell membrane and thus reduces overstimulation of the system that conducts the nerve impulse; a pathological (mostly accelerated) change in the impulse arising in the auricle is normalized. Although it does not have a positive inotropic effect, sparteine extends diastole. In cases of too low blood pressure, a favourable effect leading to normalization has been observed. In *folk medicine*, the drug is also used as a diuretic.

Side effects: Since preparations of broom may lead to an increase in the tonus of the gravid uterus, the drug is contraindicated during pregnancy. Similarly, owing to its slight tonus-increasing effect, the drug should not be employed when hypertension is present.

Making the tea: Boiling water is poured over 1–2 g of the cut drug, allowed to stand for 10 min., and then strained. A cupful is drunk up to four times a day.
1 Teaspoon = ca. 2 g.

Phytomedicines: Extracts of the herb are used in about 20 ready-made preparations

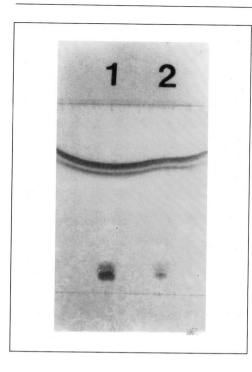

Fig. 6: TLC on 4 × 8 cm silica-gel foil
1: Broom
2: Sparteine (reference substance)
Details, see the text

Adulteration: Occasionally, confusion or adulteration with dyer's greenweed (Genistae herba, q.v.) has been noted. Its trichomes are also mostly 3-celled, but, in contrast with broom tops, mucilage cells are present in the leaf epidermis.

Literature:
[1] M. Wink et al., Plant Cell Rep. **3**, 230 (1984).
[2] M. Wink and L. Witte, Z. Naturforsch. **40C**, 767 (1985).
[3] M. Wink, L. Witte, and T. Hartmann, Planta Med. **43**, 342 (1981).
[4] M. Brum-Bousquet and P. Delaveau, Plantes Méd. Phytothérap. **15**, 201 (1981).
[5] M. Brum-Bousquet, F. Tillequin, and R.R. Paris, Lloydia **40**, 591 (1977).
[6] M. Brum-Bousquet et al., Planta Med. **43**, 367 (1981); Tetrahedron Lett. **22**, 1223 (1981).
[7] T. Kurihara and M. Kikuchi, Yakugaku Zasshi **100**, 1054 (1980); C.A. **93**, 235183 (1980).

Senecionis herba   Senecio herb

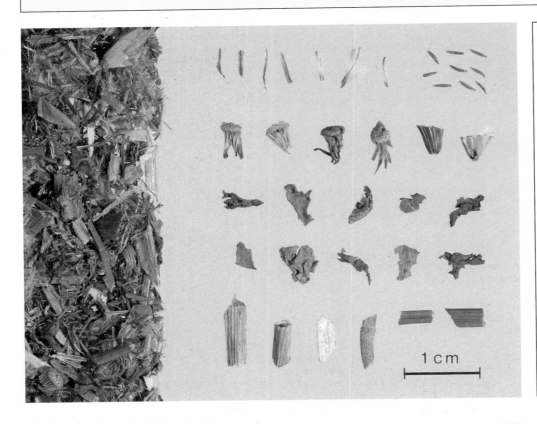

Fig. 1: Senecio herb

Description: The yellow flower-heads (with both ligulate and tubular florets) have 10–20 linear, mucronate, grass or olive green involucral bracts which are often brownish black at the tip (Fig. 3). Individual florets have a ca. 4 mm long, longitudinally striated, glabrous ovary (achene) and pappus. The margin of the green leaf fragments is finely serrate-dentate to coarsely crenate and often bristly at the edges; the lamina is glabrous or sparsely hairy. Fragments of the angular stem are green, or also have a red flush, and are glabrous or more or less hairy.

1 cm

Fig. 2: *Senecio nemorensis* L. subsp. *fuchsii* (C.C. GMEL.) DURAND

A ca. 1 m tall perennial bearing narrow leaves with a finely serrate margin. Yellow flower-heads in loose umbel-like panicles comprising tubular florets with only a few ligulate ones.

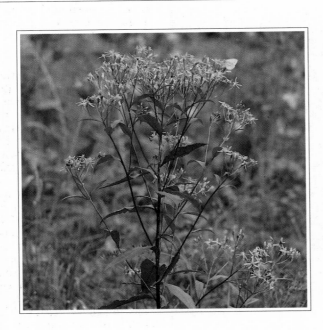

Plant source: *Senecio nemorensis* L. subsp. *fuchsii* (C.C. GMEL.) DURAND (Asteraceae).

Synonyms: Kreuzkraut, Fuchskreuzkraut, Hainkreuzkraut (Ger.). There are other (European) *Senecio* species known in German as Kreuzkraut and they are used in the same way; during the Middle Ages, they usually bore the collective name "Herba Consolidae sarracenicae". The principal species concerned are *S. vulgaris* L., groundsel (Gemeines Kreuzkraut (Ger.), Herbe à la chardonette, Feuille de Senecion (Fr.)), and *S. jacobea* L., common ragwort or St. James' wort (Jakobskreuzkraut (Ger.), Herbe St. Jacques, Herbe dorée (Fr.)).
S. aureus L., Golden Senecio or ragwort, Life root, Squaw weed (Goldkreuzkraut (Ger.), Herbe de séneçon (Fr.)) is indigenous in North America and cultivated in Europe.

Origin: Native in foothill up to alpine regions in Central Europe as far as the Caucasus. The drug comes from cultivated plants in Germany, Poland, former Czechoslovakia, Hungary, and former Yugoslavia, and partly also from the wild.

Senecionine

Fuchsisenecionine

Nemosenin A

*Extract from the German Commission
E monograph
(BAnz no. 138, dated 27.07.90)*

Uses

Senecio nemorensis subsp. *fuchsii* herb is used for diabetes mellitus, haemorrhages, high blood pressure, and for cramps and as a "uterine remedy".
Activity against diffuse mucosal haemorrhage is not fully substantiated.
Evidence for activity in the other indications listed is lacking.

Risks

S. nemorensis subsp. *fuchsii* contains varying amounts of toxic pyrrolizidine alkaloids (PA) which are known to have organotoxic, in particular hepatotoxic, effects. Carcinogenic activity, operating through a genotoxic mechanism, has been demonstrated in animal experiments.
Being in addition an inactive remedy in diabetes mellitus, it use represents a considerable health risk.

Evaluation

Since evidence of its activity is either insufficient or entirely lacking, together with its content of toxic pyrrolizidine alkaloids, the therapeutic use of *S. nemorensis* subsp. *fuchsii* cannot be justified.

Effect

Curtails bleeding time.

Constituents: Pyrrolizidine alkaloids – ca. 0.37% fuchsisenecionine and 0.007% senecionine; in other subspecies, also nemorensine, retroisosenine, and bulgarsenine. Ca. 0.1% essential oil with anhydrooplopanone, α-bisabolol, β-caryophyllene and β-caryophyllene oxide as chief components. Flavonoids: at least five flavone derivatives, rutin and quercitrin; 15 coumarin derivatives, among them aesculetin; chlorogenic acid, cynarin, fumaric acid, tannoside (0.14%); alkanes, saturated and unsaturated alkanols, fatty acids; in the rhizomes, sesquiterpene esters of the furano-eremophilane type: nemosenin A, B, C, and D, as well as senemorin.

Indications: *S. nemorensis* subsp. *fuchsii* (Fuchskreuzkraut) is considered to be a haemostyptic, which, in the form of a liquid extract, occasionally finds use in cases of capillary and arterial bleeding of different origins, especially in gynaecology in cases of menopausal bleeding and hypermenorrhoea. The activity has been confirmed in animal experiments [1]. There is also a re-duction in the bleeding in hypertrophic gingivitis [2, 3]. The active principle is unknown.
More recently, the drug has been recommended as a diabetic tea [4] – but see: **Side effects**.
In *folk medicine,* various *Senecio* species are used for menstrual disorders (dysmenorrhoea, amenorrhoea), as well as against worms and colic.

Side effects: Pyrrolizidine alkaloids with a 1,2-double bond and esterified hydroxymethyl groups are hepatotoxic, carcinogenic, and mutagenic. They are activated metabolically in the liver and rendered toxic by conversion into alkylating pyrrole derivatives which react with DNA bases and thereby bring about cross-linking of the DNA strands [5, 6, and refs. cited therein]. Senecionine has this kind of structure. In long-term toxicological experiments, it has been shown that the alkaloidal extract from *S. nemorensis* subsp. *fuchsii* has hepatotoxic, carcinogenic, and mutagenic activity [5–7]. The drug therefore has to be classified as a potential genotoxic carcinogen in man, even although the senecionine content is low. The genetic risk as compared with the toxic and carcinogenic risk appears to be slight [8]. Since diabetics usually drink teas as supportive therapy over long periods of time, weighing up the possible long-term conse-

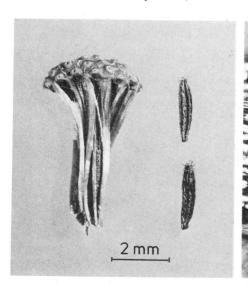
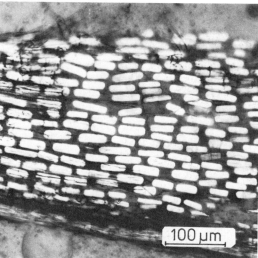

Fig. 3: Withered flower-head, showing the lanceolate involucral bracts (left) and fruit with dark spots (right)

Fig. 4: Pericarp cells with strongly birefringent contents (polarized light)

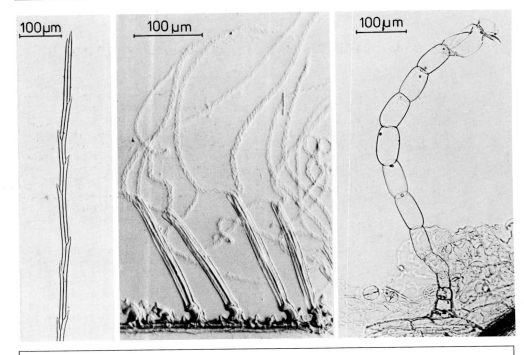

Fig. 5: Biseriate pappus hair

Fig. 6: Twinned trichomes of the fruit pericarp, showing the contents exuding in the form of spirals (chloral-hydrate mount)

Fig. 7: Multicellular covering trichome, from the leaf

Authentication: Microscopical characters to enable differentiation from other *Senecio* species have not yet been studied. A TLC method of analysis for pyrrolizidine alkaloids is given in [9].

Some microscopical features of *S. nemorensis* subsp. *fuchsii* are shown in Figs. 4–7. The contents of the epidermal cells of the ovary are strongly birefringent in polarized light (Fig. 4); the cells of the pappus hairs are biseriate; in chloral-hydrate mounts, the contents of the twinned trichomes of the ovary exude in the form of spirals (Fig. 6); the covering trichomes of the lamina consist of roundish, thin-walled cells (Fig. 7).

Note: The BHP 1983 monographs are for Jacobea (*S. jacobea* L.) with the indications: topically in arthritis, myalgia, and sciatica (after consultation), and Senecio aureus (*S. aureus* L.) with the indications: functional amenorrhoea, menopausal neurosis, and leucorrhoea (douche). Both these species appear to contain an undesirably high content of unsaturated pyrrolizidine alkaloids [11] and their use as herbal medicines ought to be discouraged.

Adulteration: Leaving aside the problems of differentiation within various *Senecio* species, adulteration is rare.

quences must lead to the rejection of senecio tea.

For a more detailed discussion concerning the adverse effects of pyrrolizidine alkaloids and *Senecio* species, see [10].

Making the tea: Boiling water is poured over 1 g of the finely cut drug and after 5–10 min strained.

1 Teaspoon = ca. 1 g.

The use is problematical, see: **Side effects**. Recent legislation introduced by the German Federal Ministry of Health prohibits herbal medicines containing unsaturated pyrrolizidine alkaloids that yield more than 1 µg internally or more than 100 µg externally per day, when used as directed. This presumably means that *S. nemorensis* subsp. *fuchsii* will no longer be a permitted ingredient in herbal medicines [cf. 11].

Phytomedicines: Only a few prepared remedies contain the drug or extracts, e.g. Senecion® (drops) as a haemostyptic and antidote in cases of dicoumarol overdosage.

Literature:
[1] B. Manstein, Ärztl. Forschung **13**, I/32-I/34 (1959).
[2] W. Klatt, Zahnärztl. Rundschau **62**, 20 (1953).
[3] E. Schmidt, Zahnärztl. Praxis **4**, 16 (1953).
[4] H. Funke, Naturheilpraxis **1978**, 253.
[5] E. Röder, Dtsch. Apoth. Ztg. **122**, 2081 (1982).
[6] H. Habs, Dtsch. Apoth. Ztg. **122**, 799 (1982).
[7] H. Habs et al., Arzneim.Forsch. **32**, 144 (1982).
[8] O. Schimmer, Dtsch. Apoth. Ztg. **123**, 1361 (1983).
[9] A.R. Mattocks, J. Chromatogr. **27**, 505 (1967).
[10] J. Westendorf, in P.G.A.M. de Smet, K. Keller, R. Hänsel, and R.F. Chandler (eds.) Adverse effects of herbal drugs, vol. 1, Springer-Verlag, Berlin, Heidelberg, New York, pp. 193, 215.
[11] In: P.G.A.M. de Smet, K. Keller, R. Hänsel, and R.F. Chandler (eds.) Adverse effects of herbal drugs, vol. 1, Springer-Verlag, Berlin, Heidelberg, New York, p. 262.

Sennae folium (DAB 10, Ph. Eur. 2), Senna leaf (BP 1988, BHP 1/1990), Senna (*USAN*; USP XXII)

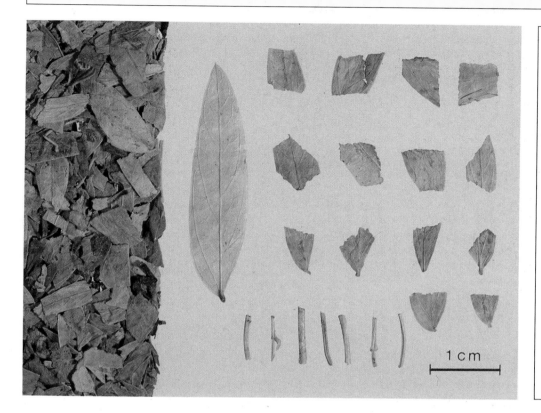

Fig. 1: Senna leaf

Description: The entire, lanceolate to narrowly lanceolate, pinnate leaflets have a short petiolule and are 2–6 cm long and 7–12 mm wide. The leaflets have an asymmetric base and a thin, stiff and brittle, light green lamina which appears as if glabrous. The leaflets are often marked with transverse or oblique lines.

Odour: Faint, characteristic.

Taste: To begin with sweetish, then bitter.

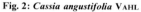

1 cm

Fig. 2: *Cassia angustifolia* VAHL

A ca. 1–1.5 m tall shrub bearing racemose inflorescences with numerous yellow, ca. 3 cm zygomorphic flowers (in contrast to the Papilionaceae, with ascending aestivation). Leaves paripinnate, with ovate-lanceolate leaflets; fruit (pods) flat, more or less reniform, brownish green and pergamentaceous, with the seeds clearly impressed.

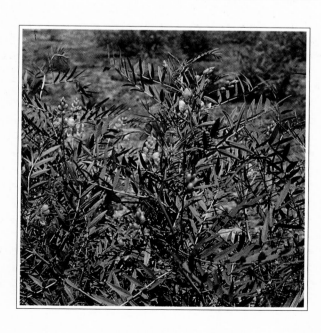

DAB 10: Sennesblätter
ÖAB: Folium Sennae
Ph. Helv. VII: Sennae folium
St. Zul. 7399.99.99

Plant sources: *Cassia angustifolia* VAHL, which furnishes so-called Tinnevelly senna, and *C. senna* L. (syn. *C. acutifolia* DEL.), which supplies so-called Alexandrian or Khartoum senna (Caesalpiniaceae).

Synonyms: Cassia leaf (Engl.), Sennesblätter (Ger.), Folioles de séné, Feuilles de séné (Fr.).

Origin: *Cassia angustifolia* is native in Arabia, but is cultivated on a large scale in southern India; *C. senna* is native in northern and north-eastern Africa and is cultivated in the valley of the Nile. Imports of the drug come mainly from India and the Sudan.
A recent account of the cultivation, processing, and trade in Tinnevelly senna (*C. angustifolia*) is given in [7].

Constituents: Ca. 3% dianthrone glycosides (the sennosides A, A$_1$, B–G) and small amounts of anthraquinone glycosides, especially aloe-emodin and rhein 8-glucosides; ca. 10% mucilage; flavonoids, especially kaempferol derivatives; naphthalene glycosides (bio-genetic precursors of the anthracene derivatives?).

Indications: Senna leaf is one of the most frequently employed plant laxatives and belongs to the group of stimulant and irritant laxatives. The drug is used in acute constipation and in all cases in which defaecation with a soft stool is required, e.g. with haemorrhoids, after anal-rectal operations, before and after abdominal operations, with anal fissures, for the evacuation of X-ray contrast media from the intestines, etc. The mechanism of action of the sennosides is fairly well understood; they are first hydrolysed by the intestinal bacteria [1–3] and then reduced to the anthrone stage, the actual active form (see also: Aloe barbadensis).

Side effects: Even with normal doses, there may be reddening of the urine (harmless) and passage of some of the anthracene derivatives into mother's milk (which may cause diarrhoea in infants).
Overdosage can lead to colicky abdominal pains and the formation of thin, watery stools.
Prolonged use should be avoided, owing to the danger of upsetting the water and electrolyte balance (loss of potassium). The drug is contraindicated in cases of ileus (intestinal obstruction) and (undiagnosed) abdominal

symptoms, and during pregnancy. As with all drugs containing anthracene derivatives, senna leaf should not be used against chronic constipation.
About possible adverse effects, see [8].

Making the tea: Warm or hot (but not boiling) water is poured over 0.5–2 g of the finely chopped drug and after 10 min. strained. Many authors also recommend macerating the drug in cold water for 10–12 hours and then straining it; the reason advanced is that, supposedly, less of the "resins", which are said to be responsible for the colicky pains, are dissolved.
In spite of the lower anthracene-glycoside content of the leaf, teas made from senna leaf are said to be stronger acting and to have more side effects than teas prepared from senna fruit. Studies show that the sen-

---

Extract from the German Commission E monograph (BAnz no. 228, dated 05. 12. 1984)

Uses

All conditions requiring an easy defaecation with a soft stool, e.g. anal fissures, haemorrhoids, after rectal-anal operations.
For emptying the bowels before X-ray investigations, as well as before and after abdominal operations. Constipation.

Contraindications

Ileus of whatever origin; during pregnancy and lactation, only after consultation with a doctor.

Side effects

None known.
With chronic use or misuse: loss of electrolytes (especially potassium), albuminuria and haematuria, deposition of pigment in the intestinal mucosa (melanosis coli), and damage to the myenteric plexus.

Interactions

With chronic use or misuse, the lack of potassium may potentiate the action of cardiotonic glycosides.

Dosage

If not otherwise prescribed: average daily dose, 20–60 mg hydroxyanthracene derivatives.

Mode of administration

Chopped drug, powdered drug, or dry extracts for infusions, decoctions, or cold macerates. Liquid and solid formulations for oral use only.

Duration of use

Anthraquinone-containing laxatives should not be taken over long periods of time.

Effects

The substances induce an active secretion of electrolytes and water into the lumen of the bowel, and inhibit the absorption of electrolytes and water in the colon. This leads to an increase in the volume of the contents of the bowel, thus raising the intraluminal pressure and stimulating peristalsis.

Sennoside A: R, R^1 = COOH (+)-form
Sennoside B: R, R^1 = COOH meso form

Sennoside C: R = COOH R^1 = CH$_2$OH (+)-form
Sennoside D: R = COOH R^1 = CH$_2$OH meso form

Sennoside A

Plants
Intestinal flora (E.coli)

Rhein anthrone

Rhein anthrone, which is believed to be the substance that induces active water secretion into the bowel and prevents its re-absorption, is formed in the colon in a reversal of the biosynthetic process by the action of hydrolytic and reducing enzymes in the bacterial flora (from: R. Hänsel and H. Haas, Therapie mit Phytopharmaka, Springer-Verlag, 1983)

nosides A and B are extracted more rapidly by hot water from the fruit than from the leaf – within 5 min., 85% and 65%, respectively. Assuming a sennoside A/B content of 2.5%, if 2 g leaf is extracted with 200 ml hot water for half-an-hour, 95 % of the glycosides is removed, which is equivalent to 48 mg sennosides A and B and thus within the recommended daily dose range of 20–60 mg. With Alexandrian senna fruit, an appropriate adjustment has to be made, to take into account the higher (5%) content of hydroxyanthracene derivatives [9].
The drug acts about 10–12 hours after being taken.
1 Teaspoon = ca. 1.5 g.

Herbal teas: The drug is available in tea bags (2 g). It is obtainable from several manufacturers under a variety of names as a monovalent preparation. To obtain senna leaf of acceptable micro-biological quality, the minimum intensity of γ-irradiation is 10 kGy, but probably such treatment is unnecessary provided the tea is prepared by hot extraction and drunk as soon as possible [10]; cf. above.
The drug is on the market as an instant tea (dry extract), and the extract is likewise a component of many instant laxative teas, e.g. Solubilax®, Depuraflux®, Dr. Klinger's Bergischer Kräutertee®, etc.
Senna leaf is a constituent of "Swedish bitters"; see the note under: Aloe capensis.

Phytomedicines: The finely chopped or powdered drug is a component of more than 80

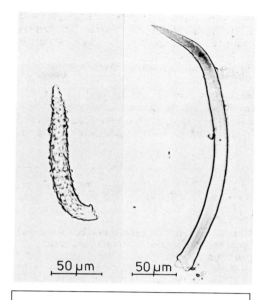

Fig. 4: Lower leaf surface of *Cassia auriculata* (adulterant) with a long and dense pubescence

prepared remedies and senna-leaf extract is present in more than 30 others. These remedies are mostly laxatives, biliary remedies, so-called "cleansing teas" of various kinds, and "slimming teas".
Among the preparations containing senna leaf and other laxative drugs available in the

UK are: Gerard House Priory Cleansing Herbs, Lanes Lustys Herbalene, and Potter's Cleansing Herbs.
Many prepared remedies have a standardized sennoside content (usually 12–22 mg sennoside B per dose) and they should be given preference over non-standardized preparations [4]. The sennosides isolated from the drug are included in prepared remedies as the calcium salts, e.g. Pursennid®, etc.
There are many combinations with bulk laxatives and with other drugs containing anthracene glycosides or digestive enzymes, e.g. Neda® Früchtwürfel (diced fruit), Kräuterlax®, Laxafix®, Cesralax®, Laxherba®, Zet 26®, etc., etc.
Among the UK products with a standardized content of sennosides are: Senade® (tablets, syrup), Bidrolar®, Primolax®, Pursennid®. Together with other laxative drugs, senna is a component of Pripsen®, Gerard House Pilewort Compound Tablets, Lanes Dual-Lax and Dual-Lax Extra Strong, and Potter's Out of Sorts Tablets, etc., etc.

Regulatory status (UK): General Sales List – Schedule 1, Table A; sennosides A and B, maximum single dose 15 mg.
Note: Sennae folium is the subject of an ESCOP proposal for a European harmonized monograph, based on the Ph. Eur. 2 monograph.

Authentication: Macro- (see: Description) and microscopically, according to the Ph.

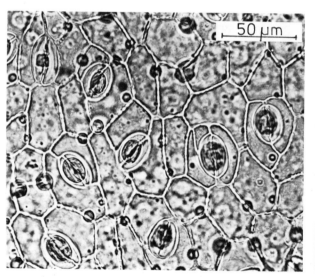

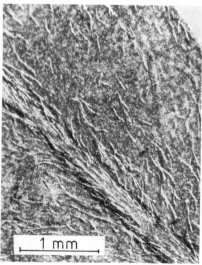

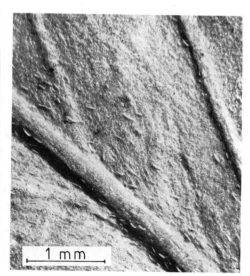

Fig. 3: Leaf epidermis with mainly paracytic stomata

Fig. 5: Lower leaf surface of *Cassia senna* with short stiff trichomes

Fig. 6: Unicellular trichomes from *Cassia senna* (left; with warty cuticle) and from *Cassia auriculata* (right; adulterant)

5.1 Uses

Constipation, all conditions in which an easy evacuation with a soft stool is desired, e.g. anal fissures, haemorrhoids, and after rectal-anal operations; for evacuating the bowels before X-ray investigations and before and after abdominal operations.

5.2 Contraindications

Preparations of senna leaves are not to be used when there is obstruction of the bowel or during pregnancy and lactation.

5.3 Side effects

When used according to the instructions, not known. With frequent or prolonged use or with overdosage, there is the possibility of an increased loss of water and salts, particularly potassium salts. Moreover, there may be excretion of protein (albuminuria) and blood (haematuria) in the urine, as well as pigmentation of the bowel mucosa (melanosis coli). Damage to the nerves of the bowel (myenteric plexus) may also occur.

5.4 Interactions with other remedies

The increased loss of potassium may potentiate the effects of cardiotonic glycosides (digitalis, strophanthus).

5.5 Dosage and Mode of administration

Warm or hot water (ca. 150 ml) is poured over $^1/_2$-1 flattened teaspoon of **Senna leaf** and after about 10 min. passed through a tea strainer. The tea can also be prepared by adding cold water and allowing it to draw for some time.

If not otherwise prescribed, a cup of the freshly made tea is drunk in the morning and/or at night before going to bed.

5.6 Duration of use

Senna-leaf tea should only be taken for a few days. For longer use, a doctor should be consulted.

Note: To help restore normal bowel function, care should be taken to ensure that the diet has plenty of roughage, that there is an adequate fluid intake, and that as much exercise as possible is taken.

5.7 Note

Store away from light and moisture.

Eur. 2 (BP 1988). The diagnostic features include the mainly paracytic stomata (Fig. 3), the unicellular, thick-walled, curved trichomes with a warty cuticle (Fig. 4), the iso-bilateral leaf structure, epidermal cells containing mucilage, vascular bundles incompletely surrounded by a sheath of fibres accompanied by rows of cells with calcium oxalate prisms, and occasional calcium oxalate clusters. The USP XXII also has detailed descriptions of the macroscopy and microscopy of the drug.

Tinnevelly and Alexandrian senna, in both powder and extract form, may be differentiated through the TLC profiles of their naphthalene glycosides [5].

TLC of the sennosides may be carried out according to the Ph. Eur. 2 (BP 1988) method. For a coloured illustration of the chromatogram, see [11].

Quantitative standards: Ph. Eur. 2, etc.: *Hydroxyanthracene glycosides*, not less than 2.5% calculated as sennoside B (M_r 863).

Foreign matter, not more than 3% other plant parts and not more than 1% other foreign matter; densely pubescent leaves (*Cassia auriculata*) must be absent. *Acid-insoluble ash*, not more than 2.5%.

Adulteration: Nowadays, very rare. The *C. auriculata* (palthé senna) leaves mentioned in the pharmacopoeias are seldom encountered. This adulterant does not contain any sennosides. It can be recognized on examination with a hand lens by the dense pubescence on the lower surface of the leaf (Fig. 5; cf. Fig. 6), and by the trichomes, which are very long (up to more than 600 μm), only slightly warty, and more sharply curved towards the tip (Fig. 4; cf. right and left). With 80% sulphuric acid, palthé senna gives a carmine-red colour – due to conversion of leuco-anthocyanidin to the oxonium salt [6].

Literature:

[1] M. Dreessen and J. Lemli, Pharm. Acta Helv. **57**, 350 (1982).

[2] M. Dreessen, H. Eyssen, and J. Lemli, J. Pharm. Pharmacol. **33**, 679 (1981).

[3] K. Kobashi, T. Nishimura, M. Kusaka, M. Hattori, and T. Namba, Planta Med. **40**, 225 (1980).

[4] H.G. Meßen, Dtsch. Apoth. Ztg. **122**, 2317 (1982).

[5] J. Lemli, J. Cuveele, and E. Verhaeren, Planta Med. **49**, 36 (1983).

[6] Kommentar DAB 10.

[7] B. Bornkessel, Dtsch. Apoth. Ztg. **131**, 171 (1991).

[8] P.F. D'Arcy, Adverse Drug React. Toxicol. Rev. **10**, 189 (1991).

[9] H. Miething, W. Boventer, and R. Hänsel, Dtsch. Apoth. Ztg. **127**, 2587 (1987).

[10] H. van Doorne, E.H. Bosch, J.H. Zwaving, and E.T. Elema, Pharm. Weekbl. (Sci. ed.) **10**, 217 (1988).

[11] H. Wagner, S. Bladt, and E.M. Zgainski, Plant drug analysis, Springer, Berlin – Heidelberg – New York – Tokyo, 1984, p. 111.

Sennae fructus acutifoliae (DAB 10, Ph. Eur. 2), Alexandrian Senna fruit (BP 1988; BHP 1990)
Sennae fructus angustifoliae (DAB 10, Ph. Eur. 2), Tinnevelly Senna fruit (BP 1988; BHP 1990)

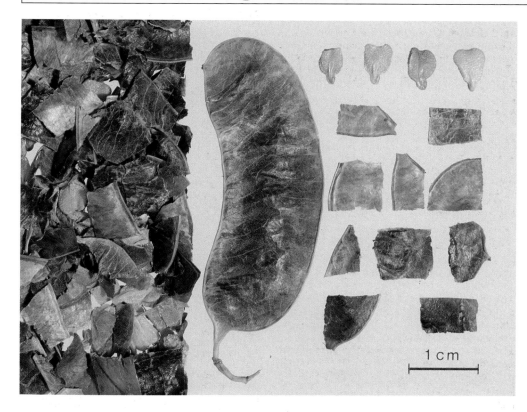

Fig. 1: Senna fruit

The flat, compressed, brownish green or greyish green, membranaceous-leathery pods are up to 5 cm long and ca. 20–25 mm (*Cassia senna*) or 15–18 mm (*Cassia angustifolia*) wide and slightly reniform. The two halves of the fruit, which adhere to each other over the whole surface, are difficult to separate. The fruit normally contain 5–7 (*C. senna*) or 7–10 seeds (*C. angustifolia*), which are more or less cordate, whitish to greyish green, and very hard, with a dimpled, reticulately ridged surface (Fig. 3).

Odour: Faint, characteristic.

Taste: Mucilaginous and sweetish, then somewhat bitter and harsh.

Fig. 2: *Cassia angustifolia* VAHL

For the description, see: Sennae folium, under Fig. 2.

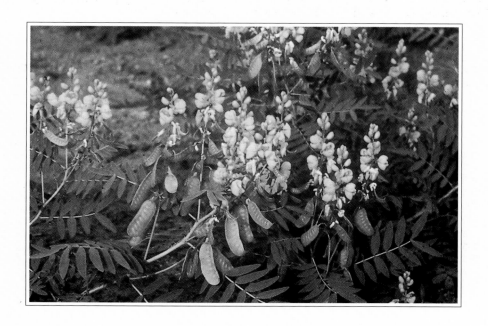

DAB 10: Alexandriner-Sennesfrüchte
Tinnevelly-Sennesfrüchte
Ph. Helv. VII: Sennae fructus acutifoliae
Sennae fructus angustifoliae
ÖAB: Fructus Sennae acutifoliae
Fructus Sennae angustifoliae
St. Zul. 1259.99.99 (Alexandriner Sennesfrüchte)
St. Zul. 1269.99.99 (Tinnevelly Sennesfrüchte)

Plant sources: *Cassia angustifolia* VAHL, which supplies Tinnevelly Senna, and *C. senna* L. (syn. *C. acutifolia* DEL.), which yields Alexandrian Senna (Caesalpiniaceae).

Synonyms: Senna pods, Cassia fruit (Engl.), Sennesfrüchte (Ger.), Gousses de séné (Fr.).

Origin: see, Sennae folium.

Constituents: A varying amount of sennosides and other anthraquinone derivatives, depending on the *Cassia* species (hence, two monographs in the Ph. Eur. 2, BP 1988, etc.; see Quantitative standards (below): Tinnevelly senna fruit ca. 3% and Alexandrian senna fruit ca. 4–5%. Like senna leaf, the main components of the mixture of anthracene derivatives are the dianthrone glycosides sennosides A-D; compounds richer in glucose (glucosennosides) are also present. The proportion of anthraquinone glycosides is smaller in the fruit than in the leaves, and the composition is different. Flavonoids, especially kaempferol derivatives, and resinous substances (?) are also present.

Indications: As for Sennae folium (q.v.). In spite of the slightly higher anthracene glycoside content (as compared with the leaf drug), the fruit drug has a somewhat gentler action (and is therefore preferred for children, for example); this depends not so much on the previously supposed absence of "resins" in the fruit, but rather on the fact that the fruit contains only a little of the (highly active) aloe-emodin glucoside.

Side effects: See, Sennae folium.

Making the tea: See, Sennae folium.
1 Teaspoon = ca. 2 g.

Herbal teas: The drug is marketed by different manufacturers under a variety of names, partly as prepared remedies, e.g. Vinco®, and partly as instant teas (dry extract from the fruit), e.g. Laxatan® Instant Abführ-Tee. An account of the manufacture of Bekunis® Instant-Tee [1] describes some of the steps taken to reduce contamination by plant-protection products and microorganisms and to standardize the product. See also p. 465.
The drug is a component of "Swedish bitters"; see the note under: Aloe capensis.

Phytomedicines: Senna fruit are available as such in the form of a powder as a prepared remedy, or in the form of an extract, e.g.

Bekunis® Kräuter Dragees (herbal dragees), Colonorm® Sirup. More often, senna fruit or extracts from them are present in combinations (more than 100 prepared remedies), e.g. Agiolax®, Laxiplant®, Depuran®, Liquidepur®, etc., etc.
UK products include Potter's Senna Tablets and various standardized preparations containing either the fruit or extracts: Seven Seas Laxative Tablets; Arkopharma Phytosenelax capsules; Manevac® (formerly Agiolax®) granules, X-Prep® liquid, and

Senokot® (perhaps the most popular UK laxative) which is available as tablets, granules, or syrup.

Regulatory status (UK): General Sales List – Schedule 1, Table A; sennosides A and B, maximum single dose 15 mg.

Authentication: Macro- (see: Description) and microscopically, following the Ph. Eur. 2 (BP 1988). The outer fruit wall has a thick cuticle, with only occasional stomata and trichomes. The inner fruit wall, the endo-

---

Wording of the package insert, from the German Standard Licence (the same wording for both drugs, except for the dosage; see *):

5.1   Uses
Constipation; all conditions in which an easy evacuation with a soft stool is required, e.g. anal fissures, haemorrhoids, and after rectal-anal operations; for emptying the bowels before operations or X-ray investigations and before and after abdominal operations.

5.2   Contraindications
Senna-fruit tea should not be used in cases of intestinal obstruction or during pregnancy and lactation.

5.3   Side effects
When used according to the instructions, not known. With frequent and prolonged use, or with overdosage, there is the possibility of an increased loss of water and salts, especially potassium salts. Moreover, there may be excretion of protein (albuminuria) and blood (haematuria) in the urine, as well as deposition of pigment in the mucosa of the bowel (melanosis coli). Damage to the nerves of the bowel (myenteric plexus) may also occur.

5.4   Interactions with other remedies
The increased loss of potassium may potentiate the effects of cardiotonic glycosides.

5.5   Dosage and Mode of administration
Warm or hot water (ca. 150 ml) is poured over half a teaspoonful* of **Senna fruit** and after 10 min. passed through a tea strainer. The tea can also be prepared by adding one teaspoonful of senna fruit to cold water and allowing it to draw for 2–3 hours. If not otherwise prescribed, a cup of the freshly prepared tea is drunk in the morning and/or at night before going to bed.

5.6   Duration of use
Senna-fruit tea should only be taken for a few days. For longer use, a doctor should be consulted.
Note: To help restore normal bowel function, care should be taken to ensure that the diet has plenty of roughage, that there is an adequate fluid intake, and that as much exercise as possible is taken.

5.7   Note
Store away from light and moisture.

* of Alexandrian senna fruit; $^{1}/_{2}$–1 flat teaspoonful of Tinnevelly senna fruit.

Fig. 3: Cordate, reticulately ridged seed

Fig. 4: Endocarp (layer of interlaced fibres) of the fruit (in polarized light)

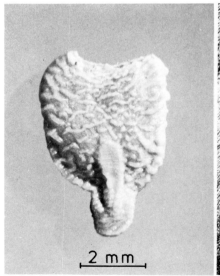

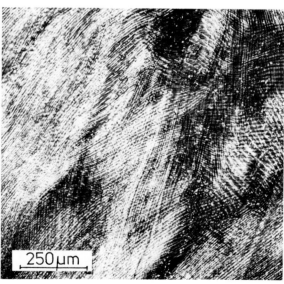

Extract from the German Commission E monograph
(*BAnz no. 228, dated 05. 12. 1984*)

The text is the same as for: Sennae folium (q.v.).

carp, consists of interlacing groups of thick-walled fibres (Fig. 4). The fruit is also readily distinguished by the nature of the seed testa (Fig. 3): in *Cassia angustifolia* mostly transverse unconnected ridges cover the surface, while in *C. senna* the ridges form a connected network. A full description of the microscopy of the powdered drugs is given in [2]. TLC examination of the sennosides may be carried out following the Ph. Eur. 2 (BP 1988); for the details, see: Sennae folium. A coloured illustration of the chromatogram is given in [3].

Quantitative standards: Ph. Eur. 2, BP 1988, etc.: *Hydroxyanthracene derivatives*, not less than 3.4% (Sennae fructus acutifoliae) or 2.2% (Sennae fructus angustifoliae) calculated as sennoside B (M_r 863). *Foreign vegetable and mineral matter*, not more than 1%. *Acid-insoluble ash*, not more than 2.0%. BHP 1/1990: Refers to the corresponding monographs in the BP 1988.

Note: Sennae fructus is also the subject of an ESCOP proposal for a harmonized European monograph, based on the Ph. Eur. 2 monograph.

Adulteration: Hardly ever occurs.

Literature:
[1] W. Silber, Dtsch. Apoth. Ztg. **131**, 349 (1991).
[2] B.P. Jackson and D.W. Snowdon, Atlas of microscopy of medicinal plants, culinary herbs and spices, Belhaven Press, London, 1990, p. 214.
[3] H. Wagner, S. Bladt, and E.M. Zgainski, Plant drug analysis, Springer, Berlin – Heidelberg – New York – Tokyo, 1984, p. 111.

Serpylli herba (DAB 10), Wild thyme, Thymus serpyllum (BHP 1983)

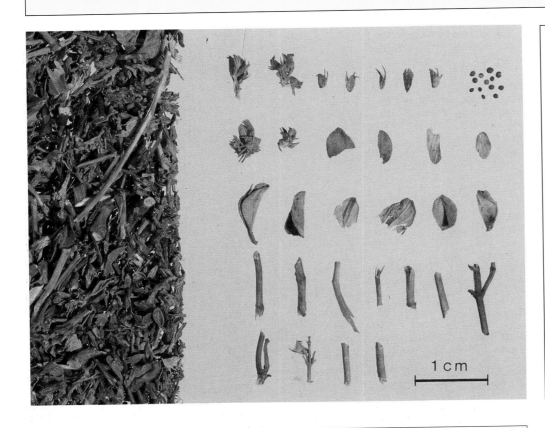

Fig. 1: Wild thyme

<u>Description:</u> The drug consists of the dried aerial parts collected at the time of flowering. The bluish violet branchlets are ca. 1 mm thick, hollow, obscurely 4-angled, and sparsely pubescent. The leaves, up to 1 cm long, are opposite in pairs and oblong to oblong-ovate, with an entire and slightly involute margin. The degree of pubescence varies, the base of the leaf is ciliate. Glandular dots can be seen with a hand lens (Fig. 3). The pink corolla is much shrivelled; the reddish violet two-lipped, tubular calyx has five teeth and a white pubescence in the throat (Fig. 3).

<u>Odour:</u> Intensely spicy.

<u>Taste:</u> Intensely spicy and aromatic, somewhat bitter.

Fig. 2: *Thymus serpyllum* L.

A low (up to 20 cm), mat-forming, scented herb or undershrub, with creeping branches. Oblong to elliptic sessile leaves with a ciliate margin. Small pink flowers grouped in more or less capitate inflorescences.

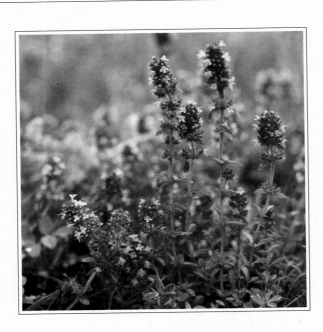

DAB 10: Quendelkraut
Ph. Helv. VI: Herba Serpylli

Plant source: *Thymus serpyllum* L., Breckland thyme (Lamiaceae); some taxonomists unite it with *T. pulegioides* L., large or larger wild thyme, as a collective species. The Flora Europaea [3] still differentiates *T. serpyllum* (2n = 24; stem pubescent all round) and *T. pulegioides* L. (2n = 28 or 30; stem 4-angled and only pubescent at the angles).
In the UK, *T. serpyllum* is very local in East Anglia [4] and the name wild thyme is usually given to the west European *T. praecox* OPIZ subsp. *arcticus* (DURAND) JALAS (syn. *T. drucei* RONNIGER) [4] or subsp. *britannicus* (RONNIGER) HOLUB [5].

Synonyms: Common thyme, Garden thyme, Mother of thyme, Serp(h)yllum, Serpolet, Quendel (Engl.), Quendel, Wilder Thymian, Feldkümmel (Ger.), Herbe de serpolet (Fr.).

Origin: According to the Flora Europaea [3], *T. serpyllum* occurs northwards from

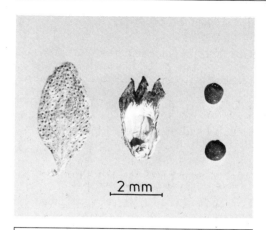

Fig. 3: *Thymus serpyllum*: leaf with numerous glandular dots (left), calyx cut open to show the white tufts of hairs (middle), and seeds (right)

Extract from the German Commission E monograph (BAnz no. 193, dated 15. 10. 1987)

Uses
Catarrh of the upper respiratory tract.

Contraindications
None known.

Side effects
None known.

Interactions with other remedies
None known.

Dosage
Unless otherwise prescribed: average daily dose, 6 g drug; preparations correspondingly.

Mode of administration
Chopped drug for infusions and other preparations for internal use.

Effects
Antimicrobial, spasmolytic.

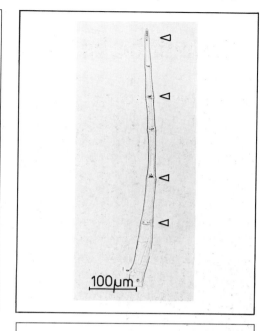

Fig. 4: Multicellular covering trichome with minute needles of calcium oxalate (*)

north-eastern France, northern Austria, and northern Ukraine, while *T. pulegioides* is native throughout most of Europe. The drug is imported from Eastern Europe.

Constituents: 0.1–0.6% essential oil, the composition of which varies widely according to the origin of the plants. Among its components are: thymol, carvacrol, *p*-cymol, linalool, cineole, α-pinene, and other terpenes; about the variation in the composition of the essential oil, see [1]. In addition, tannins (up to ca. 7%), bitter substances of unknown constitution, flavonoids, etc. [2].

Indications: Similar to genuine Thymi herba (q.v.), but less active. In *folk medicine* it is used as a stomachic, carminative, expecto-

rant, and in bladder and kidney disorders; as an aromatic; externally, for herbal cures and baths; alcoholic extracts in liniments for rheumatic pains and sprains; decoctions with milk as a diaphoretic; also as an antiseptic [2].

Making the tea: Boiling water is poured over 1.5–2 g of the finely chopped drug and after 10 min. strained. As an expectorant, several cups are drunk during the day; as a stomachic, a cup is taken before or during meals.
1 Teaspoon = ca. 1.4 g.

Phytomedicines: The drug is a component of prepared antitussives (cough teas, bronchial teas). Alcoholic extracts, together with other

plant expectorants, are present in cough drops.

Authentication: Macro- (see: Description) and microscopically. Trichomes of the following types on the leaf and stem fragments are diagnostic: (a) unicellular, short to long covering trichomes with a longitudinally striated cuticle; (b) multicellular covering trichomes with a warty cuticle and often in the corners of the cells minute calcium-oxalate needles (Fig. 4); (c) peltate glandular trichomes with 12 secretory cells (Fig. 5);

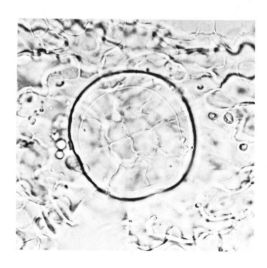

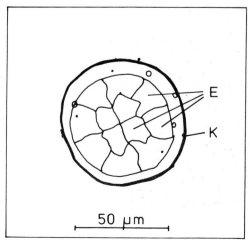

Fig. 5: Head of a peltate glandular trichome with 12 secretory cells (E) and raised cuticle (K)

chlorophyll, the parenchyma tissue also has a red pigment. Leaf fragments with the geniculate and conical trichomes typical of *Thymus vulgaris* must be absent. Cf. the BHP 1983.

The following procedure is a suitable TLC identification test:

Test solution: essential oil from 25 g drug obtained by the method for the quantitative determination of the essential oil content (but without using xylene) diluted with 10 ml ethanol.

Reference solution: 10 mg thymol dissolved in 10 ml methanol.

Loadings: 5 μl each of the test and reference solutions, as bands on silica gel.

Solvent system: toluene + ethyl acetate (97 + 3), 5 cm run.

Detection: after complete evaporation of the solvent, sprayed first with 5% ethanolic sulphuric acid, then with 1% ethanolic vanillin, followed by heating at 105 °C for 3–5 min. and immediate evaluation.

Evaluation: in daylight. <u>Test solution</u>: thymol as a bright red zone in the middle of the chromatogram. Test solution: a zone corresponding to the reference thymol zone; directly below it a violet zone and directly

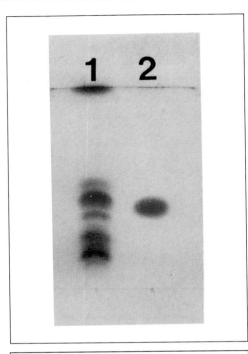

Fig. 6: TLC on 4 × 8 cm silica-gel foil

1: *Thymus serpyllum*

2: Thymol

For details, see the text

above it a bluish zone; further up, two turquoise zones (Fig. 6).

Quantitative standards: <u>DAB 10</u>: *Volatile oil*, not less than 0.3%. *Phenols (calculated as Thymol)*, not less than 0.1%. *Foreign matter*, not more than 3%. *Loss on drying*, not more than 10.0%. *Total ash*, not more than 10%. *HCl-insoluble ash*, not more than 2.0%. <u>Ph. Helv. VI</u>: *Volatile oil*, not less than 0.2%. <u>BHP 1983</u>: *Total ash*, not more than 10%. *Acid-insoluble ash*, not more than 4%.

Adulteration: Rare – mostly through inadvertent contamination with ordinary thyme (Thymi herba; q.v.), which can be detected microscopically and by TLC (see: Authentication).

Storage: Protected from moisture and light, in well-closed metal or glass (but not plastic) containers.

Literature:

[1] E. Schratz and G. Cromm, Sci. Pharm. **36**, 13, 110 (1968).

[2] Hager, vol. **6C**, p. 169 (1979).

[3] J. Jalas, in: T.G. Tutin et al. (eds.), Flora Europaea, Cambridge University Press, Cambridge – London – New York, 1972, vol. **3**, pp. 172–182.

[4] A.R. Clapham, T.G. Tutin, and D.M. Moore, Flora of the British Isles, 3rd ed., Cambridge University Press, Cambridge – London – New York, 1987, p. 407.

[5] D.J. Mabberley, The plant-book. A portable dictionary of higher plants, Cambridge University Press, Cambridge – New York – Melbourne, 1990, p. 581.

Sinapis nigrae semen (Black) Mustard seed

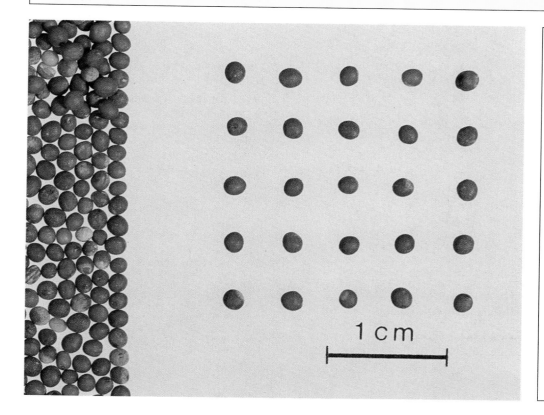

Fig. 1: (Black) Mustard seed

Description: The dark reddish brown, occasionally also paler, almost spherical seeds are 1–1.5 mm in diameter. The hilum is seen as a pale spot. With a hand lens, the surface is seen to be finely pitted (Fig. 3). Inside, the seed is yellow.

Odour: When whole, odourless; after stirring the crushed seeds with water, a smell of mustard oil quickly develops.

Taste: To begin with, mild and oily and slightly sourish; afterwards, pungently acrid.

Fig. 2: *Brassica nigra* (L.) W.D. J. KOCH

A much branched herb growing to a height of ca. 1 m and characterized by petiolate leaves pinnately divided with 2–4 blunt lobes and a large terminal segment, when on the lower part of the stem, and oblong and undivided, when on the upper part of the stem. Yellow 4-part flowers and erect follicles lying close to the stem.

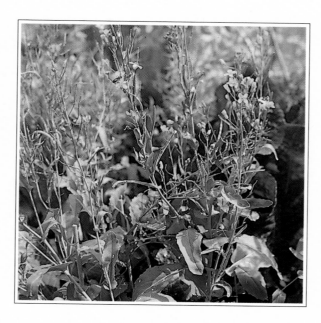

DAC 1986: Schwarze Senfsamen
ÖAB: Semen Sinapis
Ph. Helv. VII: Sinapis nigrae semen

Plant source: *Brassica nigra* (L.) W.D. J. KOCH, black mustard (Brassicaceae).

Synonyms: Semen Sinapis viridis, Semen Sinapeos (Lat.), Brown mustard (Engl.), Schwarze Senfsamen, Brauner or Grüner Senf, Holländischer or Französischer Senf (Ger.), (Graine de) Moutarde noire (Fr.).

Origin: Native in the Mediterranean region; cultivated worldwide in the temperate zones. The drug is imported from Romania, the former USSR, Turkey, China, India, and Pakistan.

Constituents: Up to 30% fixed oil; the glucosinolates (= mustard-oil glycosides) are of interest in medicine and in folk medicine. On crushing or chewing the seeds, they are hydrolysed by the enzyme myrosinase (= thioglucosidase) which inside the cells is kept in special compartments (associated

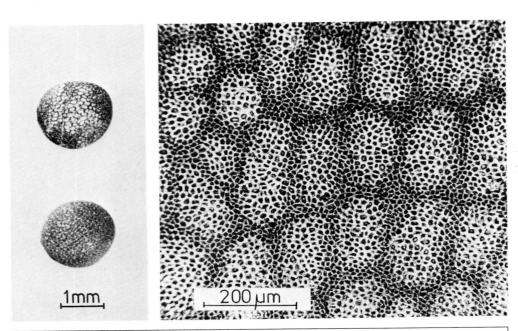

Glucosinolate
(Sinigrin) (R = −CH₂−CH=CH₂)

(Sinalbin) (R = −CH₂−⟨phenyl⟩−OH) (p-Hydroxybenzyl mustard oil)

Alkyl isothiocyanate
(Allyl mustard oil)

Sinapin (Choline + Sinapic acid)

with mitochondria, among other things) separate from the glucosinolates which are localized in the vacuoles. Thus, ca. 0.7% volatile allyl mustard oil is formed from 1.0–1.2% sinigrin. [Note: In contrast, sinalbin, the glucosinolate of white mustard (Semen Erucae DAB 6 = Semen Sinapis albae, from *Sinapis alba* L.) yields the non-volatile *p*-hydroxybenzyl mustard oil.] Further, ca. 1% sinapin (=ester of choline with sinapic acid); 20% mucilage [1].

Indications: Nowadays, the medical application of mustard plasters and bandages is a rarity, since mustard oils (biogenetic or synthetic) cause particularly intense hyperaemia of the skin. Mustard plasters bring about very rapid reddening of the skin and lancing pains. Allyl mustard oil rapidly penetrates to the deeper layers of the skin and brings about inflammation.

Even so, currently, mustard-oil preparations have found renewed use in some "natural healing methods" – mustard bandages placed on the skin in revulsive treatment for acute bronchitis and bronchopneumonia: about two handfuls of ground mustard seed are stirred with *lukewarm* water to give a thick slurry. (Reminder: *hot* water, 60 °C, inactivates the enzyme.) As soon as vapour rises which irritates the eyes, the slurry is spread on to linen and placed on the part to be treated, e.g. the chest. When a strong burning sensation is felt, the bandage is removed and the skin is washed.

Mustard plasters for treating other parts of the body: these must be soaked with lukewarm water for some time in order to allow the myrosinase to act. About 5 min. after applying the plaster, the skin begins to redden and there is a considerable rise in skin temperature. The plaster must be removed within 15–30 min. at the outside (unlike capsaicin-containing plasters). The local

irritant effect lasts for 24–48 hours (details according to [2]).

In *folk medicine*, mustard preparations and mustard oils are also used in pleuritis, neuritis, in rheumatic conditions, attacks of influenza, occasionally in urinary infections, as a spice to stimulate the appetite and digestion (here, the bactericidal action of the mustard oils plays an important role).

Black mustard, even more than the milder white mustard, when ground forms the basis of the mustards used for culinary purposes (recipes in [1]).

Side effects: If mustard plasters or bandages are left too long on the site of application, blisters form, often with suppurating and poorly healing ulceration and necrosis. This is particularly the case with sensitive, predisposed patients. Mustard-oil preparations are likewise contraindicated when there is severe circulatory damage and with varicose veins and other venous disorders [2].

Making the tea: Not applicable. For preparing poultices, see: Indications.

Phytomedicines: Mustard seed are present in rubefacient plasters and poultices. Mustard oils are a component of liniments and bath additives.

Authentication: Macro- (see: Description) and microscopically, following the DAC 1986. The microscopy of the powdered drug is described and illustrated in [4]. The diagnostic features include the surface view of the testa (Fig. 4), with the palisade cells and the so-called "large cells" that shine through; these latter are not real cells and the net-like appearance is an optical effect, caused by the different heights of the palisade cells. Starch is absent or present only in traces; crystals are also absent.

A method for the TLC examination of mustard-oil drugs is set out in [5]:

Test solution: 10 g ground seeds boiled for 5 min. with 50 ml boiling methanol and

Fig. 3: Small dark-coloured seeds, showing the finely dimpled surface

Fig. 4: Surface view of the testa, showing the small, thick-walled palisade cells with their narrow lumen and the transparent network of so-called large cells

stood for 1 hour with occasional shaking, filtered, and the filtrate evaporated to 5 ml and chromatographed over cellulose powder (20 × 1 cm column); eluted with methanol – the first 20 ml rejected and the next 100 ml concentrated to ca. 1 ml at 25–30 °C under reduced pressure.

Reference solution: sinalbin mixture or sinigrin.

Loading: ca. 25 µl test solution, as a band on silica gel GF$_{254}$.

Solvent system: butan-1-ol + propan-1-ol + glacial acetic acid + water (30 + 10 + 10 + 10), 15 cm run.

Detection: sprayed with 25 % trichloracetic acid in chloroform, heated for 10 min. at 140 °C and then oversprayed with a 1:1-mixture of 1% aq. potassium hexacyanoferrate and 5% aq. iron(III) chloride.

Evaluation: in daylight; blue zones on a yellow background. Reference solution: sinigrin at Rf ca. 0.35. Test solution: depending on the concentration five or more zones, with several weak ones at higher Rf values; a zone corresponding to sinigrin; absent – a zone at Rf ca. 0.45 (characteristic of *B. alba*

extract). The quantitative determination of the mustard-oil glycosides is carried out iodometrically, following the DAC 1986.

Quantitative standards: DAC 1986: *Glucosinolates*, after enzymic hydrolysis not less than 0.6% volatile oil calculated as allyl isothiocyanate (M_r 99.2). *Foreign matter*, not more than 2%; other *Brassica* species recognized by taste, size, and colour, and by microscopical features (colourless or yellowish white or palisade cells greater than 10 µm wide).
ÖAB: *Glucosinolates*, not less than 0.7% calculated as allyl isothiocyanate (M_r 99.2). *Foreign matter*, not more than 3%; absence of *Sinapis alba* L. seeds: 1 g seed powder boiled for 5 min. with 5 ml water, filtered, and 3 drops Millon's reagent added to the filtrate should not give a red colour within 30 min. *Ash*, not more than 5.0%.
Ph. Helv. VII: the following species are permitted in addition to *B. nigra*: *B. juncea* (L.) CZERN., *B. integrifolia* (WEST) O.E. SCHULZ, and *B. cernua* (THUNB.) FORB. et HEMSL. *Glycosidic volatile oil*, not less than 0.7% calculated as allyl isothiocyanate (M_r 99.2). *Foreign matter*, not more than 3%; seeds of the same size with a smooth, or at most

punctate but not dimpled, testa (*B. alba* L.) are absent. *Sulphated ash*, not more than 6.0%.

Adulteration: Rare, with the seeds of other *Brassica* species, e.g. *Brassica juncea* (L.) CZERN., Sarepta or Romanian brown mustard, *B. cernua* MATSUM., Chinese mustard, etc. These seeds are difficult to distinguish from black mustard; the specialist literature has to be consulted and the microscopical examination necessitates the use of a polarizer [3]. However, as all these mustard seeds contain sinigrin, they are to be considered more as substitutes than as adulterants.

Literature:
[1] Hager, vol. **3**, p. 4996 (1972).
[2] R. Hänsel and H. Haas, Therapie mit Phytopharmaka, Springer, Berlin, 1984.
[3] G. Gassner, B. Hohmann, and F. Deutschmann, Mikroskopische Untersuchung pflanzlicher Lebensmittel, 5th ed., Gustav Fischer, Stuttgart, 1989.
[4] B.P. Jackson and D.W. Snowdon, Atlas of microscopy of medicinal plants, culinary herbs and spices, Belhaven Press, London, 1990, p. 22.
[5] H. Wagner, S. Bladt, and E.M. Zgainski, Plant drug analysis, Springer-Verlag, Berlin, Heidelberg, New York, Tokyo, 1984, p. 256.

Solidaginis giganteae herba   Early golden-rod herb

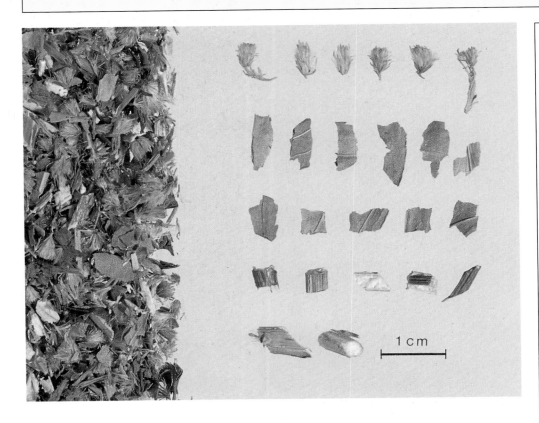

1 cm

Fig. 1: Early golden-rod herb

Description: The numerous yellow flowering heads (upper row) are also occasionally present as inflorescences in the form of unilateral, curved racemes. The ligulate florets are 4–6 mm long with the involucral bracts projecting only slightly (*Solidago gigantea*) or only 2.5–3 mm long and scarcely longer than the involucre (*Solidago canadensis*). Leaf fragments which are green on the upper surface and greyish green on the lower surface and which have a very prominent midrib are present, as are also pieces of the solid stem with their deep longitudinal grooves (bottom two rows).

Odour: Aromatic.

Taste: Weakly astringent.

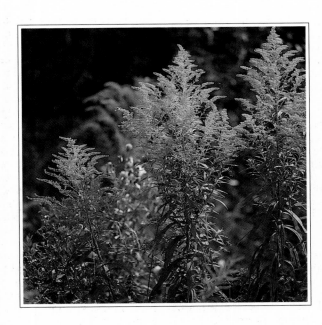

Fig. 2: *Solidago gigantea* AITON

A shrub up to 1.5 m in height, with – in contrast to that of *S. canadensis* – a glabrous stem bearing numerous lanceolate, acuminate, sessile leaves. Many flowering heads, only 5–8 mm in diameter, and arranged in panicles.

St. Zul. 1639.99.99 (Riesengoldrutenkraut)

Plant source: *Solidago gigantea* AITON, including var. *serotina* (KUNTZE) CRONQUIST (syn. *S. serotina* AITON), early golden-rod (Asteraceae) – the St.Zul. permits only this species – and *S. canadensis* L., Canadian golden-rod (Asteraceae) – the DAC 1986 permits both species.

Synonyms: Herba Solidaginis (Lat.), i.e. without differentiating the plant source, is also used for golden-rod herb (Virgaureae herba; q.v.), Herba Serotinae (Lat.), Riesengoldrutenkraut (Ger.).

Origin: Originally, native only in North America; now naturalized in Europe as a garden plant and as an escape in lowland forest and in woods along rivers; *S. canadensis* also occurs in waste places and on the banks of cuttings.
The drug comes mainly from the wild; the principal exporting countries are former Yugoslavia, Hungary, Poland, and Bulgaria.

Constituents: Flavonoids, among which kaempferol, rhamnetin, isorhamnetin, quercetin and their 3-*O*-rutinosides [1], isoquercitrin, astragalin, afzetin (= kaempferol 3-rhamnoside). Saponins: the principal components of the bisdesmoside mixture from *S. gigantea*, the gigantea saponins 1–4, have the aglycone bayogenin coupled with up to 10 sugars (which include D-apiose, D-chinovose (6-desoxyglucose), D-xylose, D-galactose, D-glucose, L-rhamnose, and arabinose), the principal chain being doubly branched. The main bisdesmosides isolated from *S. canadensis*, the canadensis saponins 1–8, have closely related structures – bayogenin is again the aglycone and it is coupled with up to nine sugars [2, 3, 19]. The saponin complex in the two species is thus very similar [4], but differs from that of Virgaureae herba (golden-rod herb) which contains saponins based on the aglycone polygalacic acid [5]; moreover, their content of both saponin and flavonoid is higher [6, 7]. Diterpenes: in *S. canadensis* one diterpene acid and three diterpenes of the labdane type [8]; in *S. gigantea*, the diterpene butenolides 6-desoxy-solidago-lactone IV-18,19-olide and its 2β-hydroxyl derivative (clerodane type), which have not been found in *S. canadensis* and *S. virgaurea* [9]. Essential oil: *S. canadensis*, flowers 1.7%, leaves 0.9%, stems 0.2%, comprising 85% hydrocarbons and 15% oxygenated compounds [10], which include caryophyllene oxide [8], cyclocolorenone, *ar*-curcumene, γ-salinene, β-caryophyllene; *S. gigantea*, among the components germacrene D, α-pinene, limonene,

bornyl acetate [11]. Phenol-carboxylic acids: chlorogenic, hydroxycinnamic, and caffeic acids and their glucose esters; tannins. Polysaccharides: a β-1,2-fructosan with a chain length of 12–20 units, as well as a mixture of acidic polysaccharides with an identical sugar composition: 23.5% uronic acids, 25% D-galactose, 21.5% L-rhamnose, 15% L-arabinose, 5% D-xylose, 4% L-fucose, and 2% D-mannose [12]. The phenolic glycosides leiocarposide and virgaureoside A, which are present in golden-rod (q.v.), have not been detected in early golden-rod [13].

Indications: Like Virgaureae herba (q.v.), the drug is used to increase the amount of urine in cases of kidney and bladder inflammation, the flavonoids and saponins being presumed to be the active substances. Early golden-rod was first considered an adulterant, but has now found its way into therapeutic use as a substitute for genuine golden-rod, favoured by its higher saponin and flavonoid content. Nevertheless, the two drugs differ in their spectrum of activity. The diuretic and antiphlogistic leiocarposide is absent from early golden-rod [13] and likewise the antifungal ester saponins of polygalacic acid, the saponins of early golden-rod being found in the same test to be inactive [14]. A more precise demonstration of the action of the drug derived from early golden-rod is therefore desirable. The different findings in animal experiments regarding the diuretic activity of golden-rod, reported as being weak and also as being strong, may have arisen from the use of different drugs – golden-rod or early golden-rod.
Saponin-free extracts from early golden-rod after i.v. administration (100–300 mg/kg) in dogs had a hypotensive effect [15]. The water-soluble polysaccharides on i.p. administration had antitumour activity in the sarcoma 180 cell-strain assay [12].

Making the tea: Boiling water is poured over 1–2 teaspoonfuls of the finely chopped drug, allowed to draw for 10–15 min., and then strained. Maceration with cold water, then boiling briefly and passing while still warm through a tea strainer, is also recommended. As diuretic, a cupful is drunk three to five times a day.
1 Teaspoon = ca. 1.2 g.

Phytomedicines: It may be assumed that many of the phytomedicines mentioned under golden-rod also contain extracts from early golden-rod.

Authentication: Macro- (see: Description) and microscopically, following the DAC 1986. Leaf fragments have shining secretory

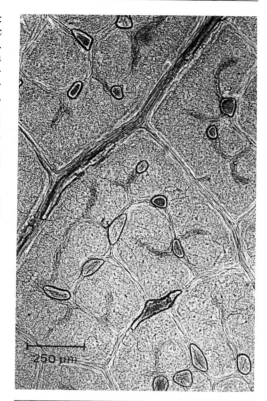

Fig. 3: Secretory glands in the mesophyll of *Solidago gigantea*

glands (Fig. 3), ca. 30–50 µm wide and 40–80 µm long (*S. gigantea*), and the lamina is densely clothed with uniseriate covering trichomes having terminal cells with oblique end walls and secretory glands in the mesophyll (*S. canadensis*). The margin at the tip of the involucral bracts has trichomes with up to 5(-6) cells and whip-like trichomes with a somewhat thicker terminal cell (*S. canadensis*) or only very occasionally distinctly polygonal and a few 2–3-celled trichomes and scarce flagellate trichomes with a thinner terminal cell (*S. gigantea*); the tubular florets have long, slender (8–10 µm wide) papillae on the style and paired trichomes on the ovary which are less than 100 µm long (*S. canadensis*) or with broad (14–19 µm wide) papillae on the style and paired trichomes on the ovary which are up to 200 µm long (Figs. 4 and 5) with distinctly sinuate or striated cuticle (*S. gigantea*). In *S. virgaurea*, the middle wall of the paired trichomes is strongly pitted. For the microscopical differentiation of the three *Solidago* species, see [16, 17].

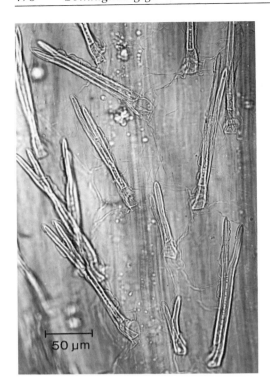

50 µm

Fig. 4: Paired trichomes from the ovary

Solvent system: ethyl acetate + anhydrous formic acid + water (88 + 6 + 6), 6 cm run.

Detection: after complete evaporation of the solvent in a current of hot air, sprayed with 1% methanolic diphenylboryloxyethylamine and then with 5% ethanolic polyethylene glycol 400.

Evaluation: in UV 365 nm light, ca. 30 min. after spraying. <u>Reference solution</u>: zones with the following approximate Rf values and fluorescence colours: rutin ca. 0.25, orange; hyperoside ca. 0.50, yellowish orange; quercitrin ca. 0.70, yellowish orange; caffeic acid ca. 0.90, blue. <u>Test solution</u>: corresponding zones; also, a blue fluorescent zone with an Rf value between those of hyperoside and quercitrin; above the quercitrin zone, two blue fluorescent zones. If *Solidago virgaurea* is present, the main zone – quercitrin – is absent (Fig. 6). See also the data in [18].

Quantitative standards: <u>St. Zul. 1639.99.99</u>: *Flavonoids* (*S. gigantea*), not less than 6.0% calculated as rutin. *Foreign matter*, not more than 1%; not more than occasional fragments of densely tomentose stem or leaf. *Loss on drying*, not more than 8.0%. *Ash*, not more than 6.0%
<u>DAC 1986</u>: *Flavonoids*, not less than 1.5%.

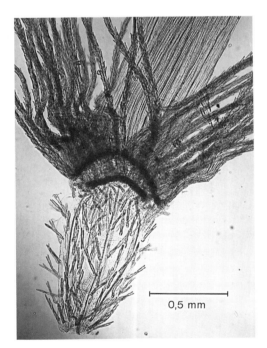

0,5 mm

Fig. 5: Ovary, showing the paired trichomes and pappus

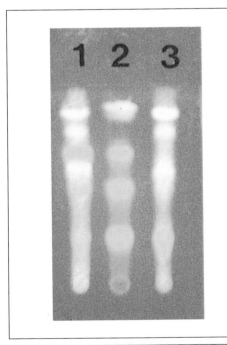

Fig. 6: TLC on 4 × 8 cm foil

1: Early golden-rod
2: Reference compounds
3: Golden-rod

For details, see the text

The following TLC method is a suitable identification test:

Test solution: 1.0 g powdered drug refluxed for 2 min. with 5 ml methanol and, after cooling, filtered.

Reference solution: 10 mg rutin and 5 mg each of hyperoside, quercitrin, and caffeic acid dissolved in 10 ml methanol.

Loadings: 2 µl test solution and 1 µl reference solution, as bands on silica gel.

Adulteration: Not uncommon. In commerce, some drugs are found which are a mixture of golden-rod and early golden-rod. Such adulteration or confusion can be established with certainty by microscopical examination. See: Authentication; see also, Virgaureae herba: Authentication. The important diagnostic features allowing differentiation are the trichomes of the leaves, the trichomes of the petals (which occur only in *Solidago virgaurea*), the paired trichomes on the ovary, and the size of the pollen [16, 17].

Literature:
[1] V.S. Batyuk and S.N. Kovalera, Khim. Prir. Soedin. **1985**, 566; C.A. **104**, 165306 (1985).
[2] G. Reznicek et al., Phytochemistry **30**, 1629 (1991).
[3] K. Hiller, G. Bader, G. Reznicek, J. Jurenitsch, and W. Kubelka, Pharmazie **46**, 405 (1991).
[4] J. Jurenitsch et al., Planta Med. **52**, 236 (1986).
[5] K. Hiller and R. Gil-Rjong, Acta Horticult. **96**(II), 91 (1980).
[6] L. Fuchs and V. Iliev, Sci. Pharm. **17**, 128 (1949).
[7] H. Schilcher, Dtsch. Apoth. Ztg. **105**, 681 (1965).
[8] F. Bohlmann et al., Phytochemistry **19**, 2655 (1980).
[9] J. Jurenitsch et al., Phytochemistry **27**, 626 (1988).
[10] S.H. Shin, Saengyak Hakhoe Chi **12**, 215 (1981); C.A. **96**, 222998 (1981).
[11] S. Fujita, Koen Yoshishu-Koryu **1979**, 203; C.A. **92**, 143284 (1979).
[12] J. Kraus, M. Martin, and G. Franz, Dtsch. Apoth. Ztg. **126**, 2045 (1986).
[13] K. Hiller and G. Fötsch, Pharmazie **41**, 415 (1986).
[14] G. Bader et al., Pharmazie **42**, 140 (1987).
[15] G. Racz, E. Racz-Kotilla, and J. Jozsa, Planta Med. **36**, 259 (1979).
[16] H. Schilcher and U. Bornschein, Dtsch. Apoth. Ztg. **126**, 1377 (1986).
[17] J. Saukel et al., Österr. Apoth. Ztg. **40**, 560 (1986).
[18] P. Rohdewald, G. Rücker, and K.-W. Glombitza, Apothekengerechte Prüfvorschriften, Deutscher Apotheker Verlag, Stuttgart, 1986, p. 725.
[19] G. Reznicek et al., Planta Med. **58**, 94 (1992).

Spiraeae flos   Meadowsweet (BHP 1/1990)

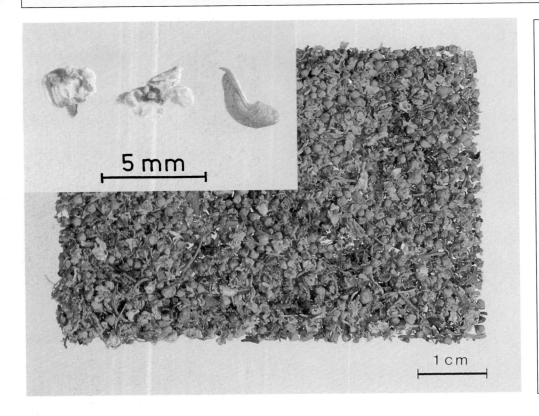

5 mm

1 cm

Fig. 1: Meadowsweet

Description: The yellowish white flowers are up to 5 mm (rarely up to 8 mm) broad. The somewhat sunken, urceolate receptacle has five small, triangular, hairy bracts, which mostly point downwards. The five petals, ca. 2–3 mm long, are obovate, abruptly mucronate, and not fused; the stamens are numerous, long, and with roundish anthers. There are 5–10 (rarely 12) small free carpels which are twisted together spirally.

In the drug, the easily shed petals predominate, along with numerous still closed flower buds (detailed illustrations: viewed from the side (left) view and from below (centre)) and occasional spiral fruits (detailed illustration (right)).

Odour: Faint, reminiscent of methyl salicylate.

Taste: Astringent and bitter.

Fig. 2: *Filipendula ulmaria* (L.) MAXIM.

A shrub found in wet localities and attaining a height of up to 2 m; many small, scented, yellowish white flowers arranged in panicles. Imparipinnate leaves with not more than five pairs of pinnae (difference from *Filipendula vulgaris*) and stipules at the leaf base.

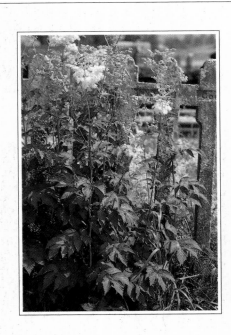

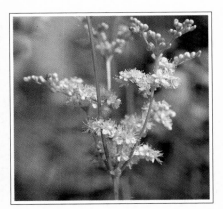

St.Zul. 1609.99.99 (Mädesüßblüten)

Plant source: *Filipendula ulmaria* (L.) MAXIM., meadowsweet Rosaceae).

Synonyms: Flores Ulmariae (Lat.), Filipendula, Meadowsweet flowers, Queen-of-the-meadow, Bridewort (Engl.), Mädesüßblüten, Spierblumen (Ger.), Fleur d'ulmaire (Fr.).

Origin: Native in Europe, but also occurring in North America. The drug is imported from both Bulgaria and former Yugoslavia.

Constituents: The drug contains ca. 0.5% flavonoids (though up to 6% total flavonoids is present in the fresh flowers), particularly spiraeoside (= quercetin 4′-glucoside) and other quercetin and kaempferol derivatives; HPLC studies show that the subsp. *ulmaria* and subsp. *denudata* (J. et C. PRESL) HAYEK have much the same flavonoid composition, with spiraeoside the main component in the flowers (and fruit) and hyperoside the principal one in the leaves and stalks [4]. The astringent taste is

Extract from the German Commission E monograph
(BAnz no. 43, dated 02. 03. 89)

Uses

In supportive treatment for chills, colds, etc.

Contraindications

None known.

Warning: Meadowsweet contains salicylates and should therefore not be used when salicylate idiosyncrasy is present.

Side effects

None known.

Interactions with other remedies

None known.

Dosage

Unless otherwise prescribed: daily dose, 2.5–3.5 g meadowsweet flowers or 4–5 g meadowsweet herb; preparations correspondingly.

Mode of administration

Chopped drug and other galenical preaprations for infusions. a cup of the infusion drunk as hot as possible several times a day.

due to the presence of hexahydroxydiphenic acid esters of glucose [1], i.e. substances related to tannins. The very small amount of essential oil in the drug is composed mainly of salicylaldehyde (ca. 75%) and phenylethyl alcohol (3%), benzyl alcohol (2%), anisaldehyde (2%), and methyl salicylate (1.5%) [2]. The odoriferous substances are present partly as glycosides [3], e.g. spiraein (salicylaldehyde primveroside).

Indications: Chiefly as a diaphoretic for colds, chills, etc., but particularly in *folk medicine* also as a diuretic. Meadowsweet is employed as well for treating rheumatism of the muscles and joints and against arthritis, but exclusively in *folk medicine*.

Making the tea: Boiling water is poured over 3–6 g of the chopped drug and after 10 min. passed through a tea strainer. A cupful is drunk several times a day.
1 Teaspoon = ca. 1.4 g.

Phytomedicines: Some mixed herbal teas as remedies for influenza, rheumatism, and kidney-bladder teas contain meadowsweet as a component. Extracts of meadowsweet are present in only a few prepared remedies. Among the UK multi-ingredient products containing meadowsweet or extracts of it are Potter's Acidosis (tablets) and Indigestion Mixture (liquid).

Authentication: Macro- (see: Description) and microscopically. The carpels and the outer epidermis of the sepals have numerous anomocytic stomata and unicellular, some-

Fig. 4: Fragment of a sepal, showing unicellular curved trichomes

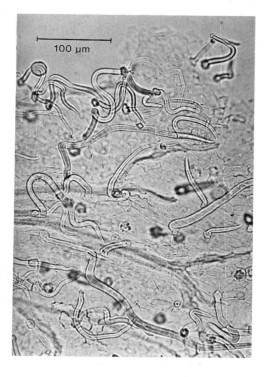

Fig. 5: Prismatic crystals, from the ovary

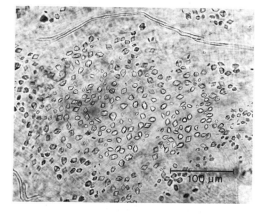

Fig. 6: Endothecium, showing stellate ridges of thickening

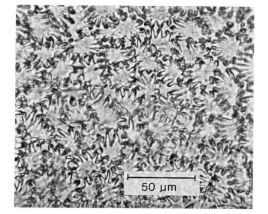

what curved, thick-walled, pointed trichomes which are 50–150 µm long (Fig. 4). In the mesophyll of the sepals there are many cluster crystals of calcium oxalate and in the ovaries prismatic crystals. The endothecium has stellate thickening (Fig. 6). The pollen grains are spherical and smooth, with three pores. See also the BHP 1/1990. A suitable TLC identification test is as follows:

Test solution: 1 g powdered drug refluxed for 10 min. with 10 ml methanol and then filtered warm.

Reference solution: 1 mg each of hyperoside, quercetin, rutoside, and isoquercitrin, each dissolved in 2 ml methanol.

Loadings: 5 µl test solution as a band and 1 µl hyperoside and rutin reference solutions on the same starting point and quercetin and isoquercitrin reference solutions on another starting point, on silica gel.

Solvent system: ethyl acetate + anhydrous formic acid + water (80 + 8 + 12), 6 cm run.

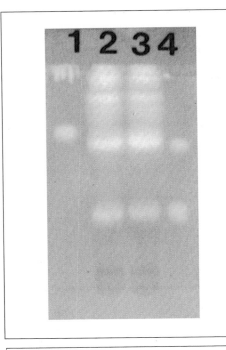

Fig. 7: TLC on 4 × 8 cm silica-gel foil

1: Isoquercitrin, quercetin
2 and 3: Meadowsweet (different origins)
4: Rutin, hyperoside

For details, see the text

Detection: after drying in a current of hot air, sprayed with 1% methanolic diphenylboryloxyethylamine and then 5% ethanolic polyethylene glycol 400; layer finally dried for a few min. in a current of warm air.

Evaluation: In UV 366 nm light. Reference solution: zones with the following approximate Rf values and fluorescence colours – rutin ca. 0.3, orange; hyperoside ca. 0.6, orange; isoquercitrin ca. 0.7, orange; quercetin ca. 0.95, yellow. Test solution: at these Rf values, a yellowish orange fluorescent band partly overlapped by green or blue fluorescent bands; directly below the rutin zone, a greenish blue fluorescent zone; at the same Rf value as isoquercitrin, an intense yellowish green fluorescent band; between the isoquercitrin and quercetin bands, a green, a blue, and two orange fluorescent bands (Fig. 7).

A method for obtaining a fingerprint chromatogram is described in the BHP 1/1990.

Quantitative standards: St.Zul. 1609.99.99: *Foreign matter*, not more than 2%; small, green, tangled, sickle-shaped fruits (from the drug plant) and flowers with a fused corolla and short filaments (elder flowers) must be absent. *Loss on drying*, not more than 10.0%. *Ash*, not more than 6.0%.

BHP 1/1990: *Water-soluble extractive*, not less than 12%. *Foreign matter*, not more than 2%. *Total ash*, not more than 8%. *HCl-insoluble ash*, not more than 2%.

Adulteration: Confusion with elder flowers (Sambuci flos, q.v.) is possible, but can be readily detected on examination with a hand lens, since elder flowers have five petals which are fused to each other. On microscopical examination, the presence of crystal sand, which is absent in meadowsweet, would be conspicuous (Sambuci flos, Fig. 4).

Storage: Kept dry and protected from light.

Literature:

[1] R.K. Gupta et al., J. Chem. Soc., Perkin Trans. **1982**, 2525.
[2] J.L. Piette and J. Lecomte, Bull. Soc. R. Sci. Liège **50**, 178 (1981); C.A. **96**, 141694 (1982).
[3] H. Thieme, Pharmazie **20**, 113 (1965).
[4] J.L. Lamaison, C. Petitjean-Freytet, and A. Carnat, Pharm. Acta Helv. **67**, 218 (1992).

Symphyti radix   Comfrey root (BHP 1/1990)

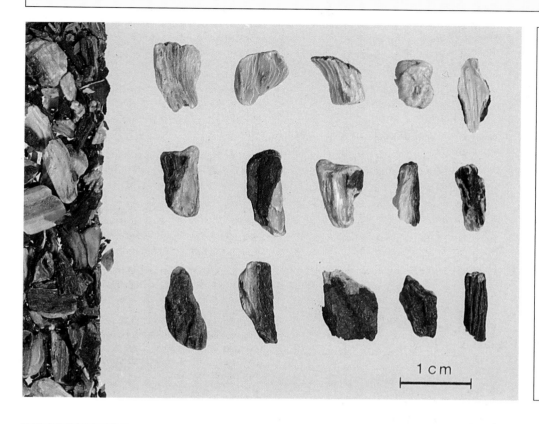

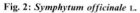
1 cm

Fig. 1: Comfrey root

<u>Description</u>: The dark brown to black pieces of root are longitudinally corrugated on the outside and they have a short fracture. The cross section shows a thin, pale-coloured cortex and a whitish to pale brown radiate xylem with broad medullary rays. With a hand lens, wide vessels, single or groups of 2–3, can be seen scattered in the rows of xylem parenchyma. Fragments of rhizome with pith may also be present.

<u>Taste</u>: Mucilaginous, somewhat sweetish and slightly astringent.

Fig. 2: *Symphytum officinale* L.

A bristly perennial herb, 50–150 cm in height; leaves long and narrowing at the ends, with a coarse reticulate venation. Yellowish white or violet-red campanulate corolla.

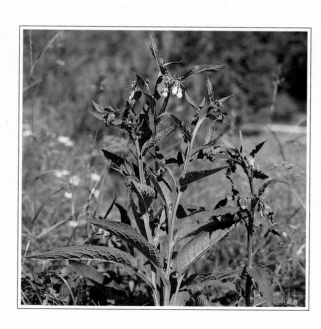

Plant source: *Symphytum officinale* L., common comfrey (Boraginaceae).

Synonyms: Consolidae radix (Lat.), Symphytum root (Engl.), Beinwellwurzel (Ger.), Racine de (grand) consoude (Fr.).

Origin: Native throughout almost the whole of Europe and in the east as far as Siberia; as an escape from cultivation, naturalized in North America. The drug comes from cultivated plants.
Other *Symphytum* species are cultivated for use as animal feed and green manure (*S. asperum* LEPECH., known as Russian, rough, or blue comfrey; *S. × uplandicum* NYMAN) and as a vegetable (*S. peregrinum* LEDEB.).
The drug is imported from Bulgaria, Poland, Romania, and Hungary. It is also obtained from the UK, northern Europe, and the USA.

Constituents: Ca. 0.6–0.8% allantoin; ca. 0.02–0.07% pyrrolizidine alkaloids: intermedine, acetylintermedine, lycopsamine, acetyllycopsamine, symphytine, and in materials from some sources also echimidine,

	R^1	R^2	R^3	R^4
Intermedine	OH	H	H	H
Acetylintermedine:	OH	H	Acetyl	H
Lycopsamine:	H	OH	H	H
Acetyllycopsamine:	H	OH	Acetyl	H
Symphytine:	H	OH	Tigloyl	H
Echimidine:	H	OH	Angeloyl	OH

all these also being partly present as *N*-oxides; ca. 4–6% tannins; abundant mucilage (fructans); starch; triterpenes (isobauerenol) and sterols (sitosterol); depsides of dehydrocaffeic acid (="lithospermic acid"); ca. 1–3% asparagine; amino acids (including γ-aminobutyric acid).

Indications: Externally in the form of poultices and pastes as an anti-inflammatory in damage to the periosteum, inflammation of the joints, arthritic swellings, for promoting callus formation in fractures, inflammation of the tendinous sheaths, arthritis, dislocations, contusions, haematomas, in thrombophlebitis, phlebitis, mastitis, parotitis, and glandular swellings, as well as for the treatment of poorly healing wounds and furuncles. Decoctions are given as a mouth rinse and gargle in periodontitis, pharyngitis, and angina (utilizing, among other things, emollient action of mucilage and astringent effect of the tannins). Internally, the drug is given for gastritis and stomach and intestinal ulcers (see: Side effects).
In *folk medicine,* the drug is used additionally against rheumatism, bronchitis, pleuritis, and as an antidiarrhoeic (tannin, mucilage). Allantoin is one of the active principles of the drug – it promotes granulation and tissue regeneration. A few reports on the anti-tumour effects of specially prepared extracts [1] or on the activity of these extracts in liver cirrhosis [2] are (at least at the present time) without relevance to the therapeutic uses of

Extract from the German Commission E monograph (BAnz no. 138, dated 27.07.90)

Uses

Externally: contusions, sprains, and dislocations.

Contraindications

None known.

Warning: The drug should only be applied to the intact skin; a doctor should be consulted before using it during pregnancy.

Side effects

None known.

Interactions with other remedies

None known.

Dosage

Unless otherwise prescribed: ointments or other preparations for external use containing 5–20% of the drug; preparations correspondingly.
The daily dose applied must not contain more than 100 μg pyrrolizidine alkaloids with a 1,2-unsaturated necine residue, including their *N*-oxides.

Mode of administration

Comminuted drug, extracts, freshly expressed plant juice for semi-solid preparations and poultices for external use.

Duration of use

Not longer than 4–6 weeks in a year.

Effects

Anti-inflammatory, promoting callus formation, antimitotic.

the drug and require confirmation through more extensive studies.
The rise in aminopyrine-*N*-demethylase acitvity [3] observed after feeding the drug to rats does not allow any conclusions to be drawn about the therapeutic suitability of the drug.
In rats, *Symphytum*-leaf extracts have been shown to have wound-healing and mild analgesic activity [4] and rosmarinic acid has been isolated as an active anti-inflammatory constituent [5].

Side effects: In *long-term studies*, it has been demonstrated in rats that the pyrrolizidine alkaloids present in the drug are hepatotoxic, carcinogenic, and mutagenic [6–8; there further literature; see also: Senecionis herba]. Acetylintermedine and acetyllycopsamine have proved to be mutagenic in somatic Drosophila cells at a concentration of 5×10^{-3}M [9]. The drug must therefore be recognized as a potentially genotoxic carcinogen in man. However, the genetic risk from the pyrrolizidine alkaloids as against their toxic potential appears to be of minor importance [10].

A normal cup of the tea may contain up to 8.3 mg alkaloid [11]. *Lengthy internal use is to be discouraged*, since possible damaging effects cannot then be excluded. Only slight absorption occurs on external use. After putting an alcoholic extract on rats, corresponding to a dose of 194 mg of an alkaloid/alkaloid *N*-oxide mixture per kg body weight, between 0.1 and 0.4% alkaloid was excreted in the urine, mainly as *N*-oxide. Oral administration for the same length of time led to a 20–50 times greater excretion in the urine [12].
For further discussion of the pyrrolizidine alkaloids present in comfrey and of their possible adverse effects, see [13–16].
A recent review on the toxicity of comfrey [16] concludes that: "[the] balance of benefit to risk is no longer acceptable for conditions such as catarrh; gastrointestinal disorders such as cholecystitis; rheumatic disorders such as arthritis and gout; and as an anti-haemorrhagic in conditions such as haematuria." See also [15].
Comfrey has now been banned in Australia and its use is restricted in New Zealand. In the UK, oral medicinal preparations containing comfrey have been withdrawn.

Making the tea: Boiling water is poured over 5–10 g of the finely chopped or coarsely powdered drug and after 10–15 min. passed through a tea strainer. A cupful is drunk two or three times a day, but not during a prolonged period (see: Side effects).
For external use, instead of a paste of the fresh roots as a poultice, a 1 : 10 decoction will serve.
1 Teaspoon = ca. 4 g.

Herbal teas: None. A paste of the roots for use as a poultice is available commercially under various brand names (see also: Phytomedicines).

Phytomedicines: Comfrey root or extracts prepared from it are present especially in various prepared analgesics and anti-rheumatics (10) and antiphlogistics (3), and also in an antitussive and expectorant (1), skin remedy (1), antiphlebitis remedy (1), and circulation-stimulating remedy (1), and alterative (1). The Kytta specialities are well-known preparations, particularly Kytta-Plasma®-Umschlagpaste (poultice paste) and Kytta-Salbe® (ointment).
Potter's Comfrey Ointment is a UK product containing an extract of comfrey root.
Note: The BHP 1983 also has a monograph on Symphytum leaf which includes indications that are much the same as those listed for Symphytum root, with the addition of antirheumatic and anti-inflammatory applications. The leaf is reported to have a lower

content of pyrrolizidine alkaloids than the root [14, 15]. Nevertheless, its indiscriminate use as a health food remains a matter for concern. A high level of consumption as a salad is five or six leaves a day and at ca. 1 mg alkaloid/leaf could mean an intake of up to ca. 0.1 mg/kg body weight for an adult – a level which is within the toxic range for causing liver disease [16].

Authentication: Macro- and microscopically according to the DAC 1986. See also the BHP 1/1990.
The DAC 1986 also has the following TLC method for detecting allantoin:

Test solution: 1.0 g powdered drug refluxed with 25 ml 70% aqueous ethanol and, after cooling, filtered.

Reference solution: 25 mg allantoin in 25% 70% aqueous ethanol.

Loadings: 10 µl each of the test and reference solutions, on silica gel.

Solvent system: methanol, 10 cm run.

Detection: after evaporation of the solvent, sprayed with 4-dimethylaminobenzaldehyde solution (1 g in 20 ml conc. hydrochloric acid, diluted to 100 ml with ethanol), followed by blowing hot air (hair drier) over the plate.

Evaluation: Reference and Test solutions: yellow allantoin spot in the upper third of the chromatogram.
About the TLC quantitative estimation of the total content of retronecine-type alkaloids, including the more polar N-oxides, in Symphytum tincture, see [17].

Quantitative standards: DAC 1986: *Swelling index*, not less than 8 (the presence of roots from other cultivated *Symphytum* species cannot be excluded in this way).
BHP 1/1990: *Water-soluble extractive*, not less than 45%. *Loss on drying*, not more than 12%. *Foreign matter*, not more than 2%. *Total ash*, not more than 10%. *HCl-insoluble ash*, not more than 4%.

Adulteration: Rarely occurs. However, in Canada, it appears that many products on the market, labelled simply "comfrey" or "common comfrey", contain echimidine (considered to be the most toxic of the comfrey pyrrolizidine alkaloids) and must therefore have come from *S. asperum* or *S. × uplandicum* [15]. Proper identification of the *Symphytum* species used in herbal drugs is thus seen to be extremely important, and often in the published literature it is not possible to say which species is being discussed.

Literature:
[1] K. Hirosaki, Japan. Patent 78, 88312, dated 03. 08. 1978; C.A. **89**, 186068 (1978).
[2] K. Hirosaki, Japan. Patent 78, 127811, dated 08. 11. 1978; C.A. **90**, 76557 (1979).
[3] J.B. Garret et al., Toxicol. Lett. **10**, 183 (1982).
[4] R.S. Goldman, P.C. D. de Freitas, and S. Oga, Fitoterapia **56**, 323 (1985).
[5] L. Gracza, H. Koch, and E. Löffler, Arch. Pharm. (Weinheim) **318**, 1090 (1985).
[6] E. Röder, Dtsch. Apoth. Ztg. **122**, 2081 (1982).
[7] P. Stengel, H. Wiedenfeld, and E. Röder, Dtsch. Apoth. Ztg. **122**, 851 (1982).
[8] R. Schoental, Toxicol. Lett. **10**, 323 (1982).
[9] U. Graf et al., Mutat. Res. **120**, 233 (1983).
[10] O. Schimmer, Dtsch. Apoth. Ztg. **123**, 1361 (1983).
[11] J.N. Roitman, Lancet **1** (no. 8226), 944 (1981); C.A. **95**, 92071 (1981).
[12] J. Brauchli, J. Lüthy, U. Zweifel, and C. Schlatter, Experientia **38**, 1085 (1982).
[13] P.F. D'Arcy, Adverse Drug React. Toxicol. Rev. **10**, 189 (1991).
[14] J. Westendorf, in P.A.G.M. de Smet, K. Keller, R. Hänsel, and R.F. Chandler, Adverse effects of herbal drugs, vol. 1, Springer, Berlin, Heidelberg, New York, 1992, pp. 219, 262.
[15] D.V.C. Awang, Herbal Gram no. **25**, p. 20 (1991).
[16] K.A. Winship, Adverse Drug React. Toxicol. Rev. **10**, 47 (1991).
[17] U. Zweifel and J. Lüthy, Pharm. Acta Helv. **65**, 165 (1990).

Taraxaci radix cum herba

Dandelion root (BHP 1/1990), Dandelion herb (BHP 1/1990), Dandelion root and herb

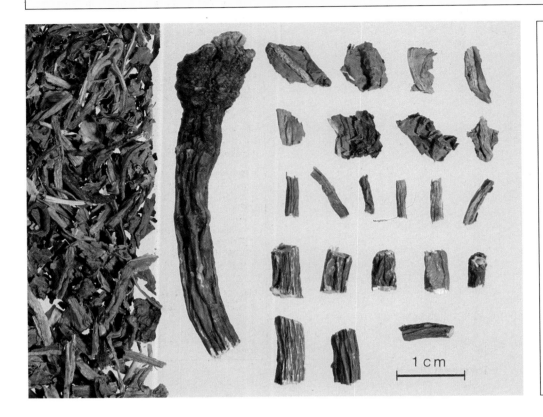

Fig. 1: Dandelion root and herb

Description: The drug consists of the dried, entire dandelion plant, harvested before the flowering period. The dark brown to blackish pieces of root have coarse longitudinal wrinkles on the outside. In transverse section, there are several concentric zones with tangentially connected brown laticifers in the broad greyish white to brownish cortex (Fig. 3). The darker cambial zone surrounds a lemon-yellow porous, but not radiate xylem, which in some fragments may also be fissured. The fracture is cartilaginous and short, not fibrous. There are also leaf fragments, which may be glabrous or villous and often with a violet-coloured midrib, reddish violet petiole fragments, unripe inflorescences, and only occasional yellow ligulate flowers with a white pappus.

Odour: Faint and characteristic.

Taste: Somewhat bitter.

Fig. 2: *Taraxacum officinale* WEBER

A cosmopolitan in meadows and along roadsides with a stout taproot and runcinate, basal leaves. The flowering heads consisting only of ligulate flowers, the white pappus enabling the achenes to float in the air. Latex present throughout the plant.

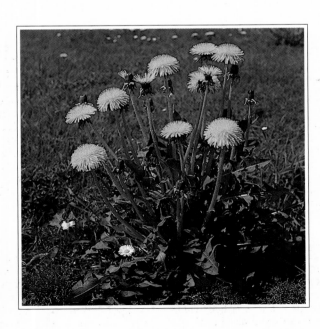

DAC 1986: Löwenzahn
ÖAB: Radix Taraxaci
St. Zul. 1139.99.99

Plant source: *Taraxacum officinale* WEBER, dandelion (Asteraceae).

Synonyms: Radix et Folia Dentis leonis, Taraxaci folium (Lat.), Taraxacum leaf and Taraxacum root. (Engl.), Löwenzahnkraut, Löwenzahnwurzel (Ger.), Racine et herbe de dent de lion, Racine et herbe de pissenlit (Fr.).

Origin: Native throughout the northern hemisphere, with many varieties and microspecies; introduced into South America. The drug is collected from both wild and cultivated plants. The main suppliers are Bulgaria, former Yugoslavia, Romania, Hungary, and Poland; it is also obtained in the UK.

Constituents: The bitter substances called taraxacin in the older literature have now been identified [1–3]. They are eudesmanolides which have not been found anywhere

Tetrahydroridentin B

Taraxacolide β-D-glucoside

Taraxinic acid β-D-glucoside

Taraxacoside

Taraxasterol: R = H
Arnidiol   R = OH

ψ-Taraxasterol R = H
Faradiol   R = OH

else: tetrahydroridentin B and taraxacolide β-D-glucopyranoside, and the likewise new germacranolides: taraxic β-D-glucopyranoside and 11,13-dihydrotaraxic acid β-D-glucopyranoside, as well as the *p*-hydroxyphenylacetic acid derivative taraxacoside [3]. The supposed lactucapicrin has not been found. Triterpenes: taraxasterol (= α-lactucerol), ψ-taraxasterol (= isolactucerol), their acetates and their 16-hydroxyl derivatives (arnidiol and faradiol), β-amyrin. Sterols: sitosterol, stigmasterol; carotenoids: xanthophylls; flavonoids: apigenin and luteolin 7-glucosides; caffeic acid; carbohydrates (root): ca. 1.1% mucilage. In spring, ca. 18% sugar (fructose), ca. 2% inulin, rising to as much as 40% in the autumn. Also worth mentioning is the high potassium content (in the herb up to 4.5%).

Indications: As a mild choleretic, diuretic, appetite-stimulating bitter, and as an adjuvant in liver and gall-bladder disorders, and digestive complaints, especially the incomplete digestion of fat.

In *folk medicine*, the drug is considered to be a "blood purifier" and is employed as a mild laxative, for treating arthritic and rheumatic complaints, as well as eczema and other skin conditions. Besides the tea, the pressed sap from the fresh plant is used. In spring, the freshly gathered leaves are much appreciated as a salad (so-called "spring cure"), particularly in the Latin countries. The roots harvested in the autumn (when rich in inulin) are roasted and used as a substitute for coffee.

Indications of the cholagogic and diuretic actions of the drug are to be found in older animal [4–7] and clinical [7, 8] studies. Fluid extracts have recently been shown to have a diuretic and saluretic action in the rat [10]. Their effect was equal to that of furosemide tested at the same time and stronger than that of other plant diuretics (including Equiseti herba, Juniperi fructus). After daily administration of the fluid extract, rats and mice exhibited a weight loss of ca. 30%, in parallel with the diuresis; toxic effects were not observed. Although so far no pharmacological studies have been carried out with the isolated sesquiterpene lactones, according to available knowledge about the actions of this kind of bitter substance (see: Arnicae flos), they are likely to be the main active constituents of the drug. The unusually high potassium content may also play a part in the diuretic effect [10].

There is a more recent Commission E monograph on *Taraxaci herba* (Löwenzahnkraut).

Side effects: Nothing is known about any side effects on therapeutic use. Frequent contact with dandelions, especially the latex, may occasionally give rise to contact dermatitis [11], perhaps due to taraxic acid glucoside with its α-methylene-γ-lactone structure.

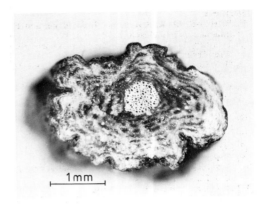

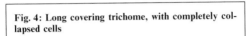
Fig. 3: Fragment of a root, showing the whitish cortex with numerous concentric brownish zones (laticifers)

1mm

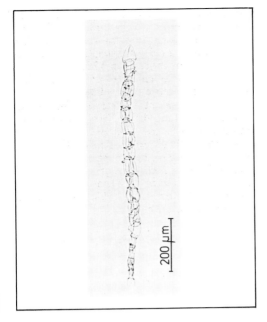

200 μm

Making the tea: 1–3 g of the finely chopped drug is put into cold water, boiled for a short time, and after 10 min. passed through a tea strainer.
1 Teaspoon = ca. 1.2 g.

Fig. 4: Long covering trichome, with completely collapsed cells

Phytomedicines: The drug is present in about 50 prepared cholagogues and biliary remedies, e.g., Aristochol®, Galleb® (drops), Hepagallin®, Neurochol® (dragees), etc., also in urological remedies, gastrointestinal remedies, laxatives, roborants and tonics, etc.
Dandelion root/leaf or extracts are included in a range of UK products, e.g. Gerard House Herbal Powder No. 8, Waterlax Tablets, Golden Seal Compound Tablets; Potter's Boldo Aid to Slimming (tablets), Out of Sorts Tablets, Stomach Mixture (liquid); Seven Seas Laxative Tablets; etc.

Regulatory status (UK): Root, General Sales List – Schedule 1, Table A.

Authentication: Macro- and microscopically, following the DAC 1986, where there is a detailed description of the anatomical characters. See also the BHP 1/1990 and [12]. Particularly diagnostic are the long, mostly collapsed, thin-walled covering trichomes of the leaves (Fig. 4).
Histochemical detection of the inulin (placed in 20% ethanolic 1-naphtholsulphuric acid, on adding one drop of 96% sulphuric acid, the inulin dissolves with a deep violet colour) and mucilage (placed in Indian ink, the mucilage forms bright haloes; in 0.15% methylene blue, the mucilage forms violet-blue globules) can be carried out.
The DAC 1986 also has a method for the TLC examination of the methanol extract of the drug; however, the conclusions to be drawn from the procedure set out are questionable and details of the method are not given here.

Extract from the German Commission E monograph (BAnz no. 162, dated 29.08.92)

Clinical information

Uses
Lack of appetite, dyspeptic complaints such as a feeling of distension and flatulence.

Contraindications
Obstruction of the biliary tract, empyema of the gall bladder; ileus; when gallstones are present, only after consultation with a physician.
After contact with the latex, contact allergies, brought about by sesquiterpene lactones, have been noted. Investigations and observations concerning preparations of the drug are not available.

Side effects
None known.

Special precautions for use
None known.

Use during pregnancy and lactation
None known.

Interactions with other remedies
None known.

Dosage
Unless otherwise prescribed: 3× daily, 4–10 g drug; 3× daily, 4–10 g liquid extract 1:1 in 25% alcohol.

Mode of administration
Comminuted drug for infusions and liquid formulations for internal use.

Duration of use
Not limited.

Overdosage
None known.

Special warnings
None known.

Effects on drivers and the use of machines
None known.

Wording of the package insert, from the German Standard Licence:

6.1 Uses
Biliary disorders, gastrointestinal complaints such as a feeling of distension and flatulence, and digestive complaints; to stimulate diuresis.

6.2 Contraindications
Inflammation or obstruction of the bile duct; intestinal obstruction.

6.3 Dosage and Mode of administration
Ca. 1–2 teaspoonfuls of **Dandelion root and herb** are boiled for a short time with water (ca. 150 ml) and after ca. 15 min. passed through a tea strainer.
Unless otherwise prescribed, a cup of the freshly prepared infusion is drunk morning and evening.

Duration of use
Dandelion preparations may be used for periods of up to 4–6 weeks.

Note
Store protected from light and moisture.

Quantitative standards: <u>DAC 1986</u>: *Water-soluble extractive*, not less than 30.0%. *Foreign matter*, not more than 2%; see also: Adulteration. *Loss on drying*, not more than 11%. *Ash*, not more than 17%.
<u>ÖAB</u>: *Bitterness value (root)*, not less than 100. *Ash*, not more than 9.0%.
<u>BHP 1/1990</u>: Root – *Water-soluble extractive*, not less than 40%. *Foreign matter*, not more than 1%. *Loss on drying*, not more than 15%. *Total ash*, not more than 12%. *HCl-insoluble ash*, not more than 3.5%.
Leaf – *Water-soluble extractive*, not less than 20%. *Foreign matter*, not more than 2%. *Total ash*, not more than 15%. *HCl-insoluble ash*, not more than 4%.

Note: There are ESCOP proposals for European harmonized monographs on Taraxaci folium and Taraxaci radix.

Adulteration: In practice, very rare. Admixture with *Leontodon* species, especially *L. autumnalis* L., autumn hawkbit, recognizable from the flower buds which have a sessile pappus consisting of feathery (branched) hairs. On rare occasions, the root drug may be adulterated with the roots of *Cichorium intybus* L., wild chicory, the transverse section of which shows only a narrow cortex and a wide, and owing to the presence of broad medullary rays, distinctly radiate xylem.

Literature:
[1] R. Hänsel, M. Kartarahardia, J.-T. Huang, and F. Bohlmann, Phytochemistry **19**, 857 (1980).
[2] T. Kuusi, H. Pyysalo, and K. Autio, Lebensmit.-Wiss. Technol. **18**, 347 (1985).
[3] H.W. Rauwald and J.-T. Huang, Phytochemistry **24**, 1557 (1985).
[4] J. Büssemaker, Arch. Exp. Pathol. Pharmakol. **181**, 512 (1936).
[5] J. Büssemaker, Pharm. Ztg. **82**, 851 (1937).
[6] M.R. Bonsmann, Arch. Exp. Pathol. Pharmakol. **199**, 376 (1942).
[7] K. Böhm, Arzneimit.-Forsch. **9**, 376 (1959).
[8] Merck's Jahresbericht **46**, 87, 138 (1932).
[9] W. Ripperger, Med. Welt **41**, 1467 (1935).
[10] E. Rácz-Kotilla, G. Rácz, and A. Solomon, Planta Med. **26**, 212 (1974).
[11] D. Janke, Hautarzt **1**, 177 (1950).
[12] B. P. Jackson and D. W. Snowdon, Atlas of microscopy of medicinal plants, culinary herbs and spices, Belhaven Press, London, 1990, p. 84.

Theae nigrae folium   Black tea

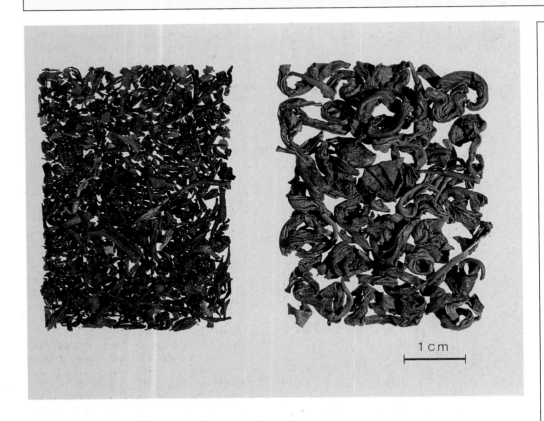

1 cm

Fig. 1: Black and (green) tea

In the production of green tea, the young leaves of the tea bush are first brought to well-ventilated chambers and allowed to "wither" (wilt). The leaves, which thus become pliable and flaccid, are rolled (or nowadays often distorted in other ways), which causes some of the cell sap to exude and the leaf structure to be partly broken down. During the "fermentation", which is the next stage, the polyphenols are converted into phlobaphenes and, at the same time, substances responsible for the aroma are formed. The leaves are then "fired" (dried) by means of hot air, sorted, and packed. In the case of green tea, the fermentation is omitted; after being harvested, the leaves are treated with steam (under pressure), thus inactivating the enzymes, and subsequently dried.

<u>Description:</u> Black tea (Fig. 1, left) consists of reddish brown to almost black, much shrivelled leaf fragments, the original shape of which can only be determined after boiling them up with water. The better qualities consist of the leaf buds and are finely pubescent on the lower surface (hand lens). The margin is finely serrate and the tip of each tooth has a small glandular trichome.
Green tea (Fig. 1, right) consists of greenish yellow to brownish green leaf fragments, the structure of which can be more readily observed.

<u>Odour:</u> Black tea faintly aromatic; green tea practically no smell.

<u>Taste:</u> Astringent, bitter.

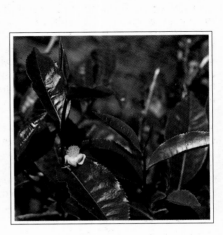

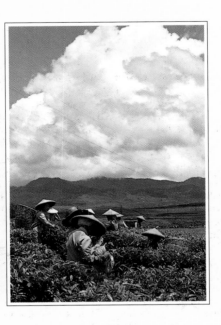

Fig. 2: *Camellia sinensis* (L.) KUNTZE

Oblong-ovate, dark green, shiny leaves, with a distinctly serrate margin. Scented flowers, up to 3 cm in diameter, with 5–6 white petals and numerous yellow stamens, appearing singly.

Fig. 3: *Camellia sinensis* (L.) KUNTZE

In cultivation, the up to 15 m high shrub is kept low as a much branched bush; only the young shoots are more or less densely pubescent. These are picked by hand and give the best quality tea.

Plant source: *Camellia sinensis* (L.) KUNTZE (syn. *Thea sinensis* L.), tea (Theaceae).

Synonyms: Schwarzer Tee, Russischer Tee, Chinesischer Tee (Ger.), Théier (Fr.).

Tea is marketed in many different grades under a great variety of names which give some idea of the origin or quality of the product. It may be classified according to the country of origin (China, Ceylon, Indonesian, Rwandan, etc.) or the district of origin (Darjeeling, Assam, Enshu, Dimbula, etc.) or the grade or size of the processed leaf (flowery pekoe (FP), pekoe (P), souchong (S), broken orange pekoe (BOP), etc.) or by manufacturing process ("fermented" (black), "unfermented" (green), and "semi-fermented" (oolong or pouchong)).

Origin: The original home of the tea plant is believed to be western Yunnan (sinensis group) and the warmer parts of Assam, Burma to Vietnam and southern China (assamica group). Long cultivated in China, it has been cultivated on a large scale in Indonesia since the 18th century and in India and Sri Lanka since the 19th century; it has also also been planted in the higher regions (500–2000 m) of other countries with a mild climate and high rainfall. The drug is imported from the countries mentioned and also from other tropical or subtropical regions where it is grown.

Constituents: 1. Methylxanthines: caffeine (theine), up to 4%, together with smaller amounts of theobromine and theophylline (the data in the literature vary considerably), as well as traces of adenine and xanthine; the methylxanthines are partly combined with tannins. Caffeine is biosynthesized in the young leaves during the early develop-

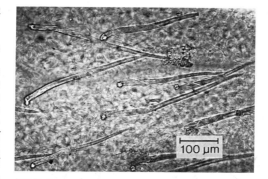

Fig. 4: Unicellular, thick-walled trichomes

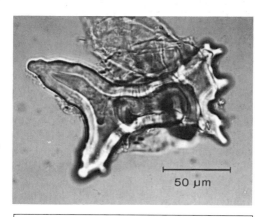

Fig. 5: Irregular and branched idioblast from the tea leaf

Theophylline: $R^1 = CH_3$, $R^2 = CH_3$, $R^3 = H$
Theobromine: $R^1 = H$, $R^2 = CH_3$, $R^3 = CH_3$
Caffeine: $R^1 = CH_3$, $R^2 = CH_3$, $R^3 = CH_3$

Theanine

ment of the shoot, the limiting factor being the induction and repression of various methyltransferases [9].

2. Polyphenols, especially tannins: mainly catechol tannins, depending on the cultivar and the age of the leaf between 10 and 20%; many individual components have been isolated, e.g. (−)-epicatechol, 4-gallocatechol, and other catechol gallates; flavan-3-ols and flavan-3,4-diols, as well as dimeric theaflavins and oligomeric procyanidins (thearubigenins), phenolic carboxylic acids such as gallic and chlorogenic acids, etc.

3. The flavour and aroma substances form a complex mixture in which the components may be present in both free and glycosidically-bound forms. The latter represent a variable but large proportion of the total, depending on the variety of tea; some of these components arise during the withering and fermentation stages and it implies that glycosylating enzymes are then still functional. Among the flavour substances present in combined form are such alcohols as hex-3-en-1-ol, benzyl alcohol, and 2-phenylethanol, as well as linalool in black tea and geraniol in green tea [10]. In the "essential oil", there are mainly monoterpene aldehydes and alcohols; more than 300 compounds have been detected by GC. Theanine, the 5-ethylamide of glutamic acid, is a characteristic component of the amino-acid spectrum of tea; it can also be used in assessing the quality [6].

4. Other constituents: abundant flavonoids (see also above), including the apigenin derivatives isoschaftoside and vicenin-3 [11]; triterpenoid saponins; hydroperoxide lyases (anti-oxidant enzymes, and potent inhibitors of lipoxygenase) [12]. The accumulation of aluminium in tea leaves and the sometimes high content of fluorine compounds in older leaves are worth noting [4].

Indications: Owing to its caffeine content, tea serves as a stimulant and because of its tannin content it can be used as an antidiarrhoeic. According to Højgaard ([5], cited from [2]), the constipating action is to be ascribed to the theophylline, which is supposed to lead to an increased absorption of fluid from the lumen of the intestine (as a result of the diuretic effect and hence resulting in extra-cellular dehydration?).

While an infusion of black tea can certainly be looked upon as a medicinally active preparation, the current legal situation is that tea, particularly scented tea, is a beverage and not a pharmaceutical product; its availability – in contrast to that of maté tea – in the German pharmacy is therefore not permitted [7, 8].

Making the tea: Boiling water is poured over a teaspoonful of tea and, depending on the purpose, covered and allowed to draw for 2–10 min. and then strained. As a stimulant, the tea should only be allowed to draw for 2 min. and several cups a day should be drunk. As an antidiarrhoeic, in supportive treatment of diarrhoea, it should be allowed to draw for 10 min. and a cup drunk 2–3 times a day.

The stimulant action is at its strongest in tea which has been allowed to brew for only a short time, since caffeine quickly dissolves in hot water. With a longer extraction (infusion) time, there is an increase in the tannins going into solution, the stimulant effect decreases (binding of the caffeine by the tannins, delaying the effect), and the antidiarrhoeic action is enhanced.

1 Teaspoon = ca. 2.5 g.

Herbal preparations: Tea bags usually contain between 1.8 and 2.2. g tea. Instant teas – tea extracts (Nestea) – are also available. Black tea is also extolled, under various phantasy names, mainly by mail-order firms, as an "effective slimming agent". It is also a component of Kneipp® Schlankheits-Unterstützungs-Tee" (tea to aid slimming).

Warning: There appears to be a significant correlation between the incidence of oesophageal cancer and the excessive consumption of certain kinds of tea containing a high proportion of condensed tannins [13].

Phytomedicines: Extractum Theae is present in the carbohydrate- and mineral salt-containing antidiarrhoeic Oralpädon®-Tabletten.

Authentication: Assessing black tea as a beverage is based primarily on the sensory (organoleptic) examination. The quality decreases as the age of the leaves increases: the caffeine and tannin contents become lower. Microscopically, besides the unicellular, thick-walled appressed trichomes of the epidermis (Fig. 4), the characteristically branched idioblasts of the mesophyll (Fig. 5) are particularly diagnostic. In the young leaf, they are rare and inconspicuous, while in the older leaf they are common. As is often the case with leaves, the pubescence decreases with age. The presence of caffeine can be easily and simply established by microsublimation.

In most European countries, the quality of tea is determined as part of the regulations that apply to the food industry. The purines can also be examined by TLC [14].

Adulteration: In the older literature, there is information about a series of adulterants or tea substitutes, e.g. willow-herb leaf tea (*Epilobium* sp.), gromwell leaf tea (*Lithospermum officinale* L.), bilberry leaf tea (*Vaccinium myrtillus* L.), Caucasian bilberry leaf tea (*Vaccinium arctostaphylos* L.), fermented bramble leaves, etc., etc.; see [1] or [3]. Nowadays, little or no adulteration takes place.

Literature:

[1] G. Gassner, B. Hohmann and F. Deutschmann, Mikroskopische Untersuchung pflanzlicher Lebensmittel, 5th ed., G. Fischer, Stuttgart, 1989.
[2] R. Hänsel and H. Haas, Therapie mit Phytopharmaka, Springer, Berlin – Heidelberg – New York – Tokyo, 1983.
[3] Hager, vol. 3, p. 636 (1972).
[4] R. Hegnauer, Chemotaxonomie der Pflanzen, Birkhäuser, Basel – Stuttgart, 1973, vol. 6, p. 499.
[5] L. Højgaard et al., Brit. Med. J. **282**, 864 (1981).
[6] K. Neumann and A. Montag, Dtsch. Lebensmittel Rundschau **79**, 160 (1983).
[7] see: Pharm. Ztg. **129**, 575 (1984).
[8] see: Pharm. Ztg. **129**, 1766 (1984).
[9] N. Fujimori, T. Suzuki, and H. Asihara, Phytochemistry **30**, 2245 (1991).
[10] N. Fischer, G. Nitz, and F. Drawert, Z. Lebensm. Unters. Forsch. **185**, 195 (1987).
[11] A. Chaboud, J. Raynaud, and G. Dellanonica, Pharm. Acta Helv. **64**, 16 (1989).
[12] K. Matsui et al., Phytochemistry **30**, 2109 (1991).
[13] J.F. Morton, in: R.W. Hemingway and J.J. Karchesy (eds.), Chemistry and significance of condensed tannins, Plenum, New York, 1989, p. 403.
[14] H. Wagner, S. Bladt, and E.M. Zgainski, Plant drug analysis, Springer-Verlag, Berlin – Heidelberg – New York – Tokyo, 1984, p. 86.

Thymi herba   (DAB 10), Thyme, Thymus vulgaris (BHP 1983)

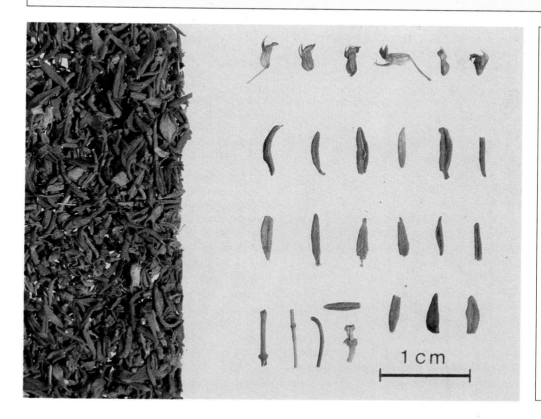

Description: The drug consists of the stripped and dried leaves and flowers. The leaves of *Thymus vulgaris* are lanceolate to ovate, with an entire and revolute margin. The upper surface is green and the lower surface is grey tomentose, with numerous glandular trichomes in depressions (Fig. 4). There are no ciliate trichomes at the base of the short petiole. Only the calices of the violet flowers are recognizable; these have a short pubescence and white bristles at the base. The leaves of *Thymus zygis* are sessile, linear-lanceolate to acicular and with an involute margin. They are green to greyish green on both sides and pubescent. At the base, there are up to 1 mm long ciliate trichomes. As with *Thymus vulgaris*, only the calices of the (white) flowers can be recognized; they are practically indistinguishable from those of *T. vulgaris*.

Odour: Aromatic, strong and characteristic.

Taste: Aromatic and somewhat pungent.

Figs. 2 and 3: *Thymus vulgaris* L.

An aromatic dwarf shrub, not winter-hard north of the Alps. Much branched, with small elliptic leaves densely pubescent on the under surface and having a revolute margin. Whorls of pale violet, dorsiventral flowers arranged in spikes or capitula.

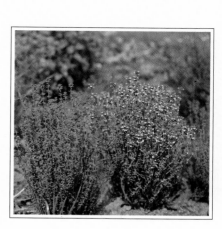

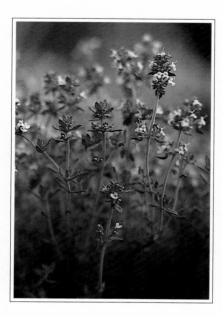

DAB 10: Thymian
ÖAB: Folium Thymi
Ph. Helv. VII: Thymi herba
St. Zul. 1329.99.99

Plant source: *Thymus vulgaris* L., common thyme, and *T. zygis* L., Spanish thyme, (Lamiaceae).

Synonyms: For Common thyme: Garden or Rubbed thyme (Engl.), Garten-Thymian, Gemeiner Thymian (Ger.), Herbe de thym vulgaire (Fr.).

Origin: *Thymus vulgaris*: native in various subspecies and forms in central and southern Europe, the Balkans, and in the Caucasus; the plant is cultivated in central Europe, East Africa, India, Turkey, Israel, Morocco, and North America [1–3]. *Thymus zygis*: native in the Iberian Peninsula; it is cultivated there and in the eastern part of Germany [2]. The drug is imported from Spain, Morocco, France, Bulgaria, and Hungary.

Constituents: 1.0–2.5% essential oil containing mainly the isomeric monoterpenes thymol (30–70%) and carvacrol (3–15%); a small proportion of the phenols in the drug is present as glucoside or galactoside. In the essential oil, there are other monoterpenes such as *p*-cymene, *γ*-terpinene, limonene, etc. [2, 3]. The composition of the oil depends to a large extent on the origin of and time of harvesting of the drug, the *γ*-terpinene and thymol contents being lower at the end of the vegetative cycle [12]. Both plant sources afford an oil of similar composition, though there are differences in the content of thymol methyl ether: in *T. vulgaris* it is ca. 1.4–2.5% and in *T. zygis* only ca. 0.3% of the oil [5]; the monoterpenes accumulate primarily in the peltate glandular trichomes [13]. There is also a chemotype of *T. vulgaris* subsp. *aestivus* (REUT. ex WILLK.) A. BOLÓS et O. BOLÓS, from Spain, which produces oil characterized mainly by the occurrence of 1,8-cineole (22%), geraniol (17%), and geranyl acetate (20%) [14]. The drug also has tannins, flavonoids, and triterpenes [2].

Indications: Because of the essential oil, internally as an expectorant and bronchospasmolytic, e.g. in acute and chronic bronchitis, whooping cough, and generally in catarrh of the upper respiratory tract; both the secretion and the transport brought about the movement of the cilia in the bronchi are enhanced [2, 6, 7]. This is caused, on the one hand, by a reflex action from the stomach, and, on the other hand, by a direct action on the bronchial mucosa, since the essential oil is partly excreted via the lungs. The antiseptic and antibacterial properties of the thymol also come into play; against many mi-

Thymol   Carvacrol

croorganisms, it is 25 times stronger than phenol, but, in contrast, because it is less soluble in water it is less injurious to the tissues [8, 9; cf. 12].
Externally, thyme is used as a hyperaemic, antibacterial, and also deodorizing agent in inflammation of the mouth and throat (as a mouthwash and gargle) and as a rubefacient in frictions, bath additives, and in pot-pourri [1].
In *folk medicine*, because of its spasmolytic action, it is an important stomachic and carminative, and it is also used as a diuretic, urinary disinfectant, and vermifuge.
Finally, thyme is also employed as a spice and in making liqueurs [1, 3].

Side effects: Normally, there is no danger attached to thyme or its preparations. But it should be noted that when thymol is used internally, e.g. as a vermifuge in *folk medicine*, in therapeutic doses (0.3–0.6 g, maximally 1.0 g), abdominal pain and temporary collapse may ensue. The internal administration of thymol is contraindicated in enterocolitis, cardiac insufficiency, and during pregnancy [10].

Making the tea: Boiling water (ca. 150 ml) is poured over ca. 1.5–2 g thyme and after 10 min. passed through a tea strainer.
1 Teaspoon = ca. 1.4 g.

Phytomedicines: The drug is a component of prepared cough teas; dry extracts and fluid extracts are present in many antitussives, Thymipin® (drops, juice, suppositories), Tussipect®, Pertussin®, Bronchicum® (all these as juice and drops), Broncholind® (drops), Perdiphen®, Equisil®, Melrosum® (syrup), Tussamag® (drops, juice, suppositories), etc., etc.

Regulatory status (UK): General Sales List – Schedule 1, Table A (thyme oil, likewise).

Authentication: Macro- (see: Description) and microscopically, following the DAB 10. See also the BHP 1983 and [15]. The diagnostic features include: the triangular trichomes, often containing fine calcium-oxalate needles, on the upper surface of the leaf (Fig. 6); the geniculate trichomes on the lower surface (Fig. 7), absent in *T. zygis*; multicellular covering trichomes; and the peltate glandular trichomes, here with 12 secretory cells (Fig. 5).
The DAB 10 TLC test of identity is as follows:

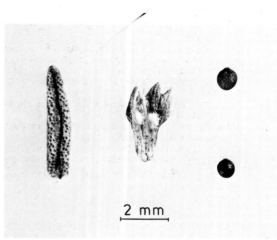

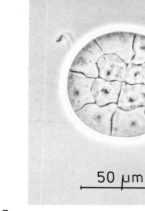

Fig. 4

Fig. 4: Lanceolate leaf, showing the revolute margin (left). Flower calyx, showing the the white bristles in the throat (centre). Ovoid, flattened seeds (right)

Fig. 7: Peltate glandular trichome with 12 secretory cells (phase-contrast photograph)

Fig. 7

Extract from the German Commission E monograph
(BAnz no. 228, dated 05. 12. 1984)

Uses
Symptoms of bronchitis and whooping cough. Catarrh of the upper respiratory tract.

Contraindications
None known.

Side effects
None known.

Interactions
None known.

Dosage
Unless otherwise prescribed: as an infusion, 1–2 g drug to a cup, several time a day as required; for poultices, a 5% infusion; as fluid extract [not less than 0.03% phenols calculated as thymol], 1–2 g.

Mode of administration
Chopped or powdered drug, liquid or dry extract, for infusions and other galenical preparations. Liquid and solid formulations for internal and external use.

Note
Combinations with other expectorant drugs may be advantageous.

Effects
Bronchospasmolytic, expectorant, antibacterial.

Test solution: 0.5 g powdered drug shaken for 2–3 min. with 5 ml dichloromethane and then filtered over ca. 2 g anhydrous sodium sylphate.

Reference solution: 2.0 mg thymol dissolved in 10 ml dichloromethane.

Loadings: 20 µl of each solution, as 2-cm bands on silica gel GF$_{254}$.

Solvent system: dichloromethane, 2 × 10 cm run.

Detection and Evaluation: in UV 254 nm light. Reference solution: the quenching thymol zone at ca. Rf 0.5. Test solution: a similar quenching zone, and directly above it a more strongly quenching zone; in the lower third several, weaker quenching zones.
Sprayed with anisaldehyde reagent and heated at 100–105 °C for 5–10 min. while under observation. Then examined in daylight. Reference solution: thymol zone sealing-wax red. Test solution: immediately below the thymol zone, at most only a faint violet zone (carvacrol); between this zone and the starting line, four coloured zones, usually of the same intensity – the uppermost zone pinkish red and below it a violet zone (cineole and linalool) and below that a brownish grey zone (borneol) and a violet to blue zone; near the solvent front, an intense reddish to greyish violet zone; other zones at the starting line.
See also [11].

Quantitative standards: DAB 10: *Volatile oil*, not less than 1.2% and not less than 0.5% phenols calculated as thymol (M_r 150.2). *Foreign matter*, not more than 10% stem fragments and not more than 2% other foreign matter. *Loss on drying*, not more than 10.0%. *Ash*, not more than 15.0%.
ÖAB: *Volatile oil*, not less than 1.5%. *Foreign matter*, not more than than 3% stem fragments. *Ash*, not more than 10.0%.
Ph. Helv. VII: *Volatile oil*, not less than 1.5% and not less than 0.5% steam-volatile phenols (calculated as thymol, M_r 150.2). *Foreign matter*, not stem fragments with a diameter greater than 1 mm and length greater than 15 mm; leaves of *T. serpyllum* absent. *Sulphated ash*, not more than 16.0%.

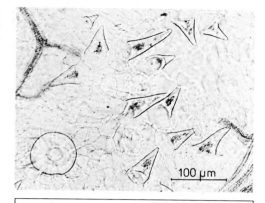

Fig. 5: Triangular trichomes with fine calcium-oxalate needles and a glandular trichome (bottom left)

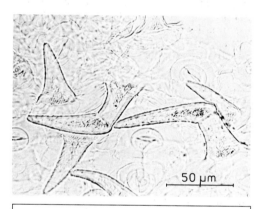

Fig. 6: Geniculate trichomes, showing the oblique, tapering, terminal cells

BHP 1983: *Foreign matter*, not more than 15% stems with a diameter up to 1 mm and stems exceeding 1 mm in diameter absent; other foreign organic matter, not more than 2%. *Total ash*, not more than 12%. *Acid-insoluble ash*, not more than 4%.

Adulteration: Rare, but admixture with wild thyme has been encountered. For its detection, see: Serpylli herba

Storage: Protected from light and moisture, in well-closed containers (not made of plastic).

Literature:
[1] Hager, vol. **6c**, p. 161 (1979).
[2] Kommentar DAB 10.
[3] V. Formácek and K.-H. Kubeczka, Essential oil analysis by capillary gas chromatography and carbon-13 NMR spectroscopy, Wiley, Chichester, 1982.
[4] E. Schratz and H. Hörster, Planta Med. **19**, 160 (1971).
[5] W. Messerschmidt, Planta Med. **12**, 501 (1964); idem., *ibid.* **13**, 56 (1965).
[6] C.O. van den Broucke and J.A. Lemli, Planta Med. **41**, 129 (1981).
[7] W. Müller-Limmroth and H.H. Fröhlich, Fortschr. d. Medizin **98**, 95 (1980).
[8] D. Patáková and M. Chládek, Pharmazie **29**, 140 (1974).
[9] G. Frölich, Naturheilpraxis **35**, 1118 (1982).
[10] H. Braun and D. Frohne, Heilpflanzenlexikon für Ärzte und Apotheker, G. Fischer Verlag, Stuttgart – New York, 1987.
[11] P. Pachaly, Dünnschichtchromatographie in der Apotheke, 2nd ed., Wissenschaftliche Verlagsgesellschaft, Stuttgart, 1983.
[12] G. Vampa et al., Plantes Méd. Phytothérap. **22**, 195 (1988).
[13] T. Yamaura, S. Tanakam and M. Tabata, Phytochemistry **28**, 741 (1989).
[14] A. Amparo Blázquez and M. Carmen Zafra-Polo, Pharmazie **45**, 802 (1990).
[15] B.P. Jackson and D.W. Snowdon, Atlas of microscopy of medicinal plants, culinary herbs and spices, Belhaven Press, London, 1990, p. 234.

Tiliae flos   (DAB 10), Lime tree flower (BHP 1990)

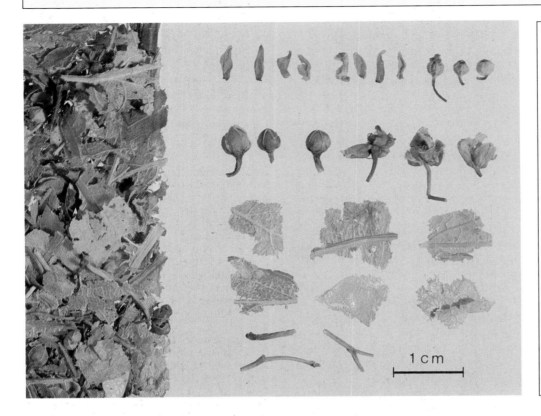

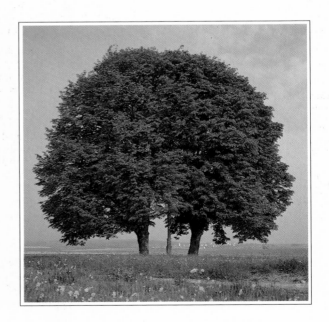

Fig. 1: Lime tree flower

<u>Description:</u> The fragments of pale yellowish green entire bracts with a distinct reticulate nervature, which are partly fused with the flower stalk, are characteristic. There are also yellowish white flowers with five sepals and five free petals, numerous stamens, and a densely pubescent superior ovary (Fig. 4). Occasionally, buds are also present.

<u>Odour:</u> Characteristic and faintly aromatic.

<u>Taste:</u> Sweetish, mucilaginous, pleasant.

Figs. 2 and 3: *Tilia cordata* MILL.

Small-leaved lime – trees growing to a height of 30 m, with glabrous cordate leaves with a serrate margin and brown hairs in the angles of the nerves on the lower surface (white hairs in the large-leaved lime). 5-merous, greenish yellow, scented flowers, with numerous stamens and a relatively large, pubescent ovary, grouped together in cymes (5–10 in the small-leaved lime and 2–5 in the large-leaved lime), and stalks fused with the accompanying bract.

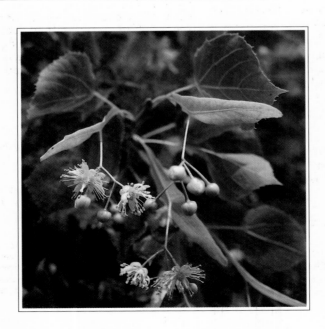

DAB 10: Lindenblüten
ÖAB: Flos Tiliae
Ph. Helv. VII: Tiliae flos
St. Zul. 1129.99.99

Plant sources: *Tilia cordata* MILLER, small-leaved lime, and *T. platyphyllos* Scop., large-leaved lime (Tiliaceae).

Synonyms: Tilia, Lime or Linden flowers (Engl.); Lindenblüten, *T. cordata*: Winter-, Stein-, Spät-, or Waldlinde; *T. platyphyllos*: Sommer-, Gras- or Frühlinde (Ger.); Fleur de tilleul (Fr.).

Origin: Native throughout Europe; it is also planted. The drug comes partly from China and partly also from the Balkans (former Yugoslavia, Bulgaria, Romania) and Turkey.

Constituents: Slightly more than 1% flavonoids, principally quercetin glycosides (rutin, hyperoside, quercitrin, isoquercitrin, a rhamnoxyloside, and a 3-gluco-7-rhamnoside) and also kaempferol glycosides (astragalin, its 6″-p-coumaric acid ester tiliroside, the 3-gluco-7-rhamnoside, and the 3,7-dirhamnoside). Ca. 10% of a complex

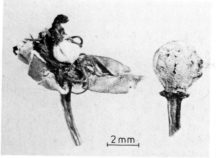
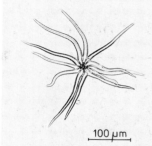
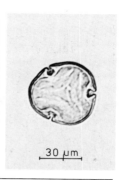

Fig. 4: A single flower (left) and a pubescent fruit (right)

Fig. 5: Stellate trichome

Fig. 6: Tricolpate pollen grain

mucilage [1, 2], mainly arabino-galactans. Leucoanthocyanidins. Caffeic, p-coumaric, and chlorogenic acids. Ca. 0.02% essential oil containing alkanes and monoterpenes, and also farnesol, farnesyl acetate, geraniol, geranyl acetate, 2-phenylethanol, 2-phenyl-ethylbenzoic acid ester, and eugenol as odoriferous components.

Indications: To alleviate irritation of the throat in catarrh of the respiratory tract (phlegm). As a diaphoretic in feverish colds and infections for which a sweat cure is desired. Whether certain constituents are responsible for the sudorific effect, or whether it is simply a consequence of the increased intake of hot fluid, is still being debated (see: Sambuci flos).
In *folk medicine*, lime tree flower is still occasionally used as a diuretic, stomachic, antispasmodic, and sedative.

Making the tea: Boiling water is poured over 2 g of the drug, or it is put into cold water and briefly heated to boiling; after 5–10 min., the infusion is passed through a tea strainer.
1 Teaspoon = ca. 1.8 g.

Herbal preparations: Lime tree flower is available in tea bags (1–1.5 g).
Potter's Wellwoman Herbs is a UK multi-ingredient product in tea bags which includes the drug.

Phytomedicines: Extracts of lime tree flower are a component of some prepared urological remedies, antitussives, and sedatives. The drug is a component of various herbal mixtures recommended for chills, colds, etc.
Lime tree flower or an extract thereof is present in the UK products Gerard House Motherwort Compound Tablets and Potter's Wellwoman Tablets.

Authentication: Macro- and microscopically, following the DAB 10. See also the BHP 1990. The diagnostic features include the sclereids of the bracts, the tufted trichomes of the sepals, as well as the stellate trichomes of the ovary (Fig. 5). The pollen grains are 30–40 µm in diameter, spherical, and tricolpate (Fig. 6).
The DAB 10 describes identification via detection of the flavonoids extracted with methanol by means of the Shinoda magnesium/hydrochloric reaction (conversion to red-coloured anthocyanidins) and also by their TLC separation:

Extract from the German Commission E monograph (BAnz no. 164, dated 01.09.90)

Uses
Chills, colds, etc. and the associated coughs.

Contraindications
None known.

Side effects
None known.

Interactions with other remedies
None known.

Dosage
Unless otherwise prescribed: daily dose, 2–4 g drugs; preparations correspondingly.

Mode of administration
Comminuted drugs for teas and other galenical preparations for internal use.

Effects
Diaphoretic.

Wording of the package insert, from the German Standard Licence

5.1 **Uses**
Alleviation of irritation of the throat in catarrh of the respiratory tract, feverish colds, chills, etc., for which a sweat cure is desired.

5.2 **Dosage and Mode of administration**
Boiling water (ca. 150 ml) is poured over ca. 1–2 teaspoonfuls (2–4 g) of **Lime tree flower** and after about 5 min. passed through a tea strainer. Unless otherwise prescribed, one or two cups of the freshly prepared infusion is drunk as hot as possible, especially during the second half of the day.

5.3 **Note**
Store away from light and moisture.

Tiliroside

Test solution: 1.0 g powdered drug shaken with 10 ml methanol for 5 min. on the water-bath at 65 °C, cooled, and filtered.

Reference solution: 2.0 mg caffeic acid and 5 mg each of hyperoside and rutin dissolved in 10 ml methanol.

Loadings: 10 µl of each solution, as 2-cm bands on silica gel G.

Solvent system: water + anhydrous formic acid + ethyl methyl ketone + ethyl acetate (10 + 10 + 30 + 50), 15 cm run.

Detection: after drying at 100–105 °C, the still warm plate sprayed with 1% methanolic diphenylboryloxyethylamine, followed by 5% methanolic Macrogol 400.

Evaluation: after 30 min. in UV 365 nm light. Reference solution: in increasing order of Rf value, the orange-brown fluorescent zones of rutin and hyperoside and the greenish blue fluorescent zone of caffeic acid. Test solution: the main, yellowish brown to orange, fluorescent zone very slight higher than the hyperoside zone (also visible in daylight as the main zone); at about the same Rf value as rutin, another yellowish brown fluorescent zone and below it perhaps two yellow fluorescent zones; in the Rf between rutin and hyperoside, orange and yellow fluorescent zones; in the Rf range betwwen hyperoside and caffeic acid, up to five more yellow to orange fluorescent zones; very slightly below the caffeic acid zone, a blue fluorescent zone.

There is a coloured illustration of the TLC obtained in [3]. The main zone, which appears just above the hyperoside zone, has now been identified as isoquercitrin (quercetin 3-glucoside) [4].

Quantitative standards: <u>DAB 10</u>: *Swelling index*, not less than 32 (adulterants do not attain this figure); see the explanatory remarks in [5]. *Foreign matter*, not more than 2%; inflorescences with bracts on whose lower surface there are 5- to 8-branched stellate trichomes, and flowers whose corolla appears to be double because of the transformation of five anthers into corolla-like staminodes and whose stigma is not lobed or split, must be absent; at most, occasional 6-merous flowers. *Loss on drying*, not more than 12.0%. *Ash*, not more than 7.0%.
<u>ÖAB</u>: *Foreign matter*, not more than 1%. *Ash*, not more than 7.0%.
<u>Ph. Helv. VII</u>: *Swelling index*, not less than 15. *Foreign matter*, not more than 1% leaves and other foreign matter; not more than 5% flowers with spotted bracts. *Sulphated ash*, not more than 10%.
<u>BHP 1990</u>: *Water-soluble extractive*, not less than 15%. *Foreign matter*, not more than 2%. *Total ash*, not more than 12%. *HCl-insoluble ash*, not more than 4%.

Adulteration: Not infrequent, especially with the flowers of *Tilia tomentosa* MOENCH (syn. *T. argentea* DC.) and *T. × euchlora* K. KOCH (presumably a hybrid between *T. cordata* and *T. dasystyla* STEVEN), both species being

often planted as decorative trees, but in Chinese products also other species such as *T. chinensis* MAXIM. and *T. mandschurica* RUPR. These mostly have a different scent and taste. According to the ÖAB, an aqueous infusion of lime tree flower should not have an unpleasant or repulsive smell. According to the ÖAB and the Ph. Helv. VII, adulterants can be recognized microscopically by the densely pubescent bracts in, e.g. *T. americana* L. and *T. tomentosa*, and/ or by the flowers having petalaceous staminodes, e.g. *T. tomentosa*.
Some species can also be recognized by their fruits, which are almost always to be found in the drug: according to the Flora Europea, *T. cordata* has spherical and almost glabrous fruit; *T. platyphyllos* has pear-shaped fruit; *T. tomentosa* has finely tuberculate, ovoid fruit; and *T. × euchlora* has a fruit which is pointed at the ends.
The adulterants all have a lower swelling index than the official drug (see: Authentication).

Literature:
[1] G. Kram and G. Franz, Planta Med. **49**, 149 (1983).
[2] G. Kram and G. Franz, Pharmazie **40**, 501 (1985).
[3] E. Stahl and S. Juell, Dtsch Apoth. Ztg. **122**, 1951 (1982).
[4] M. Wichtl, B. Bozek, and T. Fingerhut, Dtsch. Apoth. Ztg. **127**, 509 (1987).
[5] H. Kanschat and C. Lander, Pharm. Ztg. **129**, 370 (1984).

Tormentillae rhizoma

Tormentil, Potentilla (BHP 1983)

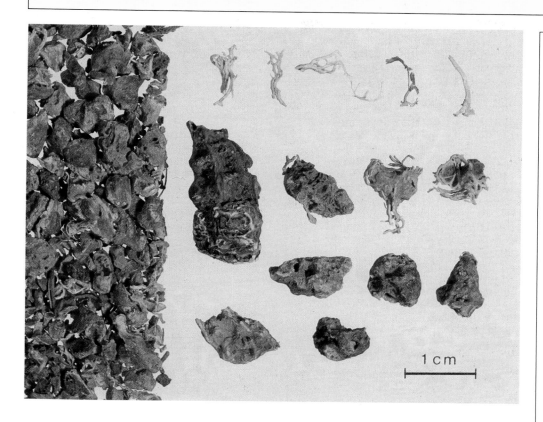

Fig. 1: Tormentil

<u>Description</u>: The drug consists of the rhizome freed from the roots. The chopped drug is made up of dark reddish brown, irregular, knobbly, very hard pieces of rhizome, which are partly covered with a very dark brown cork and whitish root scars. Some porous, broken pieces show the very pale-coloured vascular bundles leading to the roots (Fig. 3), which are sometimes present on their own.

<u>Odour</u>: Very faint, pleasant.

<u>Taste</u>: Powerfully astringent.

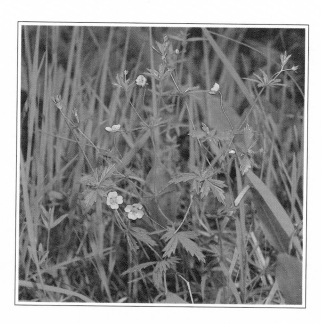

Fig. 2: *Potentilla erecta* (L.) RAEUSCH.

A low (up to 30 cm) herb with a preference for acid soils. Cut or broken surfaces of the robust rhizome rapidly become red. Stem prostrate or erect and leaves mostly 5-digitate, sessile, and with stipules. Yellow flowers with mostly 4 petals (unusual for a Rosaceae – other *Potentilla* species with 5), a good character by which to recognize the plant.

DAB 10: Tormentillwurzelstock
ÖAB: Radix Tormentillae
St. Zul. 1689.99.99

Plant source: *Potentilla erecta* (L.) RAEUSCH. (syn. *Potentilla tormentilla* STOKES), common tormentil (Rosaceae).

Synonyms: Erect cinquefoil (Engl.), Tormentillwurzelstock, Blutwurz (Ger.), Rhizome de tormentille (Fr.).

Origin: Widespread in central and northern Europe. The drug is imported from eastern European countries.

Constituents: 15% to more than 20% tannins (mainly of the catechol type), which on storage are slowly converted into phlobaphenes; besides the polymers, there is a series of monomers and dimers, e.g. flavan-3-ols and procyanidins, but catechol trimers are also known [1]. The isolation of agrimoniin, a dimeric ellagitannin [2] and the detection of gallic acid [3], ellagic acid [4], and catechol gallates [5] make it clear that at least part of the tannins belongs to the group of hydrolysable tannins.
According to [6], the content of (hydrolysable) ellagitannins is 6.2%, which, being 37% of the total tannin content of 21.6%, means that they are over-represented in the overall effect that the tannins have. Other constituents worth mentioning are: the pseudosaponin tormentoside (aglycone: the triterpene tormentillic acid), quinovic acid, phenylpropanes such as caffeic, *p*-coumaric, and sinapic acids [7], as well as traces of essential oil [8].

Indications: Because of its high tannin content, the drug is a good astringent and is used internally as an antidiarrhoeic in acute and sub-acute gastroenteritis, enterocolitis, and dysentery; externally, it is applied in inflammation of the mucous membranes of the mouth and throat as a gargle or rinse or as a paint (tincture). The drug has been proposed [9] as a substitute for Ratanhiae radix (rhatany root), as it contains an even greater proportion of tannins.
Extracts of the drug have been shown to have other pharmacological effects – anti-allergic, antihypertensive, antiviral, immunostimulant and interferon-inducing actions. It remains to be seen whether these will be of any significance as regards the medicinal uses of the drug; for a review, see [2].

Making the tea: 2–3 g of the finely chopped or coarsely drug is put into cold water and then brought to the boil for a short while; after standing for a brief period, it is passed through a tea strainer. Cold maceration is also worth while, since prolonged boiling leads to hydrolysis of the ellagitannins and reduced activity [6].
For diarrhoea, it is recommended to take 2–4 g of the powdered drug suspended in red wine. As an antidiarrhoeic, a cup of the tea or suspension in wine may be taken three or four times a day.
1 Teaspoon = ca. 4 g.

Phytomedicines: Tormentil is a component of some mixed teas, and (as the powdered drug) in prepared remedies. Extracts are present in several stomachics or antidiarrhoeics, e.g. Cefadiarrhon®, or Pasisana-Mixtur®. In remedies such as Repha-Os® Mundspray (mouth spray), or Duoform®-Balsam, extracts form one of the components.

Authentication: Macro- (see: Description) and microscopically, following the DAB 10. See also the BHP 1983. Since the drug is

very hard, it is more convenient to use some of the drug powder for the microscopy. The diagnostic features include: fragments of parenchyma with red tannin cells, moderately large clusters of calcium oxalate, vessels with lateral sieve plates, and small starch granules. The distribution of the groups of fibres and vessels is very variable. The useful and detailed description by Staesche [10] is worth consulting.
Detection of tannins: 0.1 g powdered drug is shaken with 50 ml distilled water for several min.; on adding one drop of iron(III) chloride solution, the filtrate becomes intense green or bluish green (cf. below, under: Adulteration). With vanillin/sulphuric acid, the drug particles stain red.
The DAB 10 TLC test of identity is as follows:

Test solution: 0.5 g powdered drug shaken with 10 ml water for 10 min. and filtered; filtrate extracted twice with 10 ml ethyl acetate and the combined extracts filtered over ca. 6 g anhydrous sodium sulphate; filtrate taken to dryness under reduced pressure and the residue dissolved in 1.0 ml ethyl acetate.

Reference solution: 1.0 mg cianidanol (catechol) dissolved in 1.0 ml methanol.

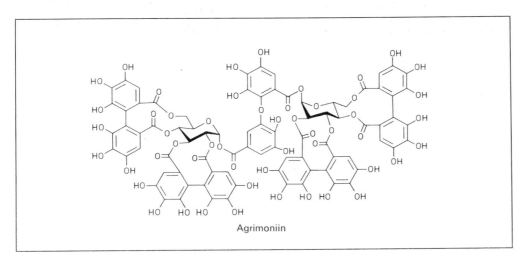

Agrimoniin

Loadings: 10 µl of each solution, as 2-cm bands on silica gel G.

Solvent system: 98% acetic acid + dichloromethane + ethyl acetate (20 + 40 + 40), 2 × 10 cm run.

Detection: after 10–15 min. at room temperature, sprayed with 0.5% aqueous Fast Blue Salt solution, the colour of the reddish zones produced being rendered more intense and taking on a reddish brown colour after exposure to conc. ammonia solution.

Evaluation: in daylight. Reference solution: the intense cianidanol (catechol) zone in the upper half. Test solution: a zone corresponding to the cianidanol zone but usually somewhat more distinct; below it, a fainter zone; in the lower half, an intense reddish brown zone; in the lower third, a few faint zones may be present.

Quantitative standards: DAB 10: *Tannin content*, not less than 15.0%. *Foreign matter*, not more than 3% root and stem fragments,

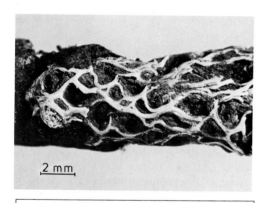

Fig. 3: Porous, broken fragment of rhizome, showing the whitish groups of fibres and vessels

2 mm

as well as rhizome with a black fracture, and not more than 2% other foreign matter. *Loss on drying*, not more than 10.0%. *Ash*, not more than 5.0%.
ÖAB: *Ash*, not more than 5%.

Adulteration: May occur, with Bistortae radix (Rhizoma Bistortae, snake root or bistort, *Polygonum bistorta* L.), a drug rhizome that also contains 15–20% tannin. The ca. 1 cm thick pieces are bent in an S-shape (whole drug) and somewhat lighter-coloured than Tormentillae rhizoma. The bark is a conspicuous feature, with its stout-walled parenchyma cells and in part large intercellular spaces and scattered thin-walled cells each containing a large cluster crystal of calcium oxalate. In contrast to tormentil rhizome, there are only occasional xylem fibres. Because of its high tannin content, some authors consider Bistortae radix as a fully equivalent substitute not only for tormentil rhizome but also for rhatany root.
Adulteration with rhizomes of *Geum* species, e.g. *G. montanum* L. is not infrequent [10].
The ÖAB requires aqueous extracts of tormentil to give a green colour with iron(III) chloride solution. Länger et al. [11,12] point

out that in practice commercial samples give a deep blue, even though microscopy and TLC examination show them to correspond with genuine herbarium material; they recommend preference for an improved DAB TLC test of identity [12].

Literature:
[1] A. Byung-Zun, Dtsch. Apoth. Ztg. **113**, 1466 (1973).
[2] K. Lund and H. Rimpler, Dtsch. Apoth. Ztg. **125**, 105 (1985).
[3] G. Schenk, K.-H. Frömming and L. Frohnecke, Arch. Pharm. (Weinheim) **10**, 453 (1957).
[4] E.C. Bate-Smith, Linn. Soc. (Bot.) **58**, 39 (1961).
[5] L.V. Selenia, R.N. Zolulya and T.N. Yakovleva, Rastit. Resur. **9**, 409 (1973); C.A. **80**, 22614 (1974).
[6] K. Lund, Dissertation Freiburg i.Br. 1986.
[7] W. Enge and K. Herrmann, Pharmazie **12**, 162 (1957).
[8] Kommentar DAB 10.
[9] W. Schier, Dtsch. Apoth. Ztg. **121**, 323 (1981).
[10] K. Staesche, Dtsch. Apoth. Ztg. **108**, 329 (1968).
[11] R. Länger, M. Kunisch, and W. Kubelka, Sci. Pharm. **59**, 34 (1991).
[12] R. Länger, K. Winter and W. Kubelka, Pharmazie **48**, 776 (1993).

Urticae fructus (semen)   Nettle fruit (seed)

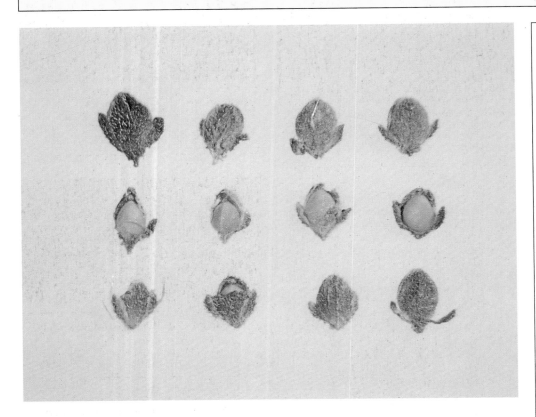

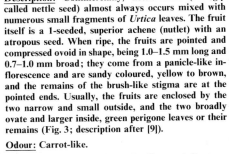

Fig. 1: Nettle fruit

Description: Commercially, nettle fruit (wrongly called nettle seed) almost always occurs mixed with numerous small fragments of *Urtica* leaves. The fruit itself is a 1-seeded, superior achene (nutlet) with an atropous seed. When ripe, the fruits are pointed and compressed ovoid in shape, being 1.0–1.5 mm long and 0.7–1.0 mm broad; they come from a panicle-like inflorescence and are sandy coloured, yellow to brown, and the remains of the brush-like stigma are at the pointed ends. Usually, the fruits are enclosed by the two narrow and small outside, and the two broadly ovate and larger inside, green perigone leaves or their remains (Fig. 3; description after [9]).

Odour: Carrot-like.

Taste: Not characteristic; a rancid taste indicates a drug that has been stored too long.

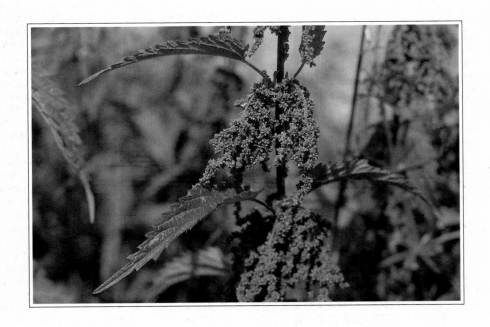

Fig. 2: Fruits of *Urtica dioica* L.

Female plants with flowering panicles giving rise to small yellowish brown fruits. Inflorescence and fructification normally longer than the petioles of the neighbouring leaves.

Plant sources: *Urtica dioica* L., common nettle (Urticaceae); occasionally, also *U. urens* L., small nettle (Urticaceae); the details below all relate to *U. dioica*.

Origin: A nitratophile ruderal plant of almost worldwide distribution. The drug is imported from south-eastern Europe, especially former Yugoslavia, but also from Bulgaria and Albania.

Synonyms: See, Urticae herba.

Constituents: The ripe fruits contain protein [1], mucilage (swelling index for the crushed drug 5–6 [2]), and fixed oil (up to 30% of the dry mass). The oil obtained by extraction with an organic solvent or by cold pressing is yellowish green to green in colour, owing to the presence of carotenoids (β-carotene, lutein, violaxanthin, etc.) and chlorophyll degradation products [4]. The few fat analyses carried out so far ([2]: here also details of the fat constants) indicate, among other things, a high linoleic acid content (up to 83% of the total fatty acids) and 0.1 to 0.2% tocopherols [5, 6].

Indications: The fruits are used principally in *folk medicine* [6]. When crushed, they are applied externally as a dressing for skin complaints and rheumatism. The fruit, or the oil (particularly the cold-pressed oil) obtained from them, are given internally as a tonic and so-called "bio-stimulant" to increase the "activity of the liver"; there is no scientific evidence for these indications. In herbals dealing with folk medicine, there are references to use of the drug in diarrhoea, biliary complaints, and as a haemostyptic, etc. Formerly, in veterinary medicine, nettle "seeds" were mixed with the feed to improve egg production by hens [7]. Giving old horses nettle fruits supposedly improved their coat so that it became more glossy. The literature occasionally mentions that the drug has galactogenic effects [6].

Making the tea: Unusual. Water is added to 2–4 g of the crushed drug, boiled, then allowed to stand for 10 mins., and strained. Recommended dosages for use as a tonic or antirheumatic are lacking.
1 Teaspoon = ca. 1.6 g.

Phytomedicines: Especially alcoholic extracts of "Semen" Urticae dioicae, as a roborant and tonic, e.g. Brennesselsamen (nettle seed) Vital-Tonikum® Grandel.

Authentication: Macroscopically (see: Description); the drug should consist of *ripe* fruits. The presence of sphaerocrystals in the testa [8] is a feature which is absent in unripe fruit. Since a comprehensive microscopical study of nettle fruit has not yet been carried out, the anatomical description by Schier [9]

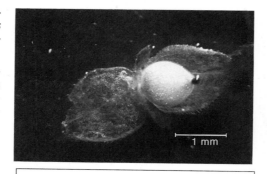

Fig. 3: Fruit, showing the two broadly ovate inner, and the two narrow and smaller outer, perigone leaves

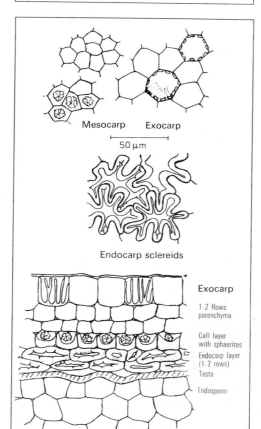

Fig. 4: Drawings showing components of the pericarp

Fig. 5: Section through the pericarp of nettle fruit

is given here. Transverse view of the fruit (Fig. 4): on the narrow side there is a hyaline edge; in polarized light, numerous sphaerocrystals light up in surface view.

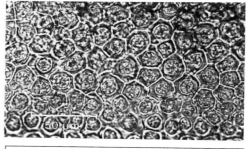

Fig. 6: Sphaerocrystals of the *ripe* fruit

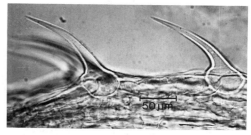

Fig. 7: Retort-shaped trichomes on the perigone leaves

With Sudan III orange-coloured papillae can be seen. Cross section of the fruit (Fig. 5): at the hyaline edge there is a thin cuticle, below which is a thin-walled exocarp and in this layer there is a scattering of cells whose anticlinal walls have ridges of thickening. The cells of the mesocarp are also thin-walled. Then follows a yellow layer of U-shaped, thickened, conical cells each containing a sphaerocrystal (Fig. 6) and below it a layer of irregularly thickened cells with intercellular spaces. The testa is fused to the endocarp and consists of reddish brown, thick-walled, lignified, tangentially elongated cells and next to it is the small-celled endosperm. – The small perigone leaves are furcate at the top. The inner and outer perigone leaves are covered with mostly 1-, rarely 2-celled trichomes which are more or less retort-shaped at the bottom and which are often curved (Fig. 7). They are thick-walled, pointed, and in the lumen occasionally there is a small granular or needle-shaped crystal; their walls shine brightly in polarized light. The cells of the epidermis are polygonal and wavy-walled, and the anomocytic stomata mostly have four subsidiary cells.

Adulteration: In practice does not occur.

Storage: Protected from light and moisture; the drug should not be kept for more than a year after harvesting, since otherwise the fat becomes rancid.

Literature:

[1] Berger, vol. **4**, p. 522 (1954).

[2] F.-C. Czygan and A. Krüger, unpublished results (1987); the swelling index was determined for eleven samples of "Semen Urticae" from different sources.

[3] R. Prögler, Fette und Seifen **48**, 541 (1936).

[4] F.-C. Czygan and A. Krüger, unpublished results (1986); the total fat was extracted in a soxhlet with light petroleum (boiling range 40–60 °C). The chloroplast pigments were estimated according to the procedure of Weber and Czygan (Arch. Mikrobiol. **84**, 243 [1972]).

[5] J.H. Schmitt, Fa. Keimdiät, Augsburg, personal communication (1987).

[6] J.H. Schmitt, Z. Naturheilkunde **30**, 74 (1979).

[7] G.A. Buchmeister, Handbuch der Drogistenpraxis, Berlin, 1911, p. 216.

[8] H. Molisch, Mikrochemie der Pflanze, Jena, 1916.

[9] W. Schier, unpublished findings (1987).

Urticae herba
Nettle herb (BHP 1/1990)

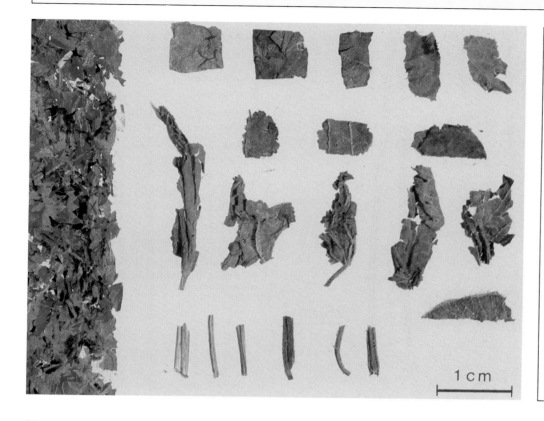

Fig. 1: Nettle herb

<u>Description:</u> The drug consists of the above-ground parts with stems not more than 3 mm thick, collected during the flowering period and dried. In the cut drug, the leaf fragments are shrivelled and often crumpled up into a ball. The upper surface is greenish black and the lower surface is pale green; there are large, scattered, erect stinging hairs (Fig. 4) and numerous small bristles; the margin of the leaf fragments is coarsely serrate and the nervature on the lower surface is distinct and prominent. Pieces of the square stem are mostly flattened, green to brown, and deeply grooved. Occasional pieces of the green flowering panicles may be present.

<u>Odour:</u> Not characteristic.

<u>Taste:</u> Not characteristic.

Fig. 2: *Urtica dioica* L., female plant

A 60–120 cm tall herb bearing ovate and acuminate leaves with a coarsely serrate margin; stinging hairs and bristles present. Flowering panicles longer than the leaf petioles (difference from *U. urens* L.).

Fig. 3: *Urtica dioica* L., male plant

Same habit as described for Fig. 2; flowers yellowish (anthers with yellow pollen grains).

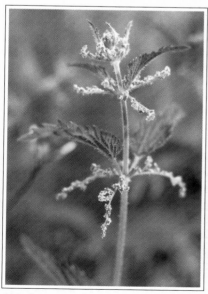

Abb. 2

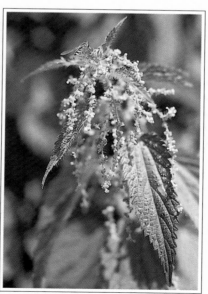

Abb. 3

DAB 10: Brennesselblätter
DAC 1986: Brennesselkraut
St. Zul.: 8599.99.99

Plant sources: Mostly *Urtica dioica* L., common nettle, but occasionally also *U. urens* L., small nettle (Urticaceae).

Synonyms: Urtica, Stinging nettle (Engl.), Brennesselkraut, Haarnesselkraut, Hanfnesselkraut (Ger.), Herbe d'ortie (Fr.).

Origin: Occurrence almost worldwide as a plant of wasteland; the drug is obtained from plants growing in the wild in central and eastern Europe (eastern part of Germany, former USSR, Bulgaria, former Yugoslavia).

Constituents: Apart from flavonoids (glycosides of quercetin, kaempferol, and rhamnetin in the flowers) [1], up till now no constituents have been found which will explain the effects ascribed to the drug. In addition to the chlorophylls a and b that are charac-

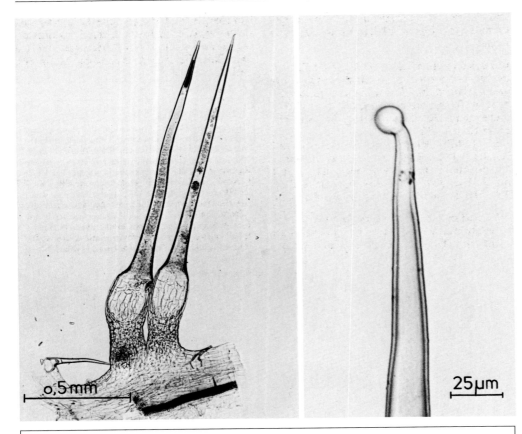

o,5 mm

25 µm

Fig. 4: Typical stinging hairs, from *Urtica dioica*

Fig. 5: Undamaged, swollen tip of the stinging hair

teristic of all green plants, chlorophyll degradation products and carotenoids (including β-carotene and xanthophylls), vitamins (among them C, B group, K_1), triterpenes and sterols (including β-sitosterol), mineral salts (among them silica, potassium salts, nitrates), other ubiquitous plant substances, e.g. formic, acetic, citric, and other acids) are also present. The detection of the glucokinins, which continue to be made responsible for the "antidiabetic" activity, is still disputed. The stinging trichomes in particular contain amines (including histamine, serotonin, choline, etc.) [2].

Indications: There are few clinically and pharmacologically assured results concerning the action and activity, and such as there are relate to the diuretic effect. Thus, nettle herb is supposed to have a favourable diuretic action, which is accompanied by considerable excretion of chlorides and urea [according to 2]. More recent studies [3] have confirmed the mild diuretic effect of the fresh sap from the herb. Treatment over a 14-day period brought about an increase in urine volume and a reduction in body weight, as well as an insignificant diminution in systolic blood pressure.

In *folk medicine*, nettle herb as a tea or as juice pressed from the fresh plant is used in many different ways [2]: internally as a "blood-forming" agent, as a diuretic in arthritis and rheumatism of the joints and muscles, "to raise enzyme production" of the glands secreting gastric juice, as a component of "anti-diabetic" teas (against the use of which there have been warnings from the medical profession [4]), to promote wound healing, in biliary complaints, externally for treating seborrhoea of the scalp and hair and against over-greasy hair. (For other folk-medicinal uses, particularly in eastern European countries, see [2].) The numerous and, in part very imprecise and wide-ranging indications for nettle herb [2] and the few

pharmacological studies carried out so far are sufficient reasons for critically appraising therapeutic practice with this drug. As a *mild diuretic*, the drug can certainly be recommended [4].

Side effects: Occasionally (rare), after taking nettle tea, allergies (cutaneous affections, oedema, oliguria, gastric irritation) have been observed.

Making the tea: 1.5 g of the finely cut drug is put into cold water and boiled for a short time, or boiling water is poured directly on to it, and after 10 mins. strained. As a diuretic, a cupful is drunk several times a day.
1 Teaspoon = ca. 0.8 g, 1 tablespoon = ca. 2.2 g.

Herbal preparations: The drug is also available in tea bags (1.0–1.8 g).

Phytomedicines: As a component of "urine-eliminating" herbal mixtures (diuretics) and so-called "blood-purifying" teas, and the fresh plant sap as a "spring cure".

Regulatory status (UK): General Sales List – Schedula 1, Table A.

Authentication: Macro- and microscopically, following the DAC 1986. See also the BHP 1/1990. The stinging hairs (Figs. 4

and 5) are characteristic, as well as the epidermal cystoliths which are up to 70 µm in length.

Quantitative standards: <u>DAC 1986</u>: *Foreign matter*, not more than 10% stem fragments and not more than 2% other foreign matter. *Loss on drying*, not more than 12%. *Ash*, not more than 20%. *Acid-insoluble ash*, not more than 4.0%.
<u>BHP 1/1990</u>: *Water-soluble extractive*, not less than 18%. *Stems above 3 mm in diameter*, not more than 2%. *Foreign matter*, not more than 2%. *Total ash*, not more than 20%. *HCl-insoluble ash*, not more than 4%.

Adulteration: The leaves of *Lamium album* L., white deadnettle, have been noted as an adulterant. These have an irregularly serrate leaf margin, and the stinging hairs and cystoliths are absent. Instead, bicellular uniseriate trichomes and short trichomes with a unicellular head are present (see: Lamii albi herba).

Literature:
[1] N. Chaurasia and M. Wichtl, Planta Med. **53**, 432 (1987).
[2] J. Lutomski and H. Speichert, Pharmazie in unserer Zeit **12**, 181 (1983).
[3] H.W. Kirchhoff, Z. Phytotherap. **4**, 621 (1983).
[4] R.F. Weiß, Herbal Medicine, Arcanum, Gothenburg, and Beaconsfield Publishers, Beaconsfield, 1988.

Urticae radix   (DAB 10), Nettle root

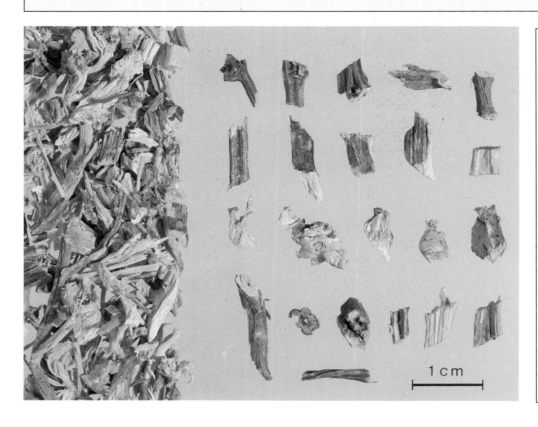

Fig. 1: Nettle root

<u>Description:</u> **The irregularly twisted, ca. 5 mm thick, greyish brown pieces of root exhibit distinct longitudinal grooves. The root is hollow in cross section and the cut surface is white; the fracture is tough and fibrous.**

<u>Odour:</u> **No characteristic smell.**

<u>Taste:</u> **No characteristic taste.**

Illustration of *Urtica dioica* L., see: Urticae herba.

1 cm

DAB 10: Brennesselwurzel

Plant sources: Mainly *Urtica dioica* L., common nettle, but occasionally also *U. urens* L., small nettle (Urticaceae).

Synonyms: Brennesselwurzel, Hanfnesselwurzel (Ger.), Racine d'ortie (Fr.), See also: Urticae herba.

Origin: Almost cosmopolitan as a plant on wasteland; the drug comes from wild plants growing in central and eastern Europe (former Yugoslavia, Bulgaria).

Constituents: The phytochemical study of nettle root has only recently begun. Following indications for the presence of β-sitosterol [1, 2] and tannins [3], recently scopoletin, β-sitosterol, β-sitosteryl 3-β-D-glucoside, and other sterols and steryl glucosides have been isolated from the drug [4, 5]. Phenylpropanes, including homovanillyl alcohol and the corresponding glucoside, as well as lignans of the relatively rare monoepoxylignan type, among them neo-olivil and deriva-tives, have been detected in the drug [6, 15, 16]. An array of polyphenols and their methyl ethers is present [16]. Several monoterpene diols in free and glucosidic form have been isolated [17]. Lectins (0.1–0.2%), the so called UDA (Urtica dioica agglutinin), and polysaccharides (both acid and neutral), as well as 9-hydroxyoctadeca-10-*trans*,12-*cis*-dienoic acid, has also been found [15].

Indications: In *folk medicine* like nettle herb, e.g. as diuretic, but also because of its tannin content as an astringent and gargle. Recently, the use of a extract of Urticae radix has been recommended in benign prostate conditions, especially for treating the congestion and associated difficulties in urination, in the early stages or stages I-IIa of benign prostate hyperplasias. The active substance(s) responsible for these effects is (are) still unknown. It is thought to interfere with testosterone metabolism by lowering the binding capacity of SHBG (sexual hormone-binding globulin), which is associated with a rise in free androgen; it may also interfere with the key enzyme aromatase, the fatty acid listed above having a weak inhibiting effect [2, 7–10, 15]. A consequence of this is supposed to be that the compensating raised metabolism in the prostate adenoma tissue is reduced, resulting in elimination of the congestion and opening of the urethral obstruction [2]. Nettle-root extracts have indeed been shown to have effects on human prostate tissue [11]. Be that as it may, the findings need to be viewed critically, for in a randomized study with Extractum Radicis Urticae [13] objectively measured parameters were not significantly improved. Although alleviation of the problems resulting from the adenoma was observed (note also the studies demonstrating a decrease in the weekly frequency of nycturia after use of a standardized Extractum Radicis Urticae [12]), this was also seen in the placebo group. More recent observations demonstrate again the positive effects in treatment of benign prostate hyperplasias [18].

It is a point of interest whether the new lignans discovered in nettle root [6] are pharmacologically active and whether they are connected with the above-mentioned effects. Lignans are known to have a wide range of activities [14]. Some of the polysaccharides are antiphlogistic and immunostimulant. The lectin mixture stimulates lymphocyte proliferation; it causes immune-induced cytotoxic activity and inhibition of prostaglandin synthesis, and as it is unusually stable to acid and heat it can be administered orally [15].

Making the tea: 1.5 g of the coarsely powdered drug is put into cold water, heated to boiling and kept boiling for ca. 1 min., then covered, and allowed to stand for 10 min., and finally strained.
1 Teaspoon = ca. 1.3 g.

Phytomedicines: In diuretic herbal mixtures; as a monovalent tea; as an extract of the fresh roots in capsules (Extractum Radicis Urticae = ERU, e.g. Bazoton®-Kapseln).

Authentication: Macro- (see: Description) and microscopically following the DAB 10. The lectin content of the lyophilisate (20–30%) can be estimated (and thus allow the possibility of standardization) by ELISA (enzyme-linked immuno-specific assay) or HPLC [15].

Adulteration: Has not so far been observed in the drug trade.

Literature:
[1] Berger, vol. **5**, p. 487 (1960).
[2] R. Hänsel and H. Haas, Therapie mit Phytopharmaka, Springer, Berlin – New York, 1984.
[3] Hager, vol. **6c**, p. 363 (1979).
[4] H. Schilcher and S. Effenberger, Dtsch. Apoth. Ztg. **126**, 79 (1986).
[5] N. Chaurasia and M. Wichtl, Dtsch. Apoth. Ztg. **126**, 81 (1986); idem., J. Nat. Prod. **50**, 881 (1987).
[6] N. Chaurasia and M. Wichtl, Dtsch. Apoth. Ztg. **126**, 1559 (1986).
[7] H. Ziegler, Fortschr. Med. **100**, 1832 (1982).
[8] U. Toschand and H. Müssiggang, euromed **23**, 334 (1983).
[9] H. Ziegler, Fortschr. Med. **101**, 2112 (1983).
[10] J. Djulepa, Mediz. Welt no. **48**, p. 49 (1983).
[11] U. Dunzendorfer, Z. Phytotherap. **5**, 800 (1984).
[12] H.-P. Stahl, Z. Allg. Med. **60**, 128 (1984).
[13] G. Schönefeld, R. Tauber, U. Rattenhuber, and H. Barth, Klin. Exper. Urologie **4**, 179 (1982).
[14] D.C. Ayres and J.D. Loike, Lignans. Chemical, biological, and clinical properties. Cambridge University Press, 1991.
[15] F. Willer, H. Wagner, and E. Schecklies, Dtsch. Apoth. Ztg. **131**, 1217 (1992).
[16] R. Kraus and G. Spiteller, Phytochemistry **29**, 1653 (1990).
[17] R. Kraus and G. Spiteller, Phytochemistry **30**, 1203 (1991).
[18] G. Rutishauser (ed.), Benigne Prostatahyperplasie, W. Zuckschwerdt-Verlag, München, Bern, Wien, New York (1992).

Uvae ursi folium   (DAB 10), Uva ursi (BHP 1/1990), Bearberry leaf

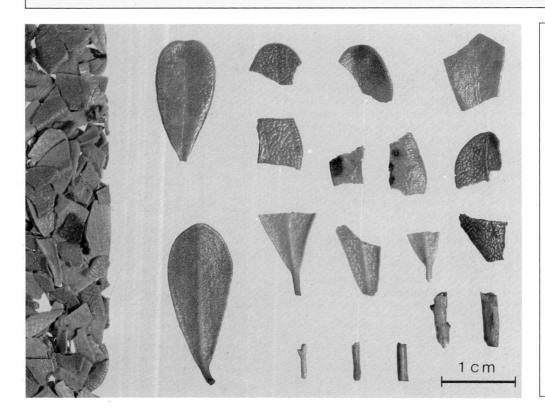

1 cm

Fig. 1: Uva ursi

Description: **The spathulate and thick, leathery, glabrous leaves are glossy green on the upper surface; they have an entire and partly revolute margin, and the venation is distinct and finely reticulate. Very young leaves are pubescent, the unicellular covering trichomes being thick-walled and mostly curved.**

Taste: **Astringent, slightly bitter.**

Fig. 2: *Arctostaphylos uva-ursi* (L.) SPRENG.
Prostrate mat-forming shrub, with evergreen leathery, spathulate leaves. Corolla urceolate and white with reddish tips.

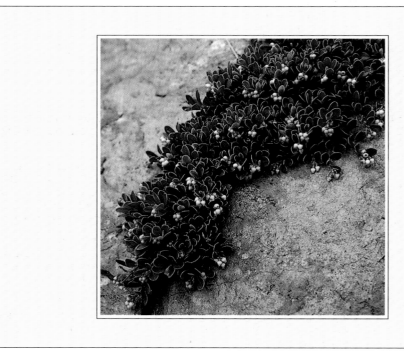

DAB 10: **Bärentraubenblätter**
ÖAB: **Folium Uvae-ursi**
Ph. Helv. VII: **Uvae ursi folium**
St. Zul.: **8299.99.99**

Plant source: *Arctostaphylos uva-ursi* (L.) SPRENG., bearberry (Ericaceae).

Synonyms: Uva-ursi, Arctostaphylos, Ptarmigan berry leaves, Bear's grape, Mountain box (Engl.), Bärentraubenblätter, Wolfsbeere, Wilderbuchs (Ger.), Feuille de busserole, Feuille de raisin d'ours (Fr.).

Origin: A low shrub distributed throughout the northern hemisphere. The drug comes entirely from wild plants growing in Spain, Italy, the Balkans, and the former USSR.

Constituents: Hydroquinone derivatives, mainly arbutin (arbutoside), hydroquinone mono-glucoside, accompanied by a varying, but mostly small, amount of methylarbutin; abundant (ca. 15–20%), of both the gallotannin and catechol types, arbutin gallic acid ester; in addition, flavonoids (especially hyperoside); triterpenes [1–3, 5, 11]; and the

Arbutin: R = H
Methylarbutin: R = CH₃

iridoid glycoside monotropein [4], as well as piceoside (*p*-hydroxyacetophenone glucoside) [5]. Phenol-carboxylic acids, mainly gallic and smaller amounts of *p*-coumaric and syringic acids, are also present [12].

Indications: As a urinary disinfectant in mild inflammatory conditions of the urinary tract and bladder. The antibacterial effect is not due to the arbutin but to the hydroquinone liberated in the urine from the metabolites, hydroquinone glucuronide and hydroquinone sulphate [6, 7]. The required slightly alkaline reaction of the urine, which only happens on infection with *Proteus vulgaris*, can be established, at least for a short period, by giving sodium hydrogen carbonate (bicarbonate); a generous plant-based diet can also contribute to formation of an alkaline urine. The aglycone of piceoside, *p*-hydroxyacetophenone, also has antibacterial activity [11].
According to R.F. Weiß [8], in the case of uva-ursi tea, "even a doctor who hardly practices phytotherapy believes he is doing the right thing in prescribing this well-known tea". The drug does not have a diuretic effect.

Side effects: Because of the high tannin content in the leaves, the tea tastes bitter and astringent, and in patients with a delicate stomach can lead to nausea and vomiting.

Making the tea: Boiling water is poured over 2.5 g of the finely cut or, better, coarsely powdered drug or cold water is added and then boiled for a short period, and after 15 min. filtered. The cold-water macerate (6–12 hours) contains the same amount of arbutin, but less tannins [9, 10].
1 Teaspoon = ca. 2.5 g.

Herbal preparations: The drug is available in tea bags. It is a component of numerous bladder and kidney teas, some of which are offered as the powdered tea, e.g. Solvefort®, Uroflux®, or as tea paste. It is also a component of the bladder and kidney tea NRF 9.1. Among the multi-ingredient products on the UK market are: Gerard House Herbal powder No. 8, Potter's Kas-bah Herb; Potter's Sciargo Herb and Wellwoman Herbs are available in tea bags.

Extract from the German Commission E monograph (BAnz no. 228, dated 05/12/1984)

Uses
For inflammatory disorders of the lower urinary tract.

Contraindications
None known.

Side effects
In patients with a delicate stomach and in children, nausea and vomiting may occur.

Interactions
Uva ursi preparations should not be given together with remedies that will lead to the production of an acid urine.

Dosage
Unless otherwise prescribed: average daily dose, 10 g cut or powdered drug, equivalent to 400–700 mg arbutin in 150 ml water, as an infusion or cold macerate. Care must be taken to ensure an alkaline urine.

Mode of administration
Cut or powdered drug, or dry extracts for infusions, cold macerates, and solid dosage forms. They are exclusively for oral use.

Duration of use
Not suitable for prolonged use without consulting a doctor.

Effects
Bacteriostatic action in alkaline (pH 8) urine, due to the hydroquinone glucuronides and hydroquinone sulphate formed in the body from arbutin. The maximum antibacterial effect is obtained about 3–4 hours after taking the drug.

Wording of the package insert, from the German Standard Licence

5.1 Uses
In supportive treatment for bladder and kidney catarrh.

5.2 Side effects
With a delicate stomach and in children, nausea and vomiting may occur.

Interactions with other remedies
Uva-ursi preparations should not be given together with remedies that will lead to the production of an acid urine.

5.4 Dosage and Mode of administration
A level teaspoonful (ca. 2 g) of powdered **Uva ursi** is boiled in water (ca. 150 ml) for 15 min. and then put through a coffee filter. The tea can also be prepared by putting the drug in cold water and allowing it to draw for several hours.

Unless otherwise prescribed, a cupful is drunk three or four times a day.
Warning: an alkaline urine should be ensured by taking a generous plant-based diet. Sodium hydrogen carbonate (bicarbonate) can be taken as a supplement.

5.5 Duration of use
Uva-ursi teas are not suitable for prolonged use without consulting a doctor.

5.6 Note
Store away from light and moisture.

Phytomedicines: Uvalysat®-Tropfen (drops) and Arctuvan®, are monovalent preparations, but there are many preparations belonging to the group urological remedies in which it is combined with other plants or synthetic components, e.g. Cystinol®, Herniol®, Nephronorm®, etc.
In the UK, uva ursi (bearberry leaf) is a component of more than 50 anti-inflammatory products [13], e.g. Seven Seas Rheumatic Pain Tablets and Backache Tablets (these latter standardized to give 3 mg arbutin), Potter's Sciargo and Potter's Tabritis (both tablets), etc.
The leaf and/or extracts from it are also in a range of multi-ingredient products, mostly diuretics, e.g. Gerard House Buchu Compound Tablets and Waterlax Tablets; Potter's Antitis Tablets, Backache Tablets, Diuretabs, Prementaid Tablets, Sciargo, etc.

Authentication: Macro- and microscopically, following the DAB 10. See also the BHP 1/1990 and [14]. A brown coloration of the leaves indicates a low arbutin content.
The DAB 10 TLC identity test is as follows:

Test solution: 0.5 g powdered drug refluxed for 10 min. with 5 ml 50% aqueous methanol, filtered hot, filter washed with the same solvent, and the volume made up to 5 ml.

Reference solution: 25 mg each of arbutin, gallic acid, and hydroquinone dissolved in 10 ml methanol.

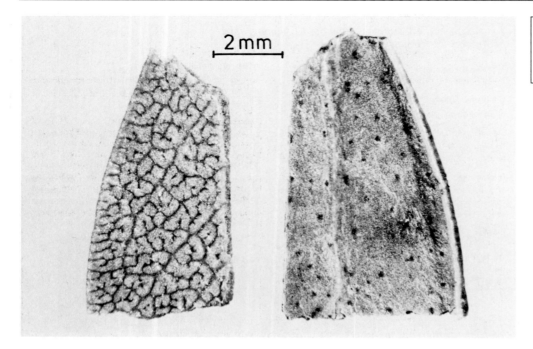

2 mm

Fig. 3: Leaf fragments from *Arctostaphylos uva-ursi* (left) and *Vaccinium vitis-idaea* (right)

Loadings: 20 µl test solution and 10 µl reference solution, as 2-cm bands on silica gel G, and dried for 5 min. in a current of cold air.

Solvent system: ethyl acetate + chloroform + anhydrous formic acid + water (60 + 19 + 12 + 9), 2 × 10 cm run.

Detection: dried at 100–105 °C until disappearance of the formic acid, then sprayed with 1% methanolic dichloroquinonechlorimide, followed by careful exposure to ammonia vapour.

Evaluation: <u>Reference solution</u>: in the lower half, the blue violet arbutin zone; in the upper half the brown to greyish brown gallic-acid zone and slightly above it the brown hydroquinone zone. <u>Test solution</u>: a strong arbutin zone possibly also containing a small amount of methylarbutin, and directly above a grey to greyish green zone (hyperoside); the gallic-acid zone easily recognized, but the brown hydroquinone zone and the blue methylhydroquinone zones only faint; some other grey or greyish blue, mostly weak, zones also present.
The BHP 1/1990 TLC procedure only gives a fingerprint chromatogram.

Quantitative standards: <u>DAB 10</u>: *Hydroquinone derivatives*, not less than 6.0% calculated as anhydrous arbutin (M_r 272.3). *Foreign matter*, not more than 3% and not more than 5% stem fragments. *Loss on drying*, not more than 10.0%. *Ash*, not more than 5.0%.

<u>ÖAB</u>: *Glycoside derivatives*, not less than 5.0% calculated as arbutin (M_r 272.3). *Discolored leaves*, not more than 1%. *Vaccinium vitis-idaea V. uliginosum*, and *Buxus sempervirens* leaves absent. *Ash*, not more than 4.0%

<u>Ph. Helv. VII</u>: *Arbutin*, not less than 8.0% (M_r 272.3). *Foreign matter*, not more than 8% stems and not more than 5% brown-coloured leaves; *Vaccinium vitis-idaea* and *Buxus sempervirens* leaves absent. *Sulphated ash*, not more than 10%.

<u>BHP 1/1990</u>: *Water-soluble extractive*, not less than 25%. *Stems*, not more than 5%. *Foreign matter*, not more than 3%. *Total ash*, not more than 5%. *HCl-insoluble ash*, not more than 1%.

Note: Uvae ursi folium is the subject of an ESCOP proposed European harmonized monograph.

Adulteration: Confusion with other ericaceous leaves, especially with the likewise arbutin-containing cowberry or red whortleberry leaves, *Vaccinium vitis-idaea* L., may occur; usually, such confusion can be easily recognized by the absence of the finely reticulate venation (Fig. 3). Cowberry leaves have paracytic stomata on the lower surface, while bearberry leaves have anomocytic stomata. Admixture can also be detected by means of the TLC method given in the DAB 8, but not by that in the DAB 10. When cowberry leaves are present, after spraying with aluminium chloride solution, the chromatogram shows yellowish green, greenish blue, and blue fluorescent spots in the middle and upper Rf regions which are not found with bearberry leaves.
In DAB 10, detection by means of aluminium chloride is no longer required. Adulteration with box leaves, from *Buxus sempervirens* L., as mentioned in the ÖAB and Ph. Helv. VII, is rarely found to occur in practice.

Literature:
[1] G. Britton and E. Haslam, J. Chem. Soc. 7312 (1965).
[2] K. Herrmann, Arch. Pharm. (Weinheim) **286**, 515 (1953).
[3] Ch. Wähner, J. Schönert, and H. Friedrich, Pharmazie **29**, 616 (1974).
[4] L. Jahodar, I. Leifertova, and M. Lisa, Pharmazie **33**, 536 (1978).
[5] G.A. Karikas, M.R. Euerby, and R.D. Waigh, Planta Med. **53**, 307 (1987).
[6] D. Frohne, Planta Med. **18**, 1 (1970).
[7] B. Kedzia et al., Med. Dosw. Mikrobiol. **27**, 305 (1975).
[8] R.F. Weiß, Herbal Medicine, Arcanum, Gothenburg, and Beaconsfield Publishers, Beaconsfield, 1988.
[9] D. Frohne, Pharm. Ztg. **125**, 2582 (1980).
[10] D. Frohne, Z. Phytotherap. **7**, 45 (1986).
[11] L. Johadár and I. Kolb, Pharmazie **45**, 446 (1990).
[12] E. Dombrowicz, R. Zadernowski, and L. Swiatek, Pharmazie **46**, 680 (1991).
[13] J.D. Phillipson and L.A. Anderson, Pharm. J. **233**, 80, 111 (1984).
[14] B.P. Jackson and D.W. Snowdon, Atlas of microscopy of medicinal plants, culinary herbs and spices, Belhaven Press, London, 1990, p. 16.

Valerianae radix

(Ph. Eur. 2), Valerian (*BAN*; BP 1988), Valerian root (BHP 1/1990)

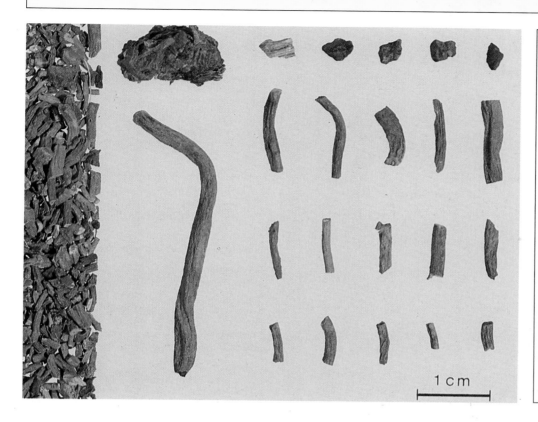

Fig. 1: Valerian root

Description: The drug consists of rhizomes, roots, and stolons. The ovoid-cylindrical, light greyish brown rhizome is about the size of a finger joint and bears many long roots. These are light to medium greyish brown, 1–3 mm thick and several cm long, and are partly covered with coarse longitudinal wrinkles. Stolons are rare in the drug – they are light greyish brown, with a somewhat gnarled appearance.

Odour: Characteristic, reminiscent of isovaleric acid.

Taste: Sweetish and spicy, somewhat bitter.

Figs. 2 and 3: *Valeriana officinalis* L., s.l.

An extremely variable 30–150 cm tall herb, with pinnate to pinnatisect leaves, comprising three subspecies connected by a series of intermediates. Terminal cymes of white or pink flowers having distinctly exserted anthers.

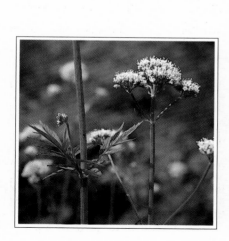

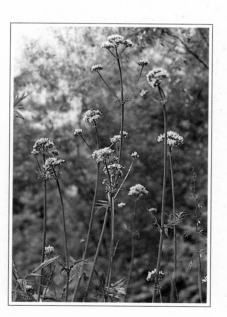

DAB 10: Baldrianwurzel
ÖAB: Radix Valerianae
Ph. Helv. VII: Valerianae Radix
St. Zul. 6199.99.99

Plant source: *Valeriana officinalis* L., s.l., common valerian (Valerianaceae).

Synonyms: Valeriana, Valeriana rhizome (Engl.), Baldrianwurzel, Katzenwurzel, Balderbrackenwurzel (Ger.), Racine de valériane (Fr.).

Origin: Native to Europe and Asia, naturalized in north-eastern America. The drug is cultivated in Holland, Belgium, France, Germany (to a small extent), eastern Europe, and in Japan and the USA.

Constituents: The drug contains 0.3–0.7% essential oil, the composition of which varies considerably according to the source [1]; usually, bornyl acetate is the main constituent, but other sesquiterpenes are always present as well (β-caryophyllene, valeranone, valerenal, etc.) [2]. Carefully dried roots, i.e. roots dried below 40 °C (pharma-

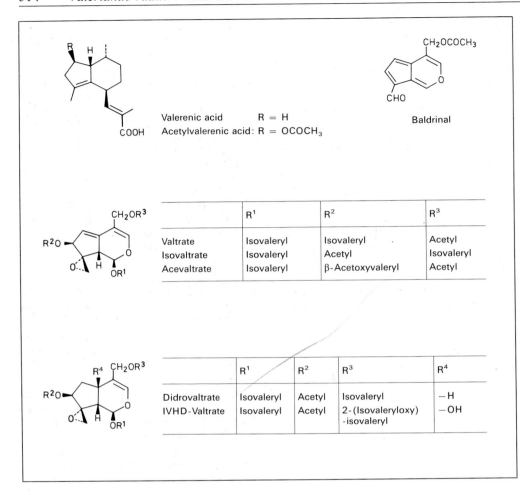

Valerenic acid   R = H
Acetylvalerenic acid: R = OCOCH₃

Baldrinal

	R¹	R²	R³
Valtrate	Isovaleryl	Isovaleryl	Acetyl
Isovaltrate	Isovaleryl	Acetyl	Isovaleryl
Acevaltrate	Isovaleryl	β-Acetoxyvaleryl	Acetyl

	R¹	R²	R³	R⁴
Didrovaltrate	Isovaleryl	Acetyl	Isovaleryl	– H
IVHD-Valtrate	Isovaleryl	Acetyl	2-(Isovaleryloxy)-isovaleryl	– OH

copoeial requirement!), contain 0.5–2% valepotriates (*valeriana epoxy-triester*), bicyclic iridoid monoterpenes. The composition of the valepotriate mixture differs greatly according to the variety [3], but quantitatively valtrate and isovaltrate generally dominate; there are also small amounts of didrovaltrate and IVHD-valtrate (isovaleryloxyhydroxydidrovaltrate) and the glycoside valerosidatum.
Valerenic and acetoxyvalerenic acids (ca. 0.08–0.3%) [4] are characteristic constituents of the official drug – they do not occur in other *Valeriana* species. Valerian root contains very small amounts (0.01–0.05%) of alkaloids such as valerianine and α-methyl pyrryl ketone.

Indications: As the authentication requirements in the pharmacopoeias indicate, views regarding the substances or groups of substances responsible for the sedative effect of the drug (and tincture) have frequently changed during the last 20 years. When Thies [5] discovered the valepotriates, it was

thought that the genuine active constituents had been found; these compounds, however, are not present in infusions and tinctures – but rather their degradation products (the so-called baldrinals) which are probably responsible (at least in part) for the sedative action [6]. The essential oil is also important in regard to the sedative effect of the drug [7] – hence the recent pharmacopoeial requirement for a minimum oil content. For a review of the constituents and biological activity of valerian, see [13].
A sharp distinction must be made between use of the drug (for the preparation of a tea or as a tincture) and use of the isolated valepotriates, e.g. in prepared medicines such as Valmane®, Baldrisedone®, which are employed more as psychostimulants than as sedatives.
The pharmacodynamic effects of a number of the individual constituents have been examined. Thus, valerenic acid is spasmolytic and muscle-relaxant [8]; valerenic acid and related sesquiterpenes inhibit the degradation of the important CNS transmitter γ-

aminobutyric acid [9]. There are now good grounds for believing that the sedative action of valepotriate-free valerian tinctures or teas is brought about by the combined action of the various constituents and degradation products already mentioned [10].
Valerian-root tea and tincture are used as a sedative in nervous tension, restlessness, difficulty in getting to sleep (only to promote sleep, not as a soporific!), and in stress and anxiety states.
On the other hand, the valepotriates or extracts standardized for their valepotriate content (usually 50 mg per dose) are used as

tranquillizers (here, it is the mono-unsaturated valepotriates, e.g. didrovaltrate, that are active) and thymoleptics (here, it is the dienes, e.g. valtrate or acevaltrate, that are active). Such preparations, which always contain a mixture of valepotriates, are usually prepared not from *Valeriana officinalis* but from other *Valeriana* species, e.g. *V. edulis* NUTT. ssp. *procera* MEYER (Mexican valerian) or *V. wallichii* DC. (Indian valerian). They usually contain fairly large amounts of didrovaltrate and isovaltrate; cf. [15]. Such preparations are employed in the treatment of psychomotor and psychosomatic problems, loss of concentration, and stress and anxiety states.

Concern has been expressed about the possible cytoxicity of the epoxide-containing (and hence potentially alkylating) valepotriates. Poor oral absorption and/or distribution of these substances may, however, be a mitigating circumstance [13]. About possible adverse effects, see [14].

Making the tea: 3–5 g of the very finely cut drug is covered with boiling water, allowed to stand for 10–15 min., and then strained. 1 Teaspoon = ca. 2.5 g.

Herbal preparations: Tea bags (mostly containing 2 g) are on the market. The drug is a component of numerous sedative and nerve teas (Species Sedativae ÖAB); aqueous drug extracts are obtainable as instant preparations, etc.

Phytomedicines: Numerous (ca. 60) ready-made hypnotics and sedatives and a few psycho-pharmaceuticals are available.

Preparations for use as tranquillizers, which have been standardized on the basis of their valepotriate content, may be distinguished from those (mostly valepotriate-free) to be employed as sedatives, which contain alcoholic extracts or spray-dried, aqueous alcoholic extracts. Valepotriate preparations include Nervipan®, etc., while valepotriate-free preparations (which are usually not designated as such) often contain extracts from other sedative plants, e.g. Hovaletten®, Plantival®, etc.

In the UK, there are more than 80 products containing valerian root and/or aqueous extracts of it, among them: Gerard House Biophylin Tablets, Gerard 99 Tablets, and Valerian Compound Tablets; Lanes Kalms and Quiet Life Tablets; Potter's Newrelax and Barefoot Brand Valerian Tablets; Seven Seas Nerve Tablets; Arkopharma Phytotranq (capsules). The drug is also a constituent of Gerard House Gladlax Tablets and of Potter's Prementaid Tablets and Wellwoman Tablets, as well as Climacteric Dellipsoids D19, Nerve Dellipsoids D16, and Sedative Tonic Dellipsoids D14.

Regulatory status (UK): General Sales List – Schedule 1, Table A.

Authentication: Macro- (see: Description) and microscopically, following the Ph. Eur. 2 (BP 1988, etc.); the microscopy of the powdered drug is described in [15]. The TLC detection of valerenic acid is the best way of verifying the absence of the roots of other *Valeriana* species, which is very difficult to establish microscopically when in the finely powdered condition.

The following method differs somewhat from that given in the Ph. Eur. 2 (BP 1988, etc.):

Test solution: 0.5 g freshly powdered drug shaken with 15 ml dichloromethane for ca. 5 min. and filtered; the filtrate carefully taken to dryness and the residue dissolved in 0.5 ml methanol.

Reference solution: authentic drug treated in the same way, or 5 mg valerenic acid dissolved in 5 ml methanol.

Loadings: 10 µl each of the test and reference solutions, as 2-cm bands on silica gel.

Solvent system: *n*-hexane + ethyl acetate (70 + 30), 5 cm run.

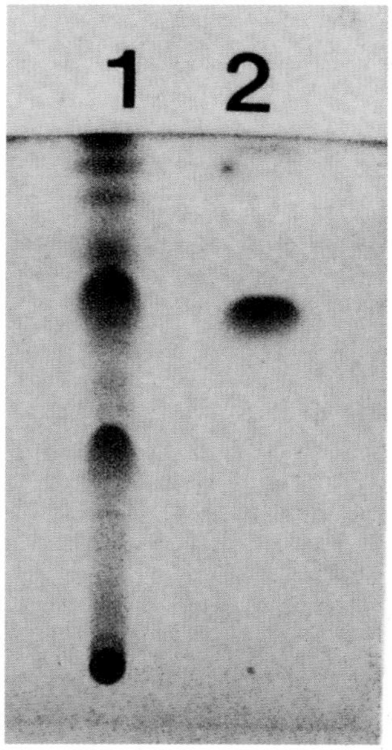

Fig. 4: TLC on 4 × 8 cm silica-gel foil

1: Valerian root
2: Valerenic acid (reference compound)

For details, see the text.

Detection: after evaporation of the solvent, sprayed with anisaldehyde reagent and heated for ca. 3 min. at 100–105 °C.

Evaluation: in daylight. Reference solution: valerenic acid, a bluish violet zone at Rf ca. 0.65. Test solution: a zone with the same colour and intensity as that of the reference solution at the same Rf; also, bluish violet zones at Rf ca. 0.4 and in the upper third between the valerenic-acid zone and the solvent front (Fig. 4).

A suitable TLC method for the valepotriates is as follows [16, 17]:

Test solution: 0.2 g powdered drug warmed at 60 °C for 5 min. with 5 ml dichloromethane and after filtration washed with a further 2 ml solvent; the residue from the combined extracts dissolved in 0.2 ml ethyl acetate or methanol.

Reference solution: 10 mg vanillin and 10 µl anisaldehyde in 10 ml methanol, or 5 mg of individual valepotriates in 5 ml methanol.

Loadings: 10 µl of each as a band on silica gel; drugs with a low valepotriate content may require a 50 µl loading of the test solution.

Solvent system: toluene + ethyl acetate (75 + 25), 15 cm run, giving higher Rf values than *n*-hexane + methyl ethyl ketone (80 + 20), 2 × 15 cm runs.

Detection and Evaluation: after removal of the solvent, sprayed with conc. hydrochloric acid + glacial acetic acid (2 + 8) and heated at 110 °C for 10 min., specific for valtrate and acevaltrate (blue zones) and didrovaltrate (brown zone); or 2,4-dinitrophenylhydrazine reagent (0.2 g in 98% acetic acid + 25% hydrochloric acid + methanol (40 + 40 + 20)) and heated at 100 °C for 5–10 min., giving grey-green or blue zones, in order of decreasing Rf value: isovaltrate/valtrate, didrovaltrate, acevaltrate, IVDH-valtrate, valtrat-hydrins, and degradation products.

Quantitative standards: Ph. Eur. 2, etc.: *Volatile oil*, not less than 0.5%. 60% *Ethanol extractive*, not less than 15.0%. *Sulphated ash*, not more than 15.0%. *Acid-insoluble ash*, not more than 7.0%.

The BHP 1/1990 requires valerian root and powdered valerian to comply with the criteria of the appropriate Ph. Eur. 2 or BP 1988 monographs.

Note: Valerianae radix is the subject of an ESCOP draft proposal for a European harmonized monograph, based on the Ph. Eur. 2 monograph.

Adulteration: Experience shows that adulteration of valerian root is not all that rare. With the whole root, such admixture is generally readily established, but with the cut drug this is almost always difficult and requires use of the microscope. Often, the adulteration is with the roots of other *Valeriana* species, but the roots of Apiaceae have also been found. A good review with illustrations of the microscopic features encountered in such falsifications is to be found in [11]. For the microscopy of Mexican valerian, see [12]. As indicated above (see: Authentication), TLC is a more reliable means of detection. Coloured illustrations of the TLC of the valepotriate mixtures in Mexican and Indian valerian, as well as in pharmaceutical preparations, are given in [16].

Storage: Protected from light; kept in a cool place, but avoiding plastic containers (presence of essential oil).

Literature

[1] R. Bos et al., Phytochemistry **25**, 133 (1986).
[2] W. Titz et al., Sci. Pharm. **51**, 63 (1983).
[3] W. Titz et al., Sci. Pharm. **50**, 309 (1982).
[4] R. Hänsel and J. Schulz, Dtsch. Apoth. Ztg. **122**, 215 (1982).
[5] P.W. Thies et al., Tetrahedron Lett. **1966**, 1155 and 1163; Tetrahedron **24**, 313 (1968).
[6] J. Veith et al., Planta Med. **52**, 179 (1986).
[7] H. Becker and J. Reichling, Dtsch. Apoth. Ztg. **121**, 1185 (1981).
[8] H. Hendriks et al., Planta Med. **42**, 62 (1981).
[9] E. Riedel, R. Hänsel and G. Ehrke, Planta Med. **46**, 219 (1982).
[10] A. Nahrstedt, Schriftenr. Bundesapothekenkammer, Wiss. Fortbild. Gelbe Reihe **1984**, 77.
[11] L. Langhammer and B. Janßen, Pharm. Ztg. **130**, 75 (1985).
[12] L. Langhammer and Chr. Belgard, Pharm. Ztg. **130**, 2653 (1985).
[13] P.J. Houghton, J. Ethnopharmacol. **22**, 121 (1988).
[14] P.F. D'Arcy, Adverse Drug React. Toxicol. Rev. **10**, 189 (1991).
[15] B.P. Jackson and D.W. Snowdon, Atlas of microscopy of medicinal plants, culinary herbs and spices, Belhaven Press, London, 1990, p. 238.
[16] H. Wagner, S. Bladt, and E.M. Zgainski, Plant drug analysis, Springer-Verlag, Berlin, Heidelberg, New York, Tokyo, 1984, p. 266.
[17] E. Stahl (ed.), Drug analysis by chromatography and microscopy, Ann Arbor Science, Ann Arbor, 1973, pp. 191 et seq.

Verbasci flos   Mullein

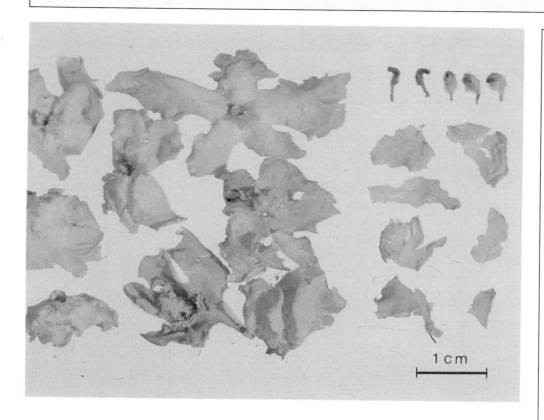

Fig. 1: Mullein flowers

<u>Description</u>: The drug consists only of the corolla and stamens. The yellow 5-part corollas have two smaller upper and three larger lower petals, all with a white tomentum; and fragments of the flowers are also present. There are occasional reddish yellow stamens with tomentose filaments and transversely attached anthers on top (the three short upper stamens of the flowers) or yellow stamens with glabrous filaments (the two long lower stamens of the flowers).

<u>Odour</u>: Faintly honey-like.

<u>Taste</u>: Sweetish and mucilaginous.

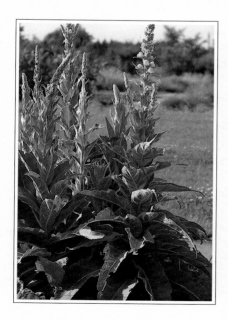

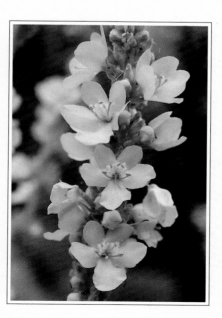

Fig. 2: *Verbascum densiflorum* BERTOL.

A tomentose biennial, up to 2 m in height, with large, greyish white, long elliptic rosette leaves and alternate stem leaves. Numerous groups of 2–5 yellow flowers arranged in long erect racemes.

Fig. 3: *Verbascum densiflorum* BERTOL.

Weakly zygomorphic 5-part flowers with a diameter of up to 5 cm; 5 stamens, the three short ones tomentose and the two long ones glabrous.

DAC 1986: Wollblumen
ÖAB: Flos Verbasci
Ph. Helv. VII: Verbasci flos

Plant sources: *Verbascum densiflorum* BERTOL. (syn. *V. thapsiforme* SCHRAD.), large-flowered mullein, and *V. phlomoides* L., orange mullein (Scrophulariaceae).

Synonyms: Flores Thapsi barbati (Lat.), Verbascum (Engl.), Wollblumen, Königskerzenblumen, Windblumen (Ger.), Fleurs de bouillon blanc, Fleurs de molène (Fr.).

Origin: Native in central, eastern, and southern Europe, Asia Minor, North Africa, and Ethiopia. The drug comes primarily from cultivated plants and is imported from Egypt, Bulgaria, and former Czechoslovakia.

Constituents: Ca. 3% mucilage, yielding after hydrolysis 47% D-galactose, 25% arabinose, 14% D-glucose, 6% D-xylose, 4% L-rhamnose, 2% D-mannose, 1% L-fucose, and 12.5% uronic acids, comprising several components, including a xyloglucan, an arabinogalactan, and an acidic much-branched arabinogalactan [1].
Iridoids: aucubin, 6β-xylosylaucubin, catalpol, 6β-xylosylcatalpol, methylcatalpol, isocatalpol, etc. [2, 3, cf. 10]; saponins (haemolytic index, ca. 350), including verbascosaponin [4, 12]; ca. 1.5–4% flavonoids, among them apigenin and luteolin, and their 7-O-glucosides, kaempferol, rutin, etc. [5, 6]; phenol-carboxylic acids, such as caffeic, ferulic, protocatechuic acids, etc. [7]; sterols;

Aucubin

Catalpol

Verbascosaponin

Digiprolactone

digiprolactone; ca. 11% invert sugar (fructose + glucose).

Indications: For chills, and coughs, etc., in which the effect is due more to the mild expectorant action of the saponins than to the soothing action (covering epithelial damage) of the small amount of mucilage that is present [1]. It has not been possible to demonstrate an effect on the mu-

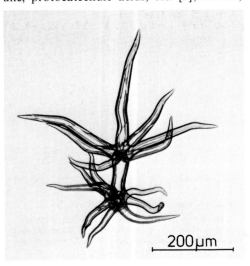

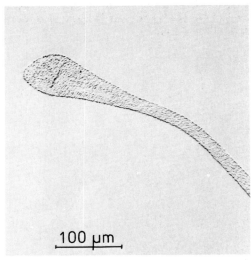

Fig. 4: Candelabra trichome from the petals

Fig. 5: Unicellular club-shaped trichome from the stamens, showing the granular cuticle

200μm

100 μm

Extract from the German Commission E monograph (BAnz no. 22a, dated 01.02.90)

Uses
Catarrh of the respiratory tract.

Contraindications
None known.

Side effects
None known.

Interactions with other remedies
None known.

Dosage
Unless otherwise prescribed: daily dose, 3–4 g drug; preparations correspondingly.

Mode of administration
Comminuted drug for infusions and other galenical preparations for internal use.

Effects
Soothing, expectorant.

co-ciliary activity of the frog ciliated epithelium [8].

In *folk medicine* the drug is also used as a diuretic and antirheumatic, as well as externally for treating wounds. The more recently identified biologically active substances (flavonoids, iridoids) appear to vindicate this application [4].

Note: The BHP 1983 monograph on Verbascum is for the dried leaves and stems of *V. thapsi* L., great mullein, with the indications: bronchitis, tracheitis, influenza with respiratory catarrh, and (topically) for inflamed mucosa. The new monograph (BHP 2/1993) will be entitled Mullein and will be on the flowers.

Making the tea: Boiling water is poured over 1.5–2 g of the finely chopped drug (or it is put into cold water and brought to the boil) and after 10–15 min. passed through a tea strainer.
1 Teaspoon = ca. 0.5 g.

Phytomedicines: Mullein is included in many mixed teas used as antitussives (cough teas, bronchial teas), e.g. Kneipp® Husten-Tee, Salus® Bronchial-Tee; extracts of the drug are also included in instant teas, e.g. Dr. Klingers Bergischer Kräutertee®, Husten- und Bronchialtee.

Authentication: Macro- (see: Description) and microscopically, following the DAC 1986. The candelabra trichomes of the corolla (Fig. 4) and the thin-walled, unicellular trichomes with a granular or sinuate-striate cuticle of the stamens (Fig. 5) are particularly diagnostic.
A suitable method for analysing the flavonoids of the drug is as follows [11, cf. 9]:

Test solution: 1 g powdered drug extracted for 5 min. with 10 ml methanol on the water-bath at 60 °C and then filtered.

Reference solutions: 0.05% solutions of rutin, chlorogenic acid, and hyperoside in methanol.

Loadings: 25–30 µl test solution and 10 µl of each reference solution, on silica gel 60 F_{254}.

Solvent system: ethyl acetate + formic acid + glacial acetic acid + water (100 + 11 + 11 + 27), 15 cm run.

Detection: sprayed with 1% methanolic diphenylboryloxyethylamine, followed by 5% ethanolic polyethylene glycol 400.

Evaluation: In UV 365 nm light. Reference solution: rutin, orange fluorescent zone at Rf ca. 0.35; caffeic acid, bluish fluorescent zone at Rf ca. 0.45; hyperoside, orange fluorescent zone at Rf ca. 0.55. Test solution: three orange fluorescent zones near the level of the reference rutin zone and above and below the level of the reference hyperoside zone (flavone glycosides); a yellowish green fluorescent zone at Rf ca. 0.6 (hesperidin); an intense yellow fluorescent zone at the solvent front (flavonoid aglycones).
An illustration of the chromatogram is to be found in [11].

Quantitative standards: DAC 1986: *Swelling index*, not less than 9. *Foreign matter*, calices and brown- coloured corollas not more than 5% and other foreign matter not more than 2%; *Loss on drying*, not more than 12%. *Ash*, not more than 6%.
ÖAB: *Discoloured flowers*, not more than 3%. *Foreign matter*, not more than 2%. *loss on drying*, not more than 10.0%. *Ash*, not more than 6.0%.

Ph. Helv. VII: *Swelling index*, not less than 12. *Foreign matter*, not more than 5% brown petals and not more than 2% calyx fragments and other foreign matter. *Loss on drying*, not more than 10.0%. *Sulphated ash*, not more than 6.0%.

Adulteration: Very rare. The flowers of other *Verbascum* species are either distinctly smaller or are conspicuous because of the presence of five equal, violet pubescent stamens.

Storage: Protected from light in well-closed containers (best over silica gel). Protection against moisture is particularly important for this drug, since otherwise it readily turns brown to dark brown because of the iridoids present.

Literature:
[1] K. Kraus and G. Franz, Dtsch. Apoth. Ztg. **127**, 665 (1987).
[2] K. Seifert et al., Planta Med. **51**, 409 (1985).
[3] L. Swiatek, O. Salama und O. Sticher, Planta Med. **45**, 153 (1982).
[4] R.Tschesche, S. Sepulveda and M.Th. Braun, Chem. Ber. **113**, 1754 (1980).
[5] V. Pápav et al., Pharmazie **35**, 334 (1980).
[6] R. Tschesche, S. Delhri and S. Sepulveda, Phytochemistry **18**, 1248 (1979).
[7] L. Swiatek, A. Kurowska and D. Rotkiewicz, Herba Pol. **30**, 173 (1984).
[8] W. Müller-Limmroth and H.-H. Fröhlich, Fortschr. d. Med. **98**, 95 (1980).
[9] P. Rohdewald, G. Rücker and K.-W. Glombitza, Apothekengerechte Prüfvorschriften, Deutscher Apotheker-Verlag Stuttgart 1986, S. 1069.
[10] L. Swiatek, B. Grabias, and P. Junior, Pharm. Weekbl. (Sci. ed.) **9**, 246 (1987).
[11] H. Wagner, S. Bladt, and E.M. Zgainski, Plant drug analysis, Springer-Verlag, Berlin, Heidelberg, New York, Tokyo, 1984, p. 178.
[12] E. Haslinger and H. Schröder, Sci. Pharm. **60**, 202 (1992).

Verbenae herba
Vervain, Verbena (BHP 1983)

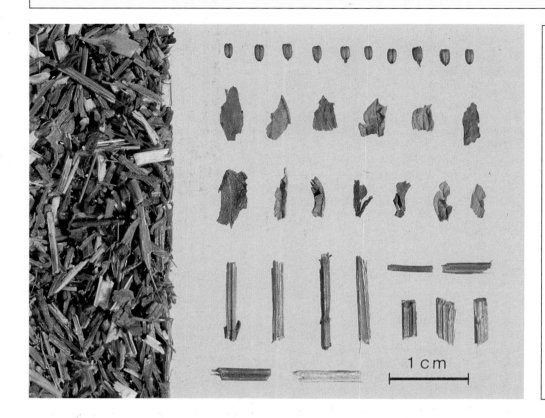

Fig. 1: Vervain

<u>Description:</u> The 4-angled, rough stem bears sessile to short-petioled, oblanceolate to rhombic, pinnatifid leaves with coarsely incised, crenate lobes. The flowers are in spikes or panicles and they have a 4–5-part calyx and an obscurely 2-lipped, 5-part, pale lilac corolla. The dehiscent fruit are brown and readily fall apart into four nutlets (Fig. 3).

<u>Taste:</u> Bitter and sharp.

Fig. 1: *Verbena officinalis* L.

A perennial herb, up to 70 cm in height. Stem woody at the base, leaves opposite, unevenly incised. Pale lilac flowers in 10–25 cm long spikes.

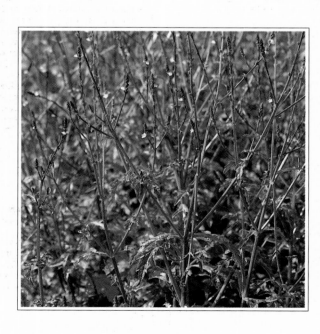

Erg. B. 6: Herba Verbenae

Plant source: *Verbena officinalis* L., vervain (Verbenaceae).

Synonyms: Vervain herb (Engl.), Eisenkraut, Taubenkraut (Ger.), Herbe de vervaine officinale, Herbe à tous les maux (Fr.).

Origin: A scattered to widely distributed weed in all the temperate regions of the earth. The drug is collected from the wild in south-eastern Europe.

Constituents: 0.2–0.5% iridoid glycosides (verbenalin, hastatoside); caffeic-acid derivatives such as verbascoside; traces of essential oil; bitter substances (? possibly identical with the iridoids); some mucilage.

Indications: Almost exclusively in *folk medicine* as a diuretic, as an astringent for poorly healing wounds and in fever, as a galactagogue, as an expectorant in chronic bronchitis, and as an antirheumatic. There are very few pharmacological or clinical

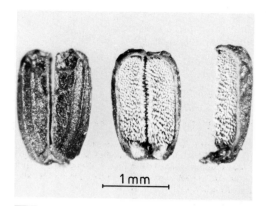

Fig. 3: **Dehiscent fruit, breaking up into four nutlets**

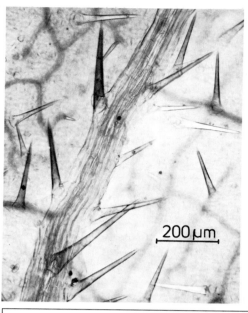

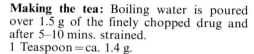

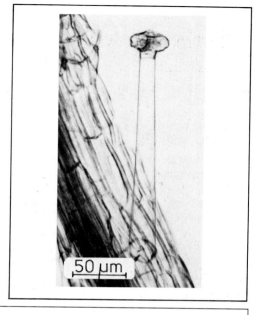

Fig. 4: **Stiff bristles, present on both leaf surfaces**

Fig. 5: **Longer, glandular trichomes, occurring especially over the veins of the leaf**

findings reported for this drug; on the other hand, the iridoids have been tested in experimental animals and shown to have antiphlogistic, analgesic, and weak parasympathomimetic activities. Verbenalin is said to have antitussive activity [1].

At the Peking Medical College it has been established that Herba Verbenae acts as a synergist to prostaglandin E_2. There, the possibility of using vervain preparations to induce abortion has been discussed (C. A. **82**, 149650 [1975]).

Extracts of vervain are antithyrotropic; some constituents attach themselves to the TSH receptor or combine with TSH [2].

Making the tea: Boiling water is poured over 1.5 g of the finely chopped drug and after 5–10 mins. strained.
1 Teaspoon = ca. 1.4 g.

Herbal preparations: The drug is also available in tea bags (1.5 g); checking for the correct content is sometimes advisable.

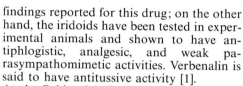

Verbenalin (= Cornin)

Hastatoside

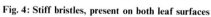

Verbascoside

Extract from the German Commission E monograph
(BAnz no. 22a, dated 01. 02. 90)

Uses

Vervain preparations are used for the following indications: disorders and complaints involving the mucous membranes of the mouth and throat, such as angina and neck pains, for respiratory complaints such as coughs, asthma, whooping cough, also for aches, cramps, exhaustion, nervous disorders, digestive upsets, liver and biliary disorders, jaundice, disorders and complaints involving the kidneys and lower urinary tract, for menopausal complaints, irregular periods, for promoting the secretion of milk during lactation, also for rheumatic disorders, arthritis, metabolic upsets, "greensickness" [chlorosis, anaemia], "water retention" [oedema], and externally for poorly healing wounds, sores, and burns.

Risks

None known.

Evaluation

Since activity in the indications listed has not been substantiated, therapeutic application of the drug cannot be recommended.

Because of its secretolytic action, it is possible that the drug can contribute positively to the activity of established combinations for use in catarrh of the upper respiratory tract. However, the contribution to such preparations must be specifically determined.

Effect

Secretolytic.

Phytomedicines: The drug is a component of herbal mixtures with widely differing indications, corresponding to the uses in *folk medicine*.

Among the UK products containing the herb are Potter's Newrelax and Prementaid (both tablets) and· Seven Seas Catarrh Tablets.

Regulatory status (UK): General Sales List – Schedule 1, Table A.

Authentication: Macro- (see: Description) and microscopically. The up to 500 µm long, unicellular, thick-walled trichomes are characteristic (Fig. 4); they are found particularly at the leaf margin and over the veins on the lower surface of the leaf; the base of the trichome is surrounded by a single ring of domed, spherical epidermal cells. Ca. 200 µm long glandular trichomes (Fig. 5) and short glandular trichomes with a 4-celled head are also present. See the BHP 1983 for a detailed description of the microscopy of the powdered drug.

Quantitative standards: Erg. B. 6: Ash, not more than 12%.

BHP 1983: *Foreign organic matter*, not more than 2%. *Total ash*, not more than 10%. *Acid-insoluble ash*, not more than 2%.

Adulteration: Has not been observed in the drug trade.

Literature:
[1] Ch. Kui and R. Tang, Zhongyao Tongbao **10**, 467 (1985); C.A. **104**, 203945 (1986).
[2] M. Auf'm Kolk et al., Endocrinology **116**, 1687 (1985).

Veronicae herba   Speedwell herb

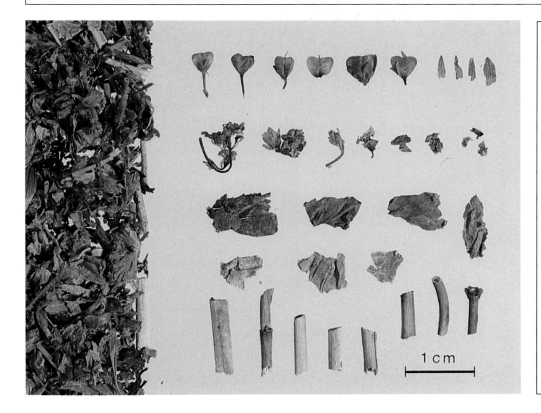

Fig. 1: Speedwell herb

<u>Description:</u> The thin, terete, brown pieces of stem have 1–2.5 cm long, obovate to lanceolate leaves with a serrate margin and with a short and rough pubescence. The small flowers are up to 5 mm long and occur in compact, many-flowered, axillary racemes; the fruit is flat and heart-shaped (upper row, Fig. 1; Fig. 3).

<u>Odour:</u> Very faintly aromatic.

<u>Taste:</u> Slightly bitter, somewhat astringent.

1 cm

Fig. 2: *Veronica officinalis* L.

A low perennial herb, up to 20 cm in height. Leaves opposite, hairy. Flowers pale blue, in erect racemes.

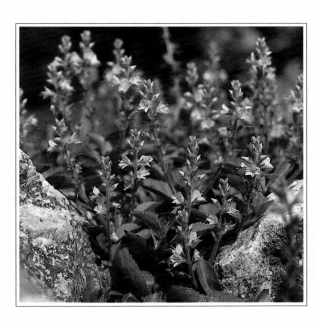

Erg. B. 6: Herba Veronicae

Plant source: *Veronica officinalis* L., heath or common speedwell (Scrophulariaceae).

Synonyms: Herba Betonicae albae (Lat.), Ehrenpreiskraut, Wundkraut (Ger.), Herbe de véronique, Herbe aux ladres (Fr.).

Origin: In light woods especially in the mountains of Europe, western Asia, and North America. Drug imports come from Bulgaria, former Yugoslavia, and Hungary.

Constituents: Ca. 0.5–1% iridoid glycosides (catalpol, veronicoside [=6-benzoylcatalpol], verproside, ladroside, etc. [1–3]); flavonoids [4] (mainly derivatives of luteolin); mannitol; tannins; chlorogenic acid, caffeic acid, etc.; triterpenes; β-sitosterol; all these substances only in in small amounts.

Indications: Only in *folk medicine*, as an expectorant in bronchitis and bronchial asthma. As a tea, also against arthritis and rheumatic complaints. Pharmacological and

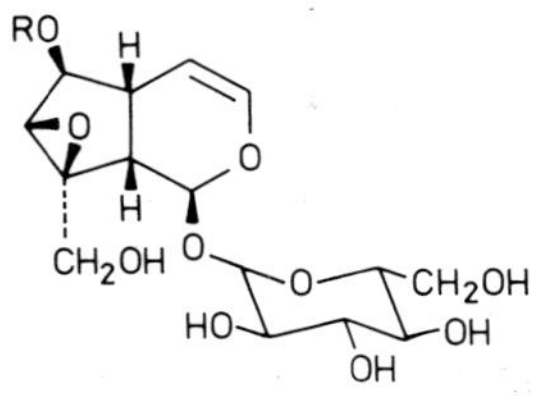

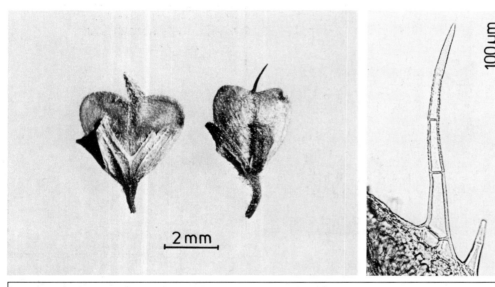

Catalpol: R = H
Veronicoside: R = Benzoyl
Verproside: R = Protocatechuic acid residue

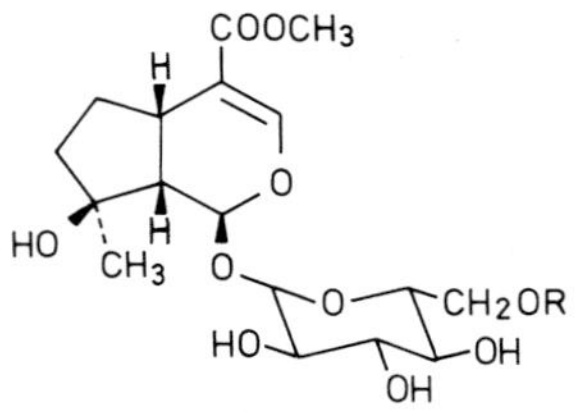

Mussaenoside: R = H
Ladroside: R = Caffeoyl

Extract from the German Commission E monograph (BAnz no. 43, dated 02. 03. 89)

Uses

Preparations of speedwell herb are used for disorders and complaints affecting the respiratory tract, gastro-intestinal tract, liver and kidneys and lower urinary tract, for arthritis, rheumatism, and rheumatic complaints, disorders of the spleen, scrofulosis, nervous hyper-irritability, for "purifying the blood", stimulating the digestion, stimulating the appetite, as tonic and diaphoretic, also externally for sweaty feet, wounds, and to promote wound healing, chronic skin complaints and itching.
Evidence for activity in the indications listed is lacking.

Risks

None known.

Evaluation

Since activity in the indications listed has not been substantiated, therapeutic use cannot be endorsed.

Fig. 3: ***Veronica officinalis*****, flat heart-shaped fruit capsules, together with the narrowly lanceolate sepals**

Fig. 4: Multicellular, thick-walled covering trichome with a rough cuticle, from the leaves

clinical evidence for these indications is lacking.

Making the tea: Boiling water is poured over 1.5 g of the finely cut drug and after 10 min. strained. As an expectorant, a cupful is drunk two or three times a day.
1 Teaspoon = ca. 1 g.

Phytomedicines: The drug is a very occasional component of herbal mixtures used as cough remedies and biliary remedies.

Authentication: Macro- (see: Description) and microscopically. On the leaves and stems there are numerous covering trichomes with a rough cuticle (Fig. 4) and glandular trichomes with a unicellular stem and a bicellular, oblong head. A suitable method for analysing the flavonoids of the drug is as follows [5]:

Test solution: 1 g powdered drug extracted for 5 min. with 10 ml methanol on the water-bath at 60 °C and then filtered.

Reference solutions: 0.05% solutions of rutin, chlorogenic acid, and hyperoside, isochlorogenic acid, and caffeic acid in methanol.

Loadings: 25–30 µl test solution and 10 µl of each reference solution, on silica gel 60 F_{254}.

Solvent system: ethyl acetate + formic acid + glacial acetic acid + water (100 + 11 + 11 + 27), 15 cm run.

Detection: sprayed with 1% methanolic diphenylboryloxyethylamine, followed by 5% ethanolic polyethylene glycol 4000.

Evaluation: in UV 365 nm light. Reference solution: rutin, orange fluorescent zone at Rf ca. 0.35; caffeic acid, bluish fluorescent zone at Rf ca. 0.45; hyperoside, orange fluorescent zone at Rf ca. 0.55; isochlorogenic and caffeic acids as bluish fluorescent zones at Rf ca. 0.8 and 0.95. Test solution: rutin zone weak; orange fluorescent zone at the solvent front more pronounced; blue fluorescent zones due partly to phenol carboxylic acid.
An illustration of the chromatogram is to be found in [5].

Quantitative standard: Erg. B. 6: *Ash*, not more than 10%.

Adulteration: In practice, rarely occurs.

Literature:

[1] O. Sticher and F.Ü. Afifi-Yazar, Helv. Chim. Acta **62**, 530, 535 (1979).
[2] F.Ü. Afifi-Yazar and O. Sticher, Helv. Chim. Acta **63**, 1905 (1980).
[3] F.Ü. Afifi-Yazar, O. Sticher, S. Useato, K. Nagajima, and H. Inouye, Helv. Chim. Acta **64**, 16 (1981).
[4] M. Tamas et al., Clujul Med. **57**, 169 (1984); C.A. **102**, 75759 (1985).
[5] H. Wagner, S. Bladt, and E.M. Zgainski, Plant drug analysis, Springer-Verlag, Berlin, Heidelberg, New York, Tokyo, 1984, p. 186.

Viburni prunifolii cortex   Black haw bark, Viburnum prunifolium (BHP 1983)

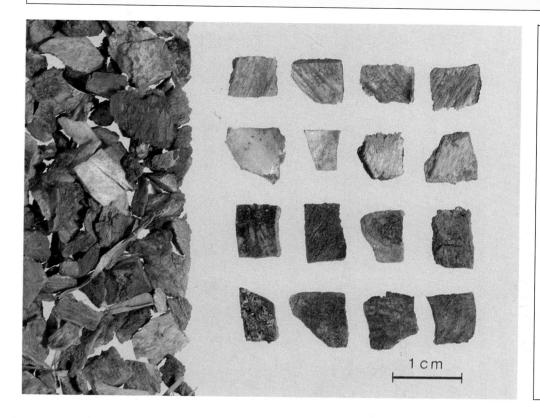

Fig. 1: Black haw bark

Description: The drug consists of the trunk and branch bark, but occasionally the root bark is also found on the market. The cut drug is greyish brown on the outside and, depending on the age, more or less covered with grey lichen and round to transverse corky nodules. The inner surface is reddish brown, smooth to slightly longitudinally striated and often attached fragments of the yellowish wood are still present. The fracture is short and coarsely granular. In the transverse section, yellow dots or spots (groups of stone cells) can be seen with a hand lens.

Odour: Characteristic, faintly tan-like.

Taste: Bitter and astringent.

Erg. B. 6: Cortex Viburni prunifolii

Plant source: *Viburnum prunifolium* L., black haw (Caprifoliaceae).

Synonyms: Sweet viburnum, American sloe, Stagbush (Engl.), Schneeballbaumrinde (Ger.), Écorce de Viburnum (Fr.).

Origin: Native in North America; planted as a decorative bush in Europe. The drug is imported from the USA.

Constituents: Amentoflavone (a biflavone); triterpenes: α- and β-amyrin, oleanolic and ursolic acids and their acetates; sitosterol; coumarins: scopoletin, scopolin, aesculetin; arbutin (?); chlorogenic, isochlorogenic, and salicylic acids and salicoside (?) (=salicin); fatty acids and low-molecular weight organic acids; alkanes; ca. 2% tannis.

Indications: Black haw bark is considered to be a uterine spasmolytic and is used to calm and alleviate uterine pain, thus in menstrual disorders (dysmenorrhoea and amenorrhoea). There have been reports by several groups describing *in-vivo* and *in-vitro* experiments demonstrating the spasmolytic action on the musculature of the uterus, which also takes place after oral administration [incl.

Amentoflavone

Aesculetin: $R^1 = R^2 = -H$
Scopoletin: $R^1 = H, R^2 = -CH_3$
Scopolin: $R^1 = $ Glucose, $R^2 = -CH_3$

1–3, where there is further literature]. The active principle is still unknown. According to [4], the methanolic extract contains at least four substances which supposedly act directly on the musculature of the uterus and not as sympathomimetics. Scopoletin and aesculetin are also active as musculotropic spasmolytics [1, 2].

In *folk medicine*, the drug is also employed in treating morning sickness and menopausal complaints. Use as a contraceptive has also been recorded [5].

Making the tea: Boiling water is poured over 1.0 g of the finely chopped drug and after 10 min. passed through a tea strainer. As a spasmolytic, mainly for dysmenorrhoea, a cup of the infusion two or three times a day.

1 Teaspoon = ca. 1.2 g.

Phytomedicines: The drug is seldom used.

Authentication: Macro- (see: Description) and microscopically. See also the BHP 1983. The cork consists of thin-walled, tabular cells with a brown content; the parenchyma of the primary phloem is stout-walled and tangentially elongated, and it is occasionally interspersed with small stone cells. At the boundary of the secondary phloem, there are isolated, heavily thickened, lignified fibres, which also often occur in groups. Only older pieces of bark have secondary phloem and in it there are groups of stone cells and both uniseriate and biseriate medullary rays, the cell contents of which are stained brownish red with caustic potash. The somewhat thickened parenchyma cells contain starch and tannin (green colour with iron(III) chloride). In longitudinal section, septate fibres with clusters or, more rarely single, crystals of calcium oxalate can be seen.

Adulteration: Occasionally, pieces of the bark of *Viburnum opulus* L., guelder rose, are found; they cannot be distinguished macroscopically or microscopically with certainty from the genuine drug. On the other hand, the following TLC test of purity is suitable for the purpose:

Test solution: resin and fat constituents first removed by refluxing 2 g powdered drug with 50 ml light petroleum for 15 min.; the marc then refluxed with 50 ml methanol and filtered; the filtrate concentrated to ca. 2 ml; any turbidity present does not affect the analysis.

Reference solution: 20 mg cianidanol (catechol) dissolved in 10 ml methanol.

Loadings: 4 µl test solution and 1 µl reference solution, as bands.

Solvent system: chloroform + acetone + glacial acetic acid (75 + 10 + 25), 6 cm run.

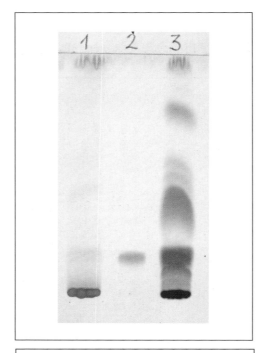

Fig. 2: TLC on 4 × 8 cm silica-gel foil

1: *Viburnum prunifolium*
2: **Catechol (reference compound)**
3: *Viburnum opulus* **(adulterant)**

For details, see the text

Detection: fluorescence under UV 366 nm light first noted, then sprayed with 1% vanillin in 20% ethanolic phosphoric acid and examined immediately in daylight.

Evaluation: in UV 366 nm light before spraying. Test solution: besides intense fluorescent zones bands in the lower third, a blue fluorescent band at Rf ca. 0.85 – absent from the *V. opulus* chromatogram. After spraying. Reference solution: a red zone at Rf ca. 0.2. Test solution: no red zones in this region, while with the adulterant at the level of the catechol zone a red zone and immediately below it a violet-grey zone band and slightly above it two reddish violet zones (Fig. 2).

A TLC produced in the same way but sprayed with 1% methanolic diphenylboryloxyethylamine, followed by 5% ethanolic polyethylene glycol 400 and examined under UV 365 nm light. Test solution: an intense green fluorescent zone (amentoflavone) at Rf ca. 0.2–0.3, absent in adulterants.

Other TLC procedures allowing the two materials to be differentiated are described in [6].

Quantitative standard: <u>BHP 1983</u>: *Ash*, not more than 3%.

Literature:
[1] L. Hörhammer, H. Wagner, and H. Reinhardt, Dtsch. Apoth. Ztg. **105**, 1371 (1965).
[2] L. Hörhammer, H. Wagner, and H. Reinhardt, Z. Naturforsch. **22b**, 768 (1967).
[3] F. Morales and J.S. Mutis, Farmacoterap. Actual **3**, 84 (1946).
[4] C.H. Jarboe, C.M. Schmidt, K.A. Nicholson, and K.A. Zirvi, Nature (London) **212**, 837 (1967).
[5] V.J. Brondegaard, Planta Med. **23**, 167 (1973).
[6] H. Wagner, S. Bladt, and E.M. Zgainski, Plant drug analysis, Springer-Verlag, Berlin, Heidelberg, New York, Tokyo, 1984, p. 122.

Violae tricoloris herba   Wild pansy Viola tricolor (BHP 1983)

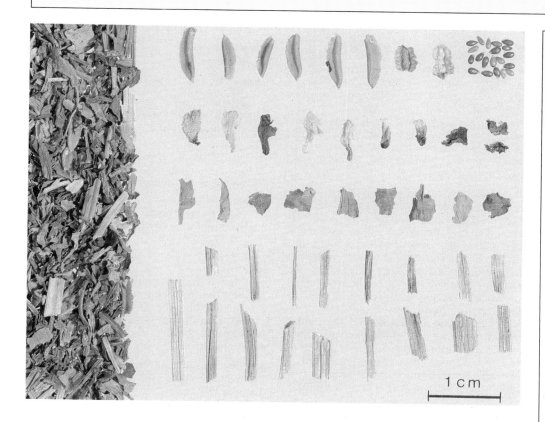

Fig. 1: Wild pansy

Description: The deep blue and bright yellow and/or pale violet to white, mostly rolled-up flowers and petals are characteristic. Often present as well are yellow to yellowish brown, closed or longitudinally dehiscent three-valved loculicidal capsules (or boat-shaped pieces of them) with numerous, pale yellow, pear-shaped seeds bearing a whitish appendix (elaiosome; Fig. 3). In addition, pieces of the thin, roundish or angular stem and pale green, much crumpled leaf fragments may be found.

Odour: Very faint, characteristic.

Taste: Mucilaginous and sweetish.

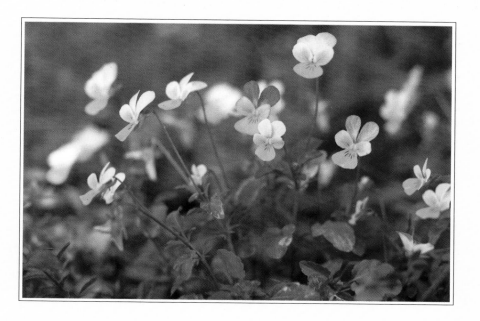

Fig. 2: *Viola tricolor* L.

A polymorphic annual to perennial species, up to 30 cm tall, with cordate to oblong-ovate, bluntly dentate leaves and pinnately divided stipules. Yellow, violet, or three-coloured, zygomorphic flowers, ca. 2 cm in diameter, provided with a short spur.

DAC 1986: Stiefmütterchenkraut
ÖAB: Herba Violae tricoloris
St. Zul. 1679.99.99

Plant source: *Viola tricolor* L. wild pansy (Violaceae).

Synonyms: Herba Jaceae, Herba Trinitatis (Lat.), Heartsease herb, Blue violet, Love-in-idleness (Engl.), Stiefmütterchenkraut, Ackerveilchen (Ger.), Herbe de pensée sauvage, Violette tricolore (Fr.).

Origin: Native in the temperate zones of Europe and Asia, in many subspecies, varieties, and forms; The sources of the drug are particularly the subsp. *vulgaris* (KOCH) OBORNÝ and subsp. *arvensis* (MURRAY) GAUDIN; the latter subsp. is more or less cosmopolitan as a weed in cornfields.

To obtain the drug, the aerial parts of the plant are collected in the wild at the time of flowering; however, it is also cultivated to some extent, e.g. in the Netherlands and France. The drug is imported from the Netherlands.

Constituents: 0.065 to ca. 0.3% salicylic acid and its derivatives such as the methyl ester

Salicylic acid methyl ester

and violutoside (= violutosin, the glucosido-arabinoside of salicylic acid methyl ester), further phenolic carboxylic acids such as *trans*-caffeic acid, *trans*- and *cis-p*-coumaric acids, gentisic acid, protocatechuic acid, etc. [1].

Ca. 10% mucilage, made up of glucose (35%), galactose (33%), arabinose (18%), and rhamnose (8%). 2.4–4.5% Tannins. Flavonoids: rutin (= violaquercitrin), violanthin, scoparin, saponarin, and the *C*-glycosides vitexin, saponaretin, orientin, and iso-orientin, and also vicenin 2. Anthocyanidin glycosides; carotenoids; violaxanthin and four geometrical isomers [2], zeaxanthin, etc.; coumarins: umbelliferone; small amounts of saponins, ascorbic acid, and α-tocopherol.

Indications: Externally and internally as an adjuvant in treating various skin conditions, such as eczema, impetigo, acne, and pruritus. The therapeutic activity in certain skin complaints has been demonstrated in animal (rat) experiments [3]. There are further indications, derived from the older *folk medicine*: catarrh of the respiratory tract, whooping cough, inflammation of the throat (gargle), and feverish chills. What the active principles are has not yet been determined. Salicylic acid and its derivatives, the so-far unidentified saponins, the flavonoids, and mucilage are all discussed in connection with the various indications listed.

In *folk medicine*, the drug is considered to be a "blood-cleansing" agent, i.e. it is supposed to deploy a metabolism-promoting action; it is therefore employed as an adjuvant for appropriate indications, as diuretic, di-

aphoretic, and purgative, as well as in rheumatism (salicylic acid?), arthritis, and arteriosclerosis. The diuretic activity is disputed. According to [4], the amount of urine is not increased, but the excretion of chloride is raised.

Making the tea: Boiling water (ca. 150 ml) is poured over 1.5 g of the finely chopped drug, or the drug is put into cold water and boiled, and strained after 10 min.
1 Teaspoon = ca. 1.2 g.

Phytomedicines: The drug and extracts prepared from it are components of some prepared antitussives, cholagogues, dermatological remedies, roborants and tonics, alteratives, and anti-phlebitis remedies.

Authentication: Macro- (see: Description) and microscopically, following the DAC 1986. See also the BHP 1983. Among the diagnostic features are: the incisor-shaped trichomes on the leaves (Fig. 4), the papillae, the bottle-shaped and humpbacked covering trichomes on the petals, the thickened endothecia shaped which are like a trefoil leaf, and the smooth pollen grains which are ca. 50 µm in diameter.

The following TLC procedure for detecting salicylic acid is similar to that given in the DAC 1986 and is a suitable identity test:

Test solution: 2.0 g powdered drug boiled for 45 min. with 20 mg sodium EDTA (which can, if desired, be omitted), and 25 ml 2N

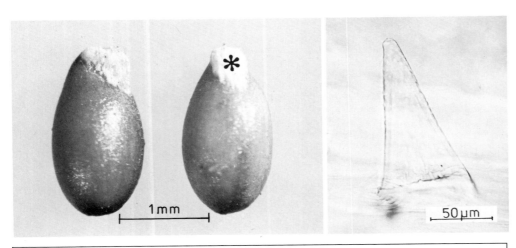

Fig. 3: Pear-shaped seeds from *Viola tricolor*, showing the small white appendage (*) or elaiosome[1]

Fig. 4: Incisor-shaped trichome with cuticular striations, from the leaf

---

[1]) A short funiculus (stalk attaching the ovule to the ovary wall or placenta) which has swollen to form an oil body.

sulphuric acid. After cooling, the filtrate extracted 3× with 40 ml chloroform and the combined chloroform phases dried over anhydrous sodium sulphate, filtered, taken to dryness, and dissolved in 2 ml ethanol.

Reference solution: 10 mg salicylic acid dissolved in 10 ml ethanol.

Loadings: 6 µl test solution and 2 µl reference solution, as bands.

Solvent system: chloroform + toluene + ether + anhydrous formic acid (60 + 60 + 15 + 5), 5 cm run.

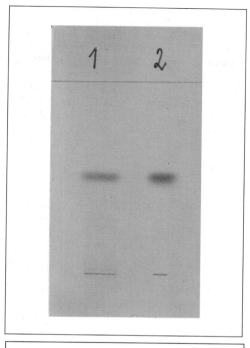

Fig. 5: TLC on 4 × 8 cm silica-gel foil
1: Wild pansy
2: Salicylic acid (reference substance)
For details, see the text

Detection: solvent removed in a current of hot air, sprayed with a 10.5% iron(III) chloride solution.

Evaluation: in daylight. Reference compound: a reddish violet zone on a brownish background. Test solution: a similar reddish violet zone at the same Rf value (Fig. 5). Both zones later turn grey.
The DAC 1986 also gives a method for determining the flavonoid content.

Quantitative standards: DAC 1986: *Flavonoids*, not less than 0.2% calculated as hyperoside (M_r 464.4). *Foreign matter*, not more than 3%. *Loss on drying*, not more than 10%. *Ash*, not more than 14%.
ÖAB: *Foreign matter*, not more than 1%. *Ash*, not more than 12.0%. *Acid-soluble ash*, not more than 1.0%.
BHP 1983: *Total ash*, not more than 15%. *Acid-insoluble ash*, not more than 4%.

Adulteration: In practice, does not occur.

Literature:
[1] T. Komorowski et al., Herba Polon. **29**, 5 (1983).
[2] P. Molnár, J. Szaboles, and L. Radics, Phytochemistry **25**, 195 (1986).
[3] Hager, vol. **6C**, p. 484 (1979).
[4] H. Vollmer and R. Weidlich, Arch Exptl. Pathol. Pharmacol. **186**, 574 (1936).

Virgaureae herba   Golden rod, Virgaurea (BHP 1983)

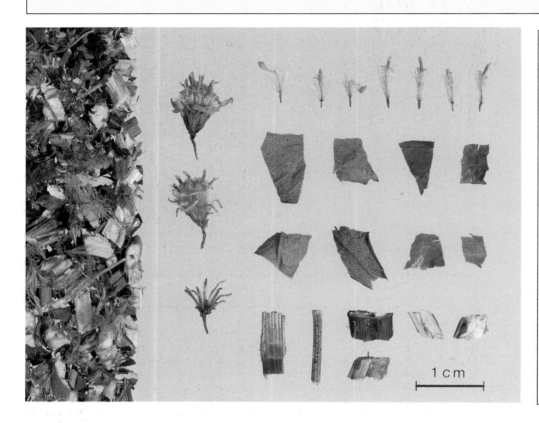

1 cm

Fig. 1: Golden rod

Description: The drug consists of the dried aerial parts of the plant harvested during the flowering period (August/October). The golden-yellow flower buds with their involucre are characteristic; the involucre is composed of membranaceous, imbricate, appressed, whitish green bracts with a glossy inner surface and a green midrib, together with peripheral ray florets and central disk florets, both with a whitish pappus. A few yellow flowers with pappus, grey to brownish grey, somewhat shrivelled leaf fragments with an entire margin and densely reticulate nervature (Fig. 3), and mostly reddish violet dark longitudinally striated pieces of stem containing pith, may also be present.

Taste: Sharp, somewhat astringent.

Fig. 2: *Solidago virgaurea* L.

A perennial herb up to 1 m in height. Lower stem leaves elliptic, with a serrate margin; the upper leaves narrow. Yellow flower-heads with 6–12 ray florets in compound racemes.

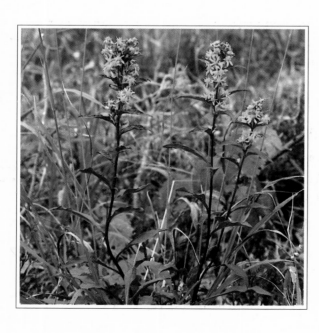

St. Zul. 1519.99.99 (Goldrutenkraut)

Plant source: *Solidago virgaurea* L., golden rod (Asteraceae); see further the section: Adulteration.

Synonyms: Herba Solidaginis virgaureae, Herba Consolidae aureae (Lat.), Goldrutenkraut, Goldwundkraut (Ger.), Herbe de verge d'or (Fr.).

Origin: Native in Europe, Asia (outside subtropical and tropical regions), North Africa, North America. The drug comes from the wild and is imported from Hungary, former Yugoslavia, Bulgaria, and Poland. For the preparation of homoeopathic remedies, it is cultivated on a small scale under contract.

Constituents: Ca. 1.4% flavonoids with quercetin, rutin, quercitrin, isoquercitrin, kaempferol, astragalin, and kaempferol 3-*O*-rutinoside (=nicotiflorin), as well as isorhamnetin and the 3-*O*-glucorhamnosides of rhamnetin, isorhamnetin, and kaempferol [1]. Anthocyanidins: cyanidin 3-

diglucoside and 3-*O*-gentiobioside (=mycocyanin). Ca. 2.4% saponins (haemolytic index, ca. 55,000; haemolytic index of the drug, 250–1000); of the eight aglycones obtained after hydrolysis, two have been identified as oleanolic acid and polygalic acid [2]. The principal components include two bisdesmosidic polygalic-acid ester saponins; they occur in the plant esterified with acetic acid and crotonic acid and combined with a tetrasaccharide at C(28), as an ester glycoside, and with β-D-glucose or β-D-glucosyl-(13)-β-D-glucoside at C(3) (=virgaureasaponins 1 and 2) [3, 4, 26]; the bisdesmosidic phenolic glycosides leiocarposide (0.08–0.48%) and virgaureoside A (0.01–0.14%) [5–7]; 12 diterpenes of the *cis*-clerodane type [8]; 0.12–0.5% essential oil; phenol-carboxylic acids: caffeic acid and its glucose ester, 0.2–0.4% chlorogenic acid and isochlorogenic acid; 10–15% catechol tannins; polysaccharides.

Indications: Because of its saponin and flavonoid content, the drug is considered to be an anti-inflammatory diuretic; owing to differing results in animal experiments, the effect is described in the literature as weak or strong. The drug is used mainly for inflammation of the bladder and kidneys and in treating kidney stones and gravel. Clinically, diuretic activity and good results in acute and chronic nephritis, as well as in oedema of renal origin, have been demonstrated [9]. In rats, leiocarposide (25 mg/kg i.p.) has been shown to have a diuretic effect [10] and, in various inflammation models, antiphlogistic and analgesic activity [11]. In the rat-paw oedema test, the saponins also exhibit an antiphlogistic effect (counter-irritation?), comparable with that of aescin [12]. The ester saponins have been shown to have an antimycotic action on human pathogenic fungi (including *Candida albicans*) which only develops fully after ester hydrolysis [13]. On the other hand, under analogous conditions, the saponin mixture from *Solidago canadensis* was completely inactive. In animal experiments, it has been demonstrated that after i.v. administration an extract had a protective effect against skin damage by X-rays; this was interpreted as being due to a reduction in capillary permeability brought about by the flavonoids [14] – hence, the inclusion of the drug in the antiphlebitis remedy Ariven®. Saponin-free extracts have a hypotensive effect in normotensive dogs and a sedative effect in mice [15]. *In vitro*, the saponins have been shown to have a spermicidal effect on human spermatozoa, supposedly due to saponins of the β-amyrin type having a particular sequence of sugars at the 28-carboxyl function [16].

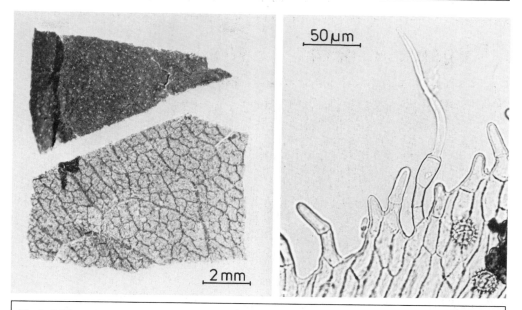

Fig. 3: *Solidago virgaurea* leaves – the darkish upper surface (above) and the paler lower surface (below) with finely reticulate venation

Fig. 4: 2–4-Celled covering trichomes with a pennant-like terminal cell (flagellate trichome) from the margin of the involucral bracts, and pollen grains with a spiny exine

In *folk medicine*, the drug is used as a so-called "blood-purifying" agent in gout, rheumatism, arthritis, eczema, and other skin conditions, like many saponin-containing drugs. Besides the diuresis, more recently a non-specific immunostimulation brought about by the saponins has been suggested as the mechanism of action [17]. Through the irritating effect of the saponins on the mucous membranes of the stomach and intestines, mild inflammation may be reduced, thereby perhaps leading to a non-specific activation of the immuno-defence system. Externally, the drug finds use as an

R = Angelicoyl: Solidagolactone II
R = Tigloyl: Solidagolactone III

Polygalic acid

Leiocarposide: R^1 = —H, R^2 = —OCH$_3$, R^3 = —O-Glucose
Virgaureoside: R^1 = -Glucose, R^2 = R^3 = —H

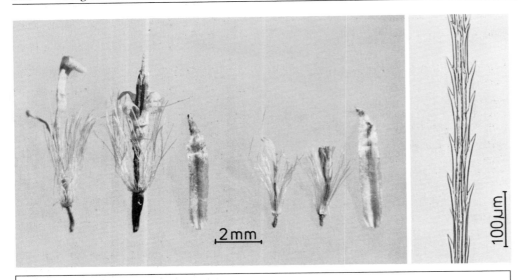

astringent (tannins) for dealing with inflammation of the mouth and throat (rinses) and poorly healing wounds.

Making the tea: Boiling water is poured over 2–3 g of the finely chopped drug or the drug is put into cold water and then boiled for a short period; after 5–10 min., the liquid is passed through a tea strainer. As a diuretic, a cupful is drunk three to five times a day. 1 Teaspoon = ca. 2 g.

Phytomedicines: The drug or extracts from it (but especially substitute drugs and their extracts, see: Adulteration) are a component of many prepared remedies, particularly urological remedies (ca. 40), e.g. Solvefort®, Rhoival®, Inconturina®, Prostamed®, etc., and also diuretics, analgesics and antirheumatics, cardiotonics, laxatives, antihypertonics, and other indications.

Authentication: Macroscopically (see: Description): the ray florets should be more than 5 mm and twice as long as the involucral bracts, which (at least the larger ones) should be more than 4 mm; the length of pappus should be mostly greater than 3 mm. Important microscopical features (see also [18]) are: the upper epidermis of leaf fragments in surface view showing almost polygonal cells with beaded walls and distinct cuticular striations; there are few stomata. Cells of the lower epidermis are sinuate to almost polygonal; there are numerous stomata mostly with 3–4 subsidiary cells (anomocytic); cuticular striations are sparse. The pubescence of the leaf surface is variable or dense. At the leaf margin, there are somewhat tortuous, distinctly striate to warty covering trichomes pointing towards the lamina and comprising (4–)5–6(–7–8) cells, 200–1000, but generally 400 μm long; white, shining excretory glands near the midrib are absent or, when present, then usually they are only 20–30 μm wide and 30–50 μm long. On the lamina and on the nerves, as well as at the margin of the involucral bracts, there are long slender tri-

chomes with 1–3 cells and a pennant-like terminal cell (Fig. 4). The ovary has ca. 300 μm long, paired trichomes with a distinctly pitted central wall. The pappus hairs consist of 3–5 rows of elongated cells (Fig. 5). 200–300 μm long biseriate glandular trichomes occur on the petals. The spherical pollen grains are ca. 25 μm in diameter with a spiny exine and three pores.

The St.Zul. prescribes the following TLC test of identity:

Test solution: 1.0 g powdered drug refluxed for 2 min. with 5 ml methanol, cooled, and filtered.

Reference solution: 5 mg each of caffeic acid, hyperoside, chlorogenic acid, and rutin dissolved in 10 ml methanol.

Loadings: 20 μl each of the test and reference solutions, as 2-cm bands on silica gel G.

Solvent system: ethyl acetate + anhydrous formic acid + water (88 + 6 + 6), 15 cm run.

Detection: after evaporation of the solvent, heated at 120 °C for a few min., and then sprayed with 1% methanolic diphenylboryloxyethylamine, followed by 5% methanolic polyethylene glycol 400.

Evaluation: in UV 365 nm light. Reference solution: at Rf ca. 0.1, the orange fluorescent rutin zone; at Rf 0.3–0.4, the pale blue fluorescent chlorogenic acid zone, with directly above it the orange fluorescent hyperoside zone; at Rf ca. 0.9, the pale blue fluorescent caffeic acid zone. Test solution: in the lower and middle Rf range, a distinct orange fluorescent rutin zone and an intense chlorogenic acid zone, with the hyperoside zone very faint or absent; in Rf range 0.8–0.9, an intense pale blue fluorescent zone; other, less intense pale blue or greenish blue fluorescent zones possibly present.

Another solvent system for the TLC separation of the flavonoids, together with an accompanying illustration of the chromatogram, is given in [19]. Details of the TLC detection of polygalic acid after hydrolysis of the saponins and partial purification of the aglycone are to be found in [20].

Quantitative standards: St.Zul. 1519.99.99: *Flavonoids*, not less than 1.5% calculated as rutin; in the identity test chromatogram (above), there should be no distinct orange to yellowish brown fluorescent zones between the hyperoside and caffeic acid zones. *Foreign matter*, not more than 1.0%; fragments of other *Solidago* species, e.g. inflorescences with unilateral racemes and a 3–5 mm long receptacle and ray florets barely projecting beyond it (*S. canadensis* L.), must not be present. *Loss on drying*, not more than 12.0%. *Ash*, not more than 8.0%.

Wording of the package insert, from the German Standard Licence:

6.1 Uses

For increasing the amount of urine in inflammation of the kidneys or bladder.

6.2 Contraindications

In chronic kidney complaints, a doctor should be consulted before using golden-rod preparations.

6.3 Dosage and Mode of administration

Boiling water (ca. 150 ml) is poured over 1–2 teaspoonfuls (3–5 g) of **Golden rod** and after 15 min. passed through a tea strainer. Unless otherwise prescribed, a cup of the infusion is drunk two to four times a day between meals.

6.4 Note

Store away from light and moisture.

Extract from the German Commission E monograph (BAnz no. 193, dated 15.10.1987)

The following text also applies to the early golden rod [Solidaginis giganteae herba].

Uses

For irrigation in cases of inflammation of the lower urinary tract, urinary calculi, and kidney gravel; for preventive treatment in cases of urinary calculi and kidney gravel.

Contraindications

None known.

Warning: no irrigation therapy when oedema resulting from cardiac or renal insufficiency is present.

Side effects

None known.

Interactions with other remedies

None known.

Dosage

Unless otherwise prescribed: average daily dose, 10 g drug; preparations correspondingly.

Mode of administration

Chopped drug for infusions and other galenical preparations for internal use.

Warning: an abundant fluid intake has to be ensured.

Effects

Diuretic, weakly spasmolytic, antiphlogistic.

BHP 1983: *Total ash*, not more than 8%. *Acid-insoluble ash*, not more than 2%. *Foreign organic matter*, not more than 2%.

Adulteration: Commercially, genuine golden rod is now almost unobtainable. Usually, as substitute, early golden rod (Fig. 6; see also: Solidaginis giganteae herba), which is derived from *S. gigantea* AIT., and *S. canadensis* L., is offered under the name Herba Solidaginis or Solidaginis giganteae herba. About the differentiation of these species, see [20–25].

Storage: Protected from light and moisture, but not in plastic containers.

Literature:

[1] V.S. Batyuk and S.N. Kovaleva, Khim. Prir. Soedin (4), 566 (1985); C.A. **104**, 165306 (1986).
[2] K. Hiller, S. Genzel, M. Murack and P. Franke, Pharmazie **30**, 188 (1975).
[3] K. Hiller, G. Bader and H.-R. Schulten, Pharmazie **42**, 541 (1987).
[4] K. Hiller, G. Bader and G. Dube, Pharmazie **42**, 744 (1987).
[5] E. Gründemann, R. Gil-Rjong and K. Hiller, Pharmazie **34**, 430 (1979).
[6] K. Hiller, G. Dube and Z. Zeigan, Pharmazie **40**, 795 (1985).
[7] K. Hiller and G. Foetsch, Pharmazie **41**, 415 (1986).
[8] A. Goswami et al., Phytochemistry **23**, 837 (1984).
[9] A. Meyer and M. Meyer, Pharmazie **5**, 82 (1950).
[10] A. Chodera et al., Acta Pol. Pharm. **42**, 199 (1985).
[11] J. Metzner, R. Hirschelmann and K. Hiller, Pharmazie **39**, 869 (1984).
[12] H.J. Jacker, G. Voigt and K. Hiller, Pharmazie **37**, 380 (1982).
[13] G. Bader et al., Pharmazie **42**, 140 (1987).
[14] H.H. Wagner, Arzneim. Forsch. **16**, 859 (1966).
[15] E. Rácz-Kotilla and G. Rácz, Planta Med. **33**, 300 (1978).
[16] B.S. Setty et al., Contraception **14**, 571 (1976).
[17] R. Hänsel, Dtsch. Apoth. Ztg. **124**, 54 (1984).
[18] P. Rohdewald, G. Rücker and K.-W. Glombitza, Apothekengerechte Prüfvorschriften, S. 725, Deutscher Apotheker Verlag Stuttgart 1986.
[19] H. Wagner, S. Bladt, and E.M. Zgainski, Plant drug analysis, Springer-Verlag, Berlin, Heidelberg, New York, Tokyo, 1984, p. 184.
[20] O.B. Genius, Dtsch. Apoth. Ztg. **120**, 1739 (1980).
[21] W. Schier, Dtsch. Apoth. Ztg. **98**, 225 (1958).
[22] L. Langhammer, Dtsch. Apoth. Ztg. **103**, 335 (1963).
[23] H. Schilcher, Dtsch. Apoth. Ztg. **105**, 681 (1965).
[24] J. Saukel, R. Ullmann, W. Bencic and J. Jurenitsch, Österr. Apoth. Ztg. **40**, 560 (1986).
[25] H. Schilcher and U. Bornschein, Dtsch. Apoth. Ztg. **126**, 1377 (1986).
[26] G. Bader, V. Wray, and K. Hiller, Phytochemistry **31**, 621 (1992).

Visci herba   (DAB 10), Mistletoe herb

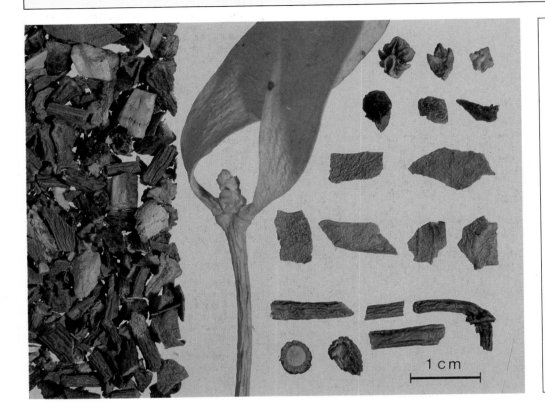

Fig. 1: Mistletoe herb

<u>Description:</u> Conspicuous features of the drug are the repeatedly forked, 2–4 mm thick, yellowish green, longitudinally wrinkled pieces of stem and the entire, stiff and leathery, lanceolate to spathulate yellowish green, sessile leaves; these latter are 2–6 cm long and 1–2 cm in width. On the other hand, most of the inconspicuous, yellowish green male and female flowers have fallen, as have also the more or less pea-size, shrivelled, yellowish white or pale reddish berries.

<u>Odour:</u> Very faint, but characteristic.

<u>Taste:</u> Bitter.

Figs. 2 and 3: *Viscum album* L.

A small, dioecious, shrubby semi-parasite with oblong, evergreen, leathery, entire leaves. The branching clearly dichasial. Inconspicuous, axillary, yellowish green, 4-part flowers, forming white sticky berries.

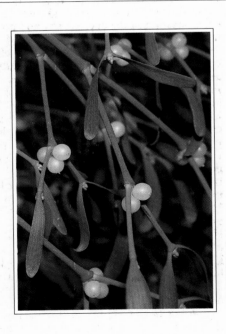

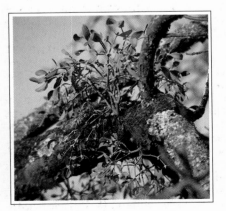

DAB 10: Mistelkraut
Erg. B. 6: Herba Visci albi

Plant source: *Viscum album* L. mistletoe (Viscaceae; formerly in Loranthaceae).

Synonyms: Folia Visci, Stipites Visci (Lat.), Viscum, European or Birdlime mistletoe (Engl.), Mistelkraut, Vogel- or Leimmistel, Hexenbesen, Drudenfuß (Ger.), Herbe de gui (Fr.).

Origin: A semi-parasite native in Europe and Asia and found on almost all deciduous trees (but not on beech); two subspecies occur only on conifers. Imports of the drug originate in Bulgaria, Turkey, former Yugoslavia, Albania, and the former USSR.

Constituents [1, 2]: Lectins (glycoproteins with the ability to bind specifically to certain sugars – galactose or *N*-acetylgalactosamine or both – and cell surfaces; 2-D electrophoresis patterns show that they each comprise a large number of isolectins which have variations in both the A and B chains [10]), some of which have been isolated in

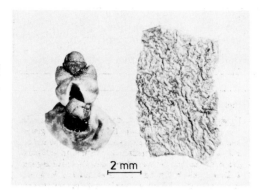

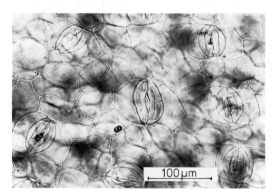

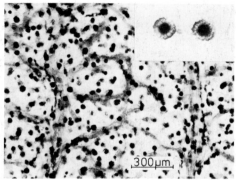

2 mm

100 μm

300 μm

Fig. 4: Conical inflorescence (left) and a leathery, wrinkled leaf fragment (right)

Fig. 5: Leaf epidermis with paracytic stomata

Fig. 6: Abundant occurrence of cluster crystals of calcium oxalate, showing (upper right) the dark centre and grey halo

Extract from the German Commission E monograph
(BAnz no. 228, dated 05. 12. 1984)

Uses

For treating degenerative inflammation of the joints by eliciting cuti-visceral reflexes following local inflammation brought about by intradermal injections. As palliative therapy for malignant tumours through non-specific stimulation.

Contraindications

Protein hypersensitivity, chronic progressive infections, e.g. tuberculosis.

Side effects

Shivering, high fever, headache, anginal problems, orthostatic circulatory disorders, and allergic reactions.

Interactions

None known.

Dosage

Unless otherwise prescribed: according to the manufacturer's instructions.

Mode of administration

Fresh plant, chopped or powdered drug for the preparation of injections.

Effects

Intradermal injection brings about local inflammation occurs which may develop into necrosis.
In animal experiments, cytostatic and non-specifically immunostimulant.

Note

The hypotensive effects and the therapeutic activity in milder forms of hypertony (threshold hypertony) needs to be checked.

pure form and about which there is a considerable amount of structural information. Proteins and polypeptides, especially the viscotoxins which are composed of 46 amino acids; 2-D gel electrophoresis reveals as many as 500 protein spots, two of which (with mol. wt. 17 000 Da) can be regarded as sex markers, since they are characteristic of male plants and occur independently of the stage of development [11]. Phenylpropanes and lignans, such as syringenin 4'-glucoside and syringaresinol 4',4''-diglucoside; caffeic-acid derivatives; flavonoids, especially derivatives of quercetin; biogenic amines (tyramine, etc.); polysaccharides, particularly galacturonans and arabinogalactans. In the leaves, the variable amount (0.9–6.6%, based on the dry wt.) of 1D-1-*O*-methyl-*muco*-inositol shows a marked increase in winter; the compound may have a crypto-protective function [12].

Indications: A clear distinction must be made between *oral* use of the drug in the form of aqueous extracts, e.g. herbal teas (as an adjuvant in the treatment of high blood pressure), and the *parenteral* use of isolated

constituents, e.g. in the form of injections. There are no real grounds for the use of mistletoe tea as a supportive measure in treating high blood pressure, in spite of the many investigations aimed at demonstrating an antihypertonic action. The results of animal experiments are contradictory and do not allow extrapolation to human medicine [1, 3]. It has indeed been shown that the isolated viscotoxins are hypotensive on parenteral administration, but they cannot be considered as the active principle since they are not absorbed orally; moreover, they are highly irritating to the skin, so much so that at high doses they even cause necrosis [4].

The lectins isolated in recent years from mistletoe, some of which are very pure, are generally composed of A and B polypeptide chains and a carbohydrate part and their principal action is a clear-cut cyototoxic effect; this has been determined for certain tumours and carcinomas (mouse ascites tumour; human tumour cells: KB and HeLa strains in tissue culture) [5–7]. Relevant investigations have shown that the polysaccharides probably participate in the working

of the lectins [8]. The different isolectin patterns alluded to above may indicate significant variation in the cytotoxicity and postulated immunomodulating potency of the lectins [10]. Helixor® has a cytostatic effect on *in-vitro* cultures of drug-resistant human acute lymphoblastic leukaemia cells [6]. Presumably, mistletoe preparations for injection, such as Iscador®, Plenosol®, Helixor®, etc., owe their efficacy to their lectin content. The scepticism with which these products are regarded, not least by the medical profession, is no doubt because their use derives from anthroposophy.

It has been established that the phenylpropanes and lignans have a significant inhibitory action towards c-AMP-phosphodiesterase [9].

However, to draw conclusions from the occurrence of the highly active viscotoxins and lectins in mistletoe and the pharmacological findings after parenteral (!) administration about the activities of mistletoe *tea*, as is done in several herbals or by irresponsible writers on health matters (extolling mistletoe *tea* as an anticancer remedy), is quite inadmissible.

Mistletoe tea is used purely *empirically* as an adjuvant in the treatment of hypertension, vertigo, and cephalic congestion. So far, rational grounds for this are lacking, since the hypotensive viscotoxins, assuming they do actually get into the tea, as already mentioned, are degraded in the gastrointestinal tract or are not absorbed intact. Patients taking mistletoe tea are advised to check their blood pressure regularly.

Side effects: See the Commission E monograph; on prolonged use, allergic reations may occur.

It has been pointed out that claims for "safety" of mistletoe products need to be verified and that a case could be made for restricting sales of such preparations [13].

Making the tea: Cold water is poured over 2.5 g of the finely chopped drug and allowed to stand at room temperature for 10–12 hours, then strained. One or two cups are drunk daily (see: Indications).
1 Teaspoon = ca. 2.5 g.

Herbal preparations: The drug is also available in tea bags (2 g).

Phytomedicines: The drug is a component of several prepared antihypertonics, e.g. Asgoviscum®, Craviscum®, Hyperidist®, Mistelan®, Mistel-Pflanzensaft (plant juice) Kneipp®, Viscysat, Antihypertonicum "Schuck", Verus®, Cardiotonics, e.g. Zirkulin® forte, etc., and sedatives; about injections, see: Indications.

Among the products available in the UK are Weleda Iscador®, Arkopharma Phytoimmuneboost (capsules), etc.

Authentication: Macro- (see: Description) and microscopically, following the DAB 10. See also the BHP 1983. The leathery, wrinkled leaf fragments, as well as the conical inflorescences (sessile cymes), are conspicuous characteristics of the cut drug (Fig. 4). On microscopical examination, the relatively large paracytic stomata (Fig. 5) and numerous cluster crystals of calcium oxalate with a sharp, grey halo (Fig. 6) are easily recognized.

TLC methods for the analysis of the flavonoids and more especially the amino acids (the pattern of which can be used for identification purposes) are to be found in [14].

2-D fingerprinting of the intrinsic mistletoe lectins would be an important step towards standardization and determining probable effectiveness of the products [10].

Quantitative standards: DAB 10: *Foreign matter*, not more than 1%. *Loss on drying*, not more than 10%. *Ash*, not more than 10%.

BHP 1983: *Water-soluble extractive*, not less than 15%. *Total ash*, not more than 10%. *Acid-insoluble ash*, not more than 2%.

Adulteration: In practice does not occur.

Literature:
[1] (a) H. Moll and H. Schmoll called Eisenwert, Mistel, Arzneipflanzen – Brauchtum – Kunstmotiv im Jugendstil, Wissenschaftliche Verlagsgesellschaft, Stuttgart, 1986; (b) P. Luther and H. Becker, Die Mistel, Springer, Berlin – Heidelberg – New York, 1987.
[2] H. Franz, Pharmazie **40**, 97 (1985).
[3] H. Becker, Dtsch. Apoth. Ztg. **126**, 1229 (1986).
[4] J. Konopa, J.M. Woynarowski, and M. Lewandowska-Gumieniak, Hoppe-Seyler's Z. Physiol. Chem. **361**, 1525 (1980).
[5] N. Bloksma et al., Planta Med. **46**, 221 (1982).
[6] M. Hülsen and F. Mechelke, Naturwissenschaften **74**, 144 (1987).
[7] P. Luther et al., Acta Biol. Med. Ger. **36**, 119 (1977).
[8] H. Heine, Z. Phytotherap. **8**, 122 (1987).
[9] H. Wagner et al., Planta Med. **52**, 102 (1986).
[10] M. Schink, D. Moser, and F. Mechelke, Naturwissenschaften **79**, 80 (1992).
[11] M. Schink and F. Mechelke, Naturwissenschaften **76**, 29 (1989).
[12] A. Richter, B. Thonke, and M. Popp, Phytochemistry **29**, 1785 (1990).
[13] L.A. Anderson and J.D. Phillipson, Pharm. J. **229**, 437 (1982).
[14] H. Wagner, S. Bladt, and E.M. Zgainski, Plant drug analysis, Springer-Verlag, Berlin, Heidelberg, New York, Tokyo, 1984, p. 286.

Zingiberis rhizoma   Ginger (*BAN*; BP 1988, BHP 1/1990)

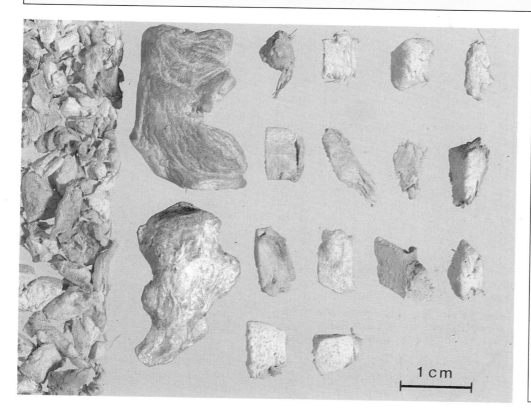

Fig. 1: Ginger

Description: The surfaces of the flattened pieces of rhizome, which branch in one plane, are peeled, leaving the remains of the cork along the narrow sides; the yellowish grey surface has fine longitudinal striations. In transverse section, there is a narrow cortex and a broad oval central stele; the vascular bundles project as short, rigid points.

Odour: Characteristic, aromatic.

Taste: Pungent and spicy.

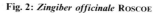
1 cm

Fig. 2: *Zingiber officinale* ROSCOE

Tropical rhizomatous plant with linear-lanceolate leaves up to more than 20 cm in length. Long flowering stems with dense inflorescences, each flower being surrounded by bracts.

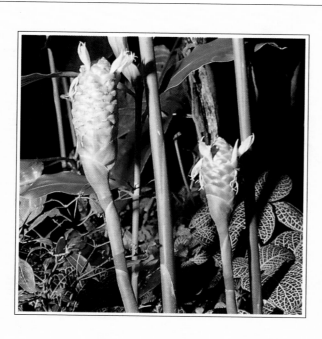

ÖAB: Radix Zingiberis
Ph. Helv. VII: Zingiberis rhizoma
DAB 6: Rhizoma Zingiberis

Plant source: *Zingiber officinale* ROSCOE, ginger (Zingiberaceae).

Synonyms: Zingiber, Jamaica ginger, Ginger root or rhizome. Ingwer, Ingberwurzel (Ger.). Gingembre (Fr.).

Origin: Cultivated in most tropical countries. There are many commercial varieties. What is considered to be the best (completely scraped) drug is that from Jamaica. Good quality (partially scraped) ginger for drug purposes also comes from Bengal and Australia. Up to 80% of present-day imports comes from China. Other parts of the world supply the drug, e.g. West Africa and South-East Asia. For further discussion of the available forms of ginger, see [6].

Constituents: 2.5–3% essential oil, the composition of which varies enormously according to the origin. Generally, but not always, sesquiterpenes predominate, e.g. (−)-zingiberene, *ar*-curcumene, *β*-bisabolone, and (*E*)-*α*-farnesene; the essential oil of Australian ginger contains mainly monoterpenes such as camphor, *β*-phellandrene, geranial, neral, and linalool, besides a small proportion of sesquiterpenes [1, 2]. Essential oil from dried Vietnamese ginger was found to consist of almost two-thirds monoterpenes (more oxygenated derivatives than hydrocarbons) and one-third sesquiterpenes (much more hydrocarbons than oxygenated derivatives); geranial (16%) was the main component and the overall composition was similar to that of a Sri Lankan variety [7]. The essential oil of fresh Japanese ginger contains mainly acyclic oxygenated monoterpenes such as neral, geraniol, geranial, and geranyl acetate; on storage, the neral/-geranial content increases to ca. 60%, arising from the conversion of geranyl into successively geraniol, geranial, and neral [8]. The non-volatile pungent principles, the gingerols and shogaols, are phenylalkanones or phenylalkanonols with different chain lengths [1]; related compounds, such as [6]-gingerdiol and analogues, are also present [9]. Other diarylheptanoids, including the gingerenones A-C, isogingerenone B, and gingerdione, have been isolated [10, 11].

Indications: Chiefly as a spice, but also as a stomachic, tonic, and digestant in sub-acid gastritis, dyspepsia, and lack of appetite. Ginger stimulates the flow of saliva, raises the tonus of the intestinal musculature, and activates peristalsis.
Powdered ginger given in a dose of 2 g is a strong anti-emetic; it is said to be better than dimenhydrinate (Dramamine®), the therapeutic dose of which is 100 mg [3]. The gingerols and shogaols are responsible for the anti-emetic effects [13].

Zingiberene

Gingerols (n = 1, 2, 3, 4, 6, 8, 10)

Shogaols (n = 3, 4, 5, 6, 8, 10)

Some of the shogaols (phenylalkanonols) have been shown to have a cardiotonic (positive inotropic) effect on the guinea-pig auricle [4].
About the inhibition of prostaglandin synthesis by the phenylalkanones, see: Galangae rhizoma.
In *folk medicine*, ginger is also in use as a carminative, expectorant, and astringent.

Making the tea: Not common, but boiling water can be poured over 0.5–1 g of the coarsely powdered drug and after 5 min. passed through a tea strainer.

As an anti-emetic, 2 g of the freshly powdered drug is taken with some fluid.
1 Teaspoon = ca. 3 g.

Phytomedicines: The powdered drug or extracts prepared from it are present in some Stomach Remedies. Zintona® capsules as an anti-emetic.
Examples of products on the UK market are Potter's Indian Brandee (liquid) and Seven

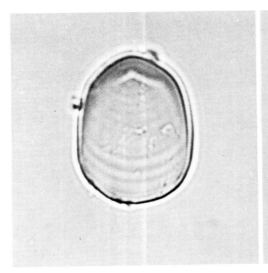
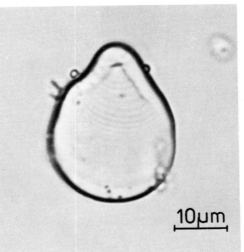

10μm

Fig. 3: **Characteristic zingiberaceous starch. Large flattened grains with a markedly excentric hilum; some grains are teat- (or muller-) shaped (right).**

Seas Ginger Tablets. Potter's Ginger Root Capsules are offered as an antimigraine preparation.

Authentication: Macro- (see: Description) and microscopically. Beneath the thin, irregular cork, there is a narrow cortex, in the parenchyma of which are numerous oil cells with a yellow or brownish yellow content; there are also small collateral vascular bundles. In the central stele as well, there are collateral vascular bundles, but here they are accompanied by septate fibres with a wide lumen; oil cells are likewise abundant in the central stele. All parenchyma cells contain characteristic starch grains: these are oblong to sub-rectangular (sack-shaped) to oval in shape and they are often drawn out into a blunt-ended point where the hilum is situated (Fig. 3); the striations are not always clearly recognizable. For the detailed microscopy of the powdered drug, see [7].

The main pungent principles can be quantitatively determined by means of TLC/HPLC [5].

Bleaching (or whitening) can be tested for as follows: on pouring dilute acetic acid over the drug, there should be no effervescence (evolution of carbon dioxide from calcium carbonate); after adding ammonium hydroxide solution and ammonium oxalate to the filtrate, there should be no cloudiness or preciptate.

Quantitative standards: <u>BP 1988</u>: 90% *Ethanol-soluble extractive*, not less than 4.5%. *Water-soluble extractive*, not less than 10.0%. *Ash*, not more than 6.0%. *Water-soluble ash*, not more than 1.7%.
<u>BHP 1/1990</u>: Ginger, as such or in powdered form, should comply with the requirements of the BP 1988.
<u>ÖAB</u>: *Volatile oil*, not less than 1.5%. *Ash*, not more than 6.0%. *Test for bleaching agents*, 2 g comminuted drug shaken for 1 min. with 20 ml 12% acetic acid and filtered; on adding 3 drops sodium sulphide soln (6 g in 35 ml glycerol diluted to 100 ml with water), there should be no change in colour.
<u>Ph. Helv. VII</u>: *Volatile oil*, not less than 1.7%. *Foreign matter*, not more than 1%; lumps of starch paste absent (boiled ginger). *Sulphated ash*, not more than 8.5%.
<u>DAB 6</u>: *Essential oil*, not less than 1.5%. *Ash*, not more than 7%.

Adulteration: The adulteration with other *Zingiber* species, described in the literature, is scarcely ever encountered in the drug trade; they would be recognized by the microscopical and TLC examination. On the other hand, drugs whitened with calcium carbonate are often met with (see: Authentication).

Storage: Protected from light and kept in a cool place (not in plastic containers).

Literature:
[1] D.J. Harvey, J. Chromatogr. **212**, 75 (1981).
[2] J. Erler et al., Z. Lebensmitt.-Unters.-Forsch. **186**, 231 (1988).
[3] D.B. Mowbrey and D.E. Clayson, Lancet **I**, 655 (1982).
[4] N. Shoji et al., J. Pharm. Sci. **71**, 1174 (1982).
[5] E. Steinegger and K. Stucki, Pharm. Acta Helv. **57**, 66 (1982).
[6] W.C. Evans, Trease and Evans' Pharmacognosy, 13th ed., Baillière Tindall, London, Philadelphia, Toronto, Sydney, Tokyo, p. 466.
[7] T.A. van Beek et al., Phytochemistry **26**, 3005 (1987).
[8] F. Sakamura, Phytochemistry **26**, 2207 (1987).
[9] H. Kikuzaki, S.-M. Tsai, and N. Nakatani, Phytochemistry **31**, 1783 (1992).
[10] K. Endo, E. Kanno, and Y. Oshima, Phytochemistry **29**, 797 (1990).
[11] H. Kikuzaki, M. Kobayashi, and N. Nakatani, Phytochemistry **30**, 3647 (1991).
[12] B.P. Jackson and D.W. Snowdon, Atlas of microscopy of medicinal plants, culinary herbs and spices, Belhaven Press, London, 1990, p. 110.
[13] T. Kawai et al., Planta Med. **60**, 17 (1994).

Indexes

List of Indications

The aim of this list is to set out the connection between certain indications frequently mentioned in the text and the herbal drugs discussed in this book. It is not, or at least not directly, intended for the layman to undertake self-medication: this is simply not possible, because, for example, the indication "for coughs" requires a different treatment depending on whether it is a dry irritating cough or whether it is a cough associated with an abundant thick sputum.

Thus, it is essential in each individual case to refer to the drug concerned in the main part of the book and to learn about the various indications (and also the side effects). However, this list gives an overview of the drugs which, for example, may be encountered in a "cough tea", a "stomach tea", a "laxative tea", etc. In mixed teas, of course, there will be drugs from other groups (in a laxative tea, besides the essential laxatives, spasmolytic or carminative herbal drugs).

The larger groups of indications are subdivided into groups with headings indicating the main type of activity. Here also, the distinction between recognized and *folk-medicinal* uses is maintained.
The order in which the herbs are listed corresponds *roughly* to their importance, with the more widely used ones being listed in the first column.

Gastrointestinal disorders

Appetite-stimulating
Digestion-stimulating
Stomachic
"Stomach tea"

wormwood
lesser centaury
gentian
bitter-orange peel
yarrow
calamus
holy thistle
bogbean
quassia
cinchona bark
condurango
red sage
white horehound
mugwort

angelica root
turmeric
unripe orange
lemon peel
rosemary
hops
Iceland moss
ginger
caraway
dandelion root, herb
Roman chamomile
star anise fruit
cinnamon

Folk medicine:

thyme
juniper berry
ramsons
basil

Spasmolytic
Antiphlogistic
"Digestive"

matricaria flower
yarrow
peppermint leaf
liquorice root
angelica root
balm
caraway
coriander
ammi visnaga fruit
galanga

marigold
mallow leaf
mallow flower
marshmallow root
butterbur leaf
agrimony
tormentil
clove
comfrey root

Folk medicine:

lavender
linseed
lovage
wild thyme
saffron
walnut leaf

Laxative
Aperient
"Laxative tea"

senna leaf
linseed
frangula bark
rhubarb
senna fruit
cascara bark
mallow flower
(aloes)

psyllium
ispaghula seed
buckthorn fruit

Folk medicine:

rose hips
blackthorn flower

Antidiarrhoeal
Astringent

rhatany root
tormentil
bilberry fruit
bramble leaf
witch hazel leaf
witch hazel bark
oak bark
wild strawberry leaf
red sage

silverweed
hemp-nettle herb
chestnut leaf
walnut leaf
lady's-mantle
agrimony

Folk medicine:

raspberry leaf
St. John's wort
avens root
horse-chestnut bark

Carminative
"Flatulence tea"

caraway
fennel
aniseed
coriander
matricaria flower
angelica root
calamus
peppermint leaf
Roman chamomile

yarrow
red sage
Greek sage
turmeric
wormwood
rosemary
cinnamon
clove
spearmint leaf

Folk medicine:

ginger
lovage
thyme
juniper berry
wild thyme
lavender
celery seed

Coughs and Chills, etc.

Secretolytic
Secretomotor
Expectorant
"Cough tea"
"Bronchial tea"

thyme
liquorice root
fennel
aniseed
ipecacuanha
plantain leaf, herb
lime tree flower
primula root
senega root
mullein
long-leaved sundew
soapwort root
eucalyptus leaf
ivy leaf
ammi visnaga fruit
meadowsweet
elecampane

burnet-saxifrage root
primula flower
quillaia
star anise fruit
clove

Folk medicine:

wild thyme
lungwort
butterbur leaf
lovage
wild pansy
white deadnettle
chestnut leaf
horse-chestnut leaf
speedwell herb
verbena
couch-grass root
orris root
knotgrass herb
elder fruit
ginger
grass flowers

Cough-alleviating
Antitussive
"Bronchial tea"
"Cough tea"

marshmallow root
mallow flower
coltsfoot
Iceland moss
mallow leaf
marshmallow leaf

Biliary disorders

Cholagogic
Cholekinetic
Choleretic
"Metabolism tea"

Javanese turmeric
boldo
peppermint leaf
helichrysum flower
turmeric
dandelion root, herb
fumitory
greater celandine
milk-thistle fruit
white horehound
yarrow

wormwood
ammi visnaga fruit
elecampane
rosemary
milk-thistle herb
butterbur leaf
balm
lavender
marigold
rhubarb

Folk medicine:

holy thistle
devil's-claw

Kidney and Bladder disorders

Diuretic
Urinary disinfectants
"Bladder tea"
"Diuretic tea"

uva ursi
rupturewort
birch leaf
restharrow root
orthosiphon leaf
equisetum
lovage
boldo
celery seed
nettle herb
celery root
elecampane
dandelion root, herb
ammi visnaga fruit
golden rod
early golden-rod herb
dyer's greenweed herb
rose hip "seeds"
corn silk

Folk medicine:

celery seed
lycopodium
juniper wood
couch-grass root
lime tree flower
kidney-bean pods
(without seeds)
burdock root
helichrysum flower
wild thyme
black currant leaf
verbena
melilot
stemless carlina root
knotgrass herb
rose hips
hemp-nettle herb
lady's-bedstraw herb
blackthorn flower
Iceland moss
devil's-claw
mullein
henna leaf

Nervous complaints

Sedatives
"Nerve tea"
"sedative tea"

valerian
balm
peppermint leaf
hops
lavender

passionflower
St. John's wort
lovage
celery seed

Folk medicine:

orange flower
lime tree flower
oats (green tops)
angelica root
saffron

Various indications, for internal and external use

Anti-inflammatory
Antiphlogistic
Antirheumatic
"Antirheumatism tea"
"Anti-inflammation tea"

willow bark
matricaria flower
arnica flower (external)
wild pansy
marigold
comfrey root (external)
fenugreek seed (external)

Folk medicine:

St. John's wort
golden rod
verbena
dandelion root, herb
celery seed
juniper wood
restharrow root
corn silk
devil's-claw
primula root
mullein
soapwort root
grass flowers (external)
nettle fruit (seed) (external)

For treating wounds, externally only

matricaria flower
arnica flower
oak bark
yarrow
Roman chamomile
St. John's wort
marigold
comfrey root
walnut leaf
fenugreek seed

Folk medicine:

golden rod
verbena
butterbur leaf
lavender
white horehound
rosemary
wild pansy
mallow leaf
mallow flower
linseed

For throat infections
Astringent
Antiseptic
"For gargling"

red sage
Greek sage
matricaria flower
Roman chamomile flower
yarrow
tormentil
rhatany root
thyme
(myrrh)
witch hazel leaf
witch hazel bark
arnica flower
plantain leaf, herb
comfrey root
burnet-saxifrage root

agrimony
stemless carlina root
elder flower

Folk medicine:

golden rod
wild pansy
caraway
avens root

For menstrual disorders

black haw bark
silverweed
matricaria flower
Roman chamomile
butterbur leaf

Folk medicine:

lady's-mantle
shepherd's purse
yarrow
elecampane
white deadnettle flower
celery seed
celery root
mistletoe herb

(Haemo)Styptic Haemostatic

shepherd's purse

Folk medicine:

yarrow
plantain leaf
equisetum
knotgrass herb
cinnamon

For so-called minor heart conditions "As heart tonic" "For circulation problems"

hawthorn leaf, flower
hawthorn berry
broom
arnica flower
balm (?)
ammi visnaga fruit (?)

Folk medicine:

primula flower

To "stimulate the flow of milk" As "galactagogue"

Folk medicine:

fennel
caraway
verbena
celery root
celery seed
Iceland moss

As "antidiabetic tea"

Folk medicine:

kidney-bean pods
(without seeds)
goat's-rue herb
bilberry leaf
red sage

Literature

A number of books are cited repeatedly in the text, i.e. Berger, Hager, the pharmacopoeias and their commentaries (see List of Abbreviations). For further reading on specific questions as well as more general topics we would also refer the reader to the following titles:

Arends J., Volkstümliche Namen der Arzneimittel, Drogen, Heilkräuter und Chemikalien, 16th edition. Springer-Verlag, Berlin-Heidelberg-New York 1971.

Braun H. and D. Frohne, Heilpflanzenlexikon für Ärzte und Apotheker, 5th edition. G. Fischer-Verlag, Stuttgart 1987.

Czygan F.-C., Biogene Arzneistoffe. Verlag F. Vieweg & Sohn, Braunschweig, Wiesbaden 1984.

Deutschmann F., B. Hohmann, E. Sprecher and E. Stahl, Pharmazeutische Biologie, Vol. 3, Drogenanalyse I: Morphologie und Anatomie, 2nd edition. G. Fischer-Verlag, Stuttgart-New York 1984.

Diener H., Arzneipflanzen und Drogen, VEB Fachbuchverlag Leipzig 1987.

Fischer R. and Th. Kartnig, Praktikum der Pharmakognosie, 5th edition. Springer-Verlag, Wien-New York 1978.

Flück H. and R. Jaspersen-Schib, Unsere Heilpflanzen, 7th edition. A. Ott-Verlag, Thun 1986.

Frohne D., Anatomisch-mikrochemische Drogenanalyse, 3rd edition. G. Fischer-Verlag, Stuttgart 1974.

Frohne D. and H. J. Pfänder, A colour atlas of poisonous plants. Wolfe Publishing, London 1984.

Hänsel R., Pharmazeutische Biologie, 2 volumes, Springer-Verlag, Berlin-Heidelberg-New York 1980.

Hänsel R. and H. Haas, Therapie mit Phytopharmaka, Springer-Verlag, Berlin-Heidelberg-New York-Tokyo 1983.

Hörhammer L., Teeanalyse, Springer-Verlag, Berlin-New York-Heidelberg 1970.

Hoppe H. A., Taschenbuch der Drogenkunde, de Gruyter-Verlag, Berlin-New York 1981.

Jackson B. P. and D. W. Snowdon, Atlas of microscopy of medicinal plants, culinary herbs and spices, Belhaven Press, London 1990.

Luckner M., Secondary Metabolism in Microorganisms, Plants and Animals. VEB Gustav Fischer Verlag Jena 1984.

Menßen H. G., Phytotherapeutische Welt, pmi-pharm & medical inform. Verlags-GmbH, Frankfurt/M. 1983.

Pachaly P., Dünnschichtchromatographie in der Apotheke. Schnelle und einfache Identifizierung gebräuchlicher Arzneistoffe, Drogen, Extrakte und Tinkturen. 2nd edition. Wissenschaftliche Verlagsgesellschaft mbH, Stuttgart 1983.

Pahlow M., Das große Buch der Heilpflanzen, Gräfe und Unzer Verlag, München 1979.

Pahlow M., Meine Heilpflanzentees, Gräfe und Unzer-Verlag, München 1981.

Poletti A., H. Schilcher and A. Müller, Heilkräftige Pflanzen in Farbe. W. Hädecke-Verlag, Weil der Stadt 1982.

Schilcher H., Kleines Heilkräuter-Lexikon, Reform-Verlag, Bad Homburg 1980.

Schneider G., Pharmazeutische Biologie, 2nd edition. Bibliograpisches Institut, Mannheim-Wien-Zürich 1985.

Stahl E. and W. Schild, Pharmazeutische Biologie, Vol. 4, Drogenanalyse II: Inhaltsstoffe und Isolierungen. G. Fischer-Verlag, Stuttgart-New York 1981.

Steinegger E. and R. Hänsel, Lehrbuch der Pharmakognosie und Phytopharmazie, 4th edition. Springer-Verlag, Berlin-Heidelberg-New York 1988.

Teuscher E., Pharmazeutische Biologie, 3rd edition. Akademie-Verlag, Berlin 1978, Lizenzausgabe F. Vieweg & Sohn Verlagsges. mbH Braunschweig, Wiesbaden 1983. Part I of the 3rd edition has since appeared in a revised version, Akademie-Verlag, Berlin 1987.

Teuscher E. and U. Lundquist, Biogene Gifte. G. Fischer Verlag, Stuttgart und New York (Lizenzausgabe) 1988.

Wagner H., Pharmazeutische Biologie, Vol. 2, Drogen und ihre Inhaltsstoffe, 4th edition. G. Fischer-Verlag, Stuttgart-New York 1988.

Wagner H., S. Bladt and E. M. Zgainski, Plant drug analysis, Springer-Verlag, Berlin-Heidelberg-New York 1984.

Weiß R. F., Herbal Medicine. Arcanum, Gothenburg, and Beaconsfield Publishers, Beaconsfield (licence edition) 1988.

Wichtl M., Die Pharmakognostisch-chemische Analyse, Akadem. Verlagsges., Frankfurt/M. 1971.

Illustration Credits

Drug photographs: Dr. H.J. Pfänder, Kiel (all)

Plant photographs:

Dr. K. von der Dunk Hemhofen	Citrus aurantium (1) Genista tinctoria (1) Plantago ovata (1) Quassia amara (1) Rubus idaeus (1) Saponaria officinalis (1) Zingiber officinale (1)
Dr. W. Förster Den Haag	Aloe ferox (1)
J. Frantz Tübingen	Sassafras albidum (2)
Dr. W. Herold Andernach	Aloe (1)
Dr. R. König Kiel	Apium graveolens (1) Cinchona pubescens (1) Citrus aurantium (1) Crocus sativus (1) Curcuma domestica (2) Galeopsis segetum (1)
H.E. Laux Biberach/Riß	Chamaemelum nobile (1) Citrus limon (1) Malva sylvestris (1) Ocimum basilicum (1) Rheum palmatum (1) Viscum album (1)
Dr. H.G. Menßen Bergheim	Cassia angustifolia (1)
I. Milas Rottenburg	Fucus vesiculosus (1)
Fa. Pharmaton Lugano	Panax ginseng (2)
Prof. Dr. W. Rauh Heidelberg	Herniaria glabra (1) Ilicium verum (2) Krameria triandra (1)
Dr. H. Sauerbier Lauchringen	Orthosiphon spicatus (1) Salvia triloba (1)
Prof. Dr. P. Schönfelder Regensburg	Alkanna tinctoria (1) Ammi visnaga (1) Apium graveolens (1) Arctium lappa (1) Pimpinella anisum (1) Polygonum aviculare (1) Trigonella foenum-graecum (1)

Prof. Dr. M. Wichtl Marburg/L.	Angelica archangelica (1) Camellia sinensis (2) Carum carvi (1) Cassia angustifolia (1) Cinnamomum sp. (1) Curcuma xanthorrhiza (2) Eucalyptus globulus (2) Glycyrrhiza glabra (1) Hamamelis virginiana (1) Hibiscus sabdariffa (1) Lavandula angustifolia (1) Levisticum officinale (1) Malva sylvestris ssp. mauritiana (1) Ononis spinosa (1) Passiflora incarnata (1) Plantago psyllium (1) Silybum marianum (1) Syzygium aromaticum (1) Thymus vulgaris (1) Verbascum densiflorum (1)
Prof. Dr. A. Vömel Ebsdorfergrund	Cinchona pubescens (1)
Prof. Dr. O.H. Volk Würzburg	Harpagophytum procumbens (2)
Dr. W. Buff Biberach/Riß	all other plants

Microphotographs:

Dr. H.J. Pfänder (233) Kiel

Dr. W. Wichtl-Bleier (79) Marburg/L.

TLC photographs:

Dr. A. Nagell (26) Hamburg
Prof. Dr. M. Wichtl (12) Marburg/L.

Dr. M. Veit (1) Würzburg

Index of Monograph Authors

The authors of the individual monographs in the German edition are given below. However, this book would not have been possible without the excellent co-operation between authors, editor and translator.

F.C. Czygan - Würzburg

Aloe

Anisi fructus

Anisi stellati fructus

Avenae herba

Basilici herba

Betulae folium

Bursae pastoris herba

Carvi fructus

Cetrariae lichen

Cinnamomi cortex

Consolidae regalis flos

Coriandri fructus

Croci stigma

Droserae longifoliae herba

Equiseti herba

Euphrasiae herba

Foeniculi fructus

Frangulae cortex

Gei urbani radix

Hamamelidis cortex

Hamamelidis folium

Harpagophyti radix

Hennae folium

Hibisci flos

Juniperi fructus

Juniperi lignum

Maydis stigma

Melissae folium

Myrrha

Paeoniae flos

Petroselini fructus

Petroselini radix

Pruni spinosae flos

Pulmonariae herba

Rhamni purshiani cortex

Rhoeados flos

Rosae pseudofructus

Rosae pseudofructus "semen"

Rosmarini folium

Rubi idaei folium

Serpylli herba

Sinapis nigrae semen

Thymi herba

Urticae fructus

Urticae herba

Urticae radix

D. Frohne - Kiel

Absinthii herba

Agrimoniae herba

Alchemillae herba

Allii ursini herba

Anserinae herba

Aurantii fructus immaturi

Aurantii pericarpium

Barosmae folium

Calami rhizoma

Castaneae folium

Centaurii herba

Chelidonii herba

Cnici benedicti herba

Condurango cortex

Curcumae longae rhizoma

Curcumae xanthorrhizae rhizoma

Farfarae folium

Fragariae folium

Fucus

Fumariae herba

Galegae herba

Gentianae radix

Marrubii herba

Mate folium

Menyanthidis folium

Myrtilli folium

Myrtilli fructus

Phaseoli pericarpium

Quassiae lignum

Quercus cortex

Rataniae radix

Rubi fruticosi folium

Theae nigrae folium

Tormentillae rhizoma

Uvae ursi folium

A. Nagell - Hamburg

Citri pericarpium

Graminis rhizoma

Meliloti herba

Menthae crispae folium

Primulae flos

Santali lignum rubri

M. Wichtl - Marburg

Alkannae radix
Althaeae folium
Althaeae radix
Aurantii flos
Boldo folium
Caryophylli flos
Cinchonae cortex
Crataegi folium cum flore
Crataegi fructus
Cucurbitae semen
Epilobii herba
Eucalypti folium
Galangae rhizoma
Galeopsidis herba
Galii veri herba
Genistae herba
Ginseng radix
Graminis flos
Herniariae herba
Hyperici herba
Ipecacuanhae radix
Iridis rhizoma
Lamii albi herba
Lavandulae flos
Lupuli strobulus
Lycopodii herba
Malvae flos
Malvae folium
Menthae piperitae folium
Nasturtii herba
Ononidis radix
Orthosiphonis folium
Passiflorae herba
Plantaginis ovatae semen
Polygalae radix
Polygoni avicularis herba
Primulae radix
Psyllii semen
Quillajae cortex
Rhamni cathartici fructus

Rhei radix
Ribis nigri folium
Salviae folium
Salviae trilobae folium
Saponariae rubrae radix
Sassfrass lignum
Scoparii herba
Sennae folium
Sennae fructus
Spiraeae flos
Valerianae radix
Verbenae herba
Veronicae herba
Visci herba
Zingiberis rhizoma

G. Willuhn - Düsseldorf

Ammeos visnagae fructus
Angelicae radix
Apii fructus
Arnicae flos
Artemisiae herba
Bardanae radix
Calendulae flos
Cardui mariae fructus
Cardui mariae herba
Carlinae radix
Chamomillae romanae flos
Echinaceae herba/radix
Foenugraeci semen
Hederae folium
Helenii rhizoma
Helichrysi flos
Hippocastani cortex
Hippocastani folium
Juglandis folium
Levistici radix
Lini semen
Liquiritiae radix
Matricariae flos

Millefolii herba
Petasitidis folium
Pimpinellae radix
Plantaginis lanceolatae folium
Salicis cortex
Sambuci flos
Sambuci fructus
Senecionis herba
Solidaginis giganteae herba
Symphyti radix
Taraxaci radix cum herba
Tiliae flos
Verbasci flos
Viburni prunifolii cortex
Violae tricoloris herba
Virgaureae herba

Subject Index

Monograph titles and the main chapters in the general section are in **bold face**.
Botanical names are given in *italics*.
Asterisks refer to formulas (plant constituents).

Because of variations in the use of singular and plural, also in the pharmacopoeias (folium, folia; flos, flores, etc.), many of the drugs appear twice in the subject index, i.e. under both forms of the name.